W9-BHS-929

Current Therapy Series

CURRENT THERAPY
IN
SPORTS MEDICINE
1 9 8 5 • 1 9 8 6

R. PETER WELSH, M.B., CH.B., F.R.C.S. (C), F.A.C.S.

Assistant Professor of Surgery
University of Toronto Faculty of Medicine
Acting Deputy Chief of Staff
Orthopaedic and Arthritic Hospital
Toronto, Ontario

ROY J. SHEPHARD, M.D. (LOND), PH.D.

Director
School of Physical and Health Education
Professor of Applied Physiology
Faculty of Medicine
University of Toronto
Toronto, Ontario

1985

B.C. DECKER INC. • Toronto • Philadelphia
THE C.V. MOSBY COMPANY • Saint Louis • Toronto • London

Publisher: **B.C. Decker Inc.**
               3228 South Service Road
               Burlington, Ontario L7N 3H8

               B.C. Decker Inc.
               P.O. Box 30246
               Philadelphia, Pennsylvania 19103

North American and worldwide sales and distribution:

               The C.V. Mosby Company
               11830 Westline Industrial Drive
               Saint Louis, Missouri 63141

In Canada: **The C.V. Mosby Company, Ltd.**
               120 Melford Drive
               Toronto, Ontario M1B 2X5

Current Therapy in Sports Medicine 1985–1986   ISBN 0-941158-33-0

© 1985 by B.C. Decker Incorporated under the International Copyright Union. All rights reserved.
No part of this publication may be reused or republished in any form without written permission of
the publisher.

Library of Congress catalog number: 85-070052

10 9 8 7 6 5 4 3 2 1

CONTRIBUTORS

FRED L. ALLMAN, Jr., M.D.

Orthopaedic Consultant Georgia Tech and Atlanta Public Schools; Director, Sports Medicine Clinic, PC Atlanta, Georgia
Overuse Injury to the Elbow in the Throwing Sports

ODED BAR-OR, M.D., F.A.C.S.M.

Professor, Department of Pediatrics, McMaster University School of Medicine; Director, Children Therapeutic Exercise and Health Centre, Chedoke-McMaster Hospitals, Hamilton, Ontario, Canada
Exercise in Childhood

LOUIS U. BIGLIANI, M.D.

Assistant Professor of Orthopaedic Surgery, Columbia University College of Physicians and Surgeons, New York, New York; Attending Orthopaedic Surgeon, New York Orthopaedic Hospital at the Columbia Presbyterian Medical Center, New York, New York and the Helen Hayes Hospital, Haverstraw, New York
Biceps Tendon Rupture in the Athlete

GUY R. BRISSON, Ph.D.

Département des Sciences de L'activité Physique, Université du Quebec à Trois-Rivières, Trois-Rivières, Quebec
Menstrual Irregularities.

KELLY D. BROWNELL, Ph.D.

Associate Professor, Department of Psychiatry, University of Pennsylvania School of Medicine, Philadelphia, Pennsylvania
Exercise in the Clinical Management of Obesity

LEONARD A. BRUNO, M.D.

Assistant Professor of Neurosurgery, University of Pennsylvania School of Medicine, Philadelphia, Pennsylvania
Head Injuries in Athletics

CHARLES R. BULL, M.D., B.Sc.(Med), F.R.C.S.(C), F.A.C.S, F.I.C.S.

Consulting Surgeon, Humber Hospital and Orthopaedic and Arthritic Hospital; Chief Medical Officer, Team Canada (Hockey); Director, Bobby Orr Sports Clinic, York University; Director, Fitness Institute Clinics, Toronto, Ontario, Canada.
Orthotic Support for the Foot
Soft Tissue Injury to the Hip and Thigh

JOHN C. CAMERON, M.D., F.R.C.S.

Lecturer, University of Toronto Faculty of Medicine; Director, Athletic Injuries Clinic, University of Toronto Faculty of Medicine; Staff Orthopaedic Surgeon, Toronto General Hospital, Toronto, Ontario, Canada
Osteochondritis Dissecans, Osteochondral Fractures, and Osteoarthritis of the Knee

GERARD J. CANNY, M.B., F.R.C.P.(C).

Assistant Professor, Department of Pediatrics, University of Toronto Faculty of Medicine; Staff Physician Division of Chest Diseases, Department of Pediatrics, Hospital for Sick Children, Toronto, Ontario, Canada
Exercise in Cystic Fibrosis

KENNETH R. CHAPMAN, M.D., M.Sc., F.R.C.P.(C), F.C.C.P.

Staff Physician and Research Associate, Division of Respiratory Medicine, Toronto Western Hospital, Toronto, Ontario, Canada
Exercise in Chronic Obstructive Lung Disease

CHRIS R. CONSTANT, M.B., B.Ch., B.A.O., F.R.C.S.(I)

Clinical Fellow of the Orthopaedic and Arthritic Hospital, Toronto, Ontario, Canada; Senior Registrar, Addenbrookes Hospital, Cambridge, England
Overuse Symptoms About the Elbow

BERNARD G. COSTELLO, M.D., F.R.C.S.(C)

Assistant Professor of Orthopaedic Surgery, McGill University Faculty of Medicine; Senior Orthopaedic Surgeon, Royal Victoria Hospital, Montreal, Quebec, Canada
Ligament Instability of the Ankle

GORDON R. CUMMING, B.Sc.(Med), M.D., F.R.C.P.(C)

Professor, Department of Pediatrics, University of Manitoba Faculty of Medicine and Children's Hospital of Winnipeg, Winnipeg, Manitoba, Canada
Exercise Tests in Pediatric Cardiology

EDWIN DALE, Ph.D.

Associate Professor, Department of Gynecology/Obstetrics, Emory University School of Medicine, Atlanta, Georgia
Exercise and Pregnancy

MARY-ANN DALZELL, B.Ph.Th., M.Sc.

Faculty Lecturer, Sports Medicine and Orthopaedics; Director, Department of Physiotherapy, Queen Elizabeth Hospital, Montreal, Quebec, Canada
The Physiotherapist's Armamentarium

LEITH G. DOUGLAS, M.D., F.R.C.S.(C), F.A.C.S.

Assistant Professor, Department of Surgery, University of Toronto Faculty of Medicine; Plastic Surgeon, Wellesley Hospital, Toronto, Ontario, Canada
Facial Injuries

BARBARA L. DRINKWATER, Ph.D.

Research Physiologist, Department of Medicine, Pacific Medical Center, Seattle, Washington
Physiological Characteristics of Female Athletes

ANTHONY D. D'URZO, B.P.H.E.

Graduate Student, Department of Community Health, University of Toronto Faculty of Medicine; Research Associate, Department of Respiratory Medicine, Toronto Western Hospital, Toronto, Ontario, Canada
Exercise in Chronic Obstructive Lung Disease

ERIC J. DUIVERMAN, M.D.

Assistant Professor, Department of Pediatric Respiratory Disease, Erasmus University and University Hospital and Sophia Children's Hospital, Rotterdam, Holland
Exercise-induced Bronchial Obstruction

BJÖRN T. EKBLOM, M.D.

Section Head, Muscle and Applied Physiology, Department of Physiology, Karolinska Institute, Stockholm, Sweden
Blood Doping and Performance
Exercise and Rheumatoid Arthritis

LAWRENCE JOHN FOLINSBEE, Ph.D.

Associate Research Physiologist, Institute of Environmental Stress, University of California, Santa Barbara, California
Air Pollution and Exercise

JOHN J. FRIM, B.Sc., M.Sc., Ph.D.

Defence Scientist, Applied Physiology Section, Biosciences Division, Defence and Civil Institute of Environmental Medicine, Department of National Defence, Toronto, Ontario, Canada
Hazards of Cold Air

THOMAS A. GENNARELLI, M.D.

Associate Professor of Neurosurgery and Clinical Director, Head Injury Research Center, University of Pennsylvania School of Medicine; Director, Neurosurgical Intensive Care Unit, Hospital of the University of Pennsylvania, Philadelphia, Pennsylvania
Head Injuries in Athletics

LAWRENCE A. GOLDING, Ph.D.

Director of Exercise Physiology, Professor of Physical Education, University of Nevada School of Medicine, Las Vegas, Nevada
Role of the Physician in Doping Control

JACK M. GOODMAN, B.P.H.E., M.Sc.

Graduate Exercise Sciences Program, Department of Community Health, University of Toronto Faculty of Medicine, Toronto, Ontario, Canada
Exercise Prescription for the Sedentary Adult

LEONARD S. GOODMAN, B.P.H.E., M.P.E.

Graduate Exercise Sciences Program, Department of Community Health, University of Toronto Faculty of Medicine, Toronto, Ontario, Canada
Exercise Prescription for the Sedentary Adult

RICHARD J. GRAY, M.D.

Associate Professor of Medicine, University of California, Los Angeles, UCLA School of Medicine; Director, Surgical Cardiology, Cedars-Sinai Medical Center, Los Angeles, California
Coronary Bypass and Exercise Prescription in Ischemic Heart Disease

ROBERT K. GRISDALE, B.A.

Research Assistant, Department of Respiratory Physiology, Hospital for Sick Children, Toronto, Ontario, Canada
Exercise in Cystic Fibrosis

JANET E. HALL, M.Sc., M.D., F.R.C.P.(C)

Endocrine Research Fellow, Massachusetts General Hospital/Harvard Medical School, Boston, Massachusetts
Females and Physical Activity

RICHARD J. HAWKINS, M.D., F.R.C.S.(C), F.A.C.S.

Clinical Associate Professor, University of Western Ontario Faculty of Medicine, London, Ontario, Canada
Shoulder Impingement Syndrome

GÖRAN A. L. HOLM, M.D.

Associate Professor of Medicine; Senior Consultant, Department of Medicine, University of Göteborg, Göteborg, Sweden
Exercise in the Treatment of Diabetes Mellitus

WILLIAM JOHN HORSEY, B.A., M.D., F.R.C.S.(C), F.A.C.S.

Professor of Surgery and Professor of Rehabilitation Medicine, University of Toronto Faculty of Medicine; Senior Neurosurgeon, St. Michael's Hospital, Toronto, Ontario, Canada
Microsurgical Lumbar Discotomy

ALAN R. HUDSON, M.B., Ch.B., F.R.C.S., (Ed), F.R.C.S.(C)

Professor and Chairman, Division of Neurosurgery, University of Toronto Faculty of Medicine, Toronto, Ontario, Canada
Head Injuries in Boxers

BRUCE R. HUFFER, M.D.

Formerly Clinical Fellow, Orthopaedic and Arthritic Hospital, Toronto, Ontario, Canada
Disorders Affecting Tendon Structures About the Ankle

CHRISTINE HUTTON, M.B., Ch.B.

Registrar, Auckland Hospital, Auckland, New Zealand
Knee Pain: Overuse Syndromes Around the Knee
Patellofemoral Arthralgia, Patellar Instability, and Chondro-malacia Patella

ROBERT S. HUTTON, Ph.D., F.A.C.S.M.

Professor of Kinesiology, University of Washington College of Arts and Sciences, Seattle, Washington
Neuromuscular Physiology

ROBERT T. HYDE, M.A.

Epidemiologist, Stanford University School of Medicine, Stanford, California
Exercise in the Primary Prevention of Ischemic Heart Disease

OMRI INBAR, Ed.D., F.A.C.S.M.

Director, Health and Fitness Assessment Center, Mor-Institute for Medical Data, Israel
Exercise in the Heat

H. PETER JAMES, M.D., F.R.C.S.(C)

Lecturer, Department of Surgery, University of Toronto Faculty of Medicine; Orthopaedic Surgeon, Active Staff, Orthopaedic and Arthritic Hospital; Consultant, Wellesley Hospital, Toronto, Ontario, Canada
Arthrography and Arthroscopy

EUGENE JANSSEN, B.S.

Exercise Biochemist, Faculty of Medicine, University of Limburg, Maastricht, The Netherlands
Exercise and Muscle Soreness

FRANK W. JOBE, M.D.

Associate Clinical Professor, Department of Ortho-paedics, University of Southern California School of Medicine; Medical Director, Los Angeles Dodgers, Los Angeles, California; Medical Director, Biomechanics Laboratory, Centinela Hospital Medical Center, Inglewood, California.
Ulnar Neuritis and Medial Collateral Ligament Instabilities in Overarm Throwers

VEIKKO KALLIO, M.D.

Rehabilitation Medicine, University of Turku; Chief and Professor, Rehabilitation Research Centre of the Social Insurance Institution, Turku, Finland
Exercise in the Secondary Prevention of Ischemic Heart Disease

FRANK I. KATCH, M.D.

Professor and Chairman, Department of Exercise Science, University of Massachusetts, Amherst, Massachusetts
Nutrition for the Athlete

JAMES F. KELLAM, B.Sc., M.D., F.R.C.S.(C)

Lecturer, University of Toronto Faculty of Medicine; Consulting Orthopaedic Surgeon, Sunnybrook Medical and Trauma Centre, Toronto, Ontario, Canada
Fractures of the Pelvis and Femur

KAREL F. KERREBIJN, M.D., Ph.D.

Professor, Department of Pediatric Respiratory Disease, Erasmus University and University Hospital and Sophia Children's Hospital, Rotterdam, Holland
Exercise-induced Bronchial Obstruction

DONALD W. KILLINGER, M.D., Ph.D., F.R.C.P.(C)

Associate Professor, Department of Medicine, University of Toronto Faculty of Medicine; Director, Division of Endocrinology, Wellesley Hospital, Toronto, Ontario, Canada
Anabolic Steroids and Health
Athletes with Menstrual Irregularities

MARCIN J. KROTKIEWSKI, M.D.

Professor of Medical Rehabilitation, Head of Department (Senior Consultant), Medical Rehabilitation, University of Göteborg; Göteborg, Sweden
Exercise in the Treatment of Diabetes Mellitus

HARM KUIPERS, M.D., Ph.D.

Exercise Physiologist, Faculty of Medicine, University of Limburg, Maastricht, The Netherlands
Exercise and Muscle Soreness

HENRY LEVISON, M.D., F.R.C.P.(C)

Professor of Pediatrics, University of Toronto Faculty of Medicine; Head, Division of Chest Diseases, Department of Pediatrics, Hospital for Sick Children, Toronto, Ontario, Canada
Exercise in Cystic Fibrosis

DONALD H. H. MACKENZIE, M.D., F.R.C.P.(C)

Associate Professor, School of Physical and Health Education, University of Toronto; Staff Physician, University Health Service, University of Toronto, Toronto, Ontario, Canada
Hazards of Diving

IAN MACNAB, M.B., Ch.B., F.R.C.S.; F.R.C.S.(C)

Professor of Surgery, University of Toronto Faculty of Medicine; Division of Orthopaedics, The Wellesley Hospital, Toronto, Ontario, Canada
Backache

LEWIS G. MAHARAM, B.A.

Student, Emory University School of Medicine, Atlanta, Georgia
Exercise and Pregnancy

JACQUES E. MARCOTTE, M.D., F.R.C.P.(C)

Fellow, Division of Chest Diseases, Department of Pediatrics, Hospital for Sick Children, Toronto, Ontario, Canada
Exercise in Cystic Fibrosis

JACK M. MATLOFF, M.D.

Assistant Clinical Professor of Surgery, University of California, Los Angeles, UCLA School of Medicine; Director, Department of Thoracic and Cardiovascular Surgery, Cedars-Sinai Medical Center, Los Angeles, California
Coronary Bypass and Exercise Prescription in Ischemic Heart Disease

VIRGIL R. MAY, Jr., M.D., F.A.C.S., A.A.O.S., C.O.A.

Clinical Professor of Orthopaedic Surgery, Virginia Commonwealth University Medical College of Virginia; Team Orthopedist, Department of Physical Education, Virginia Commonwealth University; McGuire Veterans Administration Medical Center, Richmond, Virginia
Recurrent Posterior Luxation and Dislocation of the Shoulder

JOHN A. McCULLOCH, M.D., F.R.C.S.(C)

Associate Professor, Department of Orthopaedics, Northeastern Ohio Universities College of Medicine, Rootstown, Ohio
Discolysis for Herniated Nucleus Pulposus

J. SIMON McGRAIL, M.D., M.S., F.R.C.S.(C)

Professor of Otolaryngology, University of Toronto Faculty of Medicine; Chief, ENT Department, Wellesley Hospital; Physician, Toronto Maple Leafs (Hockey) and Team Canada (Hockey), Toronto, Ontario, Canada
Ear, Nose, and Throat Injuries

LYLE J. MICHELI, M.D.

Instructor in Orthopaedic Surgery, Harvard Medical School; Director, Division of Sports Medicine, Children's Hospital Medical Centre, Boston, Massachusetts
Spinal Deformities and the Athlete

GARY W. MISAMORE, M.D.

Clinical Assistant Professor, Department of Orthopaedic Surgery, Indiana University School of Medicine, Indianapolis, Indiana
Shoulder Impingement Syndrome

ROLF MOCELLIN, M.D.

Professor, Department of Pediatric Cardiology, Universitats-Kinderklinik, Freiburg, Federal Republic of Germany
Exercise in Pediatric Cardiology

HERMAN J. NEIJENS, M.D., Ph.D.

Assistant Professor, Department of Pediatric Respiratory Disease, Erasmus University and University Hospital and Sophia Children's Hospital, Rotterdam, Holland
Exercise-induced Bronchial Obstruction

NEIL B. OLDRIDGE, Ph.D.

Professor, Departments of Physical Education and Medicine, McMaster University School of Medicine, Hamilton, Ontario, Canada
Improving Exercise Compliance

JOHN H. OLIVER, M.D., F.R.C.S.(C)

Clinical Lecturer, Department of Orthopaedics, McGill University Faculty of Medicine, Montreal, Quebec, Canada
Stress Fractures of the Lower Extremity

RALPH S. PAFFENBARGER, Jr., M.D., D.P.H.

Visiting Professor of Epidemiology, Harvard School of Public Health, Boston, Massachusetts
Exercise in the Primary Prevention of Ischemic Heart Disease

ROBERT C. PASHBY, M.D., F.R.C.S.(C)

Assistant Professor of Ophthalmology, University of Toronto Faculty of Medicine; Active Staff, Department of Ophthalmology, Toronto General Hospital and The Hospital for Sick Children, Toronto, Ontario, Canada
Ocular Injuries in Sports

THOMAS J. PASHBY, C.M., M.D., C.R.C.S.(C)

Emeritus Associate Professor of Ophthalmology, University of Toronto Faculty of Medicine; Honorary Consultant, Department of Ophthalmology, The Hospital for Sick Children, Toronto, Ontario, Canada
Ocular Injuries in Sports

MICHAEL R. PIERRYNOWSKI, B.Sc., M.Sc., Ph.D.

Assistant Professor, School of Physical and Health Education and Faculty of Medicine, University of Toronto, Toronto, Ontario, Canada.
Role of the Biomechanist in Sports Medicine

MICHAEL J. PLYLEY, B.Sc., Ph.D.

Assistant Professor, School of Physical and Health Education, Department of Community Health and Department of Physiology, University of Toronto Faculty of Medicine, Toronto, Ontario, Canada
Cardiopulmonary Physiology

ANTHONY S. REBUCK, M.D., M.B., B.S., F.A.C.P., F.C.C.P., F.R.C.P.(C)

Professor of Medicine, University of Toronto Faculty of Medicine; Head, Division of Respiratory Medicine, Toronto Western Hospital, Toronto, Ontario, Canada
Exercise in Chronic Obstructive Lung Disease

WOP J. RIETVELD, M.D., Ph.D.

Professor of Physiology and Physiological Psychology, Division of Chronobiology, University of Leiden, The Netherlands
Time-Zone Shifts and International Competition

CARTER R. ROWE, M.D.

Associate Clinical Professor (Emeritus) of Orthopaedic Surgery, Harvard Medical School; Senior Orthopaedic Surgeon, Massachusetts General Hospital, Boston, Massachusetts
Shoulder Subluxation in the Athlete

HEIKKI A. SALMI, M.D.

Docent in Internal Medicine, University of Turku, Turku, Finland; Chief of Internal Medicine, Central Military Hospital, Helsinki, Finland, Colonel, M.C., Finnish Defence Forces, Finland
Exercise in the Control of Hypertension

DHUN SETHNA, M.D.

Assistant Professor of Medicine, University of California, Los Angeles UCLA School of Medicine; Associate Cardiologist, Cedars-Sinai Medical Center, Los Angeles, California
Coronary Bypass and Exercise Prescription in Ischemic Heart Disease

ROY J. SHEPHARD, M.D.(Lond), Ph.D.

Professor, Department of Preventive Medicine and Biostatistics, University of Toronto Faculty of Medicine; Director, School of Physical and Health Education, University of Toronto, Toronto, Ontario, Canada
Principles of Exercise Testing and Fitness Assessment
Fluid and Mineral Needs
Hazards of Cold Water
Adjustment to High Altitude
Exercise and Mood State
Exercise for the Disabled: The Paraplegic

CHRISTOPHER W. SIWEK, M.D.

Attending Orthopaedic Surgeon, Susan B. Allen Memorial Hospital, El Dorado, Kansas
Quadriceps and Patellar Tendon Ruptures

JORDAN W. SMOLLER, A.B.

Research Assistant, Department of Psychiatry, University of Pennsylvania School of Medicine, Philadelphia, Pennsylvania
Exercise in the Clinical Management of Obesity

HANS STOBOY, M.D.

Professor of Physiology, Orthopädischen Klinik und Poliklinik der Freien Universität Berlin im Oskar-Helene-Heim und dem Institut für Leistungsmedizin, Berlin, Federal Republic of Germany
Effort Tolerance in Scoliosis

WILLIAM B. STRONG, M.D.

Charbonnier Professor of Pediatrics and Chief, Section of Pediatric Cardiology, Medical College of Georgia School of Medicine, Augusta, Georgia
Sickle Cell Anemia and Exercise

JOHN M. SULLIVAN, M.B., Ch.B., F.R.A.C.S.

Orthopaedic Surgeon, Waikato Hospital, Hamilton, New Zealand
Rupture of the Achilles Tendon

JOSEPH S. TORG, M.D.

Professor, Department of Orthopaedic Surgery, University of Pennsylvania Medical School; Director, University of Pennsylvania Sports Medicine Center, Philadelphia, Pennsylvania
Head Injuries in Athletics
Management of Athletic Injuries to the Cervical Spine

LARS-ERIC V. UNESTÅHL, Ph.D.

Professor in Psychology, Department of Psychology, Örebro University; Licensed Clinical Psychologist, Örebro, Sweden
Hypnosis in Conditioning the Problem Athlete

MARLEEN A. VAN BAAK, Ph.D.

Pharmacologist, Department of Pharmacology, Division of Clinical Pharmacology, University of Limburg, Maastricht, The Netherlands
Beta-adrenoceptor Blockade and Exercise

ERIC J. van der BEEK, M.D.

Staff Physician, Medical Nutritionist, Department of Human Nutrition of the Institute CIVO-Toxicology and Nutrition, TNO, Zeist, The Netherlands
Vitamins and Food Fads of Athletes

JOSEPH J. VEGSO, M.S., A.T., C.

Head Athletic Trainer, University of Pennsylvania Sports Medicine Center, Philadelphia, Pennsylvania
Management of Athletic Injuries to the Cervical Spine

FRANS T. J. VERSTAPPEN, M.D., Ph.D.

Coordinator of Education and Research in Sports Medicine, Department of Physiology, University of Limburg, Maastricht, The Netherlands
Beta-adrenoceptor Blockade and Exercise

GRAHAM R. WARD, Ph.D.

Assistant Professor, Department of Preventive Medicine and Biostatistics, University of Toronto Faculty of Medicine, Toronto, Ontario, Canada; Program Director, Variety Village Sport Training and Fitness Center, Scarborough, Ontario, Canada
Exercise and Sensory Disability

R. PETER WELSH, M.B., Ch.B., F.R.C.S.(C), F.A.C.S.

Assistant Professor of Orthopaedic Surgery, University of Toronto Faculty of Medicine, Toronto, Ontario, Canada
Dislocations of the Shoulder: Acromioclavicular and Sterno-clavicular Joints
Overuse Symptoms About the Elbow
Knee Pain: Overuse Syndromes Around the Knee
Patellofemoral Arthralgia, Patellar Instability, and Chondro-malacia Patella
Medial Ligament Instability of the Knee
Acute Injury to the Anterior Cruciate Ligament
Chronic Anterior Cruciate Ligament Instability of the Knee
Disorder Affecting Tendon Structures About the Ankle
Metatarsalgia and Other Common Foot Problems

A. M. WILEY, M.Ch., F.R.C.S., F.R.C.S.(C)

Associate Professor, Department of Surgery, Division of Orthopaedics, University of Toronto Faculty of Medicine; Division of Orthopaedic Surgery, Toronto Western Hospital, Toronto, Ontario, Canada
Shoulder Arthroscopy and Athletic Injuries

IRA N. WOLFE, B.A.

Sports Medicine Consultant, Department of Orthopaedic Surgery, Columbia Presbyterian Medical Center, New York, New York and Helen Hayes Hospital, Haverstraw, New York
Biceps Tendon Rupture in the Athlete

C. STEWART WRIGHT, M.D., F.R.C.S.(C)

Active Staff, Division of Hand Surgery, Sunnybrook Medical Centre; Staff Surgeon, Orthopaedic and Arthritic Hospital, Toronto, Ontario, Canada
Fractures and Dislocations in the Hand and Wrist
Tendon Injuries in the Hand and Wrist

PREFACE

Sports medicine as a discipline has matured and the care of the athlete occupies an important place in the delivery of health care. With fitness and health the concern of all, competitive and recreational athletes present their physicians, trainers, therapists, and coaches with an assortment of problems and disorders to diagnose and manage.

Participation in sports inevitably means that injuries will be sustained. Many maladies previously neglected or considered of little medical importance because no gross pathologic process was readily identifiable, for example myofascial strains of the lumbar spine, are now recognized as having substantial socioeconomic importance, affecting performance both in the workplace and on the sports field.

This volume brings together several areas of advancement, matching an up-to-date account of exercise physiology and applied sports medicine with details of the many maladies peculiar to the sports participant. The emphasis is on prevention and training, as well as current management procedures. The scope of the work is, we feel, quite unique: Environmental factors such as heat, cold, and altitude are discussed as well as sex, age, and concomitant medical problems ranging from diabetes to sickle cell anemia emphasizing the impact of these influences on athletic performances.

Authors have been selected for their expertise in each of these problem areas. An international group of contributors has addressed current management concepts in a clear and informative manner. We are most appreciative of their succinct contributions.

The present volume is directed particularly to those involved in the coaching, training and treatment of athletes, including orthopedists, team physicians, trainers, physical therapists, and physical educators. We hope that this and subsequent editions of *Current Therapy in Sports Medicine* will offer a regular forum for update and review of the many aspects of medicine that apply to the sportsman and sportswoman.

R. Peter Welsh
Roy J. Shephard

Toronto, 1985

CONTENTS

Head and Face Injuries

Spinal Injuries

Shoulder Injuries

Elbow, Forearm and Hand Injuries

PHYSIOLOGY AND BIOMECHANICS OF SPORT

NEUROMUSCULAR PHYSIOLOGY

ROBERT S. HUTTON, Ph.D., F.A.C.S.M.

This brief review of skeletal muscle and its neural control will consider recent trends within the context of exercise and sport sciences.

TYPES OF MOTOR UNITS

Sherrington's concept of a motor unit has been repeatedly confirmed but considerably refined at both the level of the motor neuron (neural unit) and the innervated skeletal muscle fibers (muscle unit). Functional properties of the muscle unit are well matched to the physiologic characteristics of the motor neuron. Hence, the neural and muscle unit components are viewed as homogeneous (as the term "motor unit" originally implied). Yet, as distinct tension-producing elements, motor units are divisible into at least a trimodal spectrum of faster and slower contracting populations with varying tension-producing and fatigue-resistant capacities. In the neurosciences, motor units are categorized as S (slow-twitch), FR (fast-twitch, fatigue resistant), and FF (fast-twitch, fatigable).* Scaled according to their input resistance (R_N) to excitatory current, an indication of cell size (soma size varies as the reciprocal of R_N), one finds R_N of S > FR > FF.

FF and FR motor units differ in the resistance of their respective muscle fibers to fatigue. S and FR units are distinguished according to contractile speed and their response to unfused tetani, the FR type showing a decline in tension ("sag") at lower activation frequencies over a short stimulus duration, though both fast-twitch FF and FR motor units evidence sag. Scaled according to twitch and tetanic tension, one finds FF > FR > S.

Homogeneity of neural and muscle units reflects the importance of at least two major mediating factors:

(1) trophic or neurochemical signals transmitted across neuromuscular junctions, and (2) regularity of use or disuse. A third factor, hormonal influences, has been less explored. Use/disuse involves the combined effects of recruitment (activation), frequency (rate coding), and pattern of activation (recruitment and rate coding). Conversion of the contractile properties of muscle units due, for example, to cross innervation of two different neural unit types provides evidence for neurally mediated mechanisms. Changes of metabolism and contractile speed induced by chronic electrical stimulation of muscle nerves or denervated muscle provides evidence for "pattern of use".

Recruitment and utilization pattern appear to impose phenotypic influences upon ontogenetic determinants of muscle unit type, particularly in the FR and FF groups. Fiber type conversions under natural conditions of training and extreme inactivity are of particular interest to sports physicians. These adaptations are summarized and simplified in Table 1. Note that all observations pertain to the muscle unit. It is less clear whether these changes reflect conversion of neural units, as presupposed by the concept of motor unit homogeneity.

TRAINING RESPONSES

The relative importance of neurochemical and use/disuse factors in determining motor unit type remains unresolved, if indeed these factors should be viewed as mutually exclusive. From the adaptations noted above, however, it follows that simply engaging in low resistance exercise with a high frequency of use (so-called "aerobic training") restricts skeletal muscle adaptation, skewing neuromuscular capacity to meet daily motor task demands accordingly.

Sustained changes in passive muscle length and force induce myogenic adaptive responses (for example, a decrease or increase in protein turnover), resulting in changes of fiber length and/or diameter. For example, muscles undergoing prolonged stretch or shortening tend to add or subtract, respectively, the number of sarcomeres in series, whereas, excessive loading of muscle fibers contributes to a hypertrophic response. Whether significant hyperplasia occurs is controversial, albeit unlikely. When considering the influence of joint position on myotatic contractures during immobilization, it is important to recognize that muscle tissue, as well as connective tissue, is involved in this process.

---

*Numerous additional classification schemes exist based on metabolic and physiologic properties of the muscle units or firing characteristics, after-hyperpolarization duration, and conduction velocities of motor neurons.

TABLE 1 Chronic Adaptations of Skeletal Muscle Fibers to Physiologic Conditions of Use–Disuse

Induced Change	Category and Relative Frequency of Use		
	Low Resistance (Endurance)	High Resistance (Strength)	Inactivity (Bed Rest)
Morphology			
Diameter	NC/↑–NC*	↑/NC	↓ NC?
Capillarization	↑/↑	NC/NC	↓–NC?/↓–NC?
Sarcoplasmic proteins	↑–NC†/↑	NC/NC	↓–NC†
Contractile proteins	NC/NC	↑/NC	↓/↓/–NC
Physiology			
Contractile speed	NC/NC	↓ or ↑–NC?/NC	NC/NC
Contractile tension	NC/↑–NC	↑/NC	↓/↓–NC
Fatigability	↓/↓	NC–↓?/NC	↑–NC†/↑
Metabolism			
Aerobic	↑–NC†/↑	NC/NC	↓/↓
Anaerobic	NC/NC	↑?/NC	↓–NC?/↓–NC?

* Throughout the table Fast-twitch fibers/slow-twitch fibers; ↑–increase, ↓–decrease; NC–no change; ?–controversial or no available evidence based on conditioning stimuli occurring within normal physiologic range.
† Changes may be observed in fast-twitch fibers of FR units.

Compromises must be made in immobilizing joint position and antagonistic muscle pairs after injury to avoid creating major imbalances in chronic muscle length during recovery, and if feasible, early therapy should be undertaken to promote a normal range of joint motion.

RECRUITMENT PATTERNS

Motor control of movements occurs through recruitment/de-recruitment and rate coding of motor unit populations. Since limb and axial skeletal muscles are composed of several hundred to over a thousand motor units, the process of activating the appropriate combination of motor units for purposes of movement is complex. Ontogeny and, possibly, phenotypic factors subordinate the problem of recruitment to two major mechanisms: (1) motor neuron size, and (2) synaptic organization of excitatory/inhibitory pathways to motor neurons. Recruitment/de-recruitment order is indirectly/directly proportional to cell size, respectively. Ignoring possible differences in synaptic density across motor unit types, smaller cells exhibit lower electrical stimulation thresholds due to their higher R_N, that is, local graded potentials are a product of injected current $\times R_N$. For example, the size of Ia monosynaptic excitatory postsynaptic potentials per motor unit type is scaled in the order of $S > FR > FF$.

Recruitment across motor units thus follows the order of $S > FR > FF$, or cell size. This normal pattern of use may in itself contribute to the establishment of motor unit types. Whether differences of motoneuronal excitability reflect different electrotonic properties of cell "types" is currently under investigation. This organizational scheme, called the "size principle", favors greater utilization of those motor units most resistant to fatigue, with gains of absolute muscle force and power as recruitment progresses to FF units. How fixed the size principle is remains controversial, but synaptic organiza-

tion of peripheral afferents, propriospinal pathways, and supraspinal pathways certainly could alter the balance of synaptic activity to recruit more selectively faster contracting units.

To date, few functional explanations of recruitment reversals (i.e., activation of FF > S) have been proffered. If S units were fully activated, they might kinematically constrain fast oscillatory movements (>8 c/s) owing to their relatively slow contraction and relaxation time. As the rate of switching from agonist to antagonist function increased, so would the chance of imposing a lengthening force on motor units (S units) not fully relaxed. Recruitment reversals have been demonstrated experimentally, for example, through excitation of cutaneous afferents. Recurrent inhibition via Renshaw cells (RCs) is believed directed more to S motor units than FR and FF populations. This suggests a greater inhibitory drive to smaller motoneurons as larger forces prevail. It is not known whether this organization serves the function of selective de-recruitment of S units, rate coding, or both. Since RCs, in turn, are controlled by numerous excitatory and inhibitory inputs, it has been suggested that they may control the "gain" of the synaptic input-motoneuronal output frequency. The gain would be set high (inhibitory drive to RCs) for movements demanding rapid, high-force production and low (excitatory drive to RCs) for fine coordinated movements demanding lesser and more gradual increments of tension.

FUNCTIONAL NEUROMUSCULAR STIMULATION

An understanding of recruitment order is important to clinicians employing functional neuromuscular stimulation (FNS) because even when FNS is applied directly to muscle, it selectively activates nerve branches rather than muscle fibers. Since the largest axons have the lowest electrical thresholds, FNS imposes a radical departure (FF ⟶ S) from normal recruitment patterns and provides a nonselective stimulus to motor axons. While FNS has therapeutic value in restoring bulk and force output to a muscle undergoing disuse atrophy caused by injury, surgery, or disease, the potential problems of FNS appear to outweigh possible benefits. In the few documented tests of FNS-induced strength gains, control subjects who engaged in dynamic or isometric exercises of comparable duration gained as much or more strength. The use of FNS as a means for controlling sensory feedback has received less attention. Selected patterns of FNS may also influence motoneuronal excitability and temporal sequencing of agonist-antagonist contractions.

SPEED OF CONTRACTION

Increasing the rate of recruitment by volitionally increasing the rate of muscle force production (df/dt) lowers the threshold of motor units when the onset of recruitment (electrical threshold) is expressed as a function of muscle force (overall force threshold). By increasing df/dt, as in ballistic contractions, motor units are recruited earlier, thereby activating a larger fraction of the motoneuronal pool. Owing to the inherent lag in electromechanical coupling between neural and muscle units, lowering the electrical threshold may stabilize the relative points of summation of motor unit force to total muscle force, so that the point of summation of motor unit force to total maximum force may remain unchanged. By mobilizing tension faster, the rate of recruiting S through FF motor units increases. It follows that altering the speed of movement in resistive training at submaximal loads leads to qualitative as well as quantitative differences in the motor units that are exercised, with potentially qualitative changes in adaptive responses.

MYOELECTRIC COMPONENT OF TRAINING RESPONSE

Historically, the gains of muscle strength through progressive resistance training have been attributed principally to muscle hypertrophy. Hyperplasia plays an insignificant role. Recent research has shown that increments of integrated myoelectric activity also occur in parallel with increments of muscle force, but at too early a stage to attribute to an increase of muscle fiber diameters (the larger membrane potentials of hypertrophied fibers would contribute to increased myoelectric potentials). Tested in another manner, avoiding some of the methodologic problems inherent in removal and replacement of EMG electrodes, V_1 waves (reflex myoelectric potentials during voluntary contraction, analogous to H-reflexes) normalized in terms of the maximum direct (M) response to electrical stimulation are significantly increased in strength-trained subjects and decreased following immobilization. Increases of longer latency reflexes (V_2, V_3) have also been demonstrated. Aerobically trained subjects may also demonstrate greater H-max/M-max ratios, leaving unanswered the

optimum training stimulus to induce this type of adaptation. Nevertheless, current findings suggest that chronic adaptations of stretch reflex pathways occur with training; possibly, there is a more synchronous activation of motoneural pools, thereby increasing the rate of df/dt through recruitment.

MECHANICAL INFLUENCES

Muscle tension is further influenced by the static and dynamic mechanical properties of the muscle unit at the time of activation. As predicted from the sliding filament theory of muscle contraction, there are optimal sarcomere lengths for the production of isometric force and (by extrapolation) optimal joint positions for maximum muscle torques. The optimal positions tend to be located slightly beyond mid-joint range, in a muscle lengthening direction. There are obvious implications for athletic posture in skills demanding explosive actions from a static position, as in a sprint start. Under dynamic conditions, when the muscles undergo concentric contractions (positive work), the muscle tension that is developed decreases as the rate of shortening increases. Owing largely to the series elastic properties of muscle, tension increases when supramaximal loads are imposed to produce eccentric contractions (negative work, muscle is lengthening as it attempts to contract). Though commonly explored at frequencies of complete (fused) tetanus, the nature of these mechanical responses of muscle is also stimulus frequency dependent.

Hence, the maximum tension that can be developed by a given muscle unit depends on fiber length, velocity, direction of fiber movement, and activation frequency. Assuming activation at the tetanic fusion frequency, and normalizing tension to maximum isometric force (100%), human concentric and eccentric contractions produce approximately 75 percent and 120 percent of the maximum isometric force, respectively. In dynamic performances, peak forces occur during phases of eccentric contraction or while the muscles are engaged in negative work. When negative work is followed immediately (<1.0 s) by positive work of the same muscle group, the total positive work performed (force-displacement integral) is increased, owing largely to the short-term storage and release of energy from series elastic elements. This observation forms the basis for "rebound training" or "plyometrics". Timing of the change-over in muscle function from eccentric to concentric contractions is critical, and whether optimal timing is attained owing to rebound training remains an issue. The problem is further complicated by the influence of change in total muscle length (l) on muscle stiffness (df/dl). The stiffness response is characterized by two distinct slopes, a short-range stiffness (high gain) and a secondary range of stiffness (lower gain). As dl increases, the contribution of short-range stiffness to the total amplitude of stretch decreases; thus, there is an optimum amplitude of muscle stretch for yielding the highest stiffness ratio. One is tempted to speculate that faster approaches to, and shallow gatherings at, the high jump bar, introduced years ago by the Russians, are related to these concepts. The value of rebound training remains controversial, with important physiologic factors apparently ignored in devising such workouts. Specifically, the role of stretch reflexes and tension production in plyometrics has been grossly distorted.

ACTIVATION HISTORY

Considerable attention has been focused on the effects of temperature and fatigue upon the dynamics of muscle tension, but surprisingly little attention has been paid to potentiating effects of "short-term activation history" on submaximal df/dt. A brief high-frequency contraction induces post-tetanic twitch potentiation (PTP). Expressing PTP as a multiple of pre-tetanus twitch tension, ratios as high as 2.4 can be demonstrated in principally FF and FR units. Potentiation lasts for several minutes. Potentiating frequencies need not fall outside the normal range of rate coding. An interposed maximal volitional contraction (MVC) potentiates human twitch responses for several minutes, the magnitude of this effect being % MVC and duration dependent. Higher % MVCs offer greater potentiation, with an optimal duration of approximately 10 s. The overall effect on subtetanic repetitive stimulation during PTP is an enhanced force-time integral (impulse). The mechanism is clearly myogenic, and changes of intracellular $Ca++$ transport are probably involved. The common perception of a "tuning" effect, with an increased ease of exercise during the early stages of activity, may well be associated with PTP as well as "warm-up" and other metabolic factors. One might thus consider maximum or near maximum contractions of major participating muscle groups as part of the preliminary preparation for some forms of exercise.

Stretch reflex pathways are also potentiated by brief high-intensity contractions. Possible explanations include intracapsular changes in muscle spindles and post-tetanic potentiation of monosynaptic responses at group Ia terminals in the spinal cord. Coupled with PTP of the muscle unit, these alterations facilitate the mobilization of tension during submaximal effort. These findings are at direct odds with rationale commonly given for the value of "proprioceptive neuromuscular facilitation (PNF)" as a method of improving muscle compliance (stretching a muscle immediately after a maximum contraction). From the above, maximum contraction prior to stretch would be expected to exacerbate muscle stiffness rather than increase its compliance. Electromyographic recordings from muscle undergoing PNF stretching procedures confirm this view. Myoelectric activity is greater in muscles subjected to PNF techniques. Nevertheless, acute and chronic improvements in the range of motion developed by PNF procedures appear to be at least equal to those induced by passive static stretching. Therefore, enhancing muscle compliance through a decrease of myoelectric activity does not seem a prerequisite for effective stretching. However, if a tonically active muscle is stretched, it would seem more vulnerable to injury.

CARDIOPULMONARY PHYSIOLOGY

MICHAEL J. PLYLEY, B.Sc., Ph.D.

The capacity to perform work (=force exerted× distance moved) is dependent on supplying sufficient energy at the required rate for the duration of the activity. Sources of energy for muscle contraction are designated as anaerobic and aerobic.

SUPPLY OF ENERGY

The immediate energy for muscle contraction comes from ATP, either stored in the muscle cell (6 mM/kg wet weight) or synthesized through various metabolic pathways. Although ATP within the muscle is sufficient for only one or two maximal contractions, intramuscular ATP stores are only slightly decreased during exercise. Resynthesis of ATP occurs anaerobically via the breakdown of creatine phosphate (CP) or through the breakdown of carbohydrate (either glycogen or glucose). Aerobic resynthesis of ATP occurs by oxidative phosphorylation of fat, carbohydrate, or protein. Characteristics of each of these metabolic systems are presented in Table 1.

ANAEROBIC ENERGY PRODUCTION AND UTILIZATION

The anaerobic alactic (phosphagen) system supplies energy for activities of <10 seconds duration. These activities, sometimes described as high-power output activities, require a high rate of energy turnover as work is done over a short time interval (power=work÷time). Factors limiting these activities are the rather small stores of CP in the muscle and the inability of other energy systems to supply ATP at a high rate. Although energy production is anaerobic, recovery, i.e., with the replenishment of CP stores, is an aerobic process.

There is little difference in the muscle concentrations of ATP and CP between trained and untrained individuals. CP stores increase by some 20% with interval training, but ATP stores apparently do not change.

TABLE 1   Characteristics of the Aerobic and Anaerobic Energy Systems in an Untrained Individual

Characteristic	Anaerobic System		Aerobic System
Subtype	Alactic	Lactic	
Other designations	ATP/PC, phosphagen	Glycolytic	Oxygen, oxidative phosphorylation
Fuel source	Stored ATP, PC	Stored muscle glycogen and glucose	Glycogen, glucose, fat, and protein
Enzyme system	Single enzyme	Single enzyme system	Multiple enzyme system
Metabolic by-products	ADP+ P,C	Lactic acid	$CO_2 + H_2O$
Maximum rate of ATP production (moles/minute)	3.6	1.6	1.0
Time to maximal production rate	$\cong 1$ sec	5–10 sec	2–3 min
Time limit for maximal production rate	6–10 sec	20–30 sec	3 min
Functional capacity (moles)	0.6	1.2	Theoretically unlimited
Time to exhaustion during *maximal* utilization	10 sec	30–40 sec	5–6 min
Relative contribution (%) during *maximal* efforts of:			
10 sec	50	35	15
30 sec	15	65	20
2 min	4	46	50
10 min	1	9	90
Time for 50% recovery	20–30 sec	15–20 min	5–10 min
Time for 100% recovery	3 min	1–2 hours	30–60 min
Limiting factor(s)	Depletion of creatine phosphate stores	Lactic acid accumulation resulting from production exceeding buffering capacity	Depletion of carbohydrate, inability to supply adequate oxygen, cardiovascular drift, limitation of optimal carbohydrate supply

Based on the data of Fox EL. Orthop Clin North Am 1977; 8:534–548; and from Paterson DH. *Coaching Theory Level III*. Ottawa: Coaching Association of Canada, 1981.

However, training enhances the activity of enzymes involved in anaerobic alactic energy production, namely ATPase, myokinase, and creatine phosphokinase. Improvements in the performance of an "anaerobic" athlete are most likely the result of an increased muscle mass, a higher proportion of fast-twitch fibers, and a different pattern of fiber recruitment (Table 2).

Intense activity of 30 to 40 seconds' duration mainly involves anaerobic energy production via glycolysis (see Table 1). Although the peak rate of energy production is relatively high (1.6 moles of ATP per minute), the system is inefficient, as only 3 moles of ATP can be produced from the incomplete breakdown of 180 g of glycogen (compared to 39 moles of ATP if the 180 g of glycogen were broken down aerobically). Actually, even 3 moles of ATP are never realized during such efforts, because the system fails from lactic acid accumulation after 1.0 to 1.2 moles of ATP have been produced. Failure reflects an inability to maintain intracellular pH within normal limits and the effect of pH changes on the rate of glycolysis, possibly via a rate-limiting enzyme such as phosphofructokinase. Ultimately, the factor limiting anaerobic activity is buffering capacity. Support for this view comes from studies at altitude (5500 m), where both maximal lactic acid levels and buffering capacity are at approximately 50 percent of sea level values. Recent studies have also shown that augmenting the buffering capacity by ingestion of bicarbonate enhances performance. (Note that this practice is not advocated, nor is it ethical).

Maximal blood lactate (12 to 20 mM/L) is increased following interval training; this allows a faster pace to be maintained for a longer period of time before "tying up" occurs. The higher levels of lactic acid reflect an increased buffering capacity, a greater tolerance of the effects of acidosis, and increased levels of key enzymes such as phosphorylase, phosphofructokinase, hexokinase, and the muscle form of lactate dehydrogenase. Endurance training, in contrast, decreases the activity of these enzymes, leading to lower maximal lactate values.

Children have lower maximal lactate levels (6 to 10 mM/L) than adults, possibly owing to lower muscle concentrations of phosphofructokinase. Maximal lactic acid values increase steadily between the ages of 10 and 20; this change parallels increases in creatine phosphokinase and the ratio of muscle mass: body mass. Maximal lactate values are decreased in the aged, probably as a result of a decreased muscle mass: body mass ratio or an alteration in fiber recruitment pattern (see Table 2).

The rate of lactic acid accumulation during physical activity can be decreased by reducing the rate of lactate production or by increasing the rate of lactate elimina-

TABLE 2 Characteristics of Fast-twitch and Slow-twitch Motor Units of an Untrained Individual

Characteristics	Fast-twitch Motor Unit		Slow-twitch Motor Unit
Fiber subtype	II_b	II_a	I
Other designations	White	Intermediate	Red
Size of motor unit	Large	Small	Small
Size of motor nerve	Large	Large	Small
Nerve conduction velocity	Fast	Fast	Slow
Fiber size	Large	Large	Small
Force of contraction	High	Moderate	Low
Time to maximal contraction	Fast	Fast	Slow
Ability to withstand fatigue	Low	Intermediate	High
ATPase concentration	High	High	Low
Mitochondrial enzymes	Low	Moderate	High
Glycolytic enzymes	High	High	Low
Glycogen storage	High	High	Moderate
Fat content	Low	Intermediate	High
Myoglobin content	Low	Intermediate	High
Capillary supply	Low	High	High
Recruitment pattern	Power or sprint activities	Moderate power/ endurance activities	Postural or endurance activities

tion. Decreased production at any given rate of work can be achieved by an increase of aerobic power, thereby lessening the contribution of energy from anaerobic sources. A second factor reducing the rate of lactate accumulation is the production of alanine, rather than lactic acid. This reaction is increased in the trained individual.

Major factors leading to an increased rate of lactate removal following training are: (1) an increased rate of lactic acid diffusion from the active muscles, (2) an increased muscle blood flow, and (3) an increased ability to metabolize lactate in the heart, the liver and nonworking muscle. This last change lowers blood lactate, which in turn allows a faster diffusion of lactate from the working muscle. A higher local blood flow reflects an increased capillary supply in the trained muscles and a greater cardiac output. The increased metabolism of lactate by the heart, liver, and nonworking tissues results from an increased relative blood flow and an increased level of the heart form of lactate dehydrogenase.

Increased buffering in muscle and blood allows performance to proceed at a higher sustained rate before the pH is substantially altered and "tying up" occurs.

AEROBIC ENERGY PRODUCTION AND UTILIZATION

Exercise bouts of >2 minutes duration predominantly stress the aerobic system, provided (1) the work-

TABLE 3 Physique and Maximal Aerobic Power of Male and Female Athletes

Sport	Age (yr)		Body Mass (kg)		Height (cm)		$\dot{V}_{O_2}$ max (L/min)	
	M	F	M	F	M	F	M	F
Alpine skiing	21.3	19.0	71.5	58.8	175.9	165.1	4.62	3.10
Baseball	24.5	—	85.7	—	183.2	—	4.47	—
Basketball	26.0	19.0	96.6	64.9	200.9	169.7	4.44	2.92
Canoeing/paddling	22.8	—	74.6	61.3	181.6	167.7	4.67	3.52
Cross country skiing	23.8	23.0	70.6	58.5	176.7	164.0	5.10	3.64
Cycling	24.3	20.0	73.4	58.2	180.7	166.4	5.13	3.13
Figure skating	21.0	17.0	59.6	48.6	166.9	158.8	3.49	2.38
Football	23.5	—	98.4	—	187.1	—	5.03	—
Gymnastics	22.0	17.0	69.2	53.4	178.5	161.4	3.84	2.30
Ice hockey	24.0	—	81.8	—	179.5	—	4.63	—
Orienteering	28.0	23.0	70.3	60.0	179.6	165.8	5.07	3.64
Raquetball/handball	24.5	—	80.8	—	182.7	—	4.78	—
Running	27.4	21.3	66.2	53.8	177.5	166.3	4.67	3.10
Rowing	23.7	23.0	88.3	68.0	191.5	173.0	5.84	4.10
Shotput/discus	27.0	—	109.2	—	188.4	—	4.84	—
Soccer	26.0	—	75.5	—	176.0	—	4.41	—
Speed skating	22.0	20.5	77.6	63.1	179.9	165.7	5.01	3.10
Swimming	20.9	15.7	76.7	56.5	181.0	164.3	4.52	2.54
Volleyball	25.5	—	85.0	—	189.9	—	4.78	—
Weight-lifting	26.2	—	85.0	—	173.6	—	3.84	—
Wrestling	24.2	—	75.6	—	175.9	—	4.49	—
Untrained	24.0	20.0	73.9	57.3	175.4	162.0	3.14	2.18

Based on the data of Wilmore JH. Am J Sports Med 1984; 12:120–127.

TABLE 4 Components of the Oxygen Transport System at Rest and During Maximal Exercise in Sedentary, Trained, and Well-trained Individuals of 70 kg

	Stroke volume (L/beat)	Heart rate (b/min)	Arteriovenous O_2 difference (ml/L)	$\dot{V}O_2$ (L/min)	Mean blood pressure (mmHg)	Total peripheral resistance (mmHg/L/min)
Sedentary						
At rest	0.080	75	41	0.246	95	15.8
Maximal excercise	0.110	200	137	3.014	128	5.8
Trained						
At rest	0.100	60	41	0.246	94	15.7
Maximal exercise	0.140	198	145	4.019	127	4.6
Well-trained						
At rest	0.120	50	41	0.246	93	15.5
Maximal exercise	0.180	195	155	5.441	126	3.6

(Note. SV $\times$ HR a-vo$_2$ diff = $\dot{V}O_2$ = BP $\div$ (TPR $\times$ a-vo$_2$ diff.)

ing muscles have sufficient mitochondria to meet energy requirements, (2) sufficient oxygen is supplied to the mitochondria, and (3) enzymes or intermediate products do not limit the rate of energy flux through the Krebs cycle.

The aerobic power ($\dot{V}O_2$max) of a sedentary but otherwise healthy 20-year-old male is 40 to 44 ml/min/kg. Highly trained endurance athletes achieve values of 80 to 88 ml/min/kg (Table 3). Factors that contribute to a high aerobic power include: (1) arterial oxygen content (CaO_2), (2) cardiac output ($\dot{Q}$), and (3) tissue oxygen extraction (a$-VO_2$ diff.), i.e. $\dot{V}O_2 = \dot{Q}/(a-VO_2$ diff.) max (Table 4).

Arterial oxygen content depends on (1) alveolar oxygen pressure, which is in turn a function of alveolar ventilation, (2) an adequate ventilation:perfusion ratio, (3) the absence of a diffusion limitation at the alveolar:capillary interface, and (4) the oxygen-carrying capacity of the blood, which is itself dependent on (a) hemoglobin level, (b) temperature, (c) pH, (d) oxygen pressure, and (e) the level of 2,3-diphosphoglycerate in the erythrocytes. During progressive exercise, healthy individuals maintain their arterial oxygen relatively constant at 200 ml of oxygen per liter of blood.

The oxygen consumption of working muscle may increase 60-fold during intense exercise. Since the arterial O_2 content remains relatively constant, additional O_2

requirements must be met by increasing blood flow to the active tissues. This is achieved by increasing cardiac output and/or redistributing (shunting) cardiac output to the working tissues (Table 5).

When exercising in an upright position, cardiac output increases linearly with oxygen consumption. At work rates requiring <50 percent of maximal aerobic power, the increased cardiac output is achieved by increasing both heart rate (HR) and stroke volume (SV). The increased stroke volume is the result of (1) an increased end-diastolic volume, due to a sympathetically mediated venoconstriction, (2) the action of the skeletal muscle pump, (3) a redistribution of blood flow to the working tissues, and (4) an increased myocardial contractility which decreases the end-systolic volume of the heart.

At work rates requiring <50 percent of maximal aerobic power, the increase in cardiac output is achieved solely by increasing heart rate resulting from an increased sympathetic drive plus a parasympathetic withdrawal. The linear increase in heart rate with oxygen consumption suggests some functional coupling between metabolism in the working tissues and the cardiac control centers. The linear relationship offers a basis for submaximal exercise tests to evaluate aerobic fitness and for simple methods of prescribing exercise (see chapter on Exercise Prescription).

TABLE 5 Distribution of Blood Flow at Rest and During Maximal Exercise in a 70-kg Athlete

Region of body	Mass of tissue (kg)	Blood Flow At Rest			Blood Flow During Exercise		
		(ml/min)	(ml/min/ 100 g of tissue)	(Percent of cardiac output)	(ml/min)	(ml/min/ 100 g of tissue)	(Percent of cardiac output)
Cerebral	1.5	840	56	14	840	56	3
Myocardial	0.3	240	80	4	1,200	400	4
Hepatosplanchnic	3.7	1,680	45	28	450	12	1.5
Renal	0.3	1,380	460	23	300	100	1
Skin*	2.1	480	23	8	600	28	2
Muscle	30.0	1,200	4	20	26,400	88	88
Other	31.1	180	$\cong 1$	3	150	$\cong 1$	0.5
Pulmonary	1.0	6,000	600	100	30,000	3,000	100

*At an ambient temperature of 25°C.

TABLE 6   Factors Contribution to Maintenance of Arteriolar Dilation in Muscle

↓ oxygen pressure
↑ carbon dioxide pressure
↑ hydrogen ions (↓ pH)
↑ potassium ions
↑ adenosine compounds
↑ osmolarity

TABLE 7   Factors Affecting Physical Performance

Somatic factors
  Sex
  Age
  Body dimensions
  State of health
  State of training
  Drugs
  Strength
  Fiber type distribution
Nature of the work
  Intensity
  Duration
  Technique (efficiency)
  Body position
  Mode
  Type
  Work:rest schedule
Psychic factors
  Attitude
  Motivation
Environmental factors
  Diet
  Temperature (heat and cold)
  Air pressure (hypobaric and hyperbaric)
  Air pollution
  Noise

Based on the data of Ästrand P-O, Rodahl, K. *Textbook of Work Physiology.* Toronto: McGraw-Hill Book Co, 1977: 451.

During intense exercise, muscle blood flow increases from 20 percent to >85 percent of cardiac output (see Table 5). This reflects not only an increase in cardiac output, but also a preferential redistribution of cardiac output to the working muscle at the expense of other regions, such as the splanchnic and renal vascular beds (see Table 5). There is a sympathetically mediated (cholinergic) vasodilation of the metarterioles in the working muscle coupled with an overall sympathetic vasoconstriction in nonworking tissues. Later, a local liberation of vasoactive substances (Table 6) maintains and/or augments the neutrally mediated vasodilation. Total peripheral resistance initially increases, but later falls to 30 to 40 percent of values seen at rest. Relaxation of precapillary sphincters redistributes flow through capillaries which were previously underperfused, increasing capillary surface area and decreasing the distance for diffusion of oxygen into, and for lactate out of, the muscle cells. Since the postcapillary sphincters remain constricted, the increased intracapillary pressure causes a loss of 10 to 15 percent of plasma volume to the interstitial space. The resultant hemoconcentration is beneficial in terms of oxygen-carrying capacity, but increases blood viscosity, slightly increasing resistance to flow.

The systolic blood pressure increases steadily during progressive exercise, but diastolic pressure remains stable or falls slightly; thus, mean arterial pressure increases gradually throughout effort (see Table 4).

Tissue oxygen extraction depends on (1) the rate of diffusion, influenced by (a) the gradient of Po_2 between the capillary and the cell, (b) the capillary surface area, and (c) the diffusion distance, and (2) the rate of utilization of oxygen, which depends on the levels of key enzymes in the various metabolic pathways.

The limiting factor(s) for maximal exercise has long been debated. Although it is often stated that lung function does not limit aerobic power in a healthy individual, recent evidence suggests that there may be such a limitation in elite athletes during maximal performance. Considerable argument has revolved around "central" versus "peripheral" limitations, that is, whether the supply of oxygen or its utilization ultimately limits energy production. However, the time course and pattern of training adaptations suggest that maximal blood flow and/or the distribution of blood flow within the muscle is the limiting factor.

Exercise performed with a smaller muscle mass, for example, the arm or forearm, exhibits a different pattern. At any given rate of work (either absolute or relative), heart rate and blood pressure (both systolic and diastolic) are higher, and stroke volume lower, for small muscle exercise. This is likely because the smaller muscle mass presents a higher resistance to flow and a decreased venous return.

Endurance training increases the maximal aerobic power of a sedentary individual by 15 to 25 percent, regardless of age. This rather large variation suggests the importance of "natural endowment" in determining the training response. An older individual responds in a similar fashion except that the rate of change is much slower. Maximal aerobic power peaks between the ages of 18 and 25 years, and then falls at a rate of 0.5 percent per year; both trained and sedentary individuals decline at a similar rate, although the trained person starts from a higher level.

Metabolic and circulatory adaptations to training are often specific to the trained muscles and are not fully transferable to other muscle groups. Improvements in cardiac function induced by training one muscle group can benefit the performance of other muscle groups, but the lack of the metabolic and circulatory alterations within these other muscles limit not only performance, but also the extent to which the cardiac pump can be stressed.

Many factors, both genetic and environmental, affect individual responses to a particular training program (Table 7). Important details are unfortunately still lacking. Future work will pursue these details and explore other areas to increase our knowledge of physical performance.

EXERCISE TESTS IN PEDIATRIC CARDIOLOGY

GORDON R. CUMMING, B.Sc. (Med), M.D., F.R.C.P.(C)

Exercise tests are used in pediatric cardiology to assess aerobic fitness; to observe any adverse effects of all-out exercise; to follow the course of disease, the need for, and the effect of, surgical treatment; to assess rhythm disorders that are present at rest or are induced by exercise, and the response of rhythm disorders to anti-arrhythmic drugs; and to assess children with symptoms of chest pain, dyspnea, and blackouts.

There is not much difference between the assessment of adults and children. If a cycle ergometer is used, the seat needs to be smaller and its height adjustable; many adult ergometers are unsuitable for children less than 9 years of age. Increments of work rate for children could be only 3 kpm/min or 0.5 watt per kg, so that the testing of a 10-kg child requires an ergometer with work-rate steps of only 30 kpm/min or 5 watts. Cuff sizes for blood pressure measurements should follow the recommendations of the Task Force of Blood Pressure Control in Children, 1977, with the cuff diameter covering three-quarters of the upper arm.

Adult treadmills are perfectly suitable for children. While low-profile treadmills are perhaps less frightening, we have had no trouble when children aged 3 and 4 years have exercised on a large research treadmill. Ideally, guard rails should be low for small children, but higher for older children. We used adult-sized guard rails and steadied the children as required. Safety straps are not necessary unless research is done at sprint speeds. Subjects should not be allowed to hold guard rails, because this reduces the metabolic load by an uncertain amount.

MAXIMAL OR SUBMAXIMAL TESTING

Most tests in patients with heart disease should be near maximal, if the objective is to assess fitness or the safety of vigorous activity. Submaximal tests have the drawback that a given heart rate cut-off (for example, 170 beats per min) may be maximal for some children with heart defects, but only 50 percent of maximal for other patients.

EXERCISE PROTOCOLS
Cycle Ergometer

Ergometers for young children should have an electromagnetic resistance, so that the work rate does not depend on keeping time with a metronome. Although total revolutions can be counted, the work rate may be uneven. Calibration should be performed at least yearly. Work rate is best based on body mass, rather than height or surface area. If responses to submaximal loads are of interest, test stages should last at least 3 min. If the investigator only wishes a gradual approach to near-maximal work level, then a one-minute stage duration is sufficient.

For 3-min stages, successive loads of 5, 10, 15 kpm/kg, etc., are satisfactory. A heart rate of 170 beats/min (11 kpm/kg for girls, 13.5 kpm/kg for boys) is then reached in 6 to 9 min.

With one-minute stages, the work rate can be increased by 2.5 kpm/kg per min to the maximum of 13 to 20 kpm/kg for girls and 18 to 25 kpm/kg for boys (Table 1).

When oxygen uptakes are available, there is little to choose between the various protocols. Exercise times of 5 min produce maximal heart rates of 190 beats/min, while 9-min times increase maximal heart rates to 197 beats/min without altering maximal oxygen intakes.

Graded treadmill protocols may keep a constant walking speed—about 5 km/hr and increase the grade by 2 to 5 percent every 1.0 to 3.0 min, or both the speed and grade may be increased every 2.0 to 3.0 min, with final speeds of 7 to 10 km/hr. Running yields heart rates 8 beats/min higher than walking, and maximal oxygen intakes are also up to 10 percent higher.

Children appreciate the change of pace that the variable speed programs offer. We have used the Bruce protocol (Table 2) with children down to 4 or 5 years of age. The average running speed of 5-year-old children for 800- or 1500-m races is over 8 km/hr so that they can handle the required speeds. Nevertheless, in any maximal test where the end point is exhaustion, it is challenging to ensure a truly maximal effort.

Each laboratory needs to establish its own normal values, utilizing patients without organic disease. Normals are best given in percentiles (Table 3). Body build is a major determinant of endurance in children, but a body build factor has yet to be incorporated into the tables.

TABLE 1   Progressive Cycle Ergometer Test in Children to Exhaustion

Age (years)	Maximal Work Rate (kpm/kg/min)*		Maximal Heart Rate (beats/min)†	
	Boys	Girls	Boys	Girls
5–6	17.5±5.0	16.1±5.0	189±11	191±14
7–8	21.8±5.1	19.1±5.7	193±10	196±13
9–11	23.8±3.5	18.9±4.8	198±8	194±12
12–14	21.0±4.9	17.8±4.2	197±10	194±9
15–18	21.5±5.6	16.2±2.5	193±7	196±10

* Wide range of maximal work rate (probably due to motivational problems). 1 watt = approximately 6 kpm/min.
† Large standard deviation of maximal heart rates (due to motivational problems and localized muscular fatigue). During treadmill exercise, the highest maximal heart rates are seen at ages 5–8 years.

TABLE 2   Oxygen Cost of Bruce Treadmill Test (normal subjects, stages 1–3; athletes, stages 4–7)

				Oxygen Cost ml/kg/min		
Stage	Speed km/hr	Grade %	Age 7 Yrs	Age 10 Yrs	Age 13 Yrs	Age >14 Yrs
1	2.7	10	20	19	18	17
2	4.0	12	26	26	26	25
3	5.4	14	40	37	36	34
4	6.7	16	52	50	48	46
5	8.0	18	—	59	57	56
6	8.8	20	—	—	—	63
7	9.6	22	—	—	—	70+

In patients with near-normal fitness, the first two stages can be rapidly passed through (10 to 20 sec each) without affecting the end results significantly.

Rapid Clinical Test

If a girl (any age from 4 to 20 years) cannot finish stage III of the Bruce protocol, she has a fitness level that is below normal; for a rapid test, the treadmill speed and grade can be quickly brought up to stage III. The test then requires less than 3.5 min of exercise. Stage III is also used for boys aged 4 and 5, but stage IV is substituted for boys older than age 5. Subjects not completing the 3-min test have below-normal fitness.

If subjects have had the full test before, they can be given a custom designed short test at a subsequent visit. For example, a subject previously finishing 1.0 min of stage V of the protocol can start the re-test at stage IV.

SUBJECTS WITH CARDIAC IMPAIRMENT

Subjects with mild or moderate heart disease follow the standard Bruce protocol. Subjects with myocardial disease, severe aortic stenosis, or cyanotic heart disease should start at zero degrees, 2.7 km/hr for 3 min, then 5.0 degrees and 2.7 km/hr before proceeding to the regular Bruce protocol.

Maximal Heart Rates

The earliest way to judge a laboratory's ability to obtain near maximal tests on children is to look at their maximal heart rates. Fewer than 1.0 percent of children have maximal heart rates less than 183 beats/min during treadmill testing. Mean maximal heart rates for normal children should be between 205 and 208 for children 4 to 12 years of age and 200 and 205 beats/min for youth over age 12 years. With cycle ergometer exercise, maximal heart rates are 10 beats/min lower, and for supine cycle exercise, another 15 beats/min lower.

Children in sinus rhythm with mild or moderate valve problems or septal defects have maximal heart rates within the normal range. The onus is on investigators reporting otherwise to prove that a near-maximal effort was obtained from their subjects. Children with cyanotic heart disease have reduced maximal heart rates. The rate they reach is dependent on motivation and the extent to which the physician or technologist insists on a near-maximal effort; the average in our laboratory was 178 beats/min, but I suspect that if all of these patients had made a near-maximal effort, the values would have been close to those in normal children.

Children with significant valve disease or postoperative major disease such as tetralogy of Fallot have maximal heart rates in the range of 175 to 200 (mean 188). Maximal exercise heart rates are reduced with sinus node dysfunction or interruption of atrial conduction

TABLE 3   Bruce Treadmill Test. Normal Endurance Times for Children

		Percentiles					Mean Endurance Time (min)
Age (years)	Sex	10	25	50	75	90	
4–5	M	9.5	10.5	11.5	12.5	13.5	11.5±1.5
	F	9.5	10.0	11.0	12.0	12.5	11.0±1.4
6–7	M	10.8	12.0	12.5	13.0	14.0	12.5±1.2
	F	11.0	11.5	12.3	13.0	13.5	12.3±1.2
8–9	M	12.0	12.5	13.0	13.5	15.0	13.2±1.4
	F	10.5	11.0	12.1	13.0	13.5	12.2±1.1
10–12	M	11.0	13.0	13.5	14.0	15.5	13.5±1.7
	F	10.5	11.0	12.1	13.0	13.6	12.1±1.3
13–15	M	12.0	12.9	13.8	14.9	15.5	13.8±1.4
	F	9.0	10.0	11.1	12.0	13.0	11.1±1.7
16–20	M	10.5	13.0	14.3	15.8	17.5	14.3±2.3
	F	9.2	10.3	11.1	12.3	15.0	11.6±1.7

pathways. A common example is the patient who has had the Mustard operation for transposition. Even though the rhythm appears to be sinus, maximal rates may be reduced to 175 beats/min. Patients with junctional pacemakers or more significant rhythm disturbances have reduced maximal heart rates.

Lactic Acid

The other practical criterion for defining a near-maximal effort is the blood lactate, sampled 2 to 3 min after exercise. Some investigators stab the warmed fingertip or ear lobe and obtain near arterial blood; others warm the hand and obtain dorsal vein blood. We have found sampling from the antecubital vein the least traumatic in children.

There is a tendency for post-exercise lactate levels to be higher in older children, but there is considerable overlap. Our criteria of near-maximal treadmill effort are: for children aged 10 and under, a lactate of at least 6 mM/L with a maximal heart rate over 190 beats/min, and for children over 10, a lactate of at least 8 mM/L with a maximal heart rate over 190 beats/min. On the cycle ergometer, lactates tend to be slightly higher and heart rates 5 beats/min lower.

THE EXERCISE LABORATORY

Ideally, the laboratory should be air-conditioned and maintained at 19 to 20°C and 40 to 50 percent relative humidity. Some laboratories insist on a physician's presence for all tests and the signing of an informed consent. Having allowed a trained technologist to conduct maximal exercise tests in a few thousand children with heart defects, I feel that nearly all children can be tested with the physician on 30- to 60-sec standby. Exceptions include serious rhythm disorders, aortic stenosis with anticipated gradients over 50 mmHg, and patients with myocardial disease. Patients with Marfan syndrome, severe pulmonary stenosis, and possible coronary disease also require special attention.

There is nothing to be gained by exercising children with acute illness or unbalanced chronic problems. Active carditis, uncontrolled heart failure, a rapid resting rate in patients with atrial fibrillation, and a resting blood pressure over 200/110 mmHg are all cardiovascular contraindications to testing. In other conditions such as hepatitis, nephritis, uncontrolled diabetes, and pneumonia, exercise testing serves little purpose.

Most children wear running shoes. If not, they perform best on the treadmill in bare feet.

TERMINATION OF EXERCISE TESTS IN CHILDREN

In a maximal test, the child should exercise to just short of physical collapse. Usually, when a desire to stop is expressed, he or she can be persuaded to continue for another 20 to 120 sec, or to reach a certain goal. The point of stopping is a compromise reached with the technologist.

It is rarely necessary to stop a child because of ECG changes or symptoms. We have not used ST change, but the American Heart Association recommends stopping with a 3 mm depression. Ventricular tachycardia develops in some patients with light or moderate exercise, but disappears with more intense exercise. If there are no symptoms or untoward signs, it is not necessary to halt the test.

The sudden appearance of 2:1 or complete A-V block causes distress and the patient will stop; however, development of right or left bundle branch block is usually benign. The onset of atrial fibrillation, atrial flutter, or supraventricular tachycardia usually requires the patient to stop. Frequent ventricular ectopic beats may also be a reason to stop in patients with cardiomyopathy, left ventricular problems, or aortic stenosis, but not with a mild heart defect or a structurally normal heart.

It is usually prudent to stop the test if blood pressure exceeds 250 mmHg systolic. A fall of blood pressure is seldom observed in children. If the child is obviously distressed or seems to have a poor cerebral circulation the test should be stopped, but severe cyanosis per se is not an indication for halting exercise. Arterial oxygen saturation can be monitored by ear oximeter. Some patients will not continue exercise if saturation falls to 80 percent, but others can drive their saturation below 35 percent. Generally, the less the resting saturation, the lower the patient can push the saturation during exercise.

EXERCISE ELECTROCARDIOGRAM IN CHILDREN

The main purpose of the ECG is to follow heart rate and rhythm. Some authorities recommend a 12-lead ECG, or at least leads VI, V5, and AVF, but I feel that lead CM5 provides the essential information in most tests. The simple bipolar lead saves considerable time, effort, and money. ST segment changes are recorded as in adults; at heart rates of 180 to 220 the segment is short and 50 mm/sec paper speed is required. Computerized ST analyses are prone to error at these rapid rates.

OTHER MEASUREMENTS DURING EXERCISE

In a level I exercise test, we follow work rate, heart rate, blood pressure, ECG pattern, and oxygen saturation by ear oximeter. After exercise, we measure blood lactate, and before and after exercise, peak expiratory flow rate (using either a Wright peak flow meter, or a computerized spirometer). Peak flow that declines more than 10 percent 5 min after exercise is defined as exercise-induced bronchospasm. It occurs in 6 percent of children, and occasionally explains exercise symptoms in a cardiac patient.

In a level II exercise test, which we reserve for research purposes, we add measurements of oxygen intake, carbon dioxide output, and anaerobic threshold. In young children, a flow-through system with a mask or hood has some advantages; mouthpieces sometimes shorten exercise times by 1 to 2 min. Level III exercise tests utilize arterial blood gas analyses and re-breathing cardiac output measurements. Level IV exercise tests involve intravascular catheterization with supine exercises (Table 4). Currently, we increase work load by 2.5 kpm/kg every minute to exhaustion. No problems of excessive bleeding or clot formation have been encountered with femoral catheterization. Nearly all our studies have been performed on an outpatient basis. The effects of exercise on pulmonary artery pressures, valve gradients, and aortic coarctation gradients have been studied. Indocyanine green dilution curves have measured cardiac output and quantitated intracardiac shunts. Such studies occasionally contribute to patient management, but the resting data are usually sufficient to decide on the need for surgery. After surgery, many patients still have significant abnormalities of intravascular pressures or blood flow that would not have been detected with resting measurements alone.

Catheterization for an exercise test can use the arm and a floating balloon (Swan-Ganz) catheter. Cardiac output can be determined by thermal dilution, and only venous catheterization is required.

Nuclear exercise tests are not as useful in pediatric cardiology as in adult heart disease. Thallium scans can assess regional myocardial perfusion in suspect congenital coronary artery anomalies, postoperatively if it is suspected that the surgeon has injured a coronary artery and in patients recovered from Kowasaki syndrome because of the high frequency of coronary aneurysms and potential thromboses. As in adults, thallium is injected near the point of maximal exercise, with the test continuing for another 30 to 60 sec.

Radionuclide angiography is used to assess ventricular function after repair of tetralogy of Fallot, transposition of the great arteries, large ventricular defect, or aortic stenosis. Right and left ventricular dysfunction is common in such patients, and the ejection fraction fails to increase as expected with exercise.

Echocardiography, ("M" mode, 2D or real time) provides an alternative assessment of ventricular function. Children have the advantage of thin chest walls and abdomens, and there is less chance for lung tissue to interfere than in adults. Nevertheless, exercise studies require patience and persistence. Doppler measurements of aortic and pulmonary artery blood flow are still in their infancy, but hold promise as a means of rapidly measuring flow during exercise.

SPECIFIC APPLICATIONS IN PEDIATRIC CARDIOLOGY

Aortic Stenosis

When the peak resting systolic pressure gradient across the left ventricular outflow exceeds 60 mmHg, surgery is indicated despite absence of any symptoms or ECG or radiographic changes. Patients with gradients under 30 mmHg or over 70 mmHg are usually recognized from clinical findings, rest ECG, and ultrasound

TABLE 4 Supine Ergometer Exercise During Cardiac Catheterization. Normal Values in 60 Subjects Aged 5 to 16 Years

	Boys	Girls
Rest		
Cardiac output (L/min/m²)	3.9±0.2	4.0±0.7
Stroke vol. (ml/m²)	52±6	45±6
Maximal exercise		
Cardiac output (L/min/m²)	10.1±1.8	8.6±1.8
Stroke vol. (ml/m)	56±12	46±3
Heart rate (beats/min)	170±17	174±11

measurements. It has been suggested that if the exercise ECG shows over 1.0 mm ST depression, the gradient is likely to be over 50 and catheterization should be done. In my opinion, the frequency of false-positive and false-negative ST responses in patients with mild or severe disease respectively makes the accuracy of the exercise ECG too low to be relied upon. In addition, as patients get older, ST changes tend to develop with exercise in the absence of any increase of gradient.

It has also been suggested that if the systolic pressure fails to increase more than 20 mmHg during exercise, the aortic valve gradient is likely to be more than 50 mmHg. Unfortunately, there are false-negatives and false-positives with this criterion as well, and its clinical value is borderline. If both the exercise ECG and blood pressure response are positive, catheterization is indicated, particularly if the clinical findings also support significant aortic stenosis.

Coarctation of the Aorta

If brachial artery systolic pressure is 30 mmHg above the normal range, or if arm leg systolic pressure differences immediately post-exercise exceed 30 mmHg, it has been suggested that an angiogram should be obtained to rule out significant (greater than 50%) aortic narrowing. Other studies have found no relationship between the post-exercise gradient and aortic lumen, and it remains to be proved whether the exercise tests add anything that cannot be obtained from resting data.

Arrhythmias

Heart Block. Some patients with normal sinus rhythm at rest can develop 2:1 or complete A-V block while performing intense exercise. If the ventricular rate suddenly drops from 180 to 90, these patients are acutely distressed with dyspnea, fatigue, and weakness.

In patients with congenital complete A-V block, the exercise response may assist in management, picking out candidates for pacemaker insertion. Some patients with resting rates of 40 can increase their exercise heart rates to 100 to 120 beats/min; they have normal or above-average fitness levels and usually do well. Others have peak exercise rates of only 65 beats/min and develop frequent ventricular ectopic beats during or immediately after exercise; they are candidates for pacing.

Sick Sinus Syndrome. Patients with maximal heart rates of 160 beats/min or less may have sick sinus syndrome. If symptoms suggest slow or fast dysrhythmias, Holter monitoring is indicated.

Ventricular Ectopic Beats and Ventricular Tachycardia. When ectopic beats are present at rest, they usually disappear during exercise. The same is usually true of ventricular tachycardia with a structurally normal heart.

Ventricular ectopic beats are rare during exercise, but are not rare in the first few minutes after exercise (when they are usually benign). Ventricular arrhythmias and subnormal exercise capacities usually imply significant structural or myocardial disease. Exercise testing is useful in such patients to monitor the efficacy of antiarrhythmic drugs.

Atrial Fibrillation, Atrial Flutter. These rhythms are rarely precipitated by exercise in children. In patients with atrial fibrillation at rest, exercise may be used to assess the optimal drug regimen such as Digoxin dose or the need for verapamil. Patients with flutter and 4:1 A-V block at rest may suddenly change to 2:1 conduction and then 1:1 conduction during exercise. The heart rate abruptly increases to 140, and then to 280 beats/min. This sometimes reveals "f" waves that were too small to recognize in the resting ECG.

Atrial Tachycardia. Patients with paroxysmal atrial tachycardia may develop an attack during or after near-maximal exercise.

Long QT Syndrome. QT normally shortens in proportion to exercise heart rate. Failure of the QT interval to shorten normally during exercise can unmask the long QT syndrome.

Postoperative Tetralogy, VSD, and Other Major Congenital Defects

Fitness levels range from above average to below normal. Exercise causes ventricular ectopic beats in up to 50 percent of these patients, with ventricular tachycardia in 1.0 percent. Sudden death can occur, usually in patients with poor ventricular function and resting ectopy. When exercise tolerance is good and ventricular function satisfactory, the need to control exercise-induced ventricular ectopy by antiarrhythmic drugs is less certain. Serial exercise testing documents the gradual improvement of fitness after surgery, giving reassurance that exercise activities are beneficial.

Mitral Valve Prolapse

Mild mitral valve prolapse occurs in 6 to 10 percent of all teenage girls, and perhaps 2 percent of boys. Exercise tests are needed on those cases with a history of dysrhythmia, or a grade 3 systolic murmur lasting at least half of systole. Serial tests are of value to assess antiarrhythmic therapy.

Chest Pain

In children, chest pain is usully noncardiac by history, but stress testing may reinforce the necessary reassurance of parents. Angina does occur with congenital coronary artery anomalies and premature atherosclerosis due to diabetes or hyperlipidemia. Exercise tests should be routine if total serum cholesterol is over 400 mg percent.

Juvenile Hypertension

Exercise pressures generally show a similar increment to resting values. Pressures 5 to 10 min post-exercise may drop below resting values, encouraging the hope that regular bouts of aerobic exercise may be therapeutic. Some preliminary studies have proposed that excessive increases of blood pressure with exercise identify children who will develop hypertension in later years. One immediate difficulty is that the normal range of exercise blood pressures is very wide.

Innocent Murmurs

Heart murmurs are present in 80 percent of children aged 6 years and 50 percent of children aged 12 years. Exercise tests are of no value in identifying children in whom the murmur has a structural basis such as a moderate septal defect.

EXERCISE TRAINING IN CHILDREN WITH HEART DISEASE

Children with mild heart defects can be serious athletes and train with their normal peers. After surgery for patent ductus, atrial septal defect, anomalous pulmonary veins, or pulmonary stenosis, exercise can start within a few weeks, with gradual resumption of sports activity by 2 to 3 months. After successful surgery for tetralogy of Fallot or a large ventricular septal defect, a gradual increase of activity is needed for 2 or 3 years, but with persistence an above-average exercise capacity can be developed. Children who have had corrective surgery at an early age end up with hearts that are structurally and functionally closer to normal than children whose defects were not repaired until after puberty. The younger children have the further advantage of having had their activities much less restricted. A home fitness program after heart surgery raises fitness levels above those of children not so treated. Some children must accept a residual limitation, but most can enjoy recreational exercise. Few children need written restrictions; most of those with residual disease do well by merely slowing up when they feel the need.

Differences of Exercise Responses Between Children and Young Adults

The $\dot{V}_{O_2}$ max of boys aged 6 to 10 years is the same as in young adults (on a per kilo basis), but the 6- to

10-year-old girls have higher values than adult women because they are leaner. The oxygen cost of running is 5 to 10 percent higher at any given speed in children, so that they are working at a greater percent of their $\dot{V}_{O_2}$ max. The 30 sec ergometer test shows that the maximal anaerobic power (per kg) increases in both boys (by 9%) and girls (by 12%) from age 8 to 15 years. The anaerobic threshold may be reached at a slightly higher percent of $\dot{V}_{O_2}$ max in children than in adults. Children increase their $\dot{V}_{O_2}$ more rapidly than adults at the onset of exercise. The cardiac output is a little lower than in adults at a given $\dot{V}_{O_2}$ Comparing a 6-year-old to an 18-year-old, respective maximal respiratory rates are 60- to 70/min and 45 to 50/min. The ratio of tidal volume to vital capacity is 0.45 compared to 0.58, the ventilatory equivalent is 38 vs 28, and arterial P_{CO_2} is 35 mmHg versus 40 mmHg.

PRINCIPLES OF EXERCISE TESTING AND FITNESS ASSESSMENT IN ADULTS

ROY J. SHEPHARD, M.D. (Lond), Ph.D.

This chapter will offer some comments on the principles of exercise testing in adults, relating this information to the specific needs of the fit young athlete, the middle-aged patient, and the "postcoronary" victim.

REASONS FOR FITNESS TESTING

The reasons for fitness testing are quite varied, and the required test protocol shows a corresponding variation. Young athletes are commonly submitted for quite extensive laboratory evaluation when they aspire to a position on a national team. The intent is not generally to select an oustanding competitor. Most athletes would reject the idea of "trial by machine", and in any event the precision of most physiologic tests is inadequate for gauging the outcome of events where performance differs only marginally between the best and worst competitors. Rather, the hope is to identify weaknesses in the development of an individual athlete relative to the "ideal" profile for a given sport, and to recommend specific training measures that will make good any deficiencies. Grouped data may also be useful in examining new concepts of training developed by the coach, and finally test repetition in the individual may help either tapering of training for competition or rehabilitation following injury.

The middle-aged patient may demand an exercise test from curiosity—usually to prove to himself or his spouse that he has not deteriorated as much as is generally supposed! The type of test can then be determined by the desires of the patient and the investment he is prepared to make to satisfy this curiosity. A related purpose is motivational. The physician may wish to demonstrate to a patient that heavy smoking is causing severe dyspnea with an abnormal exercise electrocardiogram, and the experience of both phenomena can indeed be a useful incentive to smoking withdrawal. Alternatively, the intent may be to show that participation in an employee fitness program has yielded substantial rewards in terms of improved physical condition; this is easily shown over the first 3 months, but unfortunately gains of test score become progressively smaller in subsequent tests, as the patients approach asymptotically to their potential maximum of condition. A third basis for testing of the middle-aged is clearance for exercise and recommendation of an appropriate exercise prescription; this will be discussed in more detail below. Finally, there may be a need to evaluate obscure exercise-induced symptoms or rehabilitation following recreational or industrial injury.

Assessment of the postcoronary patient is assuming ever-increasing importance. There is growing evidence that the amount of work a person can undertake 2 to 3 weeks after infarction provides a clear guide as to their subsequent prognosis. When more vigorous rehabilitation is contemplated (6 to 8 weeks after infarction), a stress test provides a necessary indication of the initial exercise prescription, with a warning of adverse exercise-induced changes such as ST segmental depression and premature ventricular contractions. The test can be repeated if the patient seems to be progressing well and an advance of the exercise prescription is contemplated. It may also be useful if symptoms are worsening and there appears to be an extension of the disease. Tests may be administered with and without various medications, to assess their value in improving effort tolerance. Exercise-induced symptoms may also need evaluation in the laboratory, and a formal exercise test battery may help in deciding whether a patient can return to heavy work or undertake employment where public safety is at stake (airline pilot, bus driver, or driver of an articulated truck).

TEST EQUIPMENT AND PROCEDURES

The fundamental piece of equipment for any sports physician is a method of inducing a standard work output by the patient. When testing national athletes, it is important to have a sports specific device. A swimmer, for example, is characterized not so much by a high treadmill performance, but by an ability to match this power output when swimming in the pool, or pulling against the springs of a "swim bench".

The best overall exercise device for the average patient is a treadmill. It is difficult to exceed the maximum oxygen consumption developed by all-out effort on the treadmill. Moreover, the device is machine-paced, helping motivation to a true maximum. Athletes will need to run uphill at 10 to 12 kilometers/hour to reach exhaustion, but middle-aged patients can attain the same objective by a relatively normal fast uphill walk. The main disadvantages of the treadmill are (1) capital cost (up to $30,000) (2) bulk, particularly in a small office, (3) noise, and (4) in many cases a requirement for 230-volt wiring.

The cycle ergometer provides a popular clinical alternative. Mechanically braked machines such as the Monark ergometer cost about $500, but electrically braked machines are much more expensive. The main advantage of the cycle ergometer is that the patient remains seated, allowing measurements of blood pressure and gas consumption together with blood sampling. Modifications of the ergometer allow testing of the disabled (see chapter entitled *Exercise for the Disabled: The Paraplegic*) and semirecumbent measurements during procedures such as echocardiography. The main disadvantage of cycle ergometry is that a high proportion of the total power output is derived from a single muscle group, the quadriceps. The maximum oxygen intake is thus 7 to 10 percent lower than on the treadmill (more so if there has been quadriceps wasting), and anaerobic activity begins at an atypically low fraction of maximum power output.

The simplest method of exercising a patient is to require the climbing of a standard bench at a rhythm set by a metronome or the music of a long-playing record such as the Canadian Home Fitness Test (available from Directorate of Fitness and Amateur Sport, Journal Towers, Kent at Laurier Avenue, Ottawa, Ontario). This approach is surprisingly satisfactory, provided care is taken to place both feet flat on the floor and to stand erect on the top of the bench during each stepping cycle. The rate of working is given by the product of body mass, bench height, and stepping rate. A hand support is helpful for older people, and if the cable is supported by the free hand, the electrocardiogram is easily recorded while the patient is stepping.

Many physicians encounter difficulty from a wandering ECG baseline during exercise. The problem is a varying impedance at the skin surface, and the solution is to remove the outer layer of dermis beneath the electrodes. Battery-operated dental burs with a rubber tip are now available for this purpose. Larger laboratories further improve the quality of their records by electronic devices which average 16 or 32 ECG complexes, rejecting any where a ventricular premature contraction occurs.

Standard calipers are essential for the examination of body fat. Research quality calipers are designed to exert a pressure of 10 g/mm^2 over a face area of 35 mm^2, but there are several simpler designs of caliper that are quite adequate for clinical assessment (for example, the plastic "Ponderal" skinfold caliper marketed by Servier, Nederlands b.v.).

Muscle strength has traditionally been measured by isometric dynamometers and tensiometers. A fair correlation has been claimed between the handgrip force as measured by a hand dynamometer and general body strength, but this obviously breaks down if there has been vigorous training for a sport such as tennis which has caused a local development of the wrist muscles. Sports science laboratories have more recently added various isokinetic tests (for example, Cybex II dynamometry) and isotonic tests (for example, swim bench endurance, or the maximum load that can be lifted in a sliding support to elbow height). However, clear norms have yet to be established for these newer procedures. Following injury, the restoration of lean tissue may be explored by echocardiography or soft-tissue radiography, but the dimensions thus measured are often poorly correlated with strength. If overall body mass is inadequate (as in some gymnasts and ballet dancers), it may be useful to obtain an assessment of body potassium and/or body nitrogen from a center equipped with a whole body counter.

"Static" flexibility is commonly assessed by a Dillon sit-and-reach flexometer. In essence, this consists of a vertical board against which the feet are placed, with a scale on top to measure the forward reach of the seated subject relative to the board. In some sports, dynamic flexibility is more important than the static range of motion. At present, there seems to be no alternative to attaching an electrical recording goniometer to each joint where the dynamic range of motion is of interest.

There have been various tests proposed for the measurement of anaerobic power and capacity. The simplest approach is probably to record the maximum power output on a cycle ergometer over a 5- and a 30-second interval. Anaerobic power can also be evaluated by a timed staircase sprint, while anaerobic capacity can be estimated from the endurance time of a supramaximal treadmill run (a combination of speed and load tolerated for 45 to 60 seconds).

Specialized apparatus to measure balance and to analyze filmed movements is available in many sports science laboratories.

MEASUREMENT OF MAXIMUM OXYGEN INTAKE

The maximum oxygen intake is the plateau value of oxygen transport, observed as the rate of working on a treadmill, cycle ergometer, or step test is progressively increased. It provides the best measure of a person's cardiorespiratory fitness. For most sports having a duration of several minutes to two hours, it is an important element in competitive success. Values are best expressed per kilogram of body mass, unless the body is supported when performing the activity of interest.

In a middle-aged person, the maximum oxygen

intake also provides a guide to employment prospects. Depending on situational factors (high peak loads, awkward postures, use of small muscles, high environmental temperatures), most workers can sustain an 8-hour energy expenditure that is 33 to 50 percent of maximum oxygen intake. Protection against coronary heart disease also comes through developing the type of fitness measured by maximum oxygen intake. Figures for maximum oxygen intake are finally useful in regulating exercise prescriptions for the middle-aged and the post coronary patient.

If equipment is not available to monitor oxygen consumption, the maximum oxygen intake can be approximated to within about 10 percent from the duration of a Bruce-type treadmill test. Likewise, an assessment can be made of maximum power output on the cycle ergometer, or the stepping rate attained in a progressive step test. Predictions of maximum oxygen intake from the heart rate and oxygen consumption or work rate in submaximum effort are useful in assessing the fitness of a population, but are not sufficiently accurate to be of great help in assessing the condition of the individual.

MUSCLE STRENGTH

The equipment for measuring muscle strength looks quite impressive in some instances, but the isokinetic and isotonic types of device at present lack well-developed standards of reference for either the athlete or the sedentary patient.

Isometric testing devices have been used for much longer, and extensive norms are available, particularly for handgrip force. However, many authors maintain that an almost equally useful assessment of muscularity can be obtained from lean body mass (total body mass, corrected for the percentage of body fat).

The testing of specific muscle groups nevertheless has value in assessing preparation for individual athletic events, and in following the recovery of function at a particular joint after injury. In disabled athletes, detailed assessment of muscle function is also important to their classification (see chapter entitled *Exercise for the Disabled: The Paraplegic*). Finally, in postcoronary patients, a poor development of the limb muscles may sometimes contribute to angina of effort, since a heavy afterload is imposed upon the heart by attempts to perfuse weak muscles contracting at close to their maximum force.

BODY FAT

Some laboratories make measurements of skinfold thickness at an enormous number of body sites. Female patients are often interested to know the amount of fat lost or gained from particular regions such as the hips or the thighs, but from the viewpoints of fitness, health, and athletic performance there is a law of diminishing returns as the number of measurements is increased. The commonly chosen standard sites are subscapular, suprailiac, biceps, and triceps; in a typical young man, these readings average 10 to 11 mm, while in a young woman figures are 14 to 15 mm. Both sexes typically accumulate a further 4 mm or more of fat over the adult life span. There are formulae that can predict the percentage of body fat from these readings, although the translation of the data is not particularly precise. A young man should have 14 to 16 percent body fat, and a young woman 18 to 20 percent. Endurance athletes naturally have much smaller amounts, perhaps 5 to 6 percent fat in a top male competitor, and 9 to 10 percent in a top female competitor. The only type of competition in which there is an advantage in being somewhat fat is in long-distance swimming; the fat provides both buoyancy and insulation.

Many physicians have relied on body mass as a means of assessing body composition. However, this can be quite misleading. Some tables show an increase of average body mass with age, but the increase is almost certainly fat, and the patient would be better off without it. Even if there has been no gain of body mass, an older person may have accumulated fat at the expense of muscle and a demineralization of bone. Tables of "ideal" body mass may show three columns of data for those having a slim, average, or heavy build, but such classification is quite arbitrary, and ratings are often affected by the obesity of the observer! The latest tables have attempted to counter this problem by making measurements of bone dimensions. When assessing athletes, it must be noted that a well-developed musculature can cause a person to exceed the ideal body mass, and indeed competitors in some activities such as gymnastics typically need to gain rather than lose mass.

FLEXIBILITY

A young adult can normally touch the board of the Dillon sit-and-reach apparatus, and some can reach as much as 5 cm beyond this. Women are generally more flexible than men, and scores decline by 18 to 20 percent over the adult life span.

In many sports, flexibility confers a substantial advantage. For example, swimmers have a much greater range of motion at the shoulder than does the average person. It is less clear how far this reflects training, and how far there has been a selection of individuals with a favorable anatomic form of shoulder articulation.

ELECTROCARDIOGRAPHY

The main feature of interest is an exercise-induced depression of the ST segment. A depression of 1 mm or more is associated with an increased risk of both myocardial infarction and sudden death. However, as with most clinical tests, there is difficulty in interpreting individual results, with a large number of both false-positive and false-negative findings. If a patient is asymptomatic, caution should thus be shown in stating that the exercise ECG is abnormal; it is all too easy for a doctor to create a cardiac cripple. Deep horizontal or downward ST depression at a moderate work rate is more likely to have clinical significance, and in such cases there may be value in additional investigations such as echocardiography. The number of false-positive results is reduced if such tests are restricted to high-risk patients (older individuals with some hypertension, obesity, and cigarette smoking). More sophisticated analyses which consider also the dimensions of the R wave increase the likelihood of discriminating individuals with significant myocardial ischemia.

Debate continues as to whether exercise-induced premature ventricular contractions provide any supplementary evidence of myocardial ischemia beyond that given by the ST segment. Many investigators believe that exercise PVCs are a useful sign, and that they provide an indication of individuals who are vulnerable to ventricular fibrillation.

Following myocardial infarction, it is useful to note the heart rate–systolic pressure product at which ST segmental depression, angina, and PVCs develop. A change in this threshold provides evidence of an improvement of condition with rehabilitation, or a worsening of condition with extension of disease. The exercise prescription can also be set at a ceiling of, say 10 percent below the double product inducing these adverse signs. Severe myocardial ischemia may cause a fall of cardiac stroke volume and systolic blood pressure at high work rates. This is an ominous sign, and an indication for an immediate halt to an exercise test. It is also usual to halt a test if there is increasing angina, ST depression of more than 2 mm, or more than 3 PVCs in 10 seconds of ECG recording. PVCs are particularly threatening if they are multifocal, occur early in the repolarization cycle, and appear in runs. The risk of exercise testing in an ostensibly healthy patient is extremely low, and even in postcoronary patients the risk of a cardiac emergency in a carefully conducted stress test is no greater than 1 in 10,000. Nevertheless, it is prudent to have equipment at hand for cardiac resuscitation, including a defibrillator and a cylinder of oxygen.

EXERCISE PRESCRIPTION FOR THE SEDENTARY ADULT

JACK M. GOODMAN, B.P.H.E., M.Sc.
LEONARD S. GOODMAN, B.P.H.E., M.P.E.

Exercise is regularly employed to screen for the presence of disease in asymptomatic patients, and as a modality in rehabilitation. However, relatively few practitioners prescribe exercise as a method of primary prevention in the obese, borderline hypertensive, sedentary, or borderline diabetic adult patient. Nor is the value of exercise exploited in the development of positive health behavior and the prevention of degenerative diseases.

This chapter will outline the physiologic rationale as well as the current state-of-the-art methodology of exercise prescription for sedentary adults.

CONTRAINDICATIONS AND PRECAUTIONS

Pre-exercise screening options range from the simple to the rather sophisticated, including self-administered questionnaires, medical examination, and medically supervised stress testing in a laboratory setting. Though a widely disputed matter, the use of costly, medically supervised stress testing in apparently healthy and "risk-free" patients, is not recommended. However, those with multiple primary risk factors and/or symptoms of coronary heart disease (CHD) and those who are grossly overweight and in the coronary-prone age group (males, 40–49) are encouraged to undergo such a test. It is nevertheless strongly recommended that, in conjunction with a generalized fitness assessment, healthy patients undergo a submaximal exercise test to determine functional capacity.

Absolute contraindications for exercise training, compiled from many sources (Table 1), include conditions that seriously alter the normal cardiovascular response to exercise, dangerously compromising the patient's health.

Various "relative" contraindications (Table 2) should also be considered when determining the potential benefits of exercise training relative to the associated risks, and deciding whether greater control or monitor-

TABLE 1   Absolute Contraindications for Exercise Training

Recent myocardial infarction (<6 weeks)
Unstable angina at rest
Severe sinus arrhythmias and conduction disturbances
Congestive heart failure
Aortic stenosis — severe
Diagnosed or suspected aortic aneurysm
Myocarditis or disease-induced cardiomyopathy (recent)
Thrombophlebitis, recent emboli (systemic or pulmonary)
Fever
Uncontrolled metabolic disorders
Severe exercise-induced hypertension (SBP>250; DBP>120)

TABLE 2   Relative Contraindications to Exercise Training

Frequent ectopic beats and/or uncontrolled supraventricular arrhythmias
Pulmonary hypertension, untreated
Moderate ventricular aneurysm and/or aortic stenosis
Severe myocardial obstructive syndrome
Mild cardiomyopathy
Toxemia or complicated pregnancy

ing is needed. Patients who fall into this category are advised to undergo a medically supervised test of functional capacity.

Cardiovascular risk factors should be identified during routine examination. Certain risk factors are particularly important since they may be magnified with physical activity (Table 3).

Certain conditions necessitate a supervised program in order to ensure proper monitoring and progression of the exercise prescription (Table 4).

Other conditions, both medical and environmental, call for caution in the prescription of exercise or moderation of activity (Table 5). If activity is moderated for a long period of time (>3–4 weeks), a revision of the base exercise prescription may be necessary.

INTENSITY OF EXERCISE

Intensity is the most important variable, but it is also the most difficult to determine. Early studies suggested that exercise yielding a heart rate of less than 135 beats/min had little conditioning value, some researchers setting the threshold of training response at 60 percent of the difference between resting and maximal heart rate. Others state that training should occur at a level corresponding to 50 or 60 percent of $\dot{V}o_2$ max.

Typically, intensity is expressed as a percentage of maximal heart rate, heart rate reserve (maximum minus resting), or functional capacity ($\dot{V}o_2$ max of METs). Much depends on initial fitness; unconditioned patients have a low threshold for improvement in functional capacity, whereas conditioned patients require a greater intensity. The ceiling of response also depends on initial fitness; improvements of functional capacity range from

TABLE 3   Coronary Risk Factors and the Effect of Exercise

Age	Risk increased in coronary-prone age
Family history	Increased risk if relative died while exercising
Obesity	Greater energy requirements for activity
Sedentary lifestyle	Greater energy requirements for activity
Type A personality	Overachieving may cause excessive activity
Smoking	Counteracts benefits of training
Hypertension	Increases myocardial oxygen demand

Modified from Shephard RJ: Can we identify those for whom exercise is hazardous. Sports Medicine, 1:75–86, 1984.

TABLE 4   Conditions Requiring a Supervised Program

Myocardial infarction; post-aortocoronary bypass surgery
Pacemakers — fixed rate or demand
Cardiac medication — chronotropic or inotropic
Morbid obesity in conjunction with multiple risk factors
ST-segment depression at rest
Severe hypertension
Intermittent claudication

5 to 50 percent, with unconditioned individuals showing the largest gains, owing in part to significant decreases in body fat mass.

Determining Intensity by Heart Rate

Maximal heart rate is determined, and a linear relationship between heart rate and $\dot{V}o_2$ is assumed. Intensity is then expressed as a percentage of maximal heart rate (HR_{max}), where $HR_{max} = 220 - Age$ (Table 6). Intensities of 60 to 85 percent maximal heart rate induce training, these values corresponding to approximately 60 to 80 percent functional capacity.

One serious potential error with this approach is that the predicted maximal heart rate deviates by ±15 beats/min from the actual value.

The "Karvonen" method of prescribing exercise intensity is based on heart rate reserve: $(HRR) = HR_{max} - HR_{rest}$. The training heart rate (THR) is calculated as: $THR = (.60 \text{ to } .85)(HR_{max} - HR_{rest}) + HR_{rest}$, where (.60 to .85) represents the potential range of training intensities from 60 to 85 percent. Intensity should begin at low levels, gradually increasing as fitness improves (Table 7). This method has an advantage over simple measures of maximal heart rate since the variability in resting heart rate is accounted for.

Exercise Prescription Using METS

Intensity of exercise may be prescribed in MET units (1 MET=oxygen consumption of 3.5 ml/kg per m^2)

TABLE 5   Conditions Requiring Caution in Exercise Prescription and Those Requiring Moderation of Activity

Conditions Requiring Caution in Exercise Prescription
  Viral infection or cold
  Chest pain
  Irregular heart beat
  Exercise-induced asthma
  Prolonged, unaccustomed physical activity
  Conduction disturbances (left bundle branch block, complete a-v block, biphasicular block with or without first-degree block, rare conduction syndromes)
Conditions Requiring Moderation of Activity
  Extreme heat and relative humidity
  Extreme cold, especially when strong winds are present
  Following heavy meals
  Exposure to high altitudes (>1700 meters)
  Musculoskeletal injuries

TABLE 6 Relationship Between Age and Maximal Heart Rate

Age	Max Heart Rate	85% Max	70% Max
20	200	170	140
25	195	166	137
30	190	162	133
35	185	158	129
40	180	153	126
45	175	149	123
50	170	145	119
55	165	140	115
60	160	136	112

TABLE 7 Recommended Target Heart Rates for Healthy Individuals (Assuming resting heart rate = 75)

Age	20–24	25–29	30–34	35–39	40–44	45–49	50–54	55–59
MHR*	198	193	188	183	178	173	168	163
PTHR†	186	181	177	172	168	168	158	154
ATHR‡	161	158	154	151	147	143	140	136
LTHR§	149	146	143	140	137	133	131	128

* MHR = maximal heart rate (220 − age)
† PTHR = peak training heart rate = $.9(HR_{max} - HR_{rest}) + HR_{rest}$
‡ ATHR = average training heart rate = $.7(HR_{max} - HR_{rest}) + HR_{rest}$
§ LTRH = low training heart rate = $.6(HR_{max} - HR_{rest}) + HR_{rest}$

Modified from: American College of Sports Medicine: Guidelines for Graded Exercise Testing and Exercise Prescription, 2nd Edition. Philadelphia: Lea & Febiger, 1980.

once functional capacity has been determined. This method allows only for the prescription of activities with documented metabolic costs. A range of 60 to 85 percent maximum METs (MMET) corresponds to low and peak conditioning intensities, respectively. An average training intensity may be calculated as:

$$TMET = MMET \times [\frac{60 + MMET}{100}]$$

Concurrent measurement of heart rate and metabolic rate (METs) during a graded exercise test allows interpolation of the corresponding training heart rate. Since 1 MET=4.2 kilojoules/kg/hr per m^2, energy expenditure per activity session can be also determined.

Other Methods of Determining Exercise Intensity

More sophisticated laboratory testing allows a determination of anaerobic threshold. Prescriptions for the unconditioned patient should remain well below the anaerobic threshold, since this intensity corresponds to a rapid increase in blood lactate. Better conditioned patients have a higher anaerobic threshold and can thus tolerate a greater relative intensity of training.

EXERCISE DURATION

The duration of exercise must be sufficient to increase energy expenditure by at least 1200 kilojoules (1 kilocalorie = 4.18 kilojoules).

Very short periods of exercise (5 to 10 minutes) can induce cardiovascular training if performed at very high intensity (90 to 95 percent of functional capacity), although the ideal plan for most patients is 20 to 60 minutes of continuous aerobic activity at a moderate intensity. Initially, the session should be relatively short (15 to 20 minutes), but it can be gradually extended as the individual habituates to regular activity, and as cardiovascular endurance improves.

There are several advantages of a longer exercise session. Compliance with high-intensity programs is poor, and participants sustain a high incidence of musculoskeletal injuries. In addition, fat utilization increases significantly after approximately 20 minutes of light-to-moderate exercise, enhancing body fat reduction.

FREQUENCY OF EXERCISES

The threshold for improvement of aerobic power seems to be two sessions of exercise per week, but the intensity must be relatively high for gains to occur. If frequency is reduced to once weekly, roughly half of the improvement in fitness is lost within 10 weeks.

The minimum recommended frequency for normal adults (3 to 10 METs functional capacity) is three sessions, scattered evenly through each week. This is an optimal frequency at the initial stage of an exercise program, as it allows sufficient rest for musculoskeletal adaptation between exercise bouts.

In the obese and other adults with very low functional capacities (less than 3 METs), it may be more practical to prescribe repeated sessions of 5 minutes several times per day. As functional capacity improves to 3 to 5 METs, one to two longer daily sessions can be undertaken.

As functional capacity further improves and the musculoskeletal system has adapted to increased activity, frequency can be increased to 3 or more sessions per week. However, easier days must then be included on which duration and intensity are reduced.

For attainment of optimal fitness levels, 5 days per week is sufficient. Progression from 3 to 5 days per week should occur gradually over a 4-week period, and no more than three intense sessions should occur per week. Exercising 7 days per week does not further improve aerobic power, but might serve to satisfy a perceived need for daily activity in those who have integrated exercise into their life style. On the other hand, the risk of injury becomes quite high, and many low-intensity days must be included. The exception is the obese adult; in such individuals, low-intensity sessions must be performed every day to attain the energy expenditure needed to reduce body fat.

If strength fitness or isotonic resistance training are to be incorporated into the regular aerobic exercise program, such activities should be undertaken no more than 2 or 3 days per week because a longer recuperative period is needed for heavy-resistance work.

EXERCISE MODE

Activities that utilize large muscle groups, in a rhythmic and continuous manner, are the preferred form of aerobic exercise. Theoretically, there should be no difference between modalities in terms of conditioning effect provided the criteria of intensity, frequency, and duration are met. Significant differences of heart rate response may exist, however, and strict attention must thus be paid to the energy requirements of each specific activity.

Similar cardiovascular training can be generated by jogging/running, swimming, bicycling, and cross-country skiing programs. Less intense activities such as golf, bowling, and archery offer little training stimulus, as heart rates rarely exceed 100 beats/minute. Skipping has become quite popular in recent years, although it may produce very high heart rates, and patients who are restricted to moderate exercise intensities should avoid this mode of activity. Both tennis and squash are adequate stimuli, if skill is at a sufficient level. However, squash involves rapid starts and stops, thereby increasing systemic blood pressure and myocardial O_2 demands: it should thus be prescribed only in healthy, risk-free patients.

Sustained isometric (static) activities against heavy resistance should be strongly discouraged in unconditioned, hypertensive, and coronary-prone patients. Such exercises are not aerobic activities, and there is little or no improvement of $\dot{V}O_2$ max with weight training or circuit training utilizing heavy weights.

The chosen activity should therefore be of sufficient intensity to elicit training while minimizing both musculoskeletal strain and blood pressure response. Further, the exercise must be enjoyable, providing the patient with evidence of improvement and reward, thereby facilitating motivation and compliance.

TYPE OF EXERCISE

Aerobic Activities

Both continuous and intermittent (interval) exercise can elicit a training response. The advantage of interval training (high intensity, short duration, with rest intervals) is widely recognized, and it is the form of training practiced by most endurance athletes. High-intensity exercise may be performed without significant accumulation of lactic acid, allowing high speed training and faster eventual performance times. The sedentary adult can accomplish more total work with less physiologic stress. It is advantageous to prescribe exercise on a run-walk basis initially, and as functional capacity improves, a higher energy output may be performed more continuously. Activities that are continuous and elicit a constant heart rate response (walking, jogging or running, cross country skiing, swimming, cycling) are preferred when a close control of both duration and intensity of exercise is desired. More intense interval activities (interval training, sports with an intermittent and high-intensity component) should be recommended only after an adequate period of continuous training (6 to 10 weeks).

Flexibility Activities

Flexibility exercises and calisthenics are performed during the warm-up and cool-down periods. They should be performed slowly and in a static manner (i.e., "reach and hold"). Bouncing beyond the existing range of motion is not advised since elicitation of the stretch reflex may lead to soft tissue injury.

Muscular Strength Activities

Attempts to enhance muscle strength through dynamic, high-resistance, low-repetition exercise should be strongly discouraged in patients who are unconditioned, hypertensive, or at risk of cardiovascular disease. Dynamic and static strength exercises, especially when combined with a Valsalva maneuver, may cause an excessive rise of systemic blood pressure, reducing venous return and augmenting the work of the heart by an increase of afterload. If muscular strength is required for occupational needs, low-resistance, high-repetition exercises should be prescribed, taking care to avoid breathholding.

THE EXERCISE SESSION

Every exercise session should include three components: a warm-up, an endurance phase, and a cool-down. The warm-up should last 5 to 10 minutes and should consist of light calisthenics, stretching exercises, and slow jogging or walking. Such a warm-up should help to minimize musculoskeletal injuries. Increases in muscle and general body temperature increase muscle blood flow, reduce tissue viscosity, and enhance both O_2 dissociation and enzymatic reactions (law of Arrhenius). Moreover, sudden bursts of intense exercise without warm-up may precipitate ventricular fibrillation. Vasodilatation in exercising muscle serves to reduce the work of the heart through a decrease of afterloading.

The stimulus period at the specified intensity and duration should be initiated slowly immediately ater warm-up.

A gradual cool-down lasting approximatley 5 to 10 minutes uses exercises similar to those of the warm-up period. An abrupt cessation of exercise, particularly in a warm and humid environment, may cause venous pooling and circulatory collapse, with syncope, vertigo, nausea, and possibly myocardial ischemia. Hot showers, saunas, and whirlpools should be avoided until long after the warm-down and are strongly contraindicated in patients with coronary heart disease.

MONITORING EXERCISE

Palpation of heart rate is the easiest method to monitor intensity and progression of exercise, and with appropriate instruction, palpation can be as accurate as telemetry. Self-palpation should be taught in the early stages of counseling. Wrist palpation is preferred by us to avoid the risk of reflex hypotension with overly vigorous carotid palpation.

During the first few sessions, following 3 to 5 minutes of exercise, the patient should stop and locate the wrist pulse within one second. The pulse is immediately counted for 10 seconds, and the count is multiplied by 6 to yield a minute rate (first beat counted = 0). It is imperative that the count begin rapidly because HR decreases a few seconds after exercise has stopped.

As individuals become accustomed to perceiving an appropriate effort, pulses can be counted once during and once after the stimulus period. Borg's "rating of perceived exertion" can also be used as a guide to exercise intensity in selected patients:

Borg Scale

$\left.{3 \atop 4}\right\rangle$ = extremely light

$\left.{5 \atop 6}\right\rangle$ = very light

$\left.{7 \atop 8}\right\rangle$ = light

$\left.{9 \atop 10}\right\rangle$ = rather light

$\left.{11 \atop 12}\right\rangle$ = neither light nor hard

$\left.{13 \atop 14}\right\rangle$ = rather hard

$\left.{15 \atop 16}\right\rangle$ = hard

$\left.{17 \atop 18}\right\rangle$ = very hard

19 = extremely hard

Borg scores between 12 and 17 correspond to target zone heart rates for most age groups over a normal 20 to 40-minute exercise session. Debate continues on how accurately the RPE scale correlates with heart rate, however. It seems more useful in classes than for individual exercise. The rating must be made during exercise, and not as an afterthought in the shower room.

Nevertheless, experienced participants can accurately gauge the intensity of effort by sensation alone.

PROGRESSION OF EXERCISE PRESCRIPTIONS

As greater amounts of exercise become possible, intensity, frequency, and duration should be adjusted upward. The ideal rate of progression is often difficult for the practitioner to determine. It depends on many factors; both the individual patient and the training environment must be considered when planning a progression of the exercise prescription. The American College of Sports Medicine has outlined a three-phase progression, designed to prevent musculoskeletal injuries, while allowing attainment of optimal fitness.

The initial stage covers the first to the fifth week of the training program. Stretching, light calisthenics, and low-intensity aerobics are introduced, taking care to avoid undue discomfort that could frustrate and discourage. In most cases, the aerobic phase should be begun 1 MET lower than the estimated intensity.

Objective measures of readiness to progress include: (1) a 3 to 8-beat/min decrease of heart rate during the aerobic phase of exercise, (2) voluntary adoption of a slightly faster jogging or walking pace, and (3) an improvement in functional capacity seen at exercise testing.

Subjective measures are more difficult to evaluate, but can also provide a useful guide to progression. Indicators include the level of fatigue, facial expression, breathing pattern, perceived exertion, and movement patterns.

During this phase, the aerobic session lasts 12 to 15 minutes; the participant aims to spend 800 kilojoules per session during the first week of training, and eventually the recommended 1200 kilojoules per session.

The second phase lasts from week 6 to about week 27. Duration is extended, and intensity is gradually raised from 60 to 70 to 90 percent over this phase.

If functional capacity is low, the transition from walking to jogging is best accomplished by initially using a discontinuous walk/run pattern and gradually progressing toward continuous steady-state exercise.

The third phase, the maintenance phase, is reached after 6 months of regular activity. At this point, participants are exercising at 70 to 90 percent of estimated functional capacity for at least 45 to 60 minutes, 4 or 5 times per week. Compliance-oriented goals become important in ensuring that the program continues to satisfy the participant's needs over a long-term period. Ideally, other aerobic activities should be introduced, not only for variety, but also to avoid narrow training of only a selected set of muscles.

Sample Exercise Prescriptions

This section is intended to illustrate specific examples of exercise prescriptions utilizing various methods of quantifying exercise intensity. Energy expenditure tables for various occupational and leisure activities, which are found elsewhere in this book and in numerous other sources, are indispensible for counseling your patients on the caloric expenditure of various activities.

Heart Rate

For a sedentary 46-year-old male with a resting heart rate of 78 beats/min and a heart rate of 175 beats/min, prescribe a training intensity of 60 percent HR reserve:

$$HR_{train} = HR_{rest} + 0.6 \,(HR_{max} - HR_{rest})$$

$$HR_{train} = 78 + 0.6\,(175 - 78)$$

HR_{train} = 136 beats/min 3 times a week. Start at 12 min/session for first 2 weeks, increase to 30 minutes and 75% HR reserve by end of 4th week. Mode is walking/jogging.

METs

After completing a maximal exercise test (HR_{max} = 166) a 65-kg, 50-year-old male (resting HR = 72) is found to have a $\dot{V}O_2$max of 41.5 ml/kg/min. Prescribe a training intensity of 70% of maximal $\dot{V}O_2$ or METs:

$$41.5 \div 3.5 = 11.86 \text{ METs}$$

$$\text{Training Intensity} = \frac{70 + 11.8}{100} \times 11.86$$

$$= 9.7 \text{ METs}$$

To monitor intensity, a training HR of 143 beats/min (72 + .75 [166 − 72]) should also be prescribed.

METs to speed of walking or jogging

The energy costs of walking and jogging vary greatly between 4 and 5 mph (Cunningham and Rechnitzer, Arch Phys Med Rehab 55:296, 1974). The prescribed speed in mph can be reliably estimated for three separate ranges:

$$\text{for speeds} < 4 \text{ mph} \quad v = \frac{(\text{TMETs} - 1 \text{ MET})}{.88} - 1.01$$

$$\text{for speeds } 4\text{–}5 \text{ mph} \quad v = \frac{(\text{TMETs} - 1 \text{ MET})}{3.37} + 8.51$$

$$\text{for speeds} > 5 \text{ mph} \quad v = \frac{(\text{TMETs} - 1 \text{ MET})}{1.37} - 1.85$$

$$v = \text{speed of activity (mph)}$$

$$\text{TMETs} = \text{calculated training METs}$$

In example 2, maximum METs was 11.86, and the calculated TMETs at 70% was 9.7. The third formula is used:

$$v = \frac{(9.7 - 1) - 1.85}{1.37}$$

$$v = 5.0 \text{ mph}$$

This patient should thus jog at 5.0 mph or cover 2.5 miles in 30 minutes. This represents an above-average aerobic fitness for his age and sex. The frequency can thus be extended to 3 to 5 days/week after 2 weeks at this intensity. The training HR is 137 beats/min (72 + 0.7 [166 − 72]), and values of 151 beats/min (85%) should not be exceeded as a safety check. The exercise session should be preceded by a 10-minute warm-up and a 5- to 10-minute cool-down at reduced intensities.

Stretching for the posterior muscle groups should follow toward the end of the cool-down.

An alternate method of determining *horizontal* walking and jogging speeds is to use the following formula:

walk: $\dot{V}O_2$ ml/kg/min = v (m/min) × 0.1 ml/kg/min per m/min. + 3.5 ml/kg/min (Table 8)

jog: $\dot{V}O_2$ ml/kg/min = v (m/min) × 0.2 ml/kg/min per m/min. + 3.5 ml/kg/min (Table 9)

$$v = \text{speed in m/min}$$

An example for walking speeds:
An obese 47-year-old female has a $\dot{V}O_2$max of 20.5 ml/kg/min. She will be exercising at 60% of this. What will the walking speed be for this patient?

$$0.6 \times 20.5 = 12.3 \text{ ml/kg/min}$$

Subtracting resting metabolism 12.3 − 3.5 =
$$8.8 \text{ ml/kg/min}$$

$$\frac{8.8}{0.1} = 88 \text{ m/min}$$

This patient should start with 3 or 4 sessions per day of 5 to 10 minutes of activity. After 2 weeks, she can progress to 3 sessions per week, each of 10 to 15 min duration. Subsequently, duration and intensity can be increased to 30 min/session and 70 to 80% $\dot{V}O_2$max, respectively. Cycle ergometry at the same intensity and duration can be substituted if joint or tendon pain from weight-bearing becomes a problem.

Cycle Ergometry

To calculate the metabolic cost of cycle ergometry in ml of O_2/kg/min, the following equation is utilized:

$$\dot{V}O_2 \text{ ml/min} = 10.7 \times \text{work rate (Watts)} + 300 \text{ ml.}$$

A 72.5 kg female attains a work load of 200 Watts during a fitness test in your office. What is the $\dot{V}O_2$max?

$$\dot{V}O_2\text{max (ml/min.)} = (10.7 \times 200) + 300$$

$$= 2440 \text{ ml/min.}$$

$$\dot{V}O_2\text{max (ml/kg/min)} = \frac{2440}{72.5} = 33.7 \text{ or } 9.6 \text{ METs.}$$

TABLE 8 Energy Cost of Horizontal Walking

Walking Speed	METs					
	2.3	2.5	2.9	3.3	3.6	3.9
min/mile	35	30	24	20	17.6	16
mph	1.7	2.0	2.5	3.0	3.4	3.75
m/min	45.6	53.7	67.0	80.5	91.2	100.5

TABLE 9   Engergy Cost of Horizontal Jogging

Speed	METs						
	8.6	10.2	11.7	12.5	13.3	14.8	16.3
min/mile	12:00	10:00	8.34	8:00	7.30	6.40	6:00
mph	5	6	7	7.5	8	9	10
m/min	134	161	188	201	215	241	268

SOME FINAL SUGGESTIONS

Individual patients respond at varying rates to any exercise program, and the prescription should be "dispensed" with the individual in mind. It must appeal to the patient, conforming to family, leisure, and business schedules. Monitoring of progress by training diaries and follow-up tests provides external feedback in addition to the intrinsic rewards of improved well-being and vigor. Such support and encouragement is important to compliance (See Chapter 6) and also helps in determining the effectiveness of the exercise program. Patients should be told that the early stages of exercise are the most uncomfortable, that initial improvements of fitness are rapid, but that further improvements occur much more slowly. As returns diminish, the concept of maintaining optimal fitness should be stressed, rather than continued improvement. The weakest link in an asymptomatic adult is generally the musculoskeletal system, and to avoid injury, progression of training should amount to only 5 to 10 percent increases in total volume per week, with frequent rest days each week, and a rest week each month. Training errors seem to be the primary cause of the overuse injuries seen so frequently in sports medicine, and discussed elsewhere in this text.

IMPROVING EXERCISE COMPLIANCE

NEIL B. OLDRIDGE, Ph.D.

The answer to the question, "What should our exercise program be like?" is complex, but it is also simple: there is no *one* exercise rehabilitation program to suit all situations. Each program is different, with unique patients, unique expectations, and unique facilities. There may very well be some similarities in different situations, but to expect a single model to meet the diversity of patient needs is being overly simplistic.

Many, if not all, supervised programs have a problem, to one degree or another, with patient compliance; the generally quoted figure is approximately 40 to 50 percent "dropout" of participants over 6 to 12 months. Although some patients "drop out" of formal programs to undertake no further exercise, others feel they have gained what they wanted from the supervised program and continue to exercise regularly elsewhere or on their own. At McMaster University our experience is that fully 50 percent of dropouts claim to continue their exercise after dropping out and that 66 percent of these individuals state "I gained what I wanted" as their reason for dropping out. The question, "What can I do to minimize dropouts?" is complex and needs careful evaluation. The following ideas for reducing the likelihood of dropping out of programs of exercise for patients with documented heart disease will not answer all problems, but are based upon 12 years experience with the McMaster University Cardiac Rehabilitation Program—the MacTurtles. The MacTurtle program is constantly evolving, based on what our patients, and we, believe is optimal within the limitations set by facilities, personnel, equipment and philosophy. Ideas are taken both from patient suggestions for improvement and from what has been tried in other programs, not all of which have been exercise management programs.

THE PROBLEM: RELATIVELY POOR COMPLIANCE

Management of a medical problem cannot be successful unless advice is followed. The extent to which a person's behavior coincides with medical advice is defined as compliance or adherence, and except under certain medicolegal circumstances, everybody has a right to either accept or refuse advice, medical or otherwise. Compliance with long-term medical treatment or management is a critical issue; frequently there is a marked difference between what has been prescribed and what is carried out by the patient—and this is equally true whether medication or behavioral change is prescribed. For example, only about 20 to 30 percent of hypertensives are under adequate blood pressure control; as many as 50 percent of hypertensive patients take prescribed medications for less than one year, and only about 60 to 70 percent of those who continue with medication take enough to achieve therapeutic benefit. Long-term health behavioral management programs have notoriously poor compliance rates; programs for the control of obesity commonly see dropout rates of 50 percent in year 1 and 75 percent or more by the end of year 2. The extent of the problem and the consequent lack of management effectiveness makes compliance an important issue. In exercise, the situation is further confounded by the problem of overuse injury, particularly in the early phases of the newly acquired behavior.

In reports of exercise research and service programs for the rehabilitative management of patients with coronary artery disease, the dropout rate has been variously reported to be as low as 3 percent and as high as 87 percent. While a number of factors have been identified as having an important influence upon compliance, the underlying reasons for the wide range of dropout rates are differences in program management and lack of a consistent definition of exercise compliance. Examples of possible definitions of compliance include the proportion of subjects returning for testing, the proportion of subjects attending a given proportion of exercise sessions over a given time, the proportion of subjects attending over a given time, the achievement of a certain increase in oxygen transport or decrease in body mass. By definition, those not meeting the criteria set are then dropouts or noncompliers. In other studies, the focus has been on the dropouts, defined as those missing a certain number of sessions, consecutive or total, with all other subjects considered as compliers whether or not they attended a given proportion of the sessions or achieved a certain physiologic improvement. This indeed may be appropriate if there is benefit from attending exercise sessions even if the working capacity is not significantly augmented.

The problems of comparing compliance (dropout) rates becomes even more difficult when some patients are expected to commit themselves to a program for a pre-determined period, while others attend open-ended programs with no specific commitment. Some patients are also self-referred, while others are physician referred or recruited from hospital records. Patients furthermore have different outcome expectations, for instance, becoming fit, losing weight, or increasing self-confidence by learning what to do and what not to do. Comparisons are further confounded when research studies are compared to service programs. Other factors limiting the possibility of making comparisons include the following: (1) some exercise programs are formally organized and start soon after the event while others are less structured and start later, (2) some are walking programs and others provide cycle ergometer exercise, (3) some patients have angina on exertion while others do not, and (4) some programs expect to "graduate" patients and others expect them to become long-term "clients". This last factor is further compounded if expectations become requirements. Factors affecting compliance (adherence) and dropout in long-term behavioral change programs can be summarized as (1) patient-related, (2) personnel-related, (3) facility-related, and (4) program-related.

Patient Factors

There is little consensus about the relationship between standard demographic variables and compliance with health care in general or exercise rehabilitation in particular. In studies in which a relationship between patient characteristics and compliance has been reported, other factors may also have been an influence. High self-motivation levels appear to be associated with a good exercise compliance, but the converse may not be true. Low initial self-motivation may or may not be counter-balanced by family support, by a growing self-confidence with improvement in physical condition, by enjoyment of the new experience, or by other factors that reinforce the value of the new behavior. An excess of body fat has been associated with poor compliance with exercise, but many heavier people do not join exercise programs. Smoking has been associated with an increased likelihood of dropout in the Ontario Exercise Heart Collaborative (OEHCS) 4-year exercise rehabilitation study where 58 percent of smokers (who made up 34 percent of the study population) dropped out in less than 2 years; other factors predicting dropout from this study of 733 men with myocardial infarction included blue-collar work status and the presence of angina. Blue collar workers understand less about their disease and the rehabilitative process than do white collar workers. It also makes good common sense that if exercise produces chest discomfort, the probability of dropout will be increased. In approximately 200 consecutive cardiac patients referred to the 6-month supervised MacTurtle exercise rehabilitation program, we were able to identify correctly about 3 of 4 (77%) of (1) smokers, blue-collar workers, and inactive subjects as dropouts and (2) non-smokers, white-collar workers, and active subjects as compliers (overall 55 percent compliance rate). One aspect of the MacTurtle program which differentiates it from many other exercise rehabilitation programs is that approximately 50 percent of participants are blue-collar workers. This is not because Hamilton has a particularly large proportion of blue-collar workers; perhaps there is a greater perception of the value of exercise, both among the local medical community and the community-at-large.

The major problem in using patient characteristics as predictors of exercise behavior is that human behavior is essentially unpredictable. Two factors which are important to an optimizing of patient compliance are (1) family, particularly spousal, support, and (2) satisfaction with the program personnel. A number of reports have emphasized the value of a spouse who has a positive perception of the partner's physical activity. One 2 year study of high-risk subjects carried out in the late 1960s found a good or excellent adherence in 80 percent of subjects with spousal support, compared to fair or poor adherence in 60 percent of subjects where the spouse had a neutral or negative attitude to the program. In the OEHCS, three times as many dropouts reported a perceived (or actual) lack of spousal support as reported a positive spousal attitude. This has obvious implications for compliance-improving strategies, as does the factor of participant satisfaction with the program and the personnel.

Personnel Factors

There are few data concerning the desirable characteristics of clinicians and other exercise program personnel. Results from the OEHCS indicate a 2-fold increase of drop-out rate where the patient perceived little individual attention, with an impersonal or unreceptive attitude. The general literature supports the notion of better compliance when the clinician and other personnel are perceived by patients to be warm and empathetic, to meet patient expectations, to show interest, to demonstrate concern, to give specific, individualized instructions, and to involve patients in their own management.

Facility Factors

It is difficult to alter the physical structure of an exercise facility, but there are certain features associated with better compliance. A facility that is within easy commuting distance of the patient's home or work site tends to encourage continued participation; programs offered at different times of the day promote better compliance; a variety of exercise facilities and adequate equipment are positively perceived. These factors, together with the personnel factors, offer the participant a greater sense of cooperation, flexibility, and variety, encouraging compliance.

Program Factors

Increasing complexity, longer duration, greater inconvenience, and the potential for uncomfortable side effects are all program features that have a major impact on exercise compliance. Some of these features can be changed, offering the program director the greatest potential for minimizing dropouts.

Prediction of exercise compliance remains imprecise. Certain characteristics provide some idea of the likelihood that an individual will drop out of a supervised exercise program. These characteristics do not, however, predict whether an individual will continue to exercise after either completing or dropping out of a supervised exercise program. It is difficult to change the physical structure of a facility, and in practice changes in program design, structure, and administration offer the greatest potential as methods of improving compliance. Such tactics must frequently be complemented by changed or even new attitudes on the part of those who administer the program. Too often the participant is given sole blame for poor adherence. In many cases, this is incorrect. A number of potential compliance-improving strategies should be considered. Some are simply good administrative policy and an effective use of communication skills.

COMPLIANCE-IMPROVEMENT STRATEGIES

On Entry

Measures to ensure compliance on entry include:

1. Make sure the patients know what they are undertaking and what they are expecting. The program director has a responsibility to provide as much information as possible and the patient has the right to expect this. When patients perceive that they will benefit from the program, the probability of compliance increases.

2. Introduce new patients to other patients and staff at their first session to make them feel "at home" and increase the likelihood of their returning.

3. Try to be as open as possible about risks and benefits: "We don't know that exercise will prevent another heart attack; we don't expect you to jog if you don't want to; there are potential hazards to inappropriate exercise, but we are providing you with counsel about appropriate exercise and we have emergency procedures carefully designed; we are here to provide you with answers, so ask as many questions as you wish; when we don't know the answers we will tell you that we don't know; we will not interfere with your medical management, but will consult with your physician whenever necessary; we will start out slowly and progress on an individual basis as you are the only one like you in the program; there are a number of individuals who have the same kind of problems as you and they may be able to help you, or you may be able to help them, so talk to them; this is what your exercise test tells us; we cannot exercise for you, you are going to have to take a lot of the responsibility on your own shoulders, and exercise at home."

The foregoing "strategies" are designed to provide the patient with a sense of self-confidence, of belonging to a group, and of interest in individuals on the part of the program staff, while reinforcing the concept of personal responsibility for program management. These approaches should be regular practice in any well-organized program; local circumstances will determine details, but a friendly, warm introduction, with a careful explanation of program and patient responsibilities should be viewed by the patient in a positive fashion. One of the basic tenets of our program is to try to get patients to accept personal responsibility for their exercise and other health behavior habits. We always tell the patient that our responsibility is to provide information about exercising safely and appropriately, so that personal responsibility can be assumed for exercise habits, to a degree while enrolled in the program, and certainly after "graduation". We always state our expectation of graduation within 6 months: "Your graduation is our success". Behaviors learned during those 6 months should result in changed attitudes, including a willingness to exercise alone or with one of the outreach programs.

During the Program

Compliance-improving strategies are usually methods of behavioral management. Those discussed in this chapter have been investigated at McMaster or have been investigated elsewhere and incorporated into the MacTurtle program.

Behavioral contracting. We demonstrated a 6-month compliance rate of 65 percent in subjects who signed an agreement to comply for 6 months, compared with 42 percent in control subjects (no agreement) and 20 percent in subjects who refused to sign the agreement. This is in agreement with studies of hypertensive men, in which a positive reply to the question "Do you intend taking your medication?" was the strongest predictor of compliance. Contingency contracting also improves compliance with exercise habits in healthy populations, but to our knowledge this approach has not been formally investigated in cardiac exercise programs. We now include a statement of intent to comply in our informed consent sheet and very few patients balk at signing it.

Goal-setting, Feedback, and Self-Control. We provide a 3-month target workload, based on the initial exercise test results, and encourage patients to set themselves short-term goals in the process of achieving the target workloads. We also encourage patients to initiate a request for an increase in their exercise prescription, based on their own observations of changes in their heart rate and rating of perceived exertion during submaximal effort. We provide each patient with a monthly mini-assessment form on the reverse side of their daily record (Fig. 1); patients are asked to complete three 5-minute steady-state work-bouts on the cycle ergometer at their present training load, and at 16 to 50 Watts less and 16 to 50 Watts more than their present training load. They record their own heart rate and rating of perceived exertion, plotting the heart rate/power output relationship on the graph. As soon as this is done, they take the completed graph to the program director to compare the results with the previous month's mini-assessment and

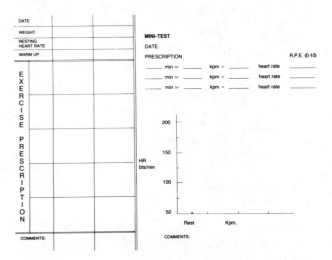

Figure 1 Acknowledgements: I would like to acknowledge the valuable contributions made by patients, students and many colleagues who have at one time or another been MacTurtles, as well as those involved in the OEHCS. Much of the investigation has been supported by the Ontario Ministry of Health, Health and Welfare, Canada, Medical Research Council, Ontario Heart Foundation and Fitness and Amateur Sport, Canada.

the previous graded exercise test results. The discussion is directed to get the patient to decide whether or not his own exercise prescription should be altered.

In our minds there is no doubt that this is an effective compliance-improving tactic. When investigating perceptions of the program, we found that 49 percent of the variance in compliance could be explained by the single variable "value of information gained from the graded exercise tests and mini-assessments". It is our firm conviction that maximizing feedback to the patients is essential in optimizing compliance. Each patient is responsible for maintaining his or her own record book, while the staff has the responsibility to discuss with the patient progress or lack of progress, making appropriate alterations in the exercise prescription in the light of these discussions.

Support. We are convinced that the support of the spouse has prime importance. Whenever possible, the spouse should be present at the exercise test, at the first exercise session, at education sessions, and at social gatherings (we try to arrange pot-luck dinners, as well as a summer activity, and a winter activity for the family each year). Because of the success of a family night program, because of requests from patients, and because we are lucky enough to have adequate facilities and leadership support (undergraduate and graduate students), we have initiated a program for spouses. This runs in conjunction with the patient program. The spouses join in the group warm-up and cool-down activities and have their own "aerobics" program. The value of this seems considerable; the compliance rate among those who participate with their spouses is 75 percent and the overall group compliance rate has improved to more than 60 percent following this innovation.

Another important support, positively perceived by the patients, is our referral system. A number of patients have specific problems unrelated to exercise. Over the years, we have developed a support system for such individuals. Programs with a special focus operate either specifically for the MacTurtle patients, or independently, accepting MacTurtle patients on a referral basis. Behavioral management programs focus—on an individual or a group basis— on coping strategies, nutrition and cooking skills, reducing smoking, stress/relaxation, and sexuality. The patients appear to be quite open in approaching us for referral, and we generally encourage spousal participation. Such programs supplement our regular 10-session education/information round-table discus-

sion series which runs alternate weeks and is designed so that new patients can fit in at any time.

COMPLIANCE AFTER GRADUATION

We have initiated outreach programs at several levels. The YMCA and YWCA accept our patients into appropriate programs. We offer a continuing exercise program at the University to all graduates (and dropouts). One group of patients contacted a local school, requested access to exercise facilities which were not being used, and with the support of one of our exercise leaders, now run their own twice-weekly program for themselves and their spouses. Some patients prefer to exercise on their own, and we provide a basic exercise prescription and program for them. All these individuals are still considered as MacTurtles, are eligible for annual exercise testing, and are invited to the various social events.

We have initiated a system of monthly return visits, where a self-monitored mini-assessment is completed and discussed as explained above. This approach was initiated following a report of the relative effectiveness of infrequent return visits by Kavanagh and colleagues. In addition, all patients are contacted for reassessment at 6 and 12 months after graduation or dropout. They remain eligible for annual reassessments thereafter, but must initiate the necessary appointment themselves. These strategies are all designed to sustain the new exercise behavior, which needs regular support and positive reinforcement.

Considerable care must be taken when motivating individuals to adopt or comply with exercise programs. Exercise has not been shown to prevent diseases such as coronary heart disease, nor has it been shown to increase longevity. These claims are inappropriate when motivating persons to become or remain, physically active. Regular exercise is associated with benefits such as an increased exercise tolerance, a more efficient cardiorespiratory system, lower body mass, favorable changes in lipoprotein profile, increased muscle tone, strength and power, increased self-confidence and "joie de vivre". Such evidence should be given to the non-exercisers. They can then make an educated decision. Once that decision is made, it becomes legitimate to incorporate various compliance-improving strategies into a program of enjoyable activities provided the strategies used are not coercive.

NUTRITION FOR THE ATHLETE

FRANK I. KATCH, M.D.

Active, exercising men and women do not require additional nutrients beyond those obtained from a balanced diet. People who eat well-balanced meals of meat, cereal, vegetables, fruit, and milk consume more than an adequate supply of vitamins to meet daily requirements. Because vitamins can be used repeatedly in metabolic reactions, the vitamin needs of athletes and other active people are generally no greater than those of sedentary people. As the level of energy expenditure increases, the amount of food required increases to maintain body mass. Competitive marathon runners, for example, consume as much as 21 megajoules of energy (5000 Calories) daily to supply the needs of their daily training. The increased food intake usually boosts the intake of vitamins and minerals, provided the person maintains a well-balanced diet. The extra energy required for exercise can be obtained from a variety of nutritious foods. Sound nutritional guidelines must be followed in planning and evaluating food intake. An optimal diet is defined as one in which the supply of required nutrients is adequate for tissue maintenance, repair, and growth. Only in the last few years has it been possible to obtain a reasonable estimate of the specific nutrient needs for men and women of various ages and body sizes, making due allowance for individual differences in digestion, storage capacity, nutrient metabolism, and daily levels of energy expenditure.

RECOMMENDED NUTRIENT INTAKE

Protein Requirement. The standard recommendation for protein intake is 0.8 g of protein per kg of body mass, which amounts to approximately 12 percent of total energy content in the typical diet. A person who weighs 75 kg would therefore need about 60 g of protein daily.

The average American consumes more than twice this protein requirement. Athletes, many of whom consume considerable quantities of food, may eat more than three times the protein requirement! There is no benefit from eating excessive protein. Muscle mass is not increased simply by eating high-protein foods. Additional energy taken in the form of protein is converted to fat and stored in the subcutaneous depots. In fact, excessive protein may be harmful because the metabolism of large quantities may place an inordinate strain on liver and renal function.

Fat Requirement. Optimal fat intake has not been firmly established because relatively little is known about human requirements for this nutrient. The amount of dietary fat varies widely according to personal taste, money spent on food, and the availability of fat-rich foods. Only about 10 percent of the energy in the average Asian diet is furnished by fat, whereas in the United States, Canada, Scandinavia, Germany, and France, fat accounts for 40 to 50 percent of energy intake. For optimal health, fat intake probably should not exceed 30 percent of the energy content of the diet. Of this 30 percent, at least half should be in the form of unsaturated fats. Even this quantity of dietary fat may be too high, especially for individuals suffering from gallbladder disease and certain cardiovascular diseases.

Attempts to eliminate "all" fat from the diet, however, are detrimental in terms of exercise performance. With low-fat diets, it is difficult to increase one's intake of carbohydrate and protein to furnish sufficient energy to maintain a stable body mass during strenuous training. Because the major essential fatty acid, linoleic acid, and many vitamins gain entrance to the body through dietary fat, a "fat-free" diet could eventually result in relative malnutrition.

Carbohydrate Requirement. How much carbohydrate should be consumed? Like fat, the prominence of carbohydrates in the diet varies widely throughout the world, depending upon factors such as the availability and relative cost of fat- and protein-rich foods. Carbohydrate-rich foods such as grains, starchy roots, and dried peas and beans are usually the cheapest foods in relation to their energy value. In the Far East, carbohydrates (mainly rice) contribute 80 percent of the total energy intake, whereas in the United States, only 40 to 50 percent of the energy requirement comes from carbohydrates. For a sedentary 70 kg person, the latter amounts to approximately 147 g of carbohydrate per day.

There seems to be no health hazard in subsisting chiefly on carbohydrates (starches), provided the essential amino acids, minerals, and vitamins are also present in the diet. In fact, the diet of the relatively primitive Tarahumara Indians of Mexico is high in complex carbohydrates (75% of energy) and fiber (19 mg/day) and correspondingly low in cholesterol (71 mg/day), fat (12% of energy), and saturated fat (2% of energy). Certain of these people are noted for their remarkable physical endurance; they reportedly run distances up to 300 km in competitive soccer-type sports events that often last several days. Their diet may be beneficial to health. Particularly notable among the Tarahumaras is the virtual absence of hypertension, obesity, and death from cardiac and circulatory complications.

If the individual is physically active, the "prudent" diet should provide at least 50 to 60 percent of energy in the form of carbohydrates, predominantly starches. In training for specific sports and prior to competition, the carbohydrate intake may even be increased above this recommended level to ensure adequate glycogen stores.

DIET AND ENDURANCE PERFORMANCE

The specific nutrient fuel for muscular contraction depends not only on exercise intensity, but also on the duration of the activity and, to some degree, on the diet of the individual. During continuous, moderate exercise, the energy for muscular contraction is provided predominantly from the body's fat and carbohydrate reserves. If exercise continues and glycogen stores in the liver and muscles are reduced, an even greater percentage of energy must be supplied by the breakdown of fat. This food nutrient is mobilized from storage sites such as adipose tissue and the liver and is delivered via the circulation to the working muscles. However, if exercise continues to the point where the glycogen stored in specific muscles is severely lowered, the performer may tire easily. It is interesting to note that glycogen is reduced only in the muscles that are actively involved in performing the exercise. Because there are no enzymes to aid the transfer of glycogen between muscles, inactive muscles conserve their glycogen stores.

Fatigue can occur during prolonged exercise, even though sufficient oxygen is available to the muscles and the potential energy from stored fat remains almost unlimited. This occurs because the relatively small amount of glycogen stored in the muscles has become depleted. If a solution of glucose and water is ingested at the point of fatigue, exercise may be prolonged for an additional period of time, but for practical purposes the muscles' "fuel tank" reads "empty" and activity becomes severely limited.

Carbohydrate Needs in Intense Training. Strenuous endurance training for activities such as distance running, swimming, cross-country skiing, or cycling can bring on a state of chronic fatigue, in which successive days of hard training become progressively more difficult. This "staleness" may be related to gradual depletion of the body's carbohydrate reserves, even though the diet contains the recommended percentage of carbohydrate. After three successive days of running 16 km a day, the glycogen in the thigh muscles can become severely depleted, even if the runner's daily food intake contains 40 to 60 percent carbohydrates. By the third day, the quantity of glycogen used is usually much less than on the first day, so that the energy for work is supplied predominantly from fat reserves.

If the diet is high in carbohydrates, liver glycogen is restored rapidly, but at least 48 hours are required to restore muscle glycogen levels after prolonged, exhaustive exercise. Some individuals may require more than 5 days to reestablish muscle glycogen levels if the diet contains only moderate amounts of carbohydrates. If long-term, strenuous exercise is to be performed on successive days, daily allowances must be adjusted to permit optimal glycogen resynthesis. In addition, at least 2 days of rest and high carbohydrate intake must be allowed to restore pre-exercise muscle glycogen levels.

Diet, Glycogen Stores, and Endurance. In the late 1930s, scientists observed that endurance performance was markedly improved simply by consuming a carbohydrate-rich diet for 3 days. Conversely, if the diet consisted predominantly of fat, endurance capability was drastically reduced. Researchers have evaluated several possible ways of increasing muscle glycogen content. In one series of experiments, subjects consumed three different diets. One diet provided the normal energy intake mainly as fat. The second diet contained the recommended daily percentages of carbohydrates, fats, and proteins. The third diet provided 82 percent of energy in the form of carbohydrates. The glycogen content, as sampled from the leg muscles of subjects fed the high-fat diet, the normal diet, and the high-carbohydrate diet averaged 0.6, 1.75, and 3.75 g of glycogen per 100 g of muscle, respectively. In addition, the endurance capacity on the high-carbohydrate diet was more than three times greater than the endurance capacity of the same subjects when fed the high-fat diet. Clearly, a simple dietary modification can alter the body's stores of carbohydrates and affect subsequent performance of prolonged submaximal exercise. These observations are important not only for the endurance athlete, but also for people who have modified their diets so that the normal, recommended percentage of carbohydrates is reduced.

Reliance on starvation diets, high-fat, low-carbohydrate diets, "liquid-protein" diets, or water diets, is counterproductive for weight control, exercise performance, optimal nutrition, and good health. The low-carbohydrate intake makes it extremely difficult to participate in vigorous physical activity or training.

Carbohydrate Loading to Increase Glycogen Reserves. This procedure of carbohydrate loading is currently "in vogue" among endurance athletes. The end result is an even greater increase of muscle glycogen than would occur with a carbohydrate-rich diet. The technique is as follows: First reduce the glycogen stores with a period of relatively long, moderate, continuous exercise. Second, deplete muscle glycogen further by maintaining a high-fat diet for several days while continuing an exercise program. Third, reduce the activity level for several days while switching to a carbohydrate-rich diet. The muscle glycogen will increase to a new, higher level. Of course, adequate daily protein, minerals, and vitamins and abundant water must also be part of the daily diet.

Glycogen supercompensation occurs only in the specific muscles exercised. In preparation for a marathon, a 20- to 30-km run is usually necessary, whereas for swimming and bicycling, moderately intense submaximal exercise for 90 minutes is required.

The combination of diet and exercise to produce glycogen packing of muscles has considerable interest for the endurance athlete, but for those who are not endurance competitors, normal levels of muscle glycogen are more than adequate to meet the energy demands of exercise. Normal levels of glycogen can usually be sustained by ingesting 50 to 60 percent of food energy as carbohydrates, but during intensive training, the carbohydrate intake should be increased.

The wisdom of repeated bouts of carbohydrate loading has yet to be verified. A severe carbohydrate overload interspersed with periods of high fat or protein intake could pose problems to people susceptible to maturity-onset diabetes or heart or kidney disease.

THE PRECOMPETITION MEAL

The main purposes of the precompetition meal are to provide adequate food energy and to ensure optimal hydration. As a general rule, foods that are high in fat content should be avoided on the day of competition, because they are digested slowly and remain in the alimentary tract longer than carbohydrates of similar energy value.

The timing of the precompetition meal does not seem important to exercise performance. However, because the main function of the meal is to provide food energy and water, a 3-hour period should be allowed for digestion and absorption by the body.

Carbohydrate or Protein? Many athletes are psychologically accustomed to, and even dependent on, a "classic" pregame meal of steak and eggs. Although this meal may be satisfying to the athlete, coach, and restaurateur, its benefits in terms of exercise performance have yet to be demonstrated. Since carbohydrates are digested and absorbed more rapidly than either proteins or fats, such food would be available for energy faster and would reduce the feeling of fullness following a meal. Furthermore, a high-protein meal elevates resting metabolism more than a high-carbohydrate meal. This heat places an additional strain on temperature regulation. Concurrently, the breakdown of protein for energy predisposes to dehydration, because the byproducts of amino acid breakdown demand large amounts of water for urinary excretion.

An equally important argument for a carbohydrate meal is its role as the main energy source for intense exercise and prolonged effort. The precompetition meal must provide adequate quantities of carbohydrate to ensure a normal blood glucose level and peak storage of liver and muscle glycogen. Although the wisdom of prolonged high carbohydrate intake, especially in the form of simple sugars, has yet to be established, it is sound nutrition to allow athletes carbohydrates in both the pre-event meal and snacks before competition.

A moderately large glucose challenge right before an endurance activity may impair performance. For example, the riding time of young men and women on a cycle ergometer was reduced 19 percent when they consumed a 300 ml solution containing 75 g of glucose 30 minutes before exercise, compared to similar trials preceded by the same volume of water or a liquid meal of protein, fat, and carbohydrate. The mobilization of free fatty acids was depressed throughout the glucose trial, thereby causing muscle glycogen stores in the muscles to be used more rapidly. This adverse response to glucose feeding is probably mediated by the inhibitory effects of an increased insulin output upon fat mobilization. If large quantities of sugars are consumed prior to competition, sufficient time must be allowed for assimilation of this nutrient and the reestablishment of metabolic and hormonal balance.

Liquid Meals. Commercially prepared liquid meals offer an alternative and seemingly effective approach to the pre-event meal. These foods are usually well balanced in nutritive value. They are high in carbohydrate, yet contain enough fat and protein to contribute to a feeling of satiety. Because they are liquid, they also boost the athlete's fluid reserves. A liquid meal is advantageous because it is digested rapidly and completely, leaving essentially no residue in the alimentary tract. This approach is especially effective during day-long meets in swimming and track, or in some tennis and basketball tournaments. In such situations, an athlete has little time (or interest) for food. Liquid meals also may be used to supplement the daily energy intake of athletes who have difficulty in maintaining or increasing body mass.

COMPUTER TECHNOLOGY TO EVALUATE NUTRITION, EXERCISE, AND BODY COMPOSITION

Application of computer technology allows accurate determinations of energy intake and exercise output based upon body composition and current state of training. The purpose is to formulate well-balanced meals and exercise programs for weight control. The creation of daily menus with the FITCOMP computer programme I helped to develop is based on the Four Food Group Plan and dietary exchange method developed by the American Dietetic Association. Unlike a prescribed food plan, the FITCOMP computerized dietary plan allows a person to select specific foods from a basic list of the most common choices. Taking into account of age, body mass, height, desired weight change, and current level of physical activity, my FITCOMP program plans nutritious meals for breakfast, lunch, and dinner over whatever time period is selected. The menu varies from day to day. The meals are balanced with respect to the intake of carbohydrate, fat, protein, vitamins, and minerals and are designed to reduce excess body mass (fat) at a safe but steady rate. The printout includes a curve of desired weight loss, daily meal plans, and 9 different beginner, intermediate, or advanced exercise programs.

The most obvious advantage of computer-generated reports is that exercise and menu planning can be based upon individual preferences, rather than standard workouts and set meal plans. It is unnecessary to make tedious calculations in order to individualize a particular plan; a typical 16-page computer report can be printed in less than 10 seconds. Interactive, computer-based technology can provide individualized reports that take into account body size, body composition, age, sex, current fitness status, and activity preference.

FLUID AND MINERAL NEEDS

ROY J. SHEPHARD, M.D. (Lond), Ph.D.

Even under relatively cold conditions, the competitive athlete loses substantial quantities of sweat. Appropriate replacement of fluid and mineral loss is thus important to both performance and safety. In discussing this topic, comment will also be made on the related issue of the wrestler who deliberately "loses weight" in preparation for a major competition.

ASSESSING FLUID NEEDS

The acute loss of fluid by sweating and humidification of expired air is determined fairly precisely by weighing a competitor before and after a game or race; a marathoner, for example, may lose 4 kg of body mass, and about 3.8 kg of this is attributable to sweating, the other 0.2 kg being due to combustion of food.

Opinions on the "safe" fluid loss have often been based on fairly sedentary exposures to a hot climatic chamber. The situation in exhausting exercise is a little different, since the combustion of perhaps 500 g of glycogen releases some 1.5 liters of bound water, and metabolism also produces 0.2 to 0.3 liter of water. There is thus no tissue dehydration until body mass has decreased by about 2 kg. However, the impact upon both performance and safe thermoregulation becomes very obvious as the next 1 to 2 kg of sweat are produced; from the performance point of view, the optimum scenario is probably to allow a 2 kg decrease of body mass.

Thirst does not usually provide a reliable guide to dehydration while exercising, and if left to their own devices, most athletes drink an inadequate volume of fluid during competition.

REPLENISHING FLUID AND MINERAL STORES

When fluid is drunk, it must be absorbed from the gastrointestinal tract if it is to help rather than hinder performance. The base rate of emptying of the stomach while exercising hard drops to about 600 ml per hour. There is thus little point in giving an athlete more than a final 500 ml drink half an hour prior to competition and then 600 ml/hour while exercising. Since thirst becomes fickle, the 600 ml is best divided into four 150-ml Dixie cups, provided at 15-minute intervals if the rules of competition allow.

There has been a vigorous market in replacement fluids for athletes, and various combinations of glucose and minerals have been added to beverages in the interests of palatability, energy, and mineral replacement. Palatability is not a major issue while competing, since normal appreciation of flavors seems distorted by exercise. The disadvantage of adding glucose and minerals is that any hyperosmotic solution further delays the empty-ing of the stomach. Up to 5% glucose is emptied as rapidly as water, and a 5% solution contributes about 120 kJ of energy per hour (30 kcal), not a very exciting bonus, but possibly enough to influence the outcome of a closely contended event. Currently, experiments are under way using various polymers of glucose, as these allow a larger amount of energy to pass the pyloric sphincter without increasing the osmotic pressure of the beverage. Most commercial beverages also contain varying concentrations of potassium and sodium ions, with a view to replacing the loss of these minerals in the sweat. It is true that sweat contains sodium and potassium, but the concentration is much lower than in the plasma. Thus, if 3 to 4 liters of sweat are secreted, there is an immediate rise in plasma concentrations of sodium and potassium. Plasma potassium is further boosted by a leakage of this mineral from the active muscles. Beverages containing sodium and potassium ions thus worsen rather than improve the ionic disturbance that develops during prolonged exercise.

Most subjects replace their water loss by drinking water, tea, soft drinks, or beer for a few hours after competing. If water is ingested at this stage, the plasma sodium and potassium will drop. However, the deficit is small relative to body pools of minerals, and is readily corrected by adding a little extra table salt to vegetables.

For most purposes, the prescription is thus simple: a pre-event drink of 500 ml, 600 ml of water per hour during competition (supplemented by 5% glucose or its polymers if glycogen stores are likely to be depleted), water ad libitum during recovery, and some extra salting of food.

If a team is staying in an unusually hot climate for an extended period, there is also some risk of chronic mineral depletion. As the salt content of the body falls, so does its water content. Blood volume is reduced, and performance deteriorates. Partly because of the mineral loss, and partly because of poor performance, the athlete becomes weak and irritable (heat neurasthenia), and confrontations with the coach may become a problem. The remedies are (1) to insist on an adequate daily salt intake (e.g., the provision of well-salted soups) and (2) to monitor compliance by keeping a daily record of body mass; a progressive decline is usually a harbinger of salt depletion. A simple check of urinary salt excretion is possible with a Fantus test, but at most major competitions the sports physician now has facilities for measuring plasma sodium concentrations in doubtful cases.

DELIBERATE WEIGHT LOSS

Some wrestlers deliberately reduce their body mass by a combination of starvation, fluid restriction, and sauna bathing in an attempt to enter a lower "weight" category than that to which they are entitled. This is undesirable on several counts.

First, it negates the principle of fair and honest competition which is the essence of good sportsmanship. Further, by pitting a heavy individual against a smaller adversary, there is an increased probability that the latter

31

will be injured. Finally, the policy is unsound on physiologic grounds, and even if the wrestler attempts rehydration after "weighing in", both cardiovascular and muscular performance are likely to remain impaired. The long-term hazards of repeated "weight reduction" are not fully analyzed, but in the young adolescent some impairment of normal growth and development seems likely from the combination of negative energy balance and restricted protein intake.

The main remedy for this abuse seems the education of both wrestlers and their coaches. In regions where the practice is prevalent, other tactics include (1) requiring medical clearance if a competitor has less than 5 percent body fat, (2) recording body mass immediately before a competition is begun, (3) maintaining a log of the "weight" categories in which a wrestler competes, (4) predicting body mass from the bone dimensions of a competitor, and (5) obtaining sophisticated measures of body composition on those suspected of flouting the rules.

VITAMINS AND FOOD FADS OF ATHLETES

ERIC J. van der BEEK, M.D.

The subject of this chapter is that group of micronutrients formerly called "vitamines". The name was introduced by the Polish biochemist Funk in 1912. It was a compilation of "-amines" because he believed such compounds belonged to the group of chemical substances called *amines* and "vit-" because they were *vital* for life. In certain matters of detail, Funk's views were not quite correct. Not all vitamins are amines. That is why, after a more or less semantic discussion, the spelling was altered to vitamins. The commonly accepted definition of vitamins today is that they are chemically unrelated substances, essential in small amounts for the maintenance of normal metabolic functions. However, they are not synthesized within the body and must therefore be furnished from exogenous sources. This definition is still somewhat incorrect in that a few organic compounds generally recognized as vitamins can be and are synthesized within the human body. Under suitable conditions, they are synthesized in amounts adequate to support normal metabolic processes. The organic synthesis of the different vitamins, which quickly became possible after their discovery, has exerted a great influence upon the combating and prevention of deficiency diseases such as beriberi, pellagra, and blindness caused by vitamin A deficiency. Because vitamins have been considered organically primitive substances, a certain amount of mysticism has surrounded their use and has led to a belief in their special properties.

Mysticism and fads of diet are probably as old as civilization itself. Food faddism is based upon an exaggerated belief in the effects of nutrition upon health and disease. Food faddists claim that nutrition is more important than science demonstrates it to be. Pharmaceutical companies take grateful advantage of both phenomena in their production of vitamin supplements.

Nutrition, especially in relation to muscular performance, is a relatively new science and it is thus particularly susceptible to distortion by fads or cults. This is not surprising, because in teaching nutrition, emphasis has traditionally been placed on the close association of good nutrition with health and poor nutrition with disease. Through that approach, the door has been opened to the idea of "supercharging" the body with nutrients that are believed to be of particular importance for the athlete. Thereby, it is hoped to raise performance beyond what would be possible on an ordinary diet. In other words, nutritionists are at least partly responsible for the misconceptions and ignorance of athletes. Obsessed with the goal of maximizing performance, and fearful that their competitors may do something to gain a decisive edge, athletes have been highly susceptible to faddish claims. Coaches are vulnerable too, and they often believe unscientific claims that performance will be improved by nutritional supplements (which they equate with vitamins). According to Ingelfinger, food faddism and other unscientific claims can be considered an expression of the arrogance of ignorance. However, it must be said that the arrogance of ignorance can be as devastating as the arrogance of expertise. While hardly ever discussed, the arrogance of ignorance or the arrogance of the antiscientific activist may be as flagrant as that of the most doctrinaire member of the conventional establishment.

VITAMINS AND VITAMIN STATUS

Most vitamins serve as essential parts of enzymes or coenzymes that are vital to the metabolism of fats and carbohydrates. Thus, although vitamins do not yield energy in themselves, they are essential to energy metabolism.

Vitamins are classified as water- or fat-soluble. The water-soluble vitamins include vitamin C (L-ascorbic acid) and the B-complex vitamins (thiamine, riboflavin, niacin, pantothenic acid, vitamin B_6, folic acid, vitamin B_{12}). These substances are not stored in the body to any appreciable amount and they must therefore be constantly supplied in the diet. When taken in excess (above requirement), they are excreted in the urine. However, there have been suggestions in recent years that large doses of water-soluble vitamins are not totally innocuous. Large doses of ascorbic acid have been associated with urinary stone formation and impaired copper absorption, while large doses of vitamin B_6 can cause sensory neuropathy. The fat-soluble vitamins (A, D, E, and K) are stored in the body, prinicpally in the liver, but also in fatty tissue. On the one hand this means that these vitamins need not be supplied every day. On the other hand, it means that excessive accumulations of these substances also can cause toxic effects.

The term vitamin status is used to define the total amount of a particular vitamin present in the body and available to catalyze normal biochemical processes. In quantifying vitamin status, biochemical data are most commonly used. These include *direct methods*: measurement of blood and/or tissue levels as well as urinary excretion; and *functional methods*: determination of the cellular activity of an enzyme which depends on a particular vitamin as coenzyme. Both approaches are currently employed in the determination of vitamin deficiencies. These same techniques also allow identification of a marginal or subclinical vitamin status, an optimal vitamin status, and a serious deficiency. A marginal vitamin status is characterized by values that deviate from statistically derived reference limits, in the absence of clinical signs or symptoms. It is not known whether such marginal status leads to any functional impairment.

INSUFFICIENT VITAMIN INTAKE

Since the early forties, there have been reports that the function of several vitamins is associated with both physical and mental performance. Particularly during World War II, extensive research was undertaken to determine the effects of various vitamins on physical working capacity. The available data indicate that physical and mental performance capacities do deteriorate with frank clinical deficiencies of water-soluble vitamins.

It is remarkable that over the last forty years, the association between physical performance capacity and vitamin intake has been investigated mainly with respect to tests of neuromuscular function and psychologic factors. Hardly any research has been done on the association with the capacity for energy output through aerobic or anaerobic processes (for instance, by measurements of aerobic power).

Mild-to-moderate vitamin deficiencies have been reported in certain sections of a number of developed countries. However, one often speculates about the functional significance of a marginal biochemical deficiency with respect to the health of a population. Up to now, evidence of a deterioration in physical performance is available only for vitamin B_1 (thiamine) and vitamin C (L-ascorbic acid), but one might theorize about detrimental effects of vitamin B_2 (riboflavin) and vitamin B_6 (pyridoxine) deficiencies.

Thiamine plays an important role in energy metabolism and in the nervous system. Specifically, it takes a key place in the oxidative decarboxylation of pyruvate to acetyl CoA, producing fuel for the Krebs cycle and thus generation of ATP. Thiamine is found in the outer layer

of seeds. Other sources include animal tissues such as meat, fish, and poultry, eggs, milk, cheese, whole grain cereals, dried beans and peas, and all vegetables.

The full biochemical function of ascorbic acid has yet to be elucidated. However, it is known to be involved in the synthesis of collagen, in the metabolic reactions of amino-acids including tyrosine, and in the synthesis of epinephrine and the glucocorticoids of the adrenal gland. Thus, vitamin C is essential to a variety of biologic oxidative processes. It is present in fresh fruits and vegetables, primarily citrus fruits such as oranges, grapefruits, and lemons. Other sources include tomatoes, potatoes, and greens. As ascorbic acid is heat-labile, it is readily destroyed by cooking.

Riboflavin functions as a coenzyme for a group of flavoproteins involved in biologic oxidation; the most common of these is flavin adenine dinucleotide (FAD). The vitamin's role appears central to oxidative reactions occurring in the mitochondria. Riboflavin is found in milk and milk products such as cheese, and in eggs, meat, and green leafy vegetables.

Vitamin B_6 is not a single substance, but rather a collective term for three naturally occurring pyridines— pyridoxine, pyridoxial, and pyridoxamine—which are metabolically and functionally related. Vitamin B_6, in the coenzyme form pyridoxal-5-phosphate (PLP), is concerned with a vast number and variety of enzyme systems, almost all of which are associated with nitrogen metabolism. Well over 60 pyridoxal phosphate-dependent enzymes are known. The best sources of vitamin B_6 are meat, poultry, fish, potatoes, whole grain products, yeast, eggs, and seeds.

We recently carried out a 12-week double-blind experiment to evaluate the possible association between marginal levels of vitamins B_1, B_2, B_6, and C and physical performance. Six healthy adult male volunteers were given a diet of normal food stuffs for 8 weeks. This provided a maximum of 30 to 35 percent of the Dutch Recommended Dietary Allowances (RDA) for the 4 vitamins. The 8 weeks were preceded and followed by a 2-week period on an identical diet, to which had been added twice the RDA of the 4 vitamins. A control group of 6 male volunteers was given the same diet, with a full intake of all vitamins during the entire period. Both groups were also given mineral and trace element supplements equal to the RDA throughout the experiment. Maximal aerobic power ($\dot{V}O_2$ max.) and anaerobic threshold (AT) were measured on a cycle ergometer, the AT being defined as the workload at which a venous blood lactate level of 4 mmol/l was reached. We were surprised to find that borderline and/or moderately deficient blood levels of all four vitamins developed within the relatively short period of 8 weeks on the deficient diet; indeed, the effect was already apparent after 4 weeks. On the other hand, a rapid improvement of vitamin status occurred with return to twice the RDA.

The marginal or deficient vitamin status was associated with a 16 percent decrease of aerobic power and a 24 percent decrease in the anaerobic threshold at the end of the vitamin-deficient period. During the 2 weeks of repletion, both measures of physical performance improved, but did not regain their initial status.

During the whole experiment, both biochemical and physical performance variables remained at rather constant levels in the control group. No changes of iron status were seen in either the deficient or the control group throughout the study, all values falling within the normal range.

Because intake of the four vitamins was manipulated simultaneously, physical performance cannot be attributed directly to a marginal biochemical status of any one dietary constituent. However, I believe that the observed decrease of anaerobic threshold is, at least partly, due to an inhibition of the thiamine-dependent pyruvate dehydrogenase complex.

Buzina followed the rehabilitation of young adolescents with subclinical ascorbic acid, riboflavin, and pyridoxine deficiencies. There was an associated increase of maximal oxygen intake, as predicted from heart rate and submaximal work load, using the Åstrand-Ryhming nomogram. Since correction of the vitamin deficiencies was associated with an improvement of iron status, it was not possible to conclude whether the increased vitamin stores or the improved iron status was responsible for the gain of aerobic power.

Nevertheless, Buzina found subsequently that after correction of concurrent subclinical riboflavin and pyridoxine deficiencies, vitamin C supplementation led to an increase in aerobic power. The iron status was adequate. In other words, the decrease of aerobic power observed in our experiment could be partly the result of low vitamin C levels.

In recent years, there have been a few studies on the vitamin status of athletes. Of all the athletes studied, 10 to 70 percent have shown abnormal values for vitamins B_1, B_2, and B_6. However, the question remains whether these alarming figures reflect an impairment of physical performance in the athletes concerned. In all of these studies, the vitamin status was assessed by in vitro stimulation of erythrocytic enzymes: transketolase, glutathione reductase, and glutamate oxaloacetate transaminase by their corresponding coenzymes: thiamine diphosphate (ThDP), flavine adenine dinucleotide (FAD), and pyridoxal-5′-phosphate (PLP). The ratio of the respective enzyme activities with and without an excess coenzyme are functional measures of vitamin B_1, B_2, and B_6 status. Regarding our short-term experiment, we believe that the usually adopted reference limits for normal vitamin status do not reflect functional limits, especially with respect to the stimulation coefficient for erythrocyte transketolase (α-ETK). In other words, it may be necessary to review critically the current reference limits of vitamin status, before embarking upon a treatment of figures instead of human beings.

VITAMIN SUPPLEMENTS

There have been numerous claims that vitamin supplements, especially B-complex vitamins, vitamin C, and vitamin E, may improve physical working capacity.

However, most studies lack a double-blind experimental design. In the absence of control subjects, it becomes difficult to discriminate the effects of time and training. The premise is advanced that athletes must have an increased demand for these vitamins, because the corresponding biochemical reactions make energy available for muscular work. Until today, there has been no experimental evidence to support this premise. However, it was observed very recently that healthy and highly active young women require more riboflavin than the 1980 Recommended Dietary Allowances (RDA) published by the U.S. Food and Nutrition Board, National Academy of Sciences–National Research Council, in order to achieve biochemical normality, because exercise increases riboflavin requirements. Impairment of physical performance was not mentioned in this report.

RDA of the United States, unlike Dutch and English RDAs, does not advocate increased vitamin allowances for physical activity. Nevertheless, it does recognize that an increased intake would result from the additional intake of food energy caused by exercise-stimulated hunger.

As already mentioned, many athletes use vitamin supplementation in an attempt to "supercharge" energy-producing reactions. Another rationale for vitamin supplementation has been a belief that large losses of vitamins occur in sweating. This idea is now disproven; body sweat is almost completely devoid of vitamins. Available evidence, based on well-controlled experiments indicates that supplementation of the diet with either single or multivitamin preparations containing B-complex vitamins, vitamin C, or vitamin E does not change physical performance in athletes who are taking a well-balanced diet.

The function and sources of the most frequently examined members of the B-complex and vitamin C have already been mentioned. Vitamin E is fat-soluble, and is a generic title for at least four tocopherols of which α-tocopherol is the most active. It appears to act as a lipid antioxidant, preventing the formation of peroxides from polyunsaturated fatty acids. Moreover, it is very closely involved with the mineral selenium during metabolism, the two substances seeming to be interdependent. Vitamin E is present in relatively high quantities in many plants, such as lettuce and peanuts, and in margarine, milk products, and wheat germ oil. Despite the lack of justification for vitamin E supplementation, this substance was number one in sales in the United States in 1978, capturing 17 percent of the vitamin market. One explanation is its assumed function as an aphrodisiac. The mythical properties as a sexual rejuvenant stem from a 1923 report that vitamin E improved the fertility of rats.

We recently completed a 4-month double-blind experiment to evaluate the effect of multivitamin-iron supplementation upon aerobic power. A total of 77 healthy free living male and female sports students participated in the trial. The supplement contained nearly all water- and fat-soluble vitamins as well as iron at levels ranging from twice the RDA for vitamin A and D to 10 times the RDA for the water-soluble vitamins, vitamin E, and iron. Only a training effect was seen, this response being demonstrated equally by supplemented and placebo groups; this result is in agreement with all other controlled experiments.

Although vitamin supplementation produces no effect when the diet is adequate, it remains possible that B-complex vitamin supplementation might be appropriate in sports with a high energy expenditure. If energy expenditure reaches 18.9 to 20.1 MJ (4500 to 5000 kcal), there is an unavoidable consumption of "empty calories", food products with low nutrient density. However, no research has yet been carried out on this subject.

In conclusion, biochemical vitamin deficiencies have more than cosmetic value: they really indicate an impaired performance capacity. However, usually employed reference limits of vitamin status need reappraisal, translating them into functional impairment limits.

The available evidence on vitamin supplementation clearly shows that there is no justification for food faddish claims, especially when an adequate diet is consumed: vitamin pills are no substitute for physical training! However, if athletes feel that they require vitamin supplementation, psychotherapeutic benefit may be derived from a daily capsule containing a few times the RDA; the excess of vitamins is simply excreted as a rather expensive urine, with no harm to the subject.

HYPNOSIS IN CONDITIONING THE PROBLEM ATHLETE

LARS-ERIC V. UNESTÅHL, Ph.D.

You have probably heard about the elite swimmer, who did not turn after his first length, having been programmed with posthypnotic suggestions that sharks were chasing him in the water. Here are some other examples. An athlete is hypnotized for the first time just before a competition. He is told to relax completely—every muscle completely relaxed—and to keep this feeling during the competition. The results: he performs badly, clearly below his real ability. Another athlete is hypnotized the day before a competition. She is told that the coming competition will be very easily handled and managed. The result: She performs badly, clearly below her real ability.

Does this imply hypnosis should not be used in sport? It can be of great value if correctly applied, but it can also be a disaster if it is intentionally or unintentionally combined with wrong techniques.

The oldest description of hypnosis goes back to 2000 BC. Modern hypnosis began with Mesmer at the end of the eighteenth century. A hundred years later, it was incorporated into medical research by Charcot and Bernheim, and some years into this century it also took a place in psychologic research.

Despite this long history, it is hard to specify just what hypnosis is. For convenience, one may discuss theories of induction, theories of the established hypnotic state, and theories of differential susceptibility to hypnosis.

Two very simple definitions are: (1) hypnosis is a state of increased concentration; and (2) hypnosis is a state of increased dissociation. At first glance, these seem contradictory, but in fact the definitions express two sides of the same coin. When you concentrate on a task, you focus on a small attention area. This means that you are less attentive to (dissociated from) everything outside this limited area.

Hypnosis is an alternative mode of consciousness with various subjective qualitative changes, characterized by restricted attention and an increased preparedness to respond to suggestions and images.

CRITERIA

Criteria of hypnosis, i.e., changes which are necessarily connected with the hypnotic state, could be (1) experiential, (2) physiologic, or (3) behavioral.

Experiential Criteria

The core of hypnosis seems to be subjective. The "A-mode of thinking" brings about many cognitive changes, which give the hypnotized person many new experiences. These are hard to measure and sometimes even difficult to describe. Paintings, poetry, metaphors, and other forms of "unscientific right-brain language" are often used to describe hypnotic experiences.

Physiologic Changes

Physiologic changes almost always appear, but they can often be related to (1) the specific method used to induce hypnosis (for instance relaxation), (2) suggestions given in hypnosis, and (3) expectations of what is going to happen. The level of activation decreases if the person is calm and relaxed, but if he is regressed back to an earlier traumatic event, the physiologic measurements often indicate an increase of activation.

Behavioral Criteria

The term "hypnosis" goes back to a Greek word for sleep, and many persons still look at hypnosis as a sleep-like state, where the hypnotized person is sitting or lying immobile with closed eyes and deeper, more relaxed breathing. This, however, is not essential. There is an important difference between passive and active hypnosis.

In one demonstration of "active hypnosis", I asked a patient with phobic problems who felt anxiety among other persons, especially new ones, to participate. She knew that she felt safe and secure when she was in a hypnotic state. While she was hypnotized, I instructed her to open her eyes and behave as usual but to remain in hypnosis. How was it possible to be sure she remained in hypnosis? One way would have been to ask her about experiential changes. Another possibility would have been to look at perceptual changes, for instance, a more limited attention area (tunnel vision). I chose to demonstrate hypnosis by using a change of pain perception after suggestions of analgesia.

HYPNOSIS AS A HEMISPHERIC SHIFT

Hypnosis is usually regarded as an altered state of consciousness or an alternative state of consciousness. I prefer the second expression, as it points at hypnosis as a "normal" alternative to the common waking state. Consciousness shifts in quantity and quality during our "waking state", and some of these shifts can be described as hypnosis-like states. Two problems with such spontaneous states are (1) the inability to use that hypnotic state in a controlled and purposeful way, and (2) the risk of negative effects, due to increased responsiveness to negative thoughts and images.

Hypnosis can most easily be described in terms of the two modes of consciousness, D-mode and A-mode (Table 1). When someone enters hypnosis there is a shift from the dominant D-mode to the alternative A-mode. This means a decrease of "left-brain" activities such as

TABLE 1 Modes of Consciousness and Sport

D–mode (dominant)	A–mode (alternative)
Logic	Insight
Analytical thinking	Synthesis
Reality — testing	Automaticity
Planning — tactics	Suggestibility
Strategies	Feel — touch — tempo
Evaluation	Intuition — creativity
Criticism	Evaluation — free information
	Positive feedback
Details — specificity	Holism — overview
Verbal instructions	Visualization
Voluntary control	Kinesthetic images
	Control by goal-programming
Thinking of future & past events	Living in the present
	Parallel processing
Time — linearity —	Non verbal understanding
serial processing	Metaphors
Verbal	Modelling
Instructor	Body language
Determination	Doer
Trying	Triggers
Effort	Effortless "Flow"

reality-testing and analytical, logical, and sequential thinking. It also means an increase of functions like imagery, suggestibility, and a holistic, integrative and simultaneous use of earlier experiences, factors of great importance in some forms of athletic performance.

IDEAL PERFORMING STATE (IPS)

In order to investigate the ideal performing state, athletes have been interviewed after peak performances. Many of their comments pointed to IPS as an alternative consciousness like hypnosis. Some of the most typical similarities were as follows.

Amnesia

Often athletes have selective or even total amnesia after a perfect performance. Elite athletes often see a direct relation between the degree of amnesia and the quality of their performance.

As a learned, automated pattern of movement is controlled by an alternative level of consciousness, the experiences and memories often remain on a more subconscious level.

Concentration—Dissociation

A more intense attentiveness to a limited number of stimuli (concentration) is accompanied by a general inattentiveness (dissociation) to every irrelevant stimulus. Expressions like "another world", "glass-room", "shell", "tunnel", and "trance" are common.

Pain Detachment

A spontaneous increase of pain tolerance seems to occur much as in hypnosis. The athlete does not have the usual feelings of exhaustion and tiredness.

Perceptual Changes

Trance-like phenomena like time-distortion or tunnel-vision are not necessary in IPS, but sometimes happen. A gymnast describes it like this: "Sometimes I can experience my performance as a dance on a film, shown in slow motion. It is a wonderful experience." A formula 1 racing-car driver suddenly experiences that he has all the time in the world to make moves which otherwise could have been impossible. The pigeon or the golf hole is now so big that there is no way you could miss.

Description of IPS

One of the best descriptions is the following. "Suddenly everything worked. I did not wonder any longer what to do or how to do it - everything was automatic. I just hooked on. Nothing could have disturbed me in that moment. I was completely involved with what was happening. I had no thoughts of doing it correctly, no thoughts of failure, no thoughts of fatigue. I felt an inner security and confidence that was tremendous. It was completely natural that I would succeed. I watched my accomplishment and enjoyed it while at the same time I was at one with it. It was a trance-like state, which I would like to experience every time, but which I probably won't experience again for a long time."

The frequency of trance experiences varies between different sports and seems related to the degree of automatization in the sport. Most athletes answer "sometimes" or "seldom", when asked to rate the frequency of trance experiences. The "hypnotic" state has special names in some sports. A basketball player talks about a "hot night", a tennis player is "playing out of his head". You "ski out of your mind" and you "lose yourself" in jogging and swimming.

One way to increase the frequency and control of this attractive state is to teach the athletes methods of inducing alternative states of consciousness.

POSTHYPNOTIC EFFECTS

Posthypnotic suggestions can be divided into 2 types: (1) suggestions for a specific response or act, and (2) suggestions for a general state, emotion, or attitude. Both types of suggestions can be released through (1) waking, (2) delay in time, and (3) stimuli which have been given signal value under hypnosis.

The effect of posthypnotic suggestion for an act limited in time ceases when the suggested act has been executed. Suggestions of type (2), on the other hand, continue to work until the effect spontaneously ceases or until a new signal is given which abolishes the effect. But every time the signal is given, the suggested effect is released again.

Before starting the concentration training, the athletes choose some behavior act, or situation that can serve as a signal (cue, trigger). This cue then receives signal value during hypnosis and is then conditioned to an earlier experience of total concentration.

Experiments with Posthypnotic Effects

Maximum Isometric Strength During Waking, Hypnotic and Posthypnotic Induced States. The maximum strength of elbow flexion and knee extension was measured during eight posthypnotic induced states. Two (high confidence and perceived task difficulty = easy) had increased strength, and the others, decreased strength compared with normal waking. By using signal-released effects as experimental tools, the experimenter can have greater control over type and degree of effects compared with real-life settings.

The Effects of Maximum Strain and/or Recovery in a Mental State. Cycling for 8 minutes (maximum heart-rate) was done in a normal state and in a mental state, combined with 20 minutes recovery in both a normal and a mental state for groups with and without IMT training. Both mental state and IMT training reduced peak lactate values and speeded recovery.

Motor Learning. Operant techniques with modification of behavior by control of its consequences have not been used much in sport. One difficulty has been finding effective reinforcers. A technique can be worked out, however, whereby a situation-related feeling, experienced under hypnosis, is separated from the situation and conditioned to a signal, for instance, a new situation or behavior.

The posthypnotic positive feeling, released every time the ball goes into the basket in penalty shooting, does not seem to enhance learning. In one experiment, two groups made emotional ratings after every shot. The "programmed" group showed stronger positive reactions after scores and stronger negative reactions after misses. However, neither group improved more than the other. Thus the immediate feedback and the "natural" positive reactions after scoring seem to give an optimal reinforcement, and additional reactions do not improve the performance further.

In another experiment, an attempt was made to create more favorable learning conditions in swimming. For the sake of more immediate feedback, underwater loudspeakers were used. A positive feeling was created and conditioned to a tone of a certain frequency. As long as the swimmers were performing correctly, the tone was on, but any fault led to a cessation of the tone, and the trainer immediately stated the necessary corrections over the microphone.

IMT training can be used regularly in motor learning in the following simple way. Before a training session, the participants use a fast relaxation procedure, after which they open their eyes and look at a perfect performance on video or film. They are instructed to experience the performance holistically, in a relaxed way, without analysis, and they are to see themselves perform. The whole procedure takes about 10 minutes.

SELF-INSTRUCTIONAL HYPNOTIC TRAINING

East European countries use hypnosis in sport. To make this approach acceptable in the West, it is important to go from an authoritarian and coach-directed style to an athlete-directed and controlled way of using self-hypnosis. It ought to be as natural for an athlete to train confidence, concentration, and emotional stability as it is for him to train conditioning, strength, and technique. Most of the psychologic skills, abilities, and attitudes necessary for facilitating a good athletic performance can be learned and automatized in the same way as the more physical athletic skills. Regular hypnotic training should thus be an integral part of general training. The major difficulty for physicians, coaches, and athletes is the lack of concrete training programs. The last part of this chapter therefore presents a systematic approach to hypnotic training.

CAREER TRAINING

A typical pattern, adopted with several Swedish national teams, is shown in Table 2.

Objectives are:

1. To increase the quality of IPS.
2. To increase the ability to reproduce, induce and control IPS.
3. To remove obstacles for a general performance improvement.
4. To remove causes for situation-related performance declines.
5. To increase the uptake of physical training by (a) improving the quality of training (model training), and (b) improving the ability for rest/recovery between training sessions.

Mental training ought to resemble physical training in the following respects:

1. Self-instructional.
2. Concrete, practically designed programs.
3. Step-by-step build-up from the basics to advanced specific skills.
4. Emphasis on acquisition, enhancement, and automatization of skills.
5. To proceed from general training in basic mental skills to more sport-specific and competition-directed training.

HYPNOTIC PREPARATION FOR COMPETITION

One of the five preparation programs starts with a regressive activation of the IPS feeling. The feeling is transferred to future competition. The rehearsal is easier to make for the individual athlete who has more controlled standard goals.

The mental preparation of a team player starts much nearer to the match, preferably 2 days before. The rehearsal can comprise:

1. Goal-programming (individual and/or team goal).
2. Rehearsal of fixed, predetermined situations.
3. Rehearsal of problem situations (individual/team-general, match-specific/match-general).
4. Tactic rehearsal (visualization of the tactic dispositions).
5. Mental planning for possible alternatives.

EVALUATIONS OF HYPNOTIC TRAINING

An investigation of 5000 Swedish athletes has shown a clear relationship between IMT training and level of competence. Of the 1980 Swedish Olympic Team, less than one-third had IMT training, but more than half of the finalists and more than two-thirds of the medalists had such training. This reflects both effects of mental training and selection factors.

Occasionally, the effects of hypnotic training appear

TABLE 2   Inner Mental Training (IMT)

Career Training	Training Content	Specific Program	Week
IMT–I: Skill acquistion	Psychotonic training	Muscular relaxation	1
			2
	Self-hypnosis	Mental relaxation	3
			4
	Activation	Activation training	5
	Concentration	Meditation	6
		Attention release	7
		Dissociation-Detachment	8
IMT–II: Motivational training	Goal-setting	Goal-awareness-inventory	9
		Goal-analysis-selection	10
		Goal-formulation-contracts	11
	Goal-programming	Ideomotor training	12
		Career goals	13
IMT–III: Applied mental training	Problem-solving	Reconditioning	14
		Systematic desensitization	15
		Thought-stopping	16
	Attitude training	Cognitive restructuring	17
		Autonomic restructuring	18
		Mastery training	19
		Self-confidence training	20

Inner Mental Preparation

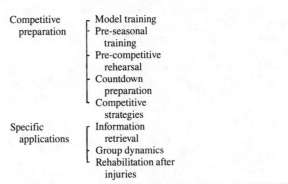

Competitive preparation	Model training Pre-seasonal training Pre-competitive rehearsal Countdown preparation Competitive strategies
Specific applications	Information retrieval Group dynamics Rehabilitation after injuries

quickly. However, more commonly the athlete has to wait a rather long time before the positive effects of mental training are identified. Mental training can even cause an initial decline in performance in the same way as can happen when athletes change to a new (and better) technique). The best results from mental training appear when the mental skills and strategies are so integrated that they become a natural way of thinking, feeling, and behaving.

A large part of the athletes' evaluations of hypnotic training concerns gains in everyday life. Reports like sleeping better, feeling calmer and more harmonious are common. Hypnotic training that teaches stress management skills, a good self-esteem, and a positive attitude to life has influences far beyond physical performance. The physical conditioning may disappear when the athletic career is over, but hypnotic training seems to create a mental conditioning that lasts for life.

HAZARDS OF COLD WATER

ROY J. SHEPHARD, M.D. (Lond), Ph.D.

Cold water presents a significant hazard during early summer boating accidents (yachting or canoeing), crashes of light aircraft, and swimming. There are early disturbances of the cardiorespiratory system, and later more general effects of hypothermia.

EARLY CARDIORESPIRATORY DISTURBANCES

The impact of very cold water on the skin surface leads to a "gasp reflex", with uncontrolled hyperventilation. If the subject is breathing through SCUBA equipment, panic may arise because of difficulty in meeting respiratory demand, whereas if the face is immersed, the aspiration of water may cause laryngospasm and asphyxia. This can be a particular problem during breath-hold dives, under conditions in which the surface water is deceptively warm; a descent that is tolerated well in warm water may become impossible if the deeper parts of a lake are cold.

If the water is very cold, rapid hyperventilation may continue, leading to hypocapnial confusion, difficulty in swimming, tetany, and an eventual loss of consciousness.

A third hazard arising from the stimulation of cold receptors on the face and over other parts of the skin surface is a sudden rise of systemic blood pressure which increases the cardiac work load, and may provoke a cardiac arrhythmia, particularly in a coronary-prone middle-aged individual.

Prophylaxis is important in avoiding these various emergencies. If the water is cool, the body should be wetted before plunging into a lake, and maneuvers that are attempted should allow more leeway than would be necessary under warm conditions. Middle-aged patients who contemplate swimming in cold water are well advised to have an exercise and/or a cold immersion electrocardiogram. Above all, no form of water activity should be undertaken without a companion who is a good swimmer and well trained in emergency procedures.

HYPOTHERMIA OF PROLONGED IMMERSION

Cerebral function begins to deteriorate when the body temperature has dropped below 35°C. At 34°C, shivering mechanisms begin to fail, accelerating the rate of cooling, and below 32°C, the situation is further worsened by a failure of mechanisms for vasoconstriction.

Early data on the rate of body cooling were obtained from the notorious Dachau "experiments". Because the victims of the concentration camps had been systematically starved, their survival in cold water was often as brief as 10 to 15 minutes. However, a typically plump North American yachtsman is likely to survive for an hour or longer. The end comes from a combination of falling cardiac output, cerebral hypoxia, cardiac arrhythmias, and drowning. There has been much discussion as to the wisdom of swimming following a boating accident. If the shore is near at hand, this is the obvious remedy, but if the distance is too great to cover in 10 to 15 minutes, it is generally better to minimize exposure to the cold water by crouching in the fetal position or huddling with a friend until rescue arrives. Swimming usually increases the rate of heat loss, since the benefit from increased metabolism is more than outweighed by stirring of the water over the body surface and a reduction of body insulation as blood flows to the active limbs.

Core temperatures are best determined by a rectal thermometer, although under field conditions one must often be content with oral readings. The medical kit for water sports should be equipped with a cold-recording rather than a standard clinical thermometer. Rectal temperatures below 35°C indicate some hypothermia, and a temperature below 32°C becomes a matter of serious concern. Profound hypothermia may cause the victim of a drowning to appear dead, with an absence of corneal, pupillary, and tendon reflexes, and undetectable pulse and breathing movements. Rewarming should thus be attempted even if a body appears lifeless.

If the temperature at rescue is over 32°C, the chances of full recovery are very good; the main point is to stop the victim from cooling further and to begin gradual rewarming. If there are multiple casualties, it is possible to attend to more serious cases once this need has been satisfied.

If no thermometer is available, severe hypothermia should be suspected if there is a clouding of consciousness, loss of coordination, or irrational behavior. Patients with severe hypothermia are very vulnerable to an attack of ventricular fibrillation. Sometimes the victim struggles, pumping cold and hyperkalemic blood into the heart. More often, the rescuer causes the problem by rough handling, forcible endotracheal intubation, unnecessary artificial ventilation or cardiac massage, and over-rapid rewarming. Unfortunately, the cold heart responds poorly to normal methods of defibrillation, so that problems are not entirely avoided by the institution of cardiac monitoring. However, the risk of ventricular fibrillation seems reduced by plasma expansion (5% dextrose saline infusion); this presumably increases cardiac output and reduces blood viscosity, both of these changes increasing coronary blood flow. An initial infusion of 300 ml is supplemented on the basis of the patient's response.

Over-rapid rewarming has two disadvantages: peripheral vasodilatation exacerbates the problem of a low cardiac output, while encouraging the return of very cold blood from the limbs to the central circulation (the so-called "after-drop" phenomenon). Some authorities thus recommend leaving the victim cold until carefully monitored rewarming can be undertaken in a hospital. Alternatively, the trunk can be warmed gently, or internal rewarming can be attempted by gentle mouth-to-mouth ventilation. The supply of oxygen heated to 40°C makes only a limited contribution to the rewarming process; given a flow of 10 L/minute, the energy input is unlikely to raise the core temperature by more than 0.3°C per hour.

The usual techniques of emergency medicine must be applied with considerable discretion. Endotracheal intubation should be avoided unless essential; local anesthesia should then be used to avoid provoking ventricular fibrillation. If artificial ventilation is needed, this also should be held below normal levels, since any tendency to alkalosis favors fibrillation. Bicarbonate was at one time suggested to counter peripheral tissue acidosis, but this is not now recommended unless there has been cardiac arrest. Oxygen is generally helpful, although it may need to be combined with ventilatory assistance, since oxygen lack is usually the stimulus to ventilation in hypothermic patients. Epinephrine should be administered only in the event of cardiac arrest.

Priority should be given to transferring cases of severe hypothermia to an intensive care unit. Here, further infusions of 5% dextrose in saline solution may be administered, solutions being heated to 43°C. Continuous monitoring of ECG, Pco_2, and Po_2 is instituted, and bicarbonate can be given if cardiac arrest has led to severe acidosis (for example, a temperature-corrected pH of less than 7.2). Discussion continues on the optimum method of rewarming—external heating (for example, immersion in a hot bath) or internal heating (heating of inspired gas, dialysate, extracorporeal circulation, or gastrointestinal infusions). Antibiotics are generally given to avoid pneumonia during the recovery period. Other potential late complications are a recurrence of the cardiac arrhythmia, hypotension, oliguria, and pulmonary edema.

HAZARDS OF COLD AIR

JOHN J. FRIM, B.Sc., M.Sc., Ph.D.

Apart from the intrinsic hazards associated with cold weather athletic activities, winter sports enthusiasts face two potentially serious health hazards of the environment—frostbite and hypothermia. Injuries often develop without the athlete's awareness of warning signs or symptoms. Profound hypothermia can result ultimately in death, while serious frostbite can lead to the equally unfortunate end points of gross disfigurement and permanent disability. Prevention of such grave consequences rests in a thorough understanding of the nature and etiology of cold injuries, along with the application of judicious foresight and common sense. In the unfortunate circumstances where cold injury occurs despite all reasonable precautions, proper treatment can minimize the extent of the tragedy.

PROTECTING THE LONG-DISTANCE SWIMMER

Swimmers who engage in events such as cross-channel or Lake Ontario swims are plainly at substantial risk of hypothermia. Accompanying persons should thus maintain close contact with the swimmer and watch carefully for signs of disturbed consciousness. Final rectal temperatures for such events are commonly in the range of 34 to 35°C.

The main protection against hypothermia is to check the escape of heat from the body. A thick layer of subcutaneous fat is one form of protection, and long-distance swimming is one sport for which no attempt should be made to reduce body fat. External applications of thick greases such as petroleum jelly also offer an appreciable advantage. While resting, they do not increase core temperature by more than 0.1°C, but when metabolism is increased tenfold by vigorous exercise, core temperatures may be 1°C higher, enough to convert serious into mild hypothermia.

A final consideration is the possibility of acclimatizing to cold. In general, human beings seem to show a hypothermic pattern of acclimatization. The reduction of shivering spares muscle glycogen and makes the use of SCUBA gear easier, but at the same time hypothermia develops more quickly than in an unacclimatized individual. On the other hand, repeated exposure to long bouts of very severe cold (as in the Korean pearl divers) apparently induces some hypertrophy of brown adipose tissue, a very active tissue that can substantially boost resting metabolism in the cold. There is also a local adaptation of skin and face to severe cold, pressor reactions becoming less severe over 5 to 10 days of repeated exposure.

THERMAL BALANCE AND COLD INJURY

The cause of cold injury, reduced to its simplest description, is a failure to maintain thermal balance at physiologically acceptable levels. Failure at the whole body level results in hypothermia, whereas excessive regional heat loss leads to localized cold injury or frostbite.

The thermoregulatory system of the body uses both physical and chemical regulation, effected through vasomotor and metabolic control, respectively, to balance heat production against heat loss.

In a cold environment, the body must often contend with the conflicting requirements of maintaining the core temperature near 37°C, while preventing cold injury to the extremities. During vigorous physical activity in relatively mild cold, metabolic heat production may be more than adequate to sustain the temperature of both core and extremities. However, at times of lesser activity, or during severe environmental conditions, heat production may be insufficient, and the body "sacrifices the extremity to save the core". While this sounds like an active and deliberate thermoregulatory decision, it is a simple consequence of physiologic thermoregulation and the thermodynamics of heat transfer to and from the tissues.

The key to reducing heat loss is to increase insulation, precisely what the thermoregulatory system does through vasoconstriction. By restricting blood flow to the skin and extremities, the body allows these tissues to cool, thereby reducing heat transfer to the environment by all avenues (conduction, convection, radiation, and evaporation). The improvement in insulation thus obtained is, however, quite limited, and amounts to a total gain of less than 1 clo of insulation.* By comparison, extra layers of clothing can provide as much as 6 clo of insulation.

The amount of insulation available from clothing is limited by how much restriction in movement the activity will allow. On the other hand, the amount of insulation required to maintain thermal balance depends on the metabolic rate and the environmental conditions. These factors are often in conflict for various sporting activities; resolution of this conflict lies in layered clothing, which can be donned or doffed as the situation demands, and in the development of newer fabrics and clothing designs that offer superior insulation with less bulk and restriction of movement.

ENVIRONMENTAL FACTORS AND COLD INJURY

Environmental thermal stress is quantified by reference to the four meteorolgic factors of humidity, temperature, wind velocity, and radiation. Unitary indices based on weighted combinations of some of these factors have been developed for hot environments, but in the cold it is simpler to describe these factors and their relationships to cold injuries independently.

Atmospheric humidity is generally low during subfreezing weather, adding to the thermal stress of the cold environment. A minor but chronic effect of this lack of moisture is a drying of exposed skin. More acutely, heat and water are lost by evaporation of moisture from the respiratory tract. The fraction of total body heat loss attributed to respiration can become quite appreciable in the cold. Absolute respiratory heat loss increases with ventilation, but since ventilatory rate is closely coupled to metabolic rate, the fraction of heat lost by breathing varies little with activity at a given temperature. Evaporation of water during exercise is not compensated without a deliberate increase of fluid intake, and it contributes significantly to dehydration in the cold.

Accumulation of moisture within clothing is a serious concern during winter sports. Most insulating materials perform best when dry, and their thermal resistance rapidly diminishes with wetting. This wetting could arise from external sources such as rain or melting snow, and suitable waterproof outer garments should be

used as appropriate. Wetting by sweat is an even more serious problem in cold climates, and physical activity should be adjusted if possible to avoid active sweating. If the metabolic rate is expected to increase substantially during a sporting activity, extra insulation should be removed to assist heat dissipation. If sweating is unavoidable, the wet garments should be removed or extra insulation added after the activity has been completed.

Temperature is the major environmental factor responsible for cold injury. It is not practicable to specify a critical temperature that delineates "safe" and "dangerous" environmental air temperatures regarding hypothermia. Avoidance of hypothermia depends upon body heat production offsetting environmental losses. There are, of course, practical limits to metabolic rate, body energy reserves, and clothing insulation. Ultimately, these factors determine tolerance and survival times under given conditions.

Since the freezing point of tissue is about $-0.3°C$, it is virtually impossible to develop frostbite at ambient temperatures above this threshold. In practice, tissue supercools somewhat before ice nucleation sets in, and the threshold air temperature for frostbite may be as low as $-10°C$. The only exception to this critical temperature guideline is a spill of cold liquid on the skin. Fuels like gasoline, kerosene, and naphtha remain liquid to well below $0°C$ and can rapidly freeze any tissue they contact. Highly volatile liquids can even cause frostbite at temperatures above $0°C$ by rapid evaporation. Rubber gloves should be worn when handling such fluids in the cold.

Next to air temperature, wind is the second most important environmental factor responsible for cold injury. While everyone is familiar with the term "windchill factor", there are several misconceptions associated with this factor.

The first is that wind can cause an object to cool to a temperature below that of the ambient air. This notion is plainly contrary to the laws of heat transfer; it probably arises from the practice of expressing the effect of wind as an equivalent temperature, several degrees below the ambient air temperature. Wind can, however, increase the rate at which an object cools, causing frostbite to develop under conditions that would pose little or no threat in the absence of wind. For the winter athlete, wind can be created in relatively still air by body movement (for instance, in skiing or riding a snowmobile).

Another misconception is that the windchill equivalent temperature describes the degree of cooling perceived by the whole body. In reality, this relative measure of cooling applies only to an inanimate object initially at $33°C$ with no insulation. The only parts of the body that even approach this condition are the exposed regions of the face and bared extremities. No account is taken of metabolic rate or clothing. The same wind speed has a much greater cooling effect on nude or lightly clad individuals than it does on well-insultated persons (assuming the clothing has a windproof outer shell).

In spite of its shortcomings, the windchill factor is still of value as a guide to outdoor activities where

---

* One clo unit provides an insulation of $0.15°C/W/m^2$. It is roughly equivalent, in practical terms, to a business suit.

exposed flesh is involved. Most windchill charts are divided into "safe" and "unsafe" zones, based upon estimated times for exposed flesh to freeze. Often, the exposed parts of the body dictate tolerance of a cold environment.

The last environmental factor to consider is radiation. All objects warmer than −273°C (absolute zero) can gain or lose heat by radiation. The net amount of heat exchanged between two objects depends upon the temperature difference between their surfaces. For well-insulated individuals in a cold environment, radiant heat losses are relatively minor, simply because the temperature difference between the surroundings and the clothing surface is small. Similarly, radiant heat loss from the body to the inner layer of clothing is minimal because of the small temperature difference between the two surfaces. Clearly, the use of "reflective" clothing over or under heavy insulation does little to reduce radiant heat loss. However, when a reflective layer is interposed between exposed warm flesh and a cold environment, or between a poorly insulated body and the environment, its effect becomes noticeable.

It is possible to gain considerable radiant heat from the sun even in the cold of winter. This raises the surface temperature of clothing, thereby reducing conductive heat loss from the body through the clothing. On sunny days, a reflective layer on the outside of clothing may be counterproductive.

OTHER EPIDEMIOLOGIC FACTORS

Age. Older persons are more likely to suffer chronic circulatory problems, making them more susceptible to cold injury. Young children, because of their small size, have a high surface area to volume ratio and lose heat at a faster rate than an adult.

Circulatory Problems. Any chronic condition (for example, Raynaud's syndrome) that interferes with the peripheral circulation predisposes to frostbite.

Fatigue. Mental fatigue and apathy can cause a neglect of warning signs, with failure to institute appropriate preventive measures. Physical fatigue compromises the defense against excessive heat loss, particularly if tissue reserves of glycogen are depleted.

Experience. Both frostbite and hypothermia can be prevented under most circumstances. When a mishap occurs (for example, getting lost, vehicle breakdown, climbing accident, or sudden weather change), persons experienced in cold survival are more likely to be dressed properly, to have extra food and clothing supplies, and to respond to the situation calmly and thoughtfully.

Race. Observations during World War II, during the Korean War, and in present-day Alaska confirm that the Negro is more susceptible to frostbite than the Caucasian.

Acclimation. Repeated exposures to cold stimuli can alter responses of the thermoregulatory system, increasing tolerance of severe conditions.

Concomitant Injury. Blood loss and shock reduce peripheral blood flow, predisposing to frostbite. After fracture, blood flow to the injured part may be limited due to severed blood vessels or constriction from bandages.

Previous Frostbite. Previous severe frostbite leaves the body more susceptible to cold injury for several years, perhaps due to slowly healing vascular and neurologic damage.

Drugs and Medication. Any drugs or medications that compromise vasomotor responses in the extremities should be used with extreme caution. Vasoconstrictors can lead to frostbite, while vasodilators predispose to hypothermia.

Alcohol. The effects of alcohol on heat exchange are controversial, but its known influence on judgment rule against its use in the cold. The percentage of frostbite and hypothermia victims who have consumed substantial amounts of alcohol prior to injury is alarmingly high.

FROSTBITE

Etiology. Frostbite occurs whenever tissue freezes, either intracellularly or extracellularly. During slow cooling, ice nucleation begins in the interstitial fluid, and cells respond to the increasing osmolality of their environment by dehydrating and shrinking. This loss of water reduces intracellular ice formation, but can cause osmotic injury to the cells. During rapid cooling, ice formation again begins extracellularly, but most cell types cannot dehydrate fast enough to avoid intracellular freezing. During rewarming, recrystallization causes the smaller ice crystals to grow disruptively, thereby inflicting physical damage upon cellular structures. Rapid rewarming generally minimizes such physical damage.

Regardless of the mechanism leading to injury, the target tissue ultimately responsible for the loss of flesh from frostbite appears to be the microcirculation. Time-lapse cinemicrography of frozen tissues has shown that the vascular system is functionally intact immediately after thawing, but that thrombi very quickly occlude the small capillaries. Electron microscopy of small blood vessels reveals extensive damage to endothelial cells. Presumably, thrombogenic agents released from these injured cells lead to clot formation with eventual total occlusion of the affected blood vessels.

Prevention. Prevention of frostbite is straightforward—avoid excessive cooling of body surface tissues. In particular, one must protect susceptible tissues such as the nose, cheeks, ears, fingers, and toes. Tissues most likely to suffer frostbite are those with a poor circulation, with a high surface area-to-volume ratio, at a distance from the body core, and with the greatest exposure to the elements. Insulation is the key to prophylaxis, but it must be used cautiously. Insulation that is excessive or constrictive can cut off the blood supply to an extremity. This is particularly true of hand and foot wear. If the source of heat is eliminated, the part cools toward ambient temperature like an inanimate object, the rate of cooling depending only upon the insulation between the tissue and the environment.

Marked blanching of the skin, numbness, loss of tactile sensation, or a sharp localized stinging (frostnip) are the first warning signs of frostbite. Rapid rewarming of the affected area with a warm hand will prevent the injury from becoming serious. However, it is then advisable to terminate the activity and seek shelter, since recurrence of the injury is highly probable.

Characterization. Frostbite injury can be graded, but the treatment for all categories is the same, since all frostbite looks identical both before and immediately after thawing. An assessment of severity can only be made in retrospect, leaving the clinician no choice but to treat all cases as severe injury.

First-degree frostbite is characterized by hyperemia and edema. After warming, the tissue becomes mottled, cyanotic, red, hot, and dry. There may be itching, burning, or a deep ache. Swelling and other symptoms may persist for several hours or even days, but the tissue usually heals with only minor peeling.

Second-degree frostbite is associated with vesicle formation, extending to the tips of the affected digits. The vesicles appear 6 to 12 hours after thawing and contain clear fluid. Only the superficial layers of the skin are affected, but after the blisters have healed, the tissue below may be very soft and sensitive to trauma.

Third-degree frostbite involves damage to the full skin thickness and to the tissue below. Vesicle formation is again present after thawing, but the blisters are filled with hemorrhagic fluid and rarely extend to the tips of the digits. Fleshy tissue loss is associated with this injury.

Fourth-degree frostbite involves injury to all tissues including bone. The development of post-thaw symptoms is slow. Vesicle formation is absent, and complete healing of the injury takes several weeks. If surgical amputation is not implemented, autoamputation of the mummified tissues occurs spontaneously.

Treatment. Provided the tissue is still frozen, the affected part is best thawed rapidly in a whirlpool bath controlled at 40°C. Water temperature should never exceed 42°C to avoid burning the already traumatized tissue. If the affected part is an ear or the nose, warm water can be poured over the injured area. Rapid warming may cause intense pain, requiring treatment with analgesics such as aspirin, Demerol, or even morphine. However, the benefit of reduced tissue loss far outweighs the drawbacks of the pain.

Warming should be terminated when thawing is complete, as indicated by the return of sensation (pain), color (red or purple), and softening of the affected area. The tissue should never be warmed above 37°C, and rapid warming should not be applied to thawed tissues. Rubbing with snow, massage, or the application of dry heat are to be avoided, since they increase tissue damage.

Severe frostbite should never be treated in the field, unless hospital facilities are hours out of reach. A frostbite victim can walk many miles on a frozen limb without incurring significant additional injury, but after thawing, such an individual becomes a stretcher case. Under no circumstances should thawing be initiated if there is a chance of refreezing, since this would greatly increase tissue loss.

Since tissue loss is mainly the result of microcirculatory failure, smoking and vasoconstrictor drugs are contraindicated. On the other hand, anything that will promote vasodilation (such as warm fluids) is beneficial. Vasodilators, chemical or surgical sympathectomies, anticoagulants, and plasma expanders have all been used to treat frostbite, but the results are somewhat controversial. This is not surprising, since it is difficult to judge the effectiveness of treatment without knowing the extent of injury prior to treatment. Many of these treatments must also be started immediately after thawing in order to be effective.

Intra-arterial reserpine (0.5 mg) injected proximal to the injured extremity just after thawing and repeated at 2- to 3-day intervals for a week produces a temporary chemical sympathectomy with few systemic side effects. Fasciotomy is being used increasingly in cases where severe edema is impeding blood flow. Infusion of low-molecular-weight dextran, because of its risks, is reserved for cases in which tissue loss is highly probable. If used, treatment should consist of Dextran 40, 1.5 g/kg IV on the first day, followed by 0.75 g/kg IV daily for 5 days. The use of heparin as an anticoagulant has had mixed success and diathermy has not been adequately researched as a possible treatment modality in frostbite.

Follow-up care after the initial thawing is centered around open treatment under sterile conditions. Whirlpool treatment with 37°C water containing a disinfectant is given for 20 to 30 minutes two or three times a day. This promotes circulation, helps control infection, alleviates pain, and debrides the wound gently. During treatment, the patient is encouraged to flex the affected joints to avoid a flexion contracture.

If tissue loss appears certain, there may be a desire to amputate early to speed recovery. However, unless the line of demarcation between live and dead tissue is clear, or unless wet gangrene has set in, surgery should be delayed as late as possible.

HYPOTHERMIA

Etiology. Hypothermia has been defined clinically as the condition of a core (rectal) temperature of 34.4°C (94°F) or lower. It arises because the body loses more heat to the environment than it produces, and can occur at ambient temperatures well above freezing.

Acute hypothermia follows a rapid loss of body heat, as during sudden immersion in cold water. The thermoregulatory system has little time to respond before metabolic rate and heart rate become severely depressed. As a result, the body is "frozen" in a physiologic state similar to that prior to cooling.

Chronic hypothermia is the result of slow body cooling, as from prolonged exposure to cold wet conditions. In this instance, the thermoregulatory system has ample time to respond. Vasoconstriction shifts fluid from the periphery to the core, and the body responds with increased diuresis. Patients with chronic hypothermia are thus often volume depleted. The body responds to the heat loss with intense shivering, but as heart rate and respiration decline, blood and oxygen supplies to the muscles decrease. Lactic acid and other metabolites accumulate in the tissues, leaving the patient acidotic. The resultant pH, electrolyte, and fluid volume disturbances become serious concerns during rewarming and treatment.

Prevention. Hypothermia is prevented by reducing heat loss to the environment. Appropriate clothing protects not only against cold, but also against wind and moisture. The usual recommendation is to wear several layers of loose clothing, topped with a windproof water-repellant shell. However, such clothing may be incompatible with an athletic activity, and many winter sports have evolved highly specialized styles of dress. In a sport such as cross-country ski racing, the clothing offers suitable protection only while the body is producing large amounts of metabolic heat, and additional clothing is required prior to and shortly after the activity has been completed. Conversely, a snowmobile suit offers excellent protection against the cold and wind while riding on the vehicle, but provides far too much insulation for the activity of building a snow shelter. Specialized clothing designed for specific activities can lead to cold injury if used inappropriately.

Often, the threat of hypothermia arises as a result of unforeseen circumstances such as getting lost, becoming injured, or falling in water. The first priority in such circumstances is to find shelter from the elements, particularly from the wind. Wet clothing should be substituted with dry, if possible. Conductive heat loss can be minimized by extra insulation, and wrapping the victim in a plastic sheet greatly reduces convective and evaporative heat losses. Additional external heat sources such as a fire, contact with a warm body (huddling), or warm fluids can further reduce cooling.

Prevention also involves recognizing the early symptoms of hypothermia. Initially, the body responds with an increase of shivering, but below a core temperature of 35°C, metabolism declines and shivering intensity wanes. With heat production now greatly reduced, the rate of body cooling increases substantially. Mental confusion, disorientation, and poor coordination are accompanied by mood changes such as depression and introversion. Simple tasks become difficult or impossible to perform. At a core temperature of about 32°C, cardiac arrhythmias may appear, and the victim may hallucinate and waver into semi-unconsciousness. Below 30°C, the victim is unconscious, with fixed, dilated pupils and no tendon reflexes.

As a rule of thumb, a person who is shivering violently but is reasonably alert may be becoming hypothermic; if shivering is weak or absent and mental confusion is profound, the patient is hypothermic and in serious danger.

Treatment. Profound hypothermia (unconsciousness; core temperature <30°C) should ideally be treated in a hospital with patient monitoring and life support equipment. Field treatment other than the prevention of additional heat loss is not recommended if hospital facilities are nearby. If prompt evacuation is not possible, or if the victim is still conscious, field treatment should be initiated immediately. Under all circumstances, gentle handling is of the utmost importance in preventing cardiac fibrillation.

After rescue, the first step in treating hypothermia is to prevent additional heat loss (seek shelter, wrap in blankets and plastic sheet, etc.). A second priority is to establish a patent airway and encourage the patient to breathe. In the field, this may involve artificial respiration (mouth-to-mouth only) at 5 to 10 breaths/minute. In the hospital, endotracheal intubation may be preferrable, but care must be taken to avoid provoking fibrillation. Administration of 100 percent warm humidified oxygen under positive pressure is helpful, taking care not to overventilate and not to burn the air passages with steam. If cardiac monitoring is available, it should be utilized.

At this point, the decision has to be made whether to treat in the field or evacuate to a hospital. A cold body has a greatly reduced metabolic demand, and a short additional time in this condition adds little further injury. In contrast, if rewarming is begun in the field, it must be continued aggressively until the patient is rewarmed and can be moved to a hospital safely. If proper facilities can be reached within 30 minutes, one should opt for evacuation.

Rapid rewarming in a bath at 40°C is recommended if the core temperature is above 32°C. If the body is colder than this, the extremities should not be immersed, since this will induce extensive vasodilation. A rush of cold peripheral blood into the body core can lower the central temperature by as much as 2°C (the "afterdrop" phenomenon), inducing ventricular fibrillation if the heart cools to 28°C. In the field, rewarming by shivering may be all that is available. Administration of warm fluids or sitting near a fire assist heat gain, although some researchers caution that this could reduce the body's sensation of the cold and thus reduce shivering.

Chronic hypothermia presents special problems during rewarming because of the altered physiologic state. Although reestablishment of a normal body temperature is mandatory, treatment should also aim at correcting body fluid volumes, blood pH, and serum electrolytes, while avoiding cardiac problems. Intravenous fluids should be started as soon as possible (difficult with a vasoconstricted body), and a blood sample should be taken for analysis of serum electrolytes, blood gases, blood pH, and serum glucose. Blood gas readings must be corrected for the patient's temperature. When rewarming is begun, physiologic changes occur rapidly, and constant monitoring and correction of physiology are essential.

Hospital rewarming techniques can be divided into internal and external methods. Internal techniques include respiratory heating, peritoneal dialysis, mediastinal irrigation, extracorporeal circulation, hemodialysis, intragastric lavage, colonic lavage, and various forms of diathermy. Disadvantages of all these methods are that they require skilled medical teams, they take valuable time to implement, and they expose the patient to a risk of infection. Those who prefer internal rewarming cite the advantages as better control of warming rate, faster rewarming, and heating only of the core, thereby facilitating cardiac output while lessening the problems associated with afterdrop. External techniques include warm baths, radiant heat, electric blankets, hot water suits, heat packs, and showers. All methods of external rewarming accentuate the afterdrop and should only be used when the core temperature exceeds 32°C. They also suppress shivering to some degree, thereby compromising natural rewarming. The advantages are that they can be applied quickly, easily, and with little intrinsic risk to the patient. Some of them can, in fact, be implemented in the field.

During rewarming, respiratory support and correction of body fluids is continued. Temperature, blood pressure, blood gases, pH, and electrolytes are monitored frequently, while the ECG is watched constantly. Atrial arrhythmias and fibrillation occur often with hypothermia, but usually correct themselves with rewarming. Drugs to treat these symptoms are ineffective in a cold body. Ventricular arrhythmias and fibrillation are more serious, and should be treated. Premature ventricular contractions can be treated with lidocaine HCl (Xylocaine). Electrical defibrillation may be ineffective until core temperature has risen above 32°C, but it should be attempted at least once even at lower temperatures. Closed chest compression or a heart-lung machine may be used instead, if a normal rhythm is not restored.

After recovery, the patient should be monitored for several days. The most frequent complications are pneumonia, renal failure, pancreatitis, and frostbite. The thermoregulatory system may also be impaired for days or weeks, and cold environments should be avoided.

The most frequent question regarding field treatment of hypothermia concerns the use of cardiopulmonary resuscitation (CPR). Most CPR training is done with mechanical models, and most experience is gained with warm bodies. The response of a cold body to such manipulation is entirely different. In particular, the muscles of the chest are stiffer, and this will alter the "feel" of the treatment. The cold heart also does not respond in the way one would expect. Finally, the decision to attempt CPR may be based upon a failure to detect respiration or a palpable pulse; however, the hypothermic body has little requirement for oxygen, and hypothermic patients have been observed with a pulse rate as low as 2 beats/minute. It is thus recommended that CPR be attempted only when cardiac monitoring is available. In this way, the function of the heart can be clearly visualized, and the need for and effectiveness of CPR can be ascertained with little doubt.

Hypothermia victims frequently show no vital signs and are often mistaken for dead. However, low body temperature by itself is not a killer, since induced hypothermia to as low as 5°C is used frequently in surgery. It is essential, therefore, to try to resuscitate any cold body before it is pronounced as dead.

EXERCISE IN THE HEAT

OMRI INBAR, Ed.D., F.A.C.S.M.

Climate plays a major and sometimes crucial role in both the exercise performance and the general well-being of the exercising individual. As Sir Adolph Abrahams has stated: "the only serious risk to life from intensive exercise comes from heat stroke". In spite of such a clear warning, sports administrators, physical educators, and coaches continue to expose athletes, school children, and soldiers to risk by arranging competitive sports events and physical activity programs under climatic conditions that present a danger of heat stroke or other heat injuries.

This chapter will review general physiologic reactions to exercise in the heat, specific environmental and human factors which may influence such reactions, critical internal and environmental conditions, and the symptoms, treatment, and possible prevention of various illnesses associated with exercise in the heat.

PHYSIOLOGIC REACTIONS TO EXERCISE IN THE HEAT

Although man is a homeotherm, his core temperature rises during steady physical exercise. In cool or comfortable air temperatures a new equilibrium level is reached within 40 to 60 minutes. The new core temperature and the rate at which it is attained are both related directly to the rate of heat production. Such rises of body temperature during exercise should not be regarded as fever or as a failure of the temperature regulatory system.

The principal means by which we lose heat during exercise or exposure to heat are: (1) restriction of blood flow through certain abdominal organs, with redirection of flow to expanded blood vessels under the skin, (2) cooling of subcutaneous blood as sweat is vaporized on the skin surface, (3) cooling of the skin surface through evaporative heat loss and (4) return of cooled blood from the skin to the central circulation.

Environmental heat reduces the thermal gradient between the environment and the skin surface, and between the skin surface and body core, thus limiting heat transfer. The main burden imposed by the combined stresses of heat and exercise falls upon the circulatory system.

In addition to delivering oxygen and other nutrients, and removing the waste products of metabolism, the circulation has the important function of heat convection, transferring heat from the exercising muscles to the skin, where it is passed to the surrounding atmosphere by radiation, convection, conduction, and evaporation. The increase in convection of heat to the skin during muscular work is effected by the opening up of previously closed capillaries and arteriovenous shunts within the skin. The opening up of skin vessels and the rise of body temperature affect both the central circulation and the regional distribution of blood flow. If submaximal exercise is performed under hot conditions, heart rate is increased and stroke volume is decreased, compared to cool conditions, but arteriovenous oxygen difference and cardiac output are virtually unchanged. Redistribution of the cardiac output under hot conditions leads to reductions in muscular, renal, and hepatic blood flow. Furthermore, diversion of cardiac output from exercising muscles to the skin under such conditions may increase anaerobic metabolism, with a rise of arterial blood lactate.

It follows that in warm to hot climates the exercising individual is at a disadvantage. Owing to added strain on the circulatory system, anaerobic metabolism begins at a lower rate of oxygen consumption and the subject becomes exhausted much earlier than when similar exercise is performed under cooler conditions. These basic reactions are modified by various environmental and personal factors, each of which must be considered in order to make an accurate evaluation of the thermal and/or physiologic responses to exercise in the heat.

ENVIRONMENTAL FACTORS

Dry Heat (Air Temperature). When an individual exercises in a hot and dry environment, cooling of the skin is brought about predominantly by evaporation of sweat. The air can absorb a considerable amount of moisture before becoming saturated. However, since heat dissipation depends upon elimination of water in perspiration, large amounts of fluid are taken out of the body, and dehydration is a distinct possibility.

Wet Heat (Humidity). When the air surrounding an individual is not only hot but also loaded with moisture, evaporative cooling is impaired. An environment in which the ambient (dry bulb) temperature is only moderately high (32°C), but relative humidity is high (85%), is considerably more stressful to both circulatory and thermoregulatory systems than an environment with a higher dry temperature (say 40°C), but a relative humidity as low as 25%.

When the air is completely saturated with water vapor (100% relative humidity) and the air temperature is higher than the skin temperature, no heat dissipation can occur. Metabolic heat then accumulates, and body temperature rises rapidly until death ensues.

It may thus be concluded that the problems in a hot, dry atmosphere are related to increased cardiovascular strain and dehydration (if water intake is insufficient). In a hot, humid climate the same problems exist, but are aggravated by a lesser ability to unload water vapor into an already loaded ambient atmosphere.

Air-Movement (Wind). For effective evaporative and convective heat loss from the skin, air movement must occur near the body surface. Even cool dry air becomes warm and wet if heat convection and evaporation are taking place. Therefore, the faster the air flow over the body, the greater the possible rate of heat loss by evaporation and convection.

When an individual is running or cycling, the added air movement over the body surface effectively enhances sweat evaporation. The greatest benefit occurs at speeds of 1 to 8 miles/hr. Running or cycling faster than 8 miles/hr could create greater heat gain than loss, since an increased metabolic rate is necessary to overcome the increased wind resistance.

When the ambient temperature rises above skin temperature, air movement around the body surface may still promote some heat loss by evaporation, but at the same time heat gain is caused through conduction and convection.

Radiation. Molecules within matter are constantly vibrating and, as a result, emit heat as electromagnetic waves. We gain heat through radiation when surrounding objects are warmer than our bodies, and vice versa. Under certain conditions (bright, sunny days, with a light background and dark clothing), radiant heating adds a tremendous burden to the overall strain imposed upon circulatory and thermoregulatory systems. Although difficult to assess accurately, it has been estimated that direct solar radiation of 4 kilojoules/cm²/min increases the effective ambient temperature by 1 to 6°C, depending on the color of clothing that is worn. An individual who sits naked on the sand during a hot and bright day may gain, through radiation, some 1200 kilojoules (kJ) within one hour.

Clothing. Clothing affects heat exchange by radiation, conduction, convection, and evaporation, and it may also increase heat production because of its mass and/or its restrictive nature.

Clothing may offer a barrier between the body surface and a radiating element, thereby protecting the body particularly from solar radiation. In this respect, light-colored clothing is much more effective than dark-colored apparel. Direct solar radiation of 4 kJ/cm²/min increases the effective ambient temperature by 1 or 2°C for light-colored clothing and by 3 to 6°C for dark colored clothing.

When the ambient temperature rises above skin temperature, evaporation becomes the only avenue of heat loss. When the skin is naked, heat vaporization is drawn from the skin itself, and the effectiveness of such evaporation in terms of body cooling is close to 100 percent. When clothing is worn, several complications arise: The efficiency of convection over the skin is reduced, and sweat is evaporated away from the skin, part of the heat of vaporization being taken from the ambient air rather than from the skin, thereby reducing the effectiveness of such evaporation.

Under all conditions, clothing impedes the outward diffusion of water vapor from the skin, to an extent which depends upon the textile used. Clothing which retards evaporation by 50 percent increases the effective temperature by as much as 7°C. Thus, clothing worn during exercise in hot climates must be selected in accordance with prevailing environmental conditions. As a general rule, bright-colored, light, and porous clothing is preferred to dark-colored, heavy, and nonporous clothing.

PERSONAL FACTORS

Metabolic Rate. Metabolic heat production is an important factor in the overall thermal response of a resting and, particularly, an exercising individual. Metabolic heat production at rest averages 6.1 kJ/min, or about 366 kJ/hr. Under most environmental conditions, 366 kJ/hr can easily be dissipated through a combination of convection, conduction, radiation, and evaporation. However, well-trained athletes may sustain an oxygen uptake up to about 6 liters/min for periods of 5 to 10 minutes. The amount of heat thus produced (some 126 kJ/min) could theoretically increase the body temperature of a 70 kg individual by some 23°C per hour, if the excess heat were not dissipated. Since the metabolic rate is closely correlated with exercise intensity, the latter plays a crucial role in thermal reactions to exercise in the heat. Thus, assuming fitness level and degree of heat acclimation to be constant, the higher the exercise intensity, the greater the overall thermal strain. However, if fitness level or degree of heat acclimation differ (the case within most populations), a similar exercise intensity (metabolic rate) will cause a varying thermal strain which depends (among other factors) on the individual's fitness and degree of heat acclimation. The key factor is, therefore, the relative rather than the absolute exercise intensity. The higher the relative exercise intensity (percentage of maximum oxygen intake) the greater the thermal strain. Thus, when supervising exercise programs in hot climates, one should take account of not only the absolute intensity of exercise, but also, and more importantly, the exercise level relative to the individual's performance capacity.

Heat Acclimation. After a few days' exposure to a hot environment, tolerance to a given heat stress increases. The major physiologic changes during heat acclimation include decrease of heart rate and body temperature at a given exercise intensity, an increase in sweat rate, a reduction of salt concentration in sweat, and an increased sensitivity of the sweating apparatus to increments of core temperature. These changes are accompanied by an improvement of subjective wellbeing and by a reduced risk of heat-related pathologies. The principal element in achieving optimal heat acclimation is exposure to high ambient temperatures while performing a physical task. In adults, merely sitting at rest, even in severe heat, does not produce the physiologic responses required for full heat acclimation. In young adults, a reasonable degree of accclimation can be reached following four to eight exposures to the combined stresses of heat and exercise. As in physical training, heat acclimation is rather specific, the best results being obtained when it is carried out under conditions of environment and work rate similar to those under which the expected task is to be performed. The carry-over

effects of heat acclimation persist for relatively short periods following heat exposure, being positively correlated with the number and length of heat exposures.

Although young children can be heat acclimatized, their rate of acclimation is physiologically slower but subjectively faster than that of young adults. The faster improvement of subjective well-being could present a health hazard by engendering a false sense of confidence and by leading a young child to be daring in performing physical exercise in the heat, despite a marked physiologic heat strain. Nevertheless, I have shown that young children can be effectively heat acclimated by either passive exposures to heat or physical training performed under neutral environmental conditions. The difference of response between young children and young adults seems attributable to age-related factors such as a lower sweat rate, different morphologic characteristics, higher adiposity level, and an immature cardiovascular system. The foregoing information has clinical importance, particularly under conditions of sudden climatic heat waves, whenever physical training is commenced during early summer, and when athletic competition or military operations are to be carried out under environmental conditions hotter than those to which the individual has been accustomed. Special attention should be paid to young children and probably to older people, particularly during the early stages of acclimation.

Physical Fitness. Among various factors affecting one's physiologic responses to exercise in heat, the maximum oxygen intake has considerable importance. Individuals with a high cardiorespiratory fitness have an advantage in terms of both exercise heat tolerance and rate of acclimation. Increased physical fitness also appears to confer a longer retention of the benefits of heat acclimation.

However, in young adults physical training that is carried out under neutral and comfortable environmental conditions cannot replace a heat acclimation program in which the combined stresses of heat and exercise are imposed. The former type of training program, while improving physical fitness and the ability to cope with increased thermal and cardiovascular strain during exercise in heat, does not bring about the physiologic (or subjective) adaptation observed following "classic" heat acclimation. It seems that the degree of heat acclimation achieved is a function of the heat stored in the body (thermal load) during each of the heat acclimation exposures. For any given population, we have found an optimal (and yet to be determined) thermal load (the end result of the combined effects of climatic and metabolic stresses). This should be maintained throughout acclimation exposures; greater or lesser loads lead to a lesser physiologic adaptation. Thus, if heat acclimation is desired but is logistically impossible, physical training at target speeds can be carried out in a cool environment while wearing sweat clothing (to increase the thermal load).

The remaining personal factors (dehydration, salt depletion, age, sex, body dimensions, and health status), although important in determining and understanding thermal and physiologic responses to exercise in the heat, are discussed elsewhere in this book.

CRITICAL TEMPERATURES

Several biometeorologic indices have been developed to assess the interactive effect of various metabolic and environmental stresses. The measured components in most of these indices include the climatic variables of air temperature, relative humidity, wind velocity, and radiation. By introduction of these measurements into complicated charts and formulas, it has been possible to estimate the integrated climatic stress and the resultant physiologic strain, thus specifying "critical temperatures" for physical activity in the heat.

These indices place relatively little emphasis on the dry bulb temperature of the ambient environment, and much more emphasis upon such items as relative humidity, radiation, and wind velocity. Three of the most popular indices are the Effective Temperature (ET), the Wet Bulb Globe Temperature Index (WBGT), and the Predicted 4-hour Sweat Production (P4SR). The first criterion (ET) is subjective, while the other two base their integrated stress evaluation upon meteorologic variables (WBGT) and sweat loss (P4SR), respectively.

Such indices fail to account for all of the factors affecting human reactions to exercise in the heat, and despite their success in reducing the number of heat casualties, in many instances they are inaccurate. Particularly lacking are heat stress indices which include exercise intensity among their measured components.

The following are some general guidelines for safe exercise in hot environments, based upon the above three heat stress indices:

For Effective Temperature (ET):
   Light work rates (up to 0.6 liters/min of oxygen consumed)—<30°C ET
   Moderate work rates (up to 1.0 liters/min of oxygen consumed)—<27.5°C ET
   Heavy work rates (up to 1.5 liters/min of oxygen consumed)—<26.5°C ET

For the Wet Bulb Globe Temperature (WBGT) Index:
   Above 26.5°C (WBGT)—utilize discretion
   Above 29.5°C (WBGT)—avoid strenuous activity
   Above 31°C (WBGT)—cease physical activity

For the Predicted 4-hour Sweat Production (P4SR):
   Up to 4.5 liters of sweat (P4SR)—Tolerable conditions for healthy young males
   Up to 3.0 liters of sweat (P4SR)—Tolerable conditions for subjects over 45 years old, untrained, unacclimatized and obese

A more sensible and reliable approach to safe performance in the heat is to use the body core temperature as an indicator of over-all strain. However, such an approach (measuring rectal temperatures) is often impractical and/or inconvenient. Conditions should be judged to be "easy" when the rectal temperature (Tre)

does not exceed 38°C; they should be considered "excessive" when Tre is higher than 39.2°C; with the Tre between these two limits, conditions should be graded as increasingly "difficult" as Tre approaches 39.2°C.

There have been recent attempts to develop models which account for the generation, dissipation and storage of heat in the body, incorporating conductive, evaporative, and radiant heat transfer, and the effects of clothing under a wide range of environmental conditions and at various levels of exercise. In the future, such models may allow the evaluation of human responses to a wide variety of ambient conditions, with specification of a maximum recommended duration of exercise under given climatic conditions, clothing, and the level of exercise.

HEAT DISORDERS—TREATMENT AND PREVENTION

Overexposure to heat not only decreases exercise performance, but also predisposes to heat disorders. It is important, therefore, that those engaged in and/or supervising physical activity in hot climates recognize the major symptoms of the various heat disorders and become familiar with methods of prevention and treatment. The various disorders can be ranked in order of increasing severity as: heat cramps, heat syncope, heat exhaustion, and heat stroke.

Heat Cramps. This is a short-term heat disorder, most common in highly trained individuals who have been training for several days in extremely hot weather. Its main cause is an excessive loss of fluid, salt, and possibly other minerals, due to failure to replace losses incurred by sweating. The cramps usually occur in muscles that have been most active, and symptoms can last for several minutes. Intravenous administration of saline solutions, together with firm massaging pressure on the cramped muscle will promptly relieve symptoms.

Heat Syncope. This is also relatively harmless. The primary cause is an unfavorable blood distribution. A large proportion of the blood volume becomes distributed to the peripheral vessels, especially in the lower extremities, through prolonged standing and/or an exercise bout which is halted abruptly. The result is a drop in blood pressure and an inadequate oxygen supply to the brain (which may lead to loss of consciousness). The major symptoms are profuse sweating and an abnormally high pulse rate. The affected individual should be placed in a horizontal position, with the legs elevated.

Heat Exhaustion. This can be a very severe heat stress disorder. It develops slowly over several days, and may lead to heat stroke if not properly treated. The victim has a body temperature of 38 to 40°C, and usually shows profuse sweating with higher than normal respiratory and pulse rates. Other usual features include nausea, headache, fatigue, confusion, drowsiness, giddiness, scant urine, frequent vomiting, and diarrhea. Medical intervention (primarily IV replacement of water and salts) and even hospitalization are often indicated, especially if symptoms persist and body mass continues to drop.

Heat Stroke. This is the most serious, and sometimes fatal, consequence of exposure to the combined stresses of heat and exercise. It can develop gradually over several days as the end result of heat exhaustion, or it can appear suddenly when heavy exercise is performed in an extremely stressful environment. The victim has a very high body temperature (41 to 43°C) and dry skin. There are usually signs of weakness, dizziness, confusion, and rapid breathing with convulsions and even coma. Immediate cooling of the body is of utmost importance. The patient should be taken into the shade, stripped, and sponged frequently with cool water to keep the skin moist, while air is blown over the body. Treatment should continue until the rectal temperature drops to 38°C. Further steps which ought to be followed include a restoration of both blood pressure (IV fluid) and acid-base balance (IV bicarbonate). Immediate diagnosis and proper treatment (especially body cooling) greatly reduce the chances of a fatal outcome.

The most frequent common denominators for all of the above heat illnesses are heat exposure, physical exercise, loss of water and salt, and storage of heat (reflected by a high internal temperature). However, the most important single factor, from a clinical standpoint, is loss of body water. Therefore, many of the acute adverse effects of heat can be avoided by simple preventive measures as follows:

1. Heat acclimation is probably the most effective method to reduce the incidence of heat disorders. It should be considered for all individuals who engage in physical exercise in the heat, but particularly for those who are moving from a cold or temperate climate to a warm or hot region, and for those who plan to start training during the summer months. We recommend a minimum of six daily exposures, each providing 2 hours of physical exercise in the heat. Work rate is progressively increased, but the final heart rate and rectal temperature are never allowed to exceed 180 beats/min and 39.2°C, respectively.

2. The severity of exercise should be reduced on hot days, cutting back on both training intensity and duration until the individual is more comfortable with the required work rate, and physiologic reactions fall within the normal range. Such an adaptation of the exercise load should take into account factors such as age, sex, level of acclimation, level of physical fitness, clothing, and health status.

3. Body mass should be recorded when training or working in extreme heat. If the cumulative loss is greater than 3 percent of initial body mass, a schedule of forced water replacement must be implemented (see chapter on fluid and mineral needs).

4. Salt must be continually replaced. A frequent intake of diluted salt solution (pinch of salt per cup) is recommended if prolonged and repeated exercise is performed in severe heat. Under milder conditions, a liberal salting of food at mealtime between workouts is sufficient to avoid a salt deficit.

ADJUSTMENT TO HIGH ALTITUDE

ROY J. SHEPHARD, M.D. (Lond), Ph.D.

Sports physicians commonly face several very practical questions when advising their patients about problems at high altitude:

1. If a competition is being organized at altitude, what is the optimum period of residence to allow in the new location?

2. Are there any drugs that can speed the process of adjustment?

3. Does an altitude training camp offer any advantage in subsequent sea-level competition?

4. Does air travel produce any of the problems of high altitude?

5. What is a safe altitude ceiling for athletic competition?

Brief answers to these questions will be provided after considering the nature of the physiologic disturbances encountered at altitude.

PHYSIOLOGY OF MODERATE ALTITUDE EXPOSURE

Athletic competitions are not held at the extreme altitudes discussed by mountaineers, experts in aviation medicine, and many early physiologists; commonly the venue is at 2000 to 3000 meters (for example, Mexico City, 2350 meters).

At 10,000 feet (3048 meters), there is 31.2 percent less oxygen delivered per unit volume of inspired air. Because of the shape of the oxygen dissociation curve, the arterial blood remains fairly completely saturated with oxygen to about 1500 meters, but thereafter its oxygen content drops steadily. Thus, in Mexico City there is a 7 to 8 percent decrease of maximum oxygen intake. During submaximum exercise, compensation is possible by a corresponding tachycardia, but during all-out effort, performance drops. The effect is less than would be predicted from maximum oxygen intake, since at 3000 meters gravitational acceleration is reduced by 0.1 percent (a particular help to jumpers, pole vaulters, hurdlers, and throwers) and a decrease of atmospheric density lowers the wind resistance encountered by a runner as much as 3.4 percent. A further advantage in equatorial countries is that temperatures are up to 20°C cooler at 3000 meters.

The immediate reactions of the body to oxygen lack are hyperventilation (which reduces alkaline reserve and thus tolerance of anaerobic events) and various fluid shifts including a hemoconcentration which helps oxygen carriage but reduces the stroke output of the heart. If the athlete remains at altitude, blood and tissue buffers are adjusted downwards to allow greater ventilation (1 week), tissue enzyme concentrations are increased (1 week), and red cell mass is increased with restoration of plasma volume (several months).

OPTIMUM PERIOD OF RESIDENCE AT ALTITUDE

Competitors who were born or have lived for many years at altitude (such as the Kenyans) plainly have an advantage in endurance events at altitude. However, if the time available for altitude adjustment is measured in weeks, there is no real agreement on the optimum schedule.

Although some authors have recommended 2 to 3 weeks of adjustment, particularly with altitudes of less than 2250 meters, there are several disadvantages to this. Specifically, training is disrupted by early reactions to altitude, there is psychologic discouragement from poor times and disturbances of sleep, and physiologic potential is waning because of a diminishing blood volume.

The optimum schedule may thus be to make a preliminary visit to the site to observe local conditions and their impact upon pacing, and then to fly in some 3 days before competing. This interval will allow recovery from both the journey and any immediate acid/base disturbance, but will not be long enough to induce a major decrease of blood volume and thus maximum cardiac output.

DRUGS TO SPEED ALTITUDE ACCLIMATIZATION

At the altitudes under discussion, no specific therapy may be required. Training schedules should be lightened temporarily, and symptomatic therapy should be given as needed for headache and sleeplessness. Carbonic anhydrase inhibiting diuretics (for example, acetazolamide, 250 mg *qid*) are best avoided. Immediate symptoms are reduced, but acclimatization is slowed and the induced fluid loss leads to a further deterioration of performance.

One useful tip is to check the hemoglobin and serum iron. A small deficit may not present a problem at sea level, but can become significant at altitude.

ARE ALTITUDE TRAINING CAMPS WORTHWHILE?

Given the outstanding performance of some Kenyan competitors, there has been interest in the possibility that sea-level residents could improve their endurance performance by attending a mountain training camp. The concept has been to time the return to sea level so that the altitude polycythemia is conserved, but body buffers are restored to a sea-level figure.

There is some theoretic possibility of gain over the period 4 to 20 days after returning to sea level, but in practice this seems to be offset by the curtailment of training at altitude. Well-trained individuals may even show a decrease of both oxygen transport and endurance performance after return from altitude. Most teams have thus abandoned this practice, although there are still occasional attempts to generate a similar erythropoiesis at sea level, either by breathing low oxygen mixtures or by tube breathing (which also adds to body carbon dioxide stores).

PROBLEMS FROM AIR TRAVEL

Large commercial aircraft are pressurized so that even on long journeys the cabin altitude does not rise above 2500 meters. Since the passengers are sitting, this causes no more than a little tachycardia.

The only likely complication is a failure to equalize pressures in the ears during descent to sea level. If the athlete then goes on to subject the eardrum to more pressure by diving, rupture may occur. Problems are most likely if there is an upper respiratory infection or allergy. If the journey cannot be postponed, a decongestant should be administered before flying, and particular care should be taken to swallow regularly during descent of the aircraft. If collapse of the inner ear passage should persist for more than a few hours after landing, arrangements should be made to catheterize the internal meatus and equalize pressures across the tympanum.

A SAFE ALTITUDE CEILING

The main dangers of altitude are mountain sickness, pulmonary edema, and a sickle cell crisis. Middle-aged recreational athletes also become more vulnerable to myocardial infarction and cardiac arrest as oxygen pressures fall.

During moderate recreational activity, the threshold altitude for mountain sickness seems about 3000 meters. However, there have been concerns that the intensive training schedules of the international competitor might lower the threshold to perhaps 2000 meters. Diagnosis of acute mountain sickness is difficult, and complaints of headache, insomnia, and a variety of gastrointestinal disturbances can readily be confused with a minor infection or food poisoning. As already noted, the condition usually resolves with no more than symptomatic treatment over the course of 2 to 3 days.

More chronic forms of mountain sickness are well recognized in climbers, but are unlikely to develop at competitive altitudes. If symptoms persist, a more likely explanation is a compounding of the initial episode with an intercurrent gastrointestinal infection, irrational fears of altitude, discouragement from poor track times, or loss of condition due to the interruption of training.

The fluid disturbances of mountain sickness can occasionally develop to an acute pulmonary edema. This is typically seen 9 to 36 hours after reaching altitude. Predisposing factors include (1) previous altitude exposure, (2) a respiratory infection, and (3) overly vigorous training on first reaching altitude. Among recreational athletes, the threshold altitude seems about 2700 meters. The condition is thus encountered at quite a number of ski resorts. The patient presents with acute dyspnea, a blood-stained watery phlegm, chest discomfort, cough, nausea, and vomiting. There are the usual physical signs of an alveolar exudate and ECG evidence of right ventricular strain, while a chest radiograph shows intense pulmonary vascular congestion with diffuse pulmonary opacities. The condition is potentially fatal, but usually responds well to bed rest, oxygen, and broad-spectrum antibiotics.

Sickle cell disease is an abnormality of both hemoglobin and red cell structure encountered almost exclusively in negroid patients. As the abnormal hemoglobin molecules become deoxygenated by exercise at altitude, they clump together, and the affected cells assume an abnormal "sickle" shape which is readily hemolyzed. There is an associated splenomegaly, and there have been several reported incidents in which black athletes have suffered a splenic rupture at altitudes of 2500 to 3500 meters. As yet, there is no satisfactory prophylaxis, other than detecting vulnerable black competitors before a crisis occurs.

High altitude problems were remarkably few when the Olympic Games were held in Mexico City (1968). Nevertheless, the Scientific Commission of the Federation Internationale de Médecine Sportive approved a resolution in 1974 urging extreme caution at altitudes in excess of 7500 feet (2286 meters), with an absolute prohibition of contests above 10,000 feet (3048 meters).

HAZARDS OF DIVING

DONALD H. H. MACKENZIE, M.D., F.R.C.P.(C)

With over four million individuals participating in recreational diving in North America and with the continued growth of the sport, it is important for physicians of all specialties to be aware of the various aspects of diving medicine.

For this discussion we agree that recreational diving should be restricted to depths not exceeding 20 to 30 meters. However, the experience and condition of the diver and the environmental conditions (for example, limited access to the surface—ice, caves, or wrecks) may influence the divemaster to establish a much shallower limit.

While there are some fundamental differences between skin diving and scuba diving, which may therefore subject each group to different maladies, most of our remarks apply to conditions common to both groups as seen in the office or a walk-in clinic. The more serious conditions which lead to diving accidents and fatalities usually require specialized attention and the expert care of a hyperbaric team. Our experience has been obtained from an enthusiastic group of sport divers, enjoying the lakes and rivers of the North American continent for more than two decades.

Most diving maladies can be prevented by application of the principles that underlie sound diving, by good judgment on the part of the diver, and by relevant medical advice. As the quality of diving instruction improves, medical counseling will become more effective in the reduction of diver-related injuries.

PRE-DIVING SCREENING

The recognition of pre-existing conditions in the potential diver cannot be overstressed. All persons considering diving should have a complete physical examination, including a chest radiograph. Sport scuba divers constitute one of the most varied groups of individuals that a doctor is asked to examine. They may range from young children to senior citizens, with or without handicaps.

ABSOLUTE CONTRAINDICATIONS TO DIVING

There are eight contraindications to diving:

1. Spontaneous pneumothorax
2. Lung cysts, definite air-trapping lesions
3. Active asthma, pulmonary infections
4. Perforated tympanum, surgically placed struts
5. Epileptic seizures, syncopal attacks
6. Drug addiction
7. Brittle diabetes (persons subject to insulin shock)
8. Claustrophobia (severe)

RELATIVE CONTRAINDICATIONS TO DIVING

Even under optimal conditions, underwater diving requires a considerable energy expenditure. When the activity becomes complicated by such variables as the environment, physical limitations, or inexperience, additional effort is needed. Hence, participants with borderline medical conditions, are at a considerable disadvantage.

Decrease of pulmonary reserve from any cause is a relative contraindication, since the work of breathing increases as one descends in water, and the breathing mixture becomes more dense.

The question of diving during pregnancy still remains unanswered. The effects of pressure upon the mother and the fetus have not been clearly identified. However, many women, including well-known scientists, have continued to dive well into the third trimester without incident. In fact, many have reported improvement of the peripheral circulation and postural distress as a result of diving during the final trimester. Complicating factors of each pregnancy should be assessed individually.

Obesity may be a problem for the diver who approaches decompression limits, since a correlation has been observed between an increased incidence of decompression sickness and a body mass 20 percent greater than actuarial height and weight charts.

COMMON DIVING MALADIES

Otitis Externa (Swimmer's Ear)

Excessive exposure to water or contact with contaminated water often leads to infection and inflammation of the external auditory canal. When the canal is inadequately cleaned and dried, the residual moisture can cause maceration of the tissue (epithelial), with pH shifts toward the alkaline side, these changes making it relatively easy for bacteria to grow. Other contributing factors include collections of ceruminous debris, seborrheic dermatitis, auditory canal exostoses and local trauma. The symptoms of swimmer's ear are itching or pain, thin and serous discharge, and crusting or flaking of skin of the ear canal. The signs are acute inflammation and swelling of the ear canal, tissue flaking at the canal opening, and extreme tenderness.

Treatment

Treatment consists of relief of pain, irrigation and cleansing of the auditory canal, specific topical antibiotics, and restoration of normal pH.

The method of choice for cleansing is irrigation with a lukewarm water solution, followed by careful drying of the canal. If perforation is suspected, suction and cotton wipes should be used instead. Adequate amounts of specific agents (e.g., antibiotic drops) should be used 3 or 4 times daily. In the advanced stages, complete obstruction of the ear canal, erythema of the adjacent pinnae, and anterior cervical lymphadenitis may occur. When swelling within the canal prevents adequate instillation of specific agents, a saturated cotton wick should be inserted. All diving and swimming should be proscribed until the infection has cleared. With such simple measures as regular cerumen removal and diligent application of prophylactic topical ear solutions (e.g., modified Burow's solution [Domeboro Otic, Miles]), otitis externa can be avoided.

Aerotitis Media (Middle Ear Barotrauma)

The most common cause of middle ear barotrauma is inadequate pressure equalization between the middle ear and the external environment. This frequently occurs when a diver does not clear the ears or if local inflammation and swelling of the eustachian tube exists (due to allergy, chronic irritation from smoking, head colds, and prolonged use of ear drops). As middle ear pressure becomes more "negative" (100 to 500 mmHg), the tympanic membrane will rupture.

The symptoms of aerotitis media are ear pain during descent, sudden relief of pain if eardrum ruptures or middle ear pressure equalizes, conductive hearing loss, and vertigo upon rupture, due to an influx of water into the middle ear. The signs are edema and hemorrhage in the middle ear mucosa and tympanum, and inflammation and collection of serous fluid and blood.

Treatment

When there is no perforation, treatment consists of (1) cessation of diving until preexisting symptoms have abated, the diver can clear both ears at the surface, and all ear symptoms have subsided; (2) systemic decongestants (Drixoral or Sudafed, three times daily), and long-acting topical nasal decongestants (Otrivin nose drops); (3) systemic antibiotics (used prophylactically); and (4) ear cleansing with a warm solution of 1.5% hydrogen peroxide should be done if there are significant amounts of blood and other debris in the canal. With perforation, treatment consists of (1) referral to an otolaryngologist; and (2) cleansing with warm 1.5% solution of hydrogen peroxide and topical ear drops containing antibiotics and steroids (Cortisporin Otic).

Occasionally, signs of negative middle ear pressure take from 2 to 24 hours to develop. In such cases, gentle air insufflation may aid the examiner in detecting a retracted and rigid tympanum.

Nasal decongestant drops are more effective than nasal sprays, but should not be used for a period longer than five days. Antihistamines are not generally indicated unless pre-existing nasal allergies are suspected.

Divers with perforated drums should be referred immediately for specialized treatment. In the interval, blood and other debris should be carefully removed from the ear with 1.5% hydrogen peroxide solution warmed to body temperature. Topical ear drops containing antibiotics and steroids are used to prevent infection and decrease inflammation following each irrigation and are continued 3 to 4 times daily until the ear is clean and dry or the ear drum has completely healed. Systemic and topical nasal decongestants may be employed to advantage. Solutions containing alcohol or strong acids should be avoided. The prophylactic use of systemic antibiotics is controversial.

Inner Ear Barotrauma (Round Window Rupture)

Round window rupture can occur in two ways. As a consequence of unrelieved middle ear barotrauma, the increasingly negative pressure differential between the inner ear and the middle ear reaches a point where the round window ruptures with leakage of perilymph. With a blocked and locked eustachian tube, forceful Valsalva efforts may result in sudden unblockage, creating an explosive blast of air into the middle ear and dislodging the round window. The latter mechanism is more common among naive, untrained skin divers. Inner ear barotrauma is far less common than middle ear barotrauma, but it is potentially more serious because it can cause permanent deafness. The symptoms of inner ear barotrauma are pain, hearing loss, and tinnitus. The signs are free hemorrhage in the middle ear, redness, swelling, and perforation of the drum.

Treatment

Treatment consists of immediate referral to an otolaryngologist and bed rest with the upper body raised to 30 degrees.

Certain factors such as nasal obstruction, nasal polyps, nasal allergy or a history of recurrent ear infections predispose to inner ear barotrauma, but the majority of cases have no underlying head or neck pathology.

Neurosensory hearing loss confirms the diagnosis. Conservative management of bed rest, with the upper body raised 30 degrees is to be recommended, although many authorities advocate immediate surgical exploration. If the patient remains asymptomatic after 10 days, return to nonstrenuous activity is permitted, with follow-up audiograms at 6 weeks and 3 months. In the absence of rupture, inner ear hemorrhage or contusion of the round window may cause similar symptoms, but hearing returns to normal. Rupture of one of the inner ear membranes is felt to have occurred if the patient has a residual hearing loss, usually notched at a particular frequency.

Patients can resume diving after the follow-up period if hearing is normal over the speech range frequency and no fistula is present.

Paranasal Sinus Barotrauma (Sinus Squeeze)

As in external ear squeeze, adequate ventilation and pressure equalization of the paranasal sinuses depend to a large degree upon nasal function. Inflammation and congestion of the nasal mucosa as well as nasal structural deformities can result in blockage of the paranasal sinus ostia. Should blockage occur while diving, swelling, engorgement, and inflammation of the sinus mucosa and collections of a transudate and hemorrhage in the cavity may occur. The symptoms of paranasal sinus barotrauma are severe pain over the involved sinus or in the upper teeth, parasthesias over the infraorbital nerve distribution, epistaxis, and purulent nasal discharge. The signs are bloody mucous discharge and tenderness over the affected sinus.

Treatment

Treatment consists of topical and systemic vasoconstrictor agents and antibiotic therapy if infection is present. Most cases of sinus squeeze recover in 5 to 10 days without serious sequelae.

External Ear Barotrauma

External ear barotrauma results from blockage of the external ear canal during descent. This blockage creates a negative pressure relative to the ambient and middle ear pressures, with resulting inflammation of the canal and tympanic membrane. The symptoms of external ear barotrauma are fullness and pain in the ear upon descent. The signs are congestion and hemorrhage in the canal and tympanum.

The common causes of external auditory canal obstruction are cerumen and other foreign bodies, the use of mechanical ear plugs, and the use of tight-fitting diving hoods. Similar problems can develop across other membranes, causing regional symptoms. Examples of these would include suit and face-mask, teeth and gastrointestinal squeeze. Lung squeeze can only occur in breath-hold dives.

Treatment

Treatment is the same as for middle ear barotrauma.

Other Conditions

Other conditions associated with diving include decompression sickness and pulmonary over-inflation syndrome. Both conditions require immediate recompression, using hyperbaric facilities. Recompression schedules and treatment tables are beyond the scope of this article.

Prevention

Physiological insight can do much to reduce diver morbidity. Only proper training and an increased awareness on the part of the medical community will continue to promote safety within this high energy activity.

Little has been said regarding diver involvement as it relates to prevention of the more serious injuries. The following recommendations should be given consideration: (1) positive equalization beginning upon descent, to decrease the likelihood of middle ear barotrauma; (2) diving in groups or with a minimum of at least one other diver; (3) regular diving medicals to detect the onset of potential physiological limitations.

The able assistance and contribution of William A. M. Boersma is gratefully acknowledged.

AIR POLLUTION AND EXERCISE

LAWRENCE J. FOLINSBEE, Ph.D.

Much of our population is located in dense urban areas which serve not only as home, workplace, and recreation area, but also as the major source of raw materials which pollute our gaseous environment. Air pollution is certainly not a new problem or one that is likely to disappear in the near future. Notable efforts have been made in recent years to retard the further degradation of air resources and, in many cases, to improve air quality; these efforts must continue. The air pollutants that are common in our urban environments include carbon monoxide, oxides of sulfur and nitrogen, ozone, hydrocarbons, and a vast array of particulates and aerosols.

The air quality criteria documents assembled by the US Environmental Protection Agency devote entire volumes to the effects of each of the aforementioned pollutants. The present chapter will focus on the effects of a few pollutants which may affect the performance of athletes, both recreational and competitive. The pollutants of major concern are ozone, sulfur dioxide, and carbon monoxide. Each of these inhaled pollutants exerts its major influence on some aspect of the oxygen transport system which is of vital concern to exercising athletes. Ozone and sulfur dioxide are airway irritants and can impair ventilation; carbon monoxide's well-known effect is to impair oxygen transport by hemoglobin.

The effects of inhaled pollutants in general depend upon the dose delivered to the target organ which is, at least in part, a function of the pollutant concentration in the inspired air and the volume of air exchanged by the lungs of the individual exposed to the pollutant. Thus a simplified method of estimating the potential exposure dose is to calculate the product of concentration × ventilation × exposure duration. Several other factors in addition to concentration and exercise ventilation are important to consider when evaluating the potential effects of pollutants. These include age, sex, smoking habits, and the presence of various forms of cardiopulmonary disease. Other factors that may alter the effects of pollutants are the temperature and humidity of the ambient air and the route of inspiration (oral vs nasal).

OZONE

Ozone (triatomic oxygen) is formed by a complex atmospheric reaction involving oxygen, nitrogen oxides, hydrocarbons, and sunlight, and it is thus designated a photochemical oxidant. It is an extremely potent airway irritant and may cause cough, tracheal or pharyngeal irritation, and pain or discomfort upon deep inspiration. Symptoms may be evident in heavily exercising individuals at concentrations in the range of 0.12 to 0.20 ppm (parts per million) and higher. Levels such as these are common in certain parts of the Los Angeles basin during the summer months.

Ozone causes measurable effects on lung function tests at concentrations as low as 0.18 ppm in individuals who exercise heavily during exposure. The lung function changes include decreased maximal inspiration (decreased inspiratory capacity) and reduced maximal expiratory flow. There may also be a modest increase in airway resistance. The maximum expiratory flow can fall to as little as 50 percent of the pre-exposure baseline level in exercising individuals exposed to 0.35 ppm O_3 (or higher). In addition, the breathing pattern during ozone exposure changes to a more rapid and shallow pattern, which is the typical (and presumably protective) response to inhalation of irritant gases.

Following a 2-hour exposure to relatively high (0.75 ppm) levels of ozone combined with mild exercise, both maximal oxygen intake and maximal expiratory flow are reduced. Such severe exposure would probably never occur in the ambient environment. Nevertheless, there are two studies in which athletes have been exposed to ozone at more commonly experienced levels (0.20 ppm) while exercising at near-competitive intensities. Several of the athletes (approximately 50% in each study) felt that they would have been unable to perform maximally if exposed to 0.20 ppm (or higher levels) throughout an endurance competition of 30 minutes or longer. The feeling of inability to perform appears to be associated mainly with the airway irritation and pain or discomfort experienced when breathing deeply. The increases in airway resistance following ozone exposure are relatively trivial in comparison to changes in breathing apparatus resistance which are necessary to impair oxygen transport and decrease endurance time.

Individuals who reside in regions such as the Los Angeles Basin may become desensitized to the irritant effects of ozone after repeated exposures. In the laboratory, 3 to 5 consecutive days of 1- to 2-hour ozone exposures are needed in order to reduce or eliminate the associated symptoms and lung function changes. With less frequent repetition of exposure in the ambient environment, the desensitization process may take considerably longer and may not occur to the same extent as it does in the laboratory. The "adaptation" effect is transitory and disappears over 5 to 10 days if there is no intervening ozone exposure. If the desensitization is acquired through regular ambient exposure, it could be more persistent, although this has not been formally studied. Another important factor in acclimating to ozone is that episodes of pollution are typically accompanied by high ambient temperatures and thus competitors must be aware of the necessity for associated heat acclimation.

It has been postulated that individuals with asthma or chronic obstructive pulmonary disease may be at greater risk from ozone exposure. This is a difficult question to answer because of considerable variability among diseased individuals, but studies to date have not verified this hypothesis. Furthermore, atopic individuals do not display increased responsiveness to ozone. However, smokers and individuals older than 35 to 40 years are less sensitive to ozone than are young nonsmokers. There have also been suggestions that women are more sensitive to the effects of ozone, but the available evidence is, as yet, equivocal.

SULFUR DIOXIDE

Sulfur dioxide (SO_2), a colorless gas, is also an airway irritant. However, at the levels typical of the urban atmosphere, SO_2 has very little effect on the lung function of "normal" individuals. A matter of concern a number of years ago was that SO_2 would interact with ozone to form SO_3, the acid anhydride of sulfuric acid, thus exposing the lungs to an aerosol of sulfuric acid. It has since been demonstrated that the mixture has no greater effect on lung function than does ozone alone. Furthermore, sulfuric acid was shown to have less effect on lung function than a comparable quantity of ozone.

The major concern with SO_2 at present is that it is a potent bronchoconstrictor in asthmatics. Asthmatics exposed to as little as 0.50 ppm SO_2 during brief periods (10 min) of heavy exercise experience marked decreases of airway conductance. This problem is exacerbated if the SO_2 is breathed in cold and/or dry air, using a mouthpiece. Cold ($-20°C$) dry air is a known broncho-constrictor in asthmatics, but the combined effects of SO_2 and cold dry air are considerably greater than the sum of the effects of each condition alone. During the less vigorous exercise of ambient exposures, the inspired air would be more likely to be inhaled via the nasal airway. In addition to its normal function of warming and humidifying the inspired air, the nasal mucosa serves as an SO_2 scrubber and thus the impact of ambient SO_2 is reduced. Interestingly, when SO_2 is present with respirable particulate matter (as it often is), the gas has greater effects in moist atmospheres. The mechanism for this effect is not clear, but it may be due in part to the adsorption of SO_2 on the moist particulate surface, enabling it to be carried to the lung periphery rather than being removed by the mucosal surfaces of the upper airways. Asthmatics who exercise outdoors in regions where SO_2 or SO_2 plus particulate pollution is prevalent should perhaps consider some prophylactic measures. Sulfur dioxide-induced bronchoconstriction can be prevented in asthmatics by the prior administration of disodium cromoglycate. The bronchoconstriction is relatively short-lasting in any event, and it is typically reversed in a few minutes without administration of bronchodilators.

Fortunately, the response to SO_2 is blunted with repeated exposure. Asthmatic patients who experience several episodes of exposure within the same day appear to develop a tolerance to the bronchoconstricting effect of the pollutant. However, this tolerance is lost by the following day.

CARBON MONOXIDE

It is well known that excessive levels of this colorless and odorless gas can be lethal. Its effects on exercise performance are less well publicized. CO reduces the ability of the hemoglobin molecule to transport oxygen by forming carboxyhemoglobin (HbCO) and causing a leftward shift of the HbO_2 dissociation curve, which restricts the unloading of oxygen at the tissue level. CO also has a strong affinity for myoglobin and the cytochromes and thus may interfere with the intracellular transport of oxygen.

An increased level of carboxyhemoglobin (>5%) in nonsmokers has been associated with a reduction both in aerobic power and in the ability to sustain heavy sub-maximal exercise. The performance of athletes may be impaired if they are required to perform prolonged exercise in atmospheres containing upward of 25 to 50 ppm CO, levels that are often reached on city streets. As with other pollutants, the magnitude of the effect of CO breathing on the level of HbCO depends upon the duration of exposure and ventilation during exposure. Furthermore, since CO is not cleared rapidly from the blood (the half time for elimination is 2–4 hr), an exposure that occurs some time prior to competition (for example, travel on congested roadways) could influence subsequent athletic endeavors. Passive smoking may also cause elevation of blood HbCO levels by 1 to 2 percent.

There is potential for an interaction between altitude and carbon monoxide exposure, since both result in hypoxemia. This could be important not only for those engaging in competition at altitude, but also for hikers and mountaineers who cook, and thus generate CO, within the confines of their tents. It has been estimated that a 3 percent increase in carboxyhemoglobin level has the same effect as a 300-meter increase in altitude.

Carbon monoxide exposure has the potential to interfere not only with maximal performance but also with more passive events that require attention and/or decision making. A number of studies suggest a deterioration in various psychomotor, behavioral, or attention-related tasks when the carboxyhemoglobin levels increase above 5 to 8 percent.

The major group at risk from carbon monoxide exposure includes patients with cardiovascular disorders such as angina pectoris or intermittent claudication. Modest elevation of HbCO (2 to 5%) in either of these patient populations is associated with impaired exercise tolerance, decreased time (i.e., exercise duration) to the onset of angina, or decreased time to the onset of ischemic leg pain. Thus individuals with ischemic cardiovascular disease should avoid carbon monoxide exposure prior to or during exercise.

COMMENT

True tests of performance are rarely achieved in the laboratory setting, and thus we must be content with various indices or models of performance. Athletes have not been exposed to measured quantities of pollutants prior to an actual performance in order to test the pollutant's effect. Since performance can only be approxi-mated in the laboratory, the true effects of these pollutants on athletes may be either over- or under-estimated by extrapolating from the laboratory data.

TIME-ZONE SHIFTS AND INTERNATIONAL COMPETITION

WOP J. RIETVELD, M.D., Ph.D.

BIOLOGICAL RHYTHMS

Cyclic physiologic rhythmicity is a fundamental property of living matter, from single cells to a complex organism such as a human patient. Periodic changes in shape and rate synchronize structure and function with periodic fluctuations in the external environment, thus facilitating integration of the individual's internal milieu.

Under constant environmental conditions, notably constant illumination, humans exhibit free-running rhythms within a period deviating somewhat from 24 hours. Free-running rhythmicity implies that an intrinsic physiologic mechanism is capable of generating self-sustained oscillations. The term circadian is restricted to those approximately 24-hour rhythms whose cyclicity persists under constant conditions.

Under experimental conditions, if light-dark cycles have a period sufficiently close to 24 hours, a person's circadian rhythms establish a constant phase relationship with the environmental regimen (for instance, a consistent one-hour lag). This results in normal entrainment when body rhythms stabilize at a period equal to that of the external synchronizing signal.

Pacemaker and entrainment mechanisms are often distinguished. The pacemaker comprises all physiologic processes essential for generating self-sustained circadian oscillations, while the entrainment mechanism is made up of an appropriate photoreceptor system and any necessary additional sensory processes.

The situation is more complex in human than in lower organisms. Experiments suggest a considerable number of hierarchically organized and possibly mutually interacting circadian oscillators. A more or less central pacemaker directly or indirectly drives other endogeneous oscillators at a lower level of the circadian organization. Hormonal and neural signals are thought to mediate the temporal coordination of rhythms during normal entrainment by controlling the phase of the rhythm in each oscillator.

The light-dark cycle is the predominant synchronizer (Zeitgeber) for most mammals. However, it is controversial whether blindness disrupts human circadian rhythms; possibly, social cues are sufficient to synchronize circadian rhythms and indeed are even more powerful than visual stimuli.

Certainly human circadian systems can be entrained by a number of Zeitgebers in addition to the light-dark cycle alone. Besides social cues, these include meal-times, work schedules and rest schedules, temperature fluctuations, and even the use of drugs (chronobiotics).

IMPORTANCE TO ATHLETIC PERFORMANCE AND SPORTS MEDICINE

Sport performance depends upon a complex interaction of physiologic and psychologic functions, including perceptual, motor, and cognitive capacities. Investigations of performance fluctuations are beset by a number of specific problems; particularly, apparent changes or fluctuations of performance may reflect fluctuations in motivation rather than a change of efficiency. A vast amount of data indicates circadian rhythms of cardiovascular and respiratory functions, and of psychomotor performance. In general, maximum values are reached during daytime hours.

Systolic and diastolic blood pressures reach maximum values about 12 hours after the mid-point of sleep. Pulse rate, stroke volume, the QRS interval of the electrocardiogram, and regional blood flow follow a similar course. Changes of body posture are not responsible, since similar rhythms are seen in patients confined to bed and taking their meals at regular 4-hour intervals. There is a close phase relationship with the sleep-wakefulness cycle, which allows the mid-point of sleep to be used as a reference point. It remains a matter of dispute whether cardiovascular rhythms have a truly endogenous component or are the result of exogenous factors like the rhythm of body temperature.

Circadian rhythms of respiration (changes of airway dimensions, respiratory frequency, and oxygen consumption) also have a time course corresponding with fluctuations of body temperature, showing minimum values in the early morning (around 6AM) and a maximum in the afternoon (around 6PM).

Circadian rhythms of psychomotor performance (like grip strength, card sorting, or mirror drawing) again present maximum and minimum values corresponding with peaks and troughs of body temperature. However, other rhythms like subjective alertness reach a maximum in the early morning hours.

Maximum oxygen intake attains significantly higher values in the daytime than at nighttime, with maximum values at about 10AM. Maximum oxygen intake coincides with the highest maximum heart rate, but the lowest heart rate occurs a bit earlier than the lowest $\dot{V}O_2$max (at about 2AM). Measurements of PWC_{170} demonstrate a mirror image of the variations in maximum oxygen intake.

Athletic performance is generally better in the afternoon (for example, running, swimming, and rowing), although in some subjects better performance is obtained in the morning hours, corresponding with the time of maximum subjective alertness. The effectiveness of training apparently depends on the timing of training sessions. Subjects trained on a treadmill for 4 weeks at different times of day (6AM to 8PM) showed a higher final PWC when trained in the late afternoon (around 5PM). The poorest response was obtained after training at 9AM.

Circadian rhythms can also affect the interpretation of clinical tests. For example, patients with Prinzmetal's angina do not suffer from cardiac pain if their physical endurance capacity is tested between 3PM and 4PM, but pain is seen with a comparable test if it is administered between 5AM and 8AM.

THE PROBLEM OF TIME-ZONE SHIFTS

Long-distance travel is commonly associated with considerable change in personal environment: shifts in local time when crossing longitudes, altered climatic conditions, and changes of season when the travel has been transequatorial. These changes occur very rapidly with modern air travel, causing special problems for both athletes and team officials. Shifts in the rest-activity cycle arise from unfavorable flight schedules and major shifts in environmental time cues after the rapid crossing of multiple time zones.

The first set of problems are similar to those encountered in shift work. The consequences, labeled "jet lag" or "transmeridian desynchronism," reflect the inability of the circadian system to adapt rapidly to the sudden shift of external synchronizers. This causes a transitory desynchronization between the body and its environment. Disturbances arise in cells and in tissues, as well as in complex behavior, in body temperature and in hormone levels, in digestion and physical fitness, in attention, in visual acuity, and in memory. The athlete's time sense becomes completely disorganized.

MECHANISMS OF RESYNCHRONIZATION

Under "normal" conditions, environmental synchronization of circadian rhythms occurs largely in response to social cues. Since all components of the temporal environment, social as well as physical synchronizers, are shifted at once, transmeridian flights favor a more rapid re-entrainment of biological rhythms than does night or shift work, where environmental and social synchronizers diverge. Nevertheless, it takes days or even weeks before the biological timing system is completely readjusted to the new environment.

The rate of resynchronization is affected by several factors, including flight direction, type of physiologic function, characteristics of time cues, and individual differences. Re-entrainment of rhythms in body temperature and psychomotor performance is faster after westbound flights and does not depend on relative direction (out- or homegoing) nor on the time of the flight (day/night flight). After a westbound flight, the shift rate of body temperature is about 60 minutes per day, whereas after an eastbound flight it is about 40 minutes per day. However, other rhythms readjust at different speeds. After a westbound flight, the shift rate for urinary noradrenaline is about 180 minutes per day, while that for psychomotor performance is 50 minutes per day. These differences in rate of adjustment lead to a transitorily abnormal phase relationship between the various body systems, a state of "internal dissociation". The relative rate of reentrainment may further be influenced by personality factors like introversion/extroversion and morning types versus evening types. Studies of shift workers have shown that evening types adapt more easily to night shifts. Older people also have greater difficulty in adapting to changes in body time.

IMPACT UPON COMPETITION AND TRAINING

The problem of jet lag is unavoidable when international contests are played all over the world. Competitors must fly from one event to another, often with a very tight time schedule. The impact upon sport performance of internal dissociation after jet lag has been beautifully documented by Sasaki. In a series of volleyball matches between Japan and the USSR, the desynchronized Soviet players lost all their games during the first few days after arrival in Japan. Thereafter, resynchronization started and was achieved in about 10 days. This was reflected in the scores. During the process of resynchronization, there were several draws. When the Soviets were fully resynchronized, they won all remaining games against the Japanese.

Some sports physicians advise athletes that are exposed to such a quick phase shift to avoid hard training for the first 3 or 4 days after arrival at their destination. During readjustment, light training may begin, but real matches or races should still be avoided. Maximum performance cannot be expected until full resynchronization has been achieved.

PRACTICAL RECOMMENDATIONS

There are a number of simple, practical ways to attenuate the effect of jet lag, for example:

1. Staying for a considerable time at the same or a neighboring time zone as the final destination.

2. Living on the local time of the destination for a considerable period before departure from the home country. This apparently easy remedy very often fails to achieve satisfactory results, as it is difficult to avoid conflicting synchronizers. The social life of the environment persists according to the home country time schedule. The situation is thus very close to that encountered by a shift worker.

3. Staying for a considerable period of time at the destination, while deliberately trying to increase the number of Zeitgebers as well as the strength of the signals.

Much of the available research has been conducted on airplane crews. Those that take part in the social life of their destination resynchronize considerably faster than those who stay in their hotel rooms. Besides light-dark alternation, social synchronizers, and the activity-rest cycle, meal timing is also a powerful entrainment signal. Indeed, in animals the availability of food can override the light-dark signal; thus nocturnal animals become diurnal if food is made available only during a few daytime hours.

Besides the timing of meals, the composition of the diet is also of major importance. Methyl-xanthines such as caffeine and theophylline (coffee and tea) shift the rhythm in a direction that is determined by the moment they are given, while high-protein and high-carbohydrate meals can activate catecholamine and indolamine metabolism. Linking these principles to careful timing of meals, Ehret has designed various diet plans for trans-atlantic flights, taking into account the times of departure and arrival as well as the flight direction.

ROLE OF THE BIOMECHANIST IN SPORTS MEDICINE

MICHAEL R. PIERRYNOWSKI, B.Sc., M.Sc., Ph.D.

Biomechanists investigate the external and internal forces which impinge upon or are generated by living structures. The external forces include gravity, fluid resistance, inertia, and forces that act on the body from animate or inanimate objects. The internal forces, generated by the muscles, are transmitted through tendons, ligaments, and bones to interact with the external environment to produce motion. To quantify these forces, biomechanists use the laws of theoretical mechanics and the mathematics of control theory and signal processing, applying these to the physiology, anatomy, neurophysiology, and anthropometry of biologic bodies.

The basic and applied nature of biomechanics research encompasses human movement problems in medicine, sport, and industry. To define the role of the biomechanist in sports medicine: he or she examines the sportsperson's activity and estimates the magnitude, direction, and duration of the forces acting on or within the biologic structures with the hope of detecting potential problems in terms of injury recognition and prevention.

In this paper, the role of the biomechanist in the sports medicine team will be addressed. Since the biomechanist is primarily concerned with the measurement of force, the significance of force in the cause of injury and how biomechanists measure these forces will be outlined. In conclusion, I shall discuss the specific information that the biomechanist can provide sport therapists, at present and in the future.

WHY SPORT INJURIES OCCUR

Both weekend sports enthusiasts and elite athletes can place extreme demands on their respective biologic systems, and damage often compels them to seek professional advice. What they almost invariably hear is that the muscle, bone, or tendon damage is primarily the result of two factors: (1) overuse and/or (2) an inherent structural fault. These are usually related, in that overuse tends to damage the weakest component in the structural chain.

Overuse syndromes are due to high-force loading plus a weak biologic structure. Cures do not necessitate decreasing the training or giving symptomatic relief (i.e., physiotherapy for muscle pain, drugs for tendinitis, fixation for stress fractures), but rather, effort must be directed to finding and correcting structural weaknesses. Otherwise, the athlete will experience a recurrence of symptoms when competition is resumed.

In sports situations, there is a considerable potential for the forces encountered by the human body to exceed the structural capacity of the tissues concerned. The reaction of the body depends to a large extent on the location of the applied force. An incomplete listing of sport injuries (muscle strain, contusion; ligament stress, rupture; bone fracture, dislocation; skin laceration; head concussion, contusion) shows the diverse consequences of a single mechanical impulse.

Injury because of impact to the body is of concern to athletes, coaches, parents, owners, and eventually sport medicine therapists who must correct the resultant damage. Many injuries could be avoided if inter-athlete contact was eliminated, the all-out nature of athletic competition was minimized, and athletes were well prepared and competently coached. Such a desirable situation is unfortunately unlikely, given the human competitive instinct and the risks individuals are willing to take in sport. Professionals such as sport biomechanists must therefore quantify the magnitude and the location of the forces encountered, offering informed suggestions on how to reduce the number of potentially injurious situations.

HOW FORCES ARE MEASURED

The direct measurement of force is of interest to biomechanists. In sports activities, the force that the athlete exerts against the physical environment (ground, water, air), equipment (balls, rackets, paddles) or opponent can often be measured by means of a force transducer, together with suitable electronic recording apparatus. Since it is often possible to measure the force exerted by the athlete on his or her equipment, Newton's Third Law reminds us that the equipment is also applying an equal and opposite force to the athlete. The magnitude and duration of these forces can be examined, especially in impact situations, and indeed such information has been used in the design of protective equipment to attenuate risk in potentially hazardous situations.

To estimate the forces acting within biologic structures, the athlete is modeled mathematically. The body is defined as a continuously changing configuration of interconnected masses; the connections are the joints and the links the main segments of the body. If reasonably accurate values can be assigned to the inertial properties (mass, moment of inertia) of individual segments, and if the spatial displacements of these segments are known as a function of time, kinetic or force-motion analyses can be performed. An important body of theory in mechanics is built on Newton's Second Law, which states that the force acting on an object causes it to accelerate in proportion to its mass. By combining kinematic data about a segmental model with a knowledge of the associated external forces acting on that model, the forces causing motion can be calculated. To estimate intrasegmental forces, each segment is separated from the others, and the muscle, ligament, and bone geometry in the vicinity of the joints is modeled. Such joint representation requires considerable simplification to solve for the unknown forces in the model. Recently, however, techniques based on neurophysiology and muscle physiology have allowed biomechanists to estimate individual muscle and ligament force-time profiles in the lower extremity.

The importance of individual muscle, ligament, and bone studies to an understanding of the causes of sports injuries is obvious, since invariably it is high magnitude forces within individual structures that cause injury. A considerable amount of data is presently available regarding the response of bone, ligament, tendon, and skin to applied forces. Knowledge of the mechanical properties of these tissues has practical importance when designing protective equipment to decrease local forces below damage thresholds.

WHAT BIOMECHANISTS CANNOT DO

The majority of biomechanical techniques developed to aid in the diagnosis and evaluation of clinical problems have yet to receive clinical acceptance. At present, biomechanical evaluations cannot diagnose between different injuries, and most of the available evaluation tools fail to meet several basic criteria. As indicated in a letter to the Journal of Biomechanics (Brand, RA, Crowninshield, RD, 1981; 14:655) a biomechanical test gains widespread clinical acceptance only if (1) it indicates the patient's functional capacity relative to his or her normal state, (2) it gives information to the physician or therapist that is not directly observable or obvious, and (3) the results are reported within the context of a physical or a physiologic model. This last criterion was expounded by A. Cappozzo in the Journal of Biomechanics (16:302, 1983); he expressed a concern that although biomechanics had advanced to the point where instrumentation was reliable and acceptable in clinical situations, conceptual models explaining why certain movements occur and specific injuries develop were still lacking. Biomechanics must evolve beyond the stage of merely gathering descriptive data; investigators must initiate a process whereby the relevant questions are asked and addressed. Only then will useful tools be available for the understanding and treatment of sports injuries.

IS THERE A ROLE?

In this paper the thesis was developed that forces of excessive magnitude caused most sport injuries. Sport biomechanists have a role in estimating the magnitude of these forces and their potential to cause injurious effects. However, biomechanists have yet to make any major contributions to the direct treatment of athletic injuries. At present, they should be seen as a support group who carry out research on the limits of athletic performance defining boundaries, which, if exceeded, cause injury. Suggestions pertaining to the design of protective equipment are offered and assistance is given in the formulation of regulations to make sport safer and more enjoyable for all participants. Moreover, such input from the sport biomechanist makes a worthwhile contribution to the prevention of sports injuries.

MEDICAL ASPECTS OF SPORTS

EXERCISE IN THE CLINICAL MANAGEMENT OF OBESITY

KELLY D. BROWNELL, Ph.D.
JORDAN W. SMOLLER, A.B.

We begin this chapter with two points. The first is that exercise can play a major role in the prevention and treatment of obesity. The second is that many obese persons do not enjoy exercise, are not good at athletic activities, and rarely continue an exercise program that they begin. Most obese persons agree with the professionals who tell them that exercise is beneficial, so the problem is more motivational than educational.

The issue of physical activity in obese persons is a major public health concern. Obesity is an important problem of modern society because of its seriousness, prevalence, and resistance to treatment. Obesity is associated with many serious medical, psychologic, and social consequences. A surprisingly high percentage of the population are at risk, somewhere between 15 and 25 percent of all adults being obese. What discourages most professionals is that the problem is so difficult to remedy. The most heroic efforts with patients yield only temporary results, and this when patients are fortunate enough to seek treatment, remain in treatment, and lose weight initially.

To strike a more optimistic note, there are promising new approaches on the scene. One recent trend is to emphasize physical activity, and as a result, its full benefits are becoming more widely known. Because attention from some researchers has been turning to the motivational factors involved in exercise adherence, there is more encouraging news to offer than ever before.

IS OBESITY A DISEASE OF INACTIVITY?

This was a question posed recently by J.S. Stern. It is important because inactivity could be either the cause or the consequence of obesity. The common belief is that obese people eat excessively, so that in the public view, physical inactivity is seldom implicated in the etiology of obesity. In contrast, some researchers have found that obese persons eat no more than peers of normal body mass*, but that they are less physically active. This controversy deserves attention, because the relative contribution of intake and expenditure in human obesity could dictate the emphasis of programs for prevention or treatment.

Studies by J. Mayer and colleagues, as early as the 1950s, first demonstrated an association between obesity and physical inactivity. For example, one study examined adolescent girls in a summer camp. Even when obese and girls of normal mass were engaged in the same type of activity, the obese girls were less active. During swimming, the obese girls floated more and swam less, and in sports like tennis, the obese girls stood more and ran less. Shortly after, studies by Mayer and others began showing no differences of food intake between obese and persons of normal body mass.

More recent studies have revealed a complex relationship between physical activity and obesity. The early studies had used self-report measures of both intake and activity. In a recent study using observational measures, food intake distinguished obese from nonobese boys, but activity did not. The literature is consistent in showing that obese adults are less active than adults of normal body mass, but the same does not appear to be true for children. This could be interpreted to show that inactivity is the consequence of excess body mass, but it is equally tempting to favor a causal theory. This issue will not be resolved soon, and so the conservative approach is to assume that exercise is important for obese persons and to emphasize it in any "weight-control" program.

BENEFITS OF EXERCISE FOR THE OBESE PERSON

Physical activity carries special benefits for the obese person. These extend far beyond the caloric expense of the exercise. Conveying this information to obese persons can increase motivation because most believe that the only reason to exercise is to "burn calories". They discover that a modest meal at a fast food restaurant can bring 5000 kJ (1200 Calories) or more, and that a great deal of exercise (e.g., 20 km of running) is necessary to expend this energy. With our patients, we recast exercise to emphasize its long-term metabolic effects rather than short-term energy expense.

In addition to energy expenditure, exercise may influence appetite, metabolic rate, nearly all the ill effects of obesity, and the preservation of lean body mass.

---

*In keeping with modern usage, the term weight has been changed to mass by the editor, with the understanding that a distinction be made between total body mass and lean mass. Mass is popularly described as weight.

Research with animals has shown that modest amounts of activity in sedentary animals can suppress appetite, although the effect varies depending on the sex of the animal and the type of activity that is undertaken. A consistent finding in both animals and humans is that basal metabolic rate declines during loss of body mass. There is some evidence that exercise may help to offset this decline. Exercise can also counteract the negative psychologic and physiologic effects of obesity (e.g., negative self-concept, diabetes, hypertension).

One of the most important benefits of physical activity may be the preservation of lean body mass. During energy restriction and loss of body mass, most people lose some lean tissue. The loss can be very large in some persons on some diets. Moreover, the loss of lean tissue is less when diet and exercise are combined than when diet alone is used.

This effect may be particularly important if body mass is regained. If the rate of increase in mass exceeds the body's ability to replace the lean tissue, increased body fat will be the consequence. As an example, a 70 kg woman may reduce to 60 kg by losing 7 kg of fat and 3 kg of lean tissue. If she returns to a mass of 70 kg, she may replace only 1 of the 3 kg of lean tissue, he remainder being added as fat. Although her mass is the same before and after this cycle, body composition has changed adversely.

The value of exercise may depend in part on whether a person's obesity is hyperplastic (excessive fat cell number) or hypertrophic (excessive cell size). Björntorp notes that fat cell number sets an upper limit for loss of body mass. Since exercise can only shrink fat cells but never eradicate them, the potential for body fat loss is greater for hypertrophic obesity. Moderately obese patients with enlarged fat cells may lose up to 20 kg with physical training, but large losses of body mass are rare in severely obese hypercellular persons.

Epidemiologic evidence underlines the utility of exercise for hypertrophic obesity. The metabolic complications of obesity (e.g., decreased glucose tolerance and hyperinsulinemia) are related to fat cell size. Exercise can alleviate these complications in many cases, thus altering several of the risk factors for cardiovascular disease. From a strictly physiologic perspective, patients with hypertrophic obesity may achieve particular benefits from exercise.

THE PROBLEM OF NONCOMPLIANCE

Most obese persons know that exercise is good for them; this notion is reinforced by health professionals and by the media. However, few obese people translate this knowledge into action. It is widely agreed among professionals that encouraging overweight persons to exercise is a major challenge. There are both physical and psychological obstacles for most patients.

Physical Barriers. The physical barriers to exercise increase with the severity of the obesity. Björntorp has reviewed several common clinical observations which corroborate this point. Severely obese patients are often plagued by locomotor diseases which make physical activity difficult to initiate or sustain. In addition, commonly observed cardiovascular and respiratory problems may present significant risks, particularly with more strenuous forms of activity. Some types of exercise pose particular problems for the obese; jogging, for example, may produce orthopedic complications by placing an extreme load on the joints and back.

The diminished heat tolerance of many obese patients is another physiologic factor which may discourage exercise. Relative to lean persons, obese individuals produce more heat during exercise and dissipate heat at a slower rate. Since the rate of heat loss decreases as the ratio of body surface area to body mass decreases, the threat of heat strain may be considerable in cases of extreme obesity. Adherence to an exercise program may be a real struggle for the patient who faces a combination of physical discomfort and a slow loss of body mass.

Psychological Barriers. The psychologic obstacles to exercise may be even more forbidding than the physical barriers. Many overweight persons have unpleasant associations with exercise. In some, this stems from childhood experiences where they were teased, selected last for teams, and discouraged from athletic activities. These impressions can be sufficiently indelible to make it difficult for some obese persons to consider joining an exercise program. Overweight adults are often self-conscious when jogging, swimming, playing tennis, and so forth. These barriers must be overcome before any significant amount of exercise is likely.

AN EXERCISE PROGRAM FOR OBESE PERSONS

Prescribing an exercise program for the obese person requires sensitivity to the physical and psychological obstacles imposed by excess body mass, and to the behavioral principles involved in encouraging changes of lifestyle. Eating and exercise habits can be firmly ingrained and can be incorporated into a person's very identity. However, these habits were learned and new habits can be learned to replace them.

In the remaining pages of this chapter, we will present the physical activity program that we prescribe for obese patients (Fig. 1). The individual application of this program requires clinical judgment, which comes from experience with patients. Their psychological state must be considered, as must their physical capacity for work. With these factors in mind, we begin with a focus on attitudes about exercise and then progress through the behavioral principles used to encourage exercise adherence.

Attitudinal Factors. One consequence of the increased popularity of exercise is that the general public has much more information about factors like the "training effect". The notion conveyed most often is that exercise must be done in large amounts in order to be beneficial. Specifically, people learn that frequency, intensity, and duration are the key factors. This—combined with the age-old philosophy that "the more it hurts, the more it helps"—has several negative effects on obese persons.

TYPE OF EXERCISE

Reduction of Body Mass

Total energy expended is primary concern. Activity may facilitate reduction of mass through direct energy expenditure, a decrease in appetite, and an increase in basal metabolism. Changes in body composition are important to consider as well as changes in body mass.

Routine Activity

1. Maximize daily walking (park some distance from destination, get on and off bus at early stop, complete errands on foot, etc.)
2. Increase use of stairs in lieu of elevators and escalators.
3. Emphasize that daily activities *are* exercise and that the cumulative effects of modest increases can be useful.

Programmed Activity

1. Movement of total body mass is best (jogging, walking, cycling, swimming, rope-jumping, and so forth).
2. Program should involve 3 to 5 sessions per week, at least 15 minutes for each session.

Cardiovascular Fitness

Improved cardiovascular fitness depends on intensity, frequency, and duration of training sessions. If exercise is sufficient to improve cardiovascular fitness, body mass and body composition will likely improve.

1. Aerobic exercises are necessary (running, brisk walking, rope jumping, cycling).
2. Intensity must be no less than 70 percent of maximum heart rate. Maximum heart rate (in beats per minute) = 220 − age.
3. Duration must not be below 15 minutes each session (or 30 minutes for walking). Benefits increase in proportion to duration, up to maximum of 45 minutes.
4. Frequency must not be below 2 days per week. Benefits increase in proportion to frequency.
5. Warm-up and cool-down periods are necessary to ensure safe cardiac response.

ADHERENCE

Poor adherence results from insufficient positive consequences (the positive consequences of exercise are remote, the negative consequences are immediate). Adherence can be improved by making physical activity more immediately rewarding. Social influence and behavioral interventions are helpful. Some persons need the structure of programmed exercise, but these regimens may lead to poor long-term adherence. Routine activity is feasible for most persons, and can be used as a precursor to more strenuous exercises. For a more detailed discussion of adherence, see the contribution of Neil Adridge, above.

Social Influence Factors

Naturally occurring social factors can improve adherence. Support from family, friends, or peers can be instrumental in making physical activity more rewarding. The nature of this social involvement is important; support persons should be active participants rather than benevolent spectators.

Spouse and Family Support

1. Emphasize importance of activity to spouse and family.
2. Describe energy equivalents of exercise as well as the distinction between routine and programmed activity.
3. Develop activities that patient and family do together.
4. Have spouse or family follow the patient's monitoring records.

Friends and Peers

1. Encourage activity with friends or other patients (buddy system).
2. Group exercise may be better than individual activity.
3. Patients can contract with others to increase activity.

Behavioral Interventions

1. Deposit/refund can improve adherence: can reward attendance in program or frequency of specific activities.
2. An exercise contract with specific terms may increase activity.
3. Self-monitoring and graphing of daily activities, energy expenditure, and body mass provide reference points for self-evaluation.
4. Feedback of physical changes is motivating. Consider resting heart rate, blood pressure, body fat, and cardiovascular endurance.

Figure 1 An exercise program for the obese person. (Adapted from Brownell KD, Stunkard AJ: Physical activity in the development and control of obesity. *In* Stunkard AJ (Ed): Obesity. Philadelphia: Saunders, 1980.

When an overweight person is motivated to exercise but learns that the training heart rate must be at 70 percent of maximum or greater, that the exercise must be taken three times per week, and that each bout must include at least 15 minutes in the target heart rate zone, the outcome is predictable. He or she is so far from attaining this goal that the exercise seems hardly worth the effort. The equation evokes images of highly trained athletes, so that feelings of inadequacy are difficult to overcome.

We present this issue to patients in order to challenge the idea of an exercise threshold. The idea that exercise must hurt, that the exerciser must perspire, or that the quantifiable conditions mentioned above must be met assumes that a person must do "enough" exercise to accrue benefits. This is absolutely counterproductive for a person at the beginning of an exercise program. Therefore, we emphasize a broad range of physical activities to replace sedentary habits. For instance, a woman might walk for 10 minutes after dinner. Instead of judging this against the standard necessary for a training effect, she is asked to compare this activity to the probable behavior that it replaces. If the option were to be supine while watching television, the walk is a positive substitute. Our philosophy is that any activity is better than no activity, and that overweight persons are saddled with the notion of an exercise threshold.

Our approach is consistent with the behavioral principle of shaping (to be discussed). Everyone must begin somewhere, even if rigorous activity is the ultimate goal. The first priority in an exercise program must be adherence, and adherence is most likely if the individual feels that exercise is enjoyable and can be beneficial even at low levels. Irrespective of the physical benefits of this low-level activity, which may not be demonstrable, the psychological benefits can be substantial. These are the benefits we seek in the early stages of a program. Exercise can be quite helpful for an overweight person even if the preferred levels of frequency, intensity, and duration are never reached.

Behavioral Principles. There are a number of principles from behavioral psychology that are relevant to exercise programs for obese patients. These include shaping, self-monitoring, feedback, and reinforcement.

The principle of shaping is to make small approximations toward a distant goal. For a person in poor physical condition, the distant goal may be regular and vigorous exercise, but small approximations toward that goal might be gradual increments in a daily walking program. Patients are instructed to focus on such intermediate steps in order to avoid the discouragement of missing a more distant goal. This relates back to the concept of the exercise threshold (discussed above). Shaping promotes the notion that *any* increase in activity is positive because it represents progress.

The first step in shaping is to establish a baseline of the individual's physical activity. For most persons, activity may consist of no more than movement in the home or occasional journeys for shopping. The first prescribed activity would thus be something the person can accomplish without pain, breathlessness, and the other factors that make activity unpleasant. It might involve 5 minutes of walking after the evening meal or in the morning. Once this has been accomplished in a comfortable fashion, minutes can be added to the total until the person is ready to progress to another form of activity. The shaping principle dictates that movement to any level of activity occurs only when the previous level has been mastered.

The second, and one of the most important behavioral principles is that of self-monitoring. This refers to the act of keeping a written record of one's behavior. In our programs, we require patients to keep "diaries" of their eating and physical activity habits. The

activity record has each person tally any but the most routine activity, including using stairs, working in the yard, and household chores. In addition to listing the behavior, the person records its duration, the time of day, location, and degree of enjoyment.

The self-monitoring record has several virtues. The first is that it provides the health professional with a base rate of activity for the individual, which is necessary for prescribing a program of gradual increases. Second, it yields valuable information on the situational determinants of activity or inactivity. Combined with records of eating, the activity records can suggest specific approaches to changing life style. If the records show that an individual consumes most of the day's food energy between dinner and bedtime and that this is a period of low activity, then scheduling several small exercise breaks during these hours could interrupt the habit of overeating. Finally, self-monitoring often serves as a cue for behavior change; the simple act of recording activity often leads to an increase in activity. It is essential that the professional check these records and acknowledge the patient's efforts.

The third behavioral principle related to activity is that of feedback. One drawback to exercise for most obese persons is that the only immediate effects are negative; the exercise is painful, time-consuming, and boring, and the loss of body mass is generally slow. Providing positive feedback is important to the success of an exercise program. This can come from an exercise chart on which the person plots the number of minutes each day devoted to exercise. The chart can be placed in a prominent location in the home, so the patient and the family can observe the gradual increases.

Feedback can also be provided by the health professional. As the level of activity increases, decreases in resting heart rate, girth measurements, and blood pressure can be pointed out to patients. Any positive information the professional can provide increases the likelihood of adherence.

The final behavioral principle related to exercise is reinforcement. Since exercise is not inherently reinforcing for obese persons, at least in the early stages of conditioning, external reinforcement must be provided to avoid the usual course of discouragement and dropout. One way to accomplish this is to enlist the aid of persons in the patient's social environment to support the activity (see Fig. 1). Another tactic is to have the patient establish a self-administered "contract" in which he or she earns special rewards (e.g., movies, clothes) for making specified changes in activity.

A powerful application of reinforcement principles is found in the deposit-refund procedure. Patients are required to deposit a sum of money prior to entering a program, and the money is returned either in a lump sum or in installments if the person satisfies the stated requirements. These might include attendance at sessions with the professional, meeting daily exercise goals, or losing a certain body mass. The deposit-refund system has greatly reduced attrition from weight loss programs. The presence or absence of the deposit seems more important than the amount, for it has symbolic value. This system will deter persons who are not motivated from joining a program, but it can help keep others in a program during periods of slow weight loss.

Life Style Versus Programmed Activity. We believe that it is important to expand our patients' concept of exercise beyond traditional activities such as jogging, swimming, calisthenics, and organized sports. These "programmed" activities are valuable, but can be combined with "life style" activities incorporated into the daily routine. Life style activities include walking and using stairs in lieu of elevators and escalators. Engaging in such activities serves as a reminder that positive changes are being made.

There are many clever ways to increase life style activity. One of our patients lived in a house with bathrooms on the first and second floors. She vowed always to use the bathroom on the other floor, so that she increased her use of the stairs. We encourage patients to disembark from a bus one stop early (to increase their walking), to use a restroom or water cooler further away than the one used typically, to stand rather than to sit, and to use stairs whenever possible. L. H. Epstein and colleagues obtained very favorable results from life style activity in obese children when it was compared with the more traditional programmed activities.

ROLE OF THE PHYSICIAN IN DOPING CONTROL

LAWRENCE A. GOLDING, Ph.D.

Physicians who are treating athletes and/or serving as team physicians are being asked questions about drugs. In order to understand doping control programs, the sports physician needs to review a history of drug use by athletes and the rationale for their usage. In addition, he should be aware of current rules, regulations, detection methods, and penalties involved in drug use.

This chapter will review the extensiveness of the drug use problem by athletes; explain the International Olympic Committee's (IOC) stand on drug use, including the present list of banned drugs and new drug-detection methods; and briefly review three major problem drugs that are widely used.

THE PROBLEM

Drug use is a major issue in the world of athletic competition. The development of sophisticated testing methods has identified a widespread usage of drugs. Intensified media coverage of major athletic events, such as the Olympic Games and the Pan American Games, has focused public attention on the problem.

The use of drugs to enhance physical performance can be traced for hundreds of years, but drug use by athletes in modern times has accelerated dramatically with the development of new drugs. During the past 25 years, its escalation has caused athletic governing bodies to formulate regulations prohibiting drug use.

The conception among athletes, coaches, and trainers is that when an athlete breaks a record or performs extraordinarily well, it is due to some magical potion

rather than to the main ingredients of championship performance: inherited characteristics, training, hard work, mental attitude, and numerous other qualities. The athlete has historically searched for the "magic ingredient" which would allow maximum performance. It is the task and the responsibility of the coach, trainer, and physician to educate the athlete in the physiology of performance and to negate the use of drugs in an attempt to gain a winning edge. The problem of drug use is even sadder when it occurs unknowingly or innocently, as in the case of the athlete who had to forfeit his gold medal at a recent Olympic Games because he was taking a prescribed drug that was on the IOC's list of banned substances.

THE OLYMPIC POSTURE

The official posture of the International Olympic Committee is that doping is prohibited. The IOC has stated that: "Doping is defined as the administration or use of substances in any form alien to the body or of physiological substances in abnormal amounts and with abnormal methods by healthy persons with the exclusive aim of attaining an artificial and unfair increase in performance in competition. Furthermore, various psychological measures to increase performance in sports must be regarded as "doping".

The official posture of the U.S. Olympic Committee and committees from other countries is the censure of drug use by their athletes. The spirit of sportsmanship, hard training, and fair play, which is the philosophic basis of all sporting groups and the foundation of the Olympic spirit, negates drug use.

During the past several years, the rules, regulations, and penalties for drug use have undergone several changes and revisions as new research has been completed and better and more reliable drug detection methods have been developed. Today, there is a well-defined, powerful, and effective drug control program in

TABLE 1   Official 1984 IOC Banned Substances

A. *Psychomotor stimulant drugs*
  amphetamine
  benzphetamine
  chlorphentermine
  cocaine
  diethylpropion
  dimethylamphetamine
  ethylamphetamine
  fencamfamin
  meclofenoxate
  methylamphetamine
  methylphenidate
  norpseudoephedrine
  pemoline (phenylisohydantoin)
  phendimetrazine
  phenmetrazine
  phentermine
  pipradol
  prolintane and related compounds

B. *Sympathomimetic Amines*
  chlorprenaline
  ephedrine
  etafedreine
  isoetharine
  isoprenaline (isoproterenol)
  methoxyphenamine
  methylephedrine and related compounds

C. *Miscellaneous Central Nervous System Stimulants*
  amiphenazole
  bemegride (methetharimide)
  caffeine*
  cropropamide**
  crolethamide**
  doxapram
  ethamivan
  leptazol
  nikethamide
  picrotoxine
  strychnine and related compounds

D. *Narcotic Analgesics*
  anileridine
  codeine
  dextromoramide
  dihydrocodeine
  dipipanone
  ethylmorphine
  heroin
  hydrocodone
  hydromorphone (dihydromorphinone)
  levorphanol
  methadone
  morphine
  oxycodone
  oxymorphone
  pentazocine
  pethidine
  phenazocine
  piminodine
  thebacon
  trimeperidine and related compounds

E. *Anabolic steroids*
  clostebol
  dehydrochlormethyltestosterone
  fluoxymesterone
  mesterolone
  methenolone
  methandienone (methandrostenolone) (Dianabol)
  methyltestosterone
  nandrolone decanoate (Deca-Durabolin)
  norethandrolone
  oxymesterone (Oranabol)
  oxymetholone
  stanozolol
  testosterone† and related compounds

* If the concentration in urine exceeds 15 μg/ml
**Components of Micoren
† If ratio of total concentration of testosterone to epi–testosterone in the urine exceeds 6.

effect, and the ban on drug use and the penalities invoked have caused a marked decrease in drug use by athletes. Officials believe that the drug control program, with its education, drug testing, and penalties, will eventually eliminate their use altogether. Dr. Kenneth Clark, Director of the Sports Medicine Division of the U.S. Olympic Committee, has said that it is no longer a matter of whether or not certain drugs work, but rather that their usage will disqualify the athlete.

Any drug on the official Olympic list of banned substances will cause the athlete to be disqualified and forfeit any medals won, and the athlete may be banned from future amateur competition. If the disqualified athlete is a participant in a team sport, the entire team may be disqualified. Even legitimate drugs prescribed by a physician for a pathologic condition, if they are on the list of banned drugs, cannot be used without penalty. In extreme instances, petitions can be made by the physician for the use of a banned drug; however, the petition must be accompanied by a history of the condition and a history of the drugs used, including dosage and frequency. The list of banned substances is constantly changing. The official 1984 IOC list of banned substances is shown in Table 1. The drugs in each major category are examples only, and do not necessarily comprise the entire list.

Many of the sympathomimetic drugs with ephedrines are found in nonprescription medicines used for upper respiratory tract infections and include common patent medicines such as: Sudafed, Nyquil, Sinutab, Allerest, Dristan, Coricidin, Contac, A.R.M., and CoTylenol.

The United States Olympic Committee has a telephone hotline which is available for physicians to call for information on particular substances or procedures.

The United States Olympic Committee Drug Control Program is equivalent to the International Olympic Committee's Doping Control Program and is "…compliant with the human rights and chain of custody expectations." The service provided by the USOC Drug Program to the national sports governing bodies is to enable urine collection at athletic events and give laboratory analyses for substances banned by the International Olympic Committee. The USOC Drug Control Program also provides educational and research information on drug use.

DRUGS AND ERGOGENIC AIDS

The use of drugs by athletes falls into two categories: street drugs and ergogenic aids.

Street Drugs. Street drugs are used by people from all segments of society to achieve some kind of emotional or physical "high". The use of drugs by athletes is in proportion to the use of drugs by the community as a whole. Because of the high visibility of athletic events, drug use by an athlete is highly publicized. Some of the more common street drugs are cocaine, marijuana, and Quaalude.

Ergogenic Aids. Ergogenic aids include a large group of substances, techniques, and applications which are commonly used by athletes in an attempt to improve performance, and which are of little concern to athletic governing bodies. Many exercise physiology textbooks discuss, in depth, the various ergogenic aids. The better known of these include bee pollen, gelatin, mineral and vitamin supplementation, protein, amino acids, wheat germ oil, yeast, alfalfa, and kelp. Other ergogenic aids that are not ingested include electric stimulation, hypnosis, massage, negatively ionized air, oxygen, and ultraviolet rays.

Almost any substance that may affect the cardiorespiratory system, serve as a fuel, combat fatigue, or act upon the muscle has been tried as an ergogenic aid. There is a serious question in most researchers' minds as to whether any of these substances improves athletic performance. Although some aids have a physiologic basis for their possible effectiveness, most studies prove that performance does not increase with their use. For example, muscle biopsy studies have shown that the muscle fiber can be supersaturated with glycogen through glycogen packing or carbohydrate loading; however, whether or not this procedure makes the difference between winning and losing is questionable. The use of *drugs* and *chemicals* as ergogenic aids is prohibited by athletic governing bodies because of possible unfair competitive advantage and the endangerment of the athlete's health.

Ergogenic drugs are used by athletes with the intent to improve performance during competition and/or to hasten recovery. Almost every drug that has been used medically to treat a pathologic condition of any organ involved in physical performance has been tried as an ergogenic aid. Typical examples are digitalis, nitroglycerine, sulfa drugs, and coramine. In addition, substances such as epinephrine, growth hormones, testosterone, and norepinephrine, which prepare the body for activity or development, have been used as ergogenic aids. The drugs that are the current focus of athletic governing bodies are the stimulants, anabolic steroids, testosterone, narcotics, pain killers, and decongestants.

DRUG TESTING

The equipment and tests involved in detecting drug use by athletes is extremely sophisticated. Urine is tested by a combination of a gas chromatograph and a mass spectrometer. Steroids, previously difficult to detect, can be isolated months after cessation of steroid-taking. How long the drug can be detected depends on the particular steroid; the dosage; whether it was taken orally or injected; whether it has an oil base; the clearance rate; and the individual's metabolic rate, size, and percent body fat. A false-positive test result is impossible, since the actual molecules of the substances are detected and measured. Some attempts have been made by athletes to use a diuretic to dilute the urine or to use sodium bicarbonate to mask the drug use. Current tests usually still detect the substance but if the pH of the urine is too alkaline or too dilute, the athlete is detained until urine of normal acidity and concentration is passed. Paraphrasing from the material provided by the USOC Sports Medicine Division, the procedure for testing is as follows:

1. When an athlete provides urine, he/she will select the container and two bottles as well as select a code number from a list.

2. The athlete pours the urine from the container into the two bottles and observes the code number application.

3. Both bottles are secured (cap and wax seal) and sent to the laboratory in a secured shipping case for analysis as Specimen A and Specimen B.

4. Specimen A is analyzed; if "positive", it is reanalyzed and confirmed.

5. If the occasion for drug testing stipulated punitive action for users, the athlete is given the opportunity to be present when Specimen B is analyzed for reconfirmation.

6. Because USOC's doping control program cannot use laboratories on the testing site as is done at the Olympics and Pan Am Games, USOC will provide a surrogate athlete representation system that the athlete can utilize if personal presence is not easily possible.

MAJOR OFFENDERS

Amphetamine. This psychostimulant is known to excite the central nervous system and has been used by athletes as an antifatigue drug, especially by those in prolonged endurance events, such as road cycle races and marathon runs. The use of amphetamine in medical practice has diminished owing to the undesirable side effects, the tendency to abuse, and the development of alternative drugs. Numerous well-controlled studies have shown that amphetamines did not improve performance, nor did they enhance performance in a fatigued athlete. One poorly controlled study on amphetamine and performance was published 15 years ago in a professional journal. This study showed improvement in performance due to amphetamine. It provided much misinformation about the ergogenic effect of the drug and has been widely criticized.

Because of its effect on the central nervous system, amphetamine is often used as an appetite appeaser or as a mood elevator. The drug has been used by athletes to get "up" for an event or performance. Since athletes need rest and sleep, this is a dangerous practice, as a depressant drug (barbiturate) is often needed to induce sleep. This cyclic pattern creates habituation. The only possible benefit of amphetamine use would be improvement of sustained attention; however, this is counterproductive. The athlete may be masking extreme fatigue, which can cause hallucinations and confusion. Although amphetamine is widely used by athletes, it serves no clinical or ethical purpose. Any use of this drug is cause for disqualification from amateur competition. The athlete who uses amphetamine must take the drug while performing; it is unlikely that he or she will use it now that it is easily and readily detected in the urine.

Anabolic Steroids and Related Drugs. Several studies have indicated that almost all champion weight-oriented athletes have taken or are taking anabolic steroids. Many books, articles, and stories have been devoted to the pros and cons of steroid use. Some studies have suggested that they produce gains of body mass, strength, and muscle bulk. An equal number of well-controlled studies have shown that these variables do not change. Weight athletes believe that steroids are effective, and popular literature contains abundant testimonial and empirical articles extolling their use.

Controlled, legitimate studies are difficult to conduct, owing to the mandate of Human Experimentation Review Boards to avoid potential contraindications and dangers of the steroids. Even well-controlled studies have been limited in dosage to two or three times the normal therapeutic dose, whereas in reality athletes may take ten to twenty times the therapeutic dosage.

There are two kinds of steroids: oral (e.g., Ethylestrenol, Stanozolol, and Methandrostenolone) and injectable (e.g., Nandrolone phenpropionate, Testosterone enanthate, aqueous testosterone, testosterone propionate, and testosterone cypionate). These are synthetic testosterone-type substances which have both an androgenic (male-producing) quality and an anabolic (building) quality. Athletes use steroids to increase their strength, size, and body mass. Several studies in the cattle industry have found that steers who were fed steroids while waiting to go to market increased in mass. Steroids have also been used in geriatric cases after debilitating illness to help patients regain their former health. This information has caused some athletes to extrapolate these findings into benefits for themselves. Considerable disagreement exists as to whether the gain of mass is due to fat or water retention as opposed to an increase of lean body mass.

There has been considerable speculation on the use of steroids by East German female swimmers. There is little doubt that females taking either anabolic steroids or testosterone will develop male secondary sex characteristics, but whether the desired increase in strength will result remains to be determined. No study on an anabolic steroid use by females will ever be done in the United States, since no responsible Human Experimentation Review Board would ever approve a study that could cause possible detrimental effects to the subjects concerned.

There is little scientific evidence that anabolic steroids aid in strength acquisition, lean body mass gain, or increased bulk, whether or not the doping is accompanied by a high protein diet. Many researchers believe that there is no difference between a placebo and the steroids in effecting strength gains.

Besides the threat to the health of the athlete, an ethical problem exists. The physician is prescribing a medication for which there is no medical need. The administration of hormones stops the body's normal production of these compounds. The risks from anabolic steroid use are insidious and require long-term study. It is now known that these drugs can impair liver function, increase blood pressure, lower sperm count, and are potentially carcinogenic for both liver and prostate. Women and young athletes have additional problems with accelerated maturity and premature closure of bone epiphyses.

Growth Hormone. As of this publication date, human growth hormone is not on the Olympic list of banned substances, because there is no way to detect its use. When a reliable test is developed, human growth hormone will be added to the banned list. Growth hormone is produced by the anterior pituitary gland and has been supposedly used by weight athletes to increase strength and muscle size. No research studies have appeared in the literature, although several athletes have claimed large gains of strength and body mass. The side effects of growth hormone are potentially more serious and extensive than the anabolic steroids. Growth hormone is a powerful anabolic agent.

ROLE OF THE PHYSICIAN

There has been a lack of interest on the part of some physicians, trainers, and coaches to take an active role in educating athletes about drug use. There are physicians, trainers, and coaches who condone drug use by competitors; some have even suggested to athletes that drugs will help their performance. There is considerable evidence to indicate that many of the banned drugs used by athletes have been prescribed or supplied by physicians. Physicians also prescribe drugs for athletes indicating a certain dosage; however, the athlete often triples or quadruples the dosage. There is a need to monitor athletic drug usage and to be aware of the contraindications and possible side effects of such usage.

Drug use by athletes is prohibited. Physicians, trainers, coaches, and sport organizers should attempt to counsel and educate athletes away from reliance on pharmaceuticals to enhance physical performance.

Athletes may take drugs because of peer pressure. Stories stating that without drugs, championship form or performance is impossible are widespread among competitors. Such attitudes and beliefs can be changed by physicians, trainers, and coaches if a concerted effort is made. Medical ethics must lead this reform. Again, it must be stated and remembered that the issue is not whether or not pharmaceuticals work, but that they are illegal and contrary to sport ethics; those taking such drugs are not allowed to compete.

ANABOLIC STEROIDS AND HEALTH

DONALD W. KILLINGER, M.D., Ph.D., F.R.C.P.(C)

The use of anabolic steroids to enhance athletic performance began in the mid 1950s. Since that time, athletes have been progressively impressed by the beneficial effects of these agents as world records improve and the male and female athletes who are successful in international competition frequently appear to have excessive muscular development. During the same period the medical community has attempted to deter the use of anabolic steroids by athletes, focusing on the potential hazards of these agents to their health. It is apparent that the health threats have been insufficient to deter athletes who have spent many years of rigorous training and who are seeking any added advantage that would make them successful in international competition. The availability of testing procedures starting in the mid 1970s and their added sophistication in the early 1980s has created an atmosphere in which athletes are afraid to forego the use of these drugs and miss qualifying for international competition, but they are also uncertain of the sophistication of the testing procedures. There is no doubt that there will be attempts made to develop anabolic agents that are not detected by current means.

It is estimated that virtually one hundred percent of the competitors in weight lifting at international competitions are either taking anabolic agents or have experimented with their use. The testing at international events in 1983 would tend to support this opinion. While the prevalence may be greatest in weight lifting, it is probable that anabolic steroids are used by the majority of competitors in events such as shot-put, discus, and other events in which strength and body mass are a predominant factor. Since there is little evidence to suggest that these agents increase maximum oxygen intake, there is no advantage to their use in events in which endurance is a major factor. However, there has been some use by sprinters to obtain a maximum effort over a short time period.

While attention has focused primarily on international olympic sports, the use of anabolic agents has also permeated professional sports where strength and weight are an asset. The use of anabolic steroids is high among professional football players and wrestlers, and it is probable that players in most sports, including basketball and hockey, have experimented with the use of these agents. Perhaps the most overt use of anabolic steroids occurs in body building, where a variety of steroid hormones including anabolic steroids and glucocorticoids are used to produce a maximum visual effect.

EFFECTS ON PERFORMANCE

The differences of opinion regarding the effects of anabolic steroids on athletic performance seem irreconcilable. The athletes are convinced that these agents produce beneficial effects, and doses from 5 to 20 times the usual prescribed limits are commonly used in the belief that they will achieve these goals. Medical scientists and physiologists involved in studies of athletes using anabolic steroids are much less enthusiastic. Of the reports available in the literature, approximately half claim some beneficial effect on muscular strength during the use of anabolic steroids, but the remaining studies have been unable to demonstrate any benefit. Many of these reports have been uncontrolled, and only four studies were double-blind. Virtually all studies suffered from one or more deficiencies including: the small number of cases tested, variations in diet, problems with cross-over design, the uneven athletic experience of the subjects tested, difficulties in measuring performance under different training conditions, and perhaps most difficult of all, the variable psychologic motivation of the subjects involved. The dosage of anabolic steroids used in virtually all of the reported studies was in the range suggested by the manufacturer and therefore much less than the range taken by the athletes on their own initiative. None of the studies reported have involved female athletes. It is unlikely that any attempt to initiate studies exposing highly motivated athletes to the doses of anabolic steroids reportedly taken by athletes would pass a human experimentation committee. It is therefore unlikely that this controversy will ever be scientifically resolved. The studies in which the most convincing evidence of body mass gain and increased strength have been reported have involved the use of high-protein diets and protein supplements along with weight training.

TYPES OF ANABOLIC STEROIDS USED

There are many preparations of anabolic steroids available, all of which are derivatives of the testosterone molecule. All agents that are orally active have either a methyl or an ethyl grouping at the 17 position. The most commonly used oral agents include methandrostenolone (Danabol, Dianabol), androstanole (Winstrol), and norethandrolone (Nilevar). All of these oral agents have some degree of hepatotoxicity, and this toxicity tends to be dose-related. The injectable forms of anabolic steroids, such as nandrolone decanoate, do not show hepatotoxicity, and for this reason parenteral forms of anabolic steroids are preferable.

Some of the side effects occurring with anabolic steroids are unique to the oral preparations and some are potential problems with all preparations. The androgenic:anabolic ratio differs somewhat between the various anabolic preparations, but all have some androgenic effects. For this reason these agents can produce masculinization in females, with hirsutism and changes in body habitus. Menstrual irregularities or amenorrhea can occur and this may be due in part to the progestational effects of some of these preparations. If administered prior to puberty, there can be acceleration in the closure of the epiphyses, with ultimate short stature. When administered to adult males even at the doses recommended by the manufacturer, all of these compounds are capable of producing a decrease in plasma testosterone and a suppression of pituitary gonadotropins. Several studies have demonstrated diminished sperm production during anabolic steroid administration. In a study using methandrostenolone at a dosage of 10 mg daily, plasma testosterone concentrations fell to levels well below the lower limit of normal by the second week of administration. Gonadotropin levels were also suppressed. Studies of the binding of testosterone to testosterone-binding globulin indicated that the anabolic steroid competed with testosterone for the binding protein, so that the amount of unbound testosterone in the serum would be much greater than expected from the determined level of total testosterone. It would appear, therefore, that the fall of plasma testosterone during the use of anabolic steroids is related both to pituitary suppression and to displacement of testosterone from the circulating binding protein. Studies of sperm counts on men taking anabolic steroids have generally indicated values below the lower limit of normal, and azospermia has been documented in some subjects. There is no evidence that testosterone production is permanently affected; after a 6-week course of anabolic steroids, sperm production and testosterone levels are back to normal within 8 weeks.

The oral agents have a relatively high degree of hepatotoxicity which increases with increasing dosage. The most common problem is a cholestatic type of jaundice; this tends to be reversible on discontinuation of treatment. Hepatocellular carcinoma following the use of anabolic steroids was first reported in 1965. There have been 12 additional cases reported since that time. Peliosis hepatis, the formation of vascular abnormalities in the liver, has been reported in over forty patients taking anabolic steroids, and this complication can be fatal. Reports of leukemia and Wilms' tumor are sporadic, and the relationship with anabolic steroids is not supported by convincing evidence.

Attempts have been made to relate these agents with atherosclerosis and hypertension, but the evidence for such an association is relatively poor. There has been some evidence of insulin resistance associated with the use of anabolic steroids, but the prevalence of this complication does not appear to be high. The problem of psychologic dependency, however, is significant, and may have a major influence upon the athletic performance of habitual users.

In general it is suggested that anabolic agents should be given in courses of 8 to 12 weeks, with at least a 12-week period between courses. The side effects on this regimen are thought to be less than those seen in individuals on continuous therapy, but the evidence for this is not compelling.

Anabolic steroids can have a striking effect upon female athletes. Androgenization resulting in hirsutism, increased muscle bulk, and deepening of the voice are relatively common, particularly when large doses have been used. Amenorrhea generally occurs during the period of steroid administration, but this appears to be reversible. It is not known whether long-term reproductive capacity is impaired by using these agents. Some of the physical features such as hirsutism disappear on discontinuance of the steroid preparation, but structural changes such as deepening of the voice are irreversible.

TESTING PROCEDURES

The ability to detect anabolic steroids and their metabolites in body fluids has been improving rapidly. Because blood sampling is considered inappropriate under the circumstances of athletic competition, testing has taken place exclusively on urine samples. Various claims have been made as to how long steroids remain detectable following cessation of administration, but there is no published information regarding such details. The current screening technique is extremely costly and time-consuming, but the effectiveness of these measures has been demonstrated in recent international competitions. Since the burden of proof resides with the testing committee, the specific metabolites of the anabolic steroid must be identified before proof of steroid intake can be substantiated. There is a very elaborate system of obtaining urine samples and labeling specimens appropriately so that there can be no doubt as to their identity. Half of the samples are preserved, so that retesting can be carried out in the event of a positive result. Samples are screened by means of radioimmunoassays. In general, two antibodies are used, one of which will recognize steroids containing a 17α-methyl grouping and a second which will detect compounds related to norethandrolone. These two antibodies will detect most of the anabolic steroids currently in use, although they do not identify the specific metabolite. Samples found to be positive on radioimmunoassay are therefore subjected to identification, using gas-liquid chromatography followed by mass spectroscopy. These procedures are capable of identifying specific chemical groupings. In order to make an absolute identification, standards are required; for this reason, the testing committee must have available to it all possible metabolites of anabolic steroids, so that appropriate standards can be incorporated into their tests. Maintaining the stock of reference compounds will undoubtedly continue to be a problem as chemical changes are made in the steroid molecule in an attempt to avoid detection.

In general, oral agents are cleared from the system more rapidly than the intramuscular preparations (which have been designed to have prolonged effect). It seems likely, therefore, that long-acting preparations could be detectable for several months after the final injection. Whether or not there are residues of these compounds within the tissues which are released over longer periods of time is nevertheless uncertain at present.

If a positive test is obtained, a repeat determination is carried out on the reserved sample with a representative of the athlete present during the entire assay procedure.

In an attempt to avoid detection while using

anabolic steroids, male athletes have given themselves synthetic testosterone; this cannot be differentiated from the endogenous product. Since exogenous testosterone tends to suppress pituitary gonadotropins, the ratio of LH to testosterone has been studied in an attempt to detect individuals who are injecting testosterone. This type of procedure is probably not of adequate sensitivity or specificity to make an unquestioned identification of exogenous testosterone administration.

The controversy as to whether anabolic steroids are capable of enhancing athletic performance beyond the levels which could have been achieved by intensive training has not yet been resolved. The athletes are convinced that the argument is academic and they point to continuing improvements of internationsl performance which they feel could only have been achieved through use of such preparations. It is evident that the attempts to dissuade athletes from using anabolic steroids because of potential health hazards have been ineffective. Moreover, the health hazards from injectable compounds are not of major significance if the medication is given appropriately. The issue is primarily a moral one, similar to that encountered with other drugs such as amphetamines, and it is only with the use of satisfactory detection techniques that the abuse of these agents will be controlled.

BETA-ADRENOCEPTOR BLOCKADE AND EXERCISE

FRANS T. J. VERSTAPPEN, M.D., Ph.D.
MARLEEN A. van BAAK, Ph.D.

Physical exercise elicits adaptations in various body functions to meet the increased metabolic rate. Autoregulatory processes, the autonomic nervous system, and the endocrine system are all involved in these adaptations. Sympathetic nervous system activity is increased during exercise, which leads to an increased release of noradrenaline and adrenaline from the sympathetic nerve endings and the adrenal medulla, respectively. Part of the effects of the increased catecholamine release is mediated via beta-adrenoceptors, which are present in various tissues and organs. Blockade of those receptors by administration of beta-adrenoceptor blocking agents thus switches off one route of regulation during exercise. However, in the interpretation of the effects of beta-blockade during exercise, it is important to keep in mind that several other regulatory mechanisms function normally and compensatory mechanisms may be activated.

BETA-ADRENOCEPTOR-MEDIATED FUNCTIONS

Beta-adrenoreceptors are involved in (1) regulating the contraction of vascular and bronchial smooth muscle cells and of heart muscle, and (2) energy substrate regulation. Concerning the role of beta-adrenoreceptors in adapting body functions to exercise we will focus on the heart, blood vessels, bronchi, liver, skeletal muscle, and adipose tissue. Beta-adrenoreceptors can be subdivided into beta-1 and beta-2 receptors. Beta-1 receptors are sensitive to both noradrenaline and adrenaline, whereas beta-2 receptors are mainly sensitive to adrenaline. Although one beta-adrenoreceptor subtype usually predominates in a given tissue, both subtypes are often found and mediate the same function. In the heart, beta-1 receptor stimulation elicits an increase of heart rate and contractile force. In the blood vessels, beta-2 receptors are found mainly in the arteries of skeletal muscle. Stimulation of these receptors causes vasodilation. Stimulation of beta-2 receptors in the bronchi also has a dilating effect. In adipose tissue, beta-1 receptors are found which, if stimulated, increase lipolysis and the release of free fatty acids (FFA) into the blood. Beta-2 receptors are involved in carbohydrate metabolism: specifically, glycogenolysis in liver and skeletal muscle is increased after beta receptor stimulation.

BETA-BLOCKADE AND EXERCISE IN HEALTHY SUBJECTS

The effects of beta-blockade during exercise depend on the type of exercise that is being performed. Below the aerobic-anaerobic transition, which occurs between 50 and 80 percent maximum oxygen intake ($\dot{V}o_2max$), depending on constitution and training status, exercise is hardly fatiguing and can be maintained for several hours. Above the so-called anaerobic threshold, endurance depends on the intensity of effort and training status. At $\dot{V}o_2max$, endurance is between 5 and 10 min, whereas higher "supramaximal" exercise can only be sustained for times varying from a couple of minutes to a few seconds.

Effects During Maximal Aerobic Exercise

Beta-blockade reduces $\dot{V}o_2max$. We found that the $\dot{V}o_2max$ of healthy subjects was reduced by 7 percent (range 0 to 20%) after a 4-week chronic treatment with a therapeutic dose of metoprolol 100 mg b.i.d. Exercise tests were performed 2 hours after the last dose, at peak plasma levels of the drug. The reduction of maximum heart rate (HRmax) was 27 percent (range 17 to 42%). Moreover, the reduction of $\dot{V}o_2max$ was correlated with the reduction of HRmax, indicating that the reduction of $\dot{V}o_2max$ is dose-dependent. Blockade by beta-1 selective blockers has a slightly less negative effect on $\dot{V}o_2max$ at the same HRmax reduction when compared with blockade by nonselective (beta-1+2) agents. The reduction of HRmax had to exceed a certain level (15 to 20%) before $\dot{V}o_2max$ began to fall. This suggests that, despite a heart rate reduction of approximately 30 beats/min, oxygen uptake by the exercising muscles is unaffected. Under normal physiologic conditions, the oxygen extraction from the blood is 85 to 90 percent at a maximal exertion, and blood flow is directed maximally to the exercising muscles; oxygen extraction thus cannot be increased. This implies that an increase of stroke volume has compensated for the reduction of HRmax, as indeed has been found in a number of studies. One possible mechanism for the increased stroke volume may be a reduced afterloading of the heart, since exercise blood pressure is reduced by beta-blockade. The increase in stroke volume is limited; thus cardiac output falls at higher degrees of beta-blockade, impairing oxygen supply to the working muscles. Ventilation during exercise is not impaired by beta-blockade in normal subjects, although asthmatic attacks may be elicited or aggravated in susceptible subjects.

Lactate acidosis within the active muscle fibers, secondary to the inadequate oxygen supply, interferes with the energy-liberating processes and/or the contractile mechanism itself, thus limiting muscle strength and continuation of the exercise. If the reduction of $\dot{V}o_2max$ after beta-blockade is due only to a decreased cardiac output, and thus reduced oxygen supply to the exercising muscles, one would anticipate a similar blood lactate concentration during maximal exercise with and without beta-blockade. However, in most studies, lower blood lactate concentrations have been found after beta-blockade. Since we found this after both beta-1 and beta-1+2 blockade, the cause does not appear to be a reduced muscle lactate production due to inhibition of beta-2 receptor-mediated glycogenolysis. Depletion of muscle or liver glycogen stores is also unlikely because of the short duration of $\dot{V}o_2max$ tests. Another possibility is that muscle lactate production is normal, but that the release of lactate from the muscles into the blood is reduced and/or lactate removal from the blood is increased. It is unlikely that the antilipolytic effect of beta-blockade interferes with maximal aerobic exercise, since free fatty acids are not an important energy source in high intensity, short duration exercise. Our conclusion is, therefore, that $\dot{V}o_2max$ is reduced after beta-blockade because of an impaired oxygen supply to the exercising muscles as a consequence of the reduction of cardiac output.

Effects During Submaximal Endurance Exercise

Endurance of submaximal exercise intensities above 50 percent $\dot{V}o_2max$ is also reduced after beta-blockade. Beta-1 selective blockers have a less negative effect than nonselective blockers. The impairment of submaximal endurance is not due to a reduced oxygen supply to the exercising muscles, since oxygen uptake is unaffected after beta-blockade. At low degrees of beta blockade, the reduction of exercise heart rate is completely compensated by an increase of stroke volume. At higher degrees of beta-blockade, cardiac output is reduced, but the oxygen supply to the exercising muscles can still be maintained by a redistribution of cardiac output and/or an increased oxygen extraction from the blood. Evidence for both adaptive mechanisms has been found.

During submaximal endurance exercise, the availability of energy substrates has decisive importance for endurance performance. The mobilization of free fatty acids from adipose tissue is regulated by beta-1 receptors, and after beta-blockade reduced blood levels of both FFA and glycerol have been found. We found that glycerol levels were reduced more after nonselective than after beta-1 selective blockade, which suggests that beta-2 receptors are also involved in lipolysis. Since the uptake of FFA by the exercising muscles depends on the arterial blood concentration, FFA supply is reduced. This situation is aggravated if muscle blood flow is reduced. The impaired availability of FFA leads to increased carbohydrate metabolism. Glycogen stores in muscle and liver are thus depleted faster, resulting in a shorter endurance.

Thus, beta-blockade leads to a reduction of submaximal endurance at intensities above the anaerobic threshold, because FFA availability is reduced and carbohydrate stores are depleted. Even symptoms of hypoglycemia may develop.

Most studies on the effects of beta-blockade during exercise have been performed after a single oral dose of a beta-blocker. Hemodynamic and metabolic effects during a progressive maximal exercise test do not differ between an acute intravenous dose of metoprolol and a 4-week chronic oral treatment. Thus no adaptations occur over this time period. In some but not all studies, people with a high proportion of slow-twitch fibers appear to be more susceptible to the adverse effects of beta blockade.

BETA-BLOCKADE AND EXERCISE IN PATIENTS

Beta-adrenoceptor blocking agents are prescribed primarily in patients with hypertension and ischemic heart disease. Only a small number of studies have been performed in hypertensive patients, but the effects during maximal and submaximal exercise appear to be similar to those in normotensive subjects. In some studies, no reduction of $\dot{V}o_2max$ has been found despite considerable reductions of HRmax. Although methodologic problems have yet to be excluded, it is theoretically possible that beta-blocker induced reductions of blood pressure improve cardiac function during exercise in hypertensive patients.

In patients with ischemic heart disease, work capacity is often limited by chest pain. Since beta-blockade reduces cardiac work rate because of the reduction in heart rate and blood pressure, a higher exercise intensity can be reached before chest pain occurs. In such patients, beta-blocker treatment improves exercise tolerance.

MUSCLE FATIGUE

An often-mentioned side effect of beta-blockers is the feeling of muscle fatigue. This feeling appears after only a few contractions. After a couple of minutes, the sensation of fatigue gradually diminishes, although it remains present. Increase of the exercise intensity elicits a similar response. The pathophysiologic mechanism behind this phenomenon is unknown. The logical explanation seems to be an impairment of blood supply and/or energy metabolism. At rest, a slight shift of skeletal muscle metabolism to the anaerobic pathway does not elicit special sensations. After moderate or heavy exercise, there are no fatigue signals from formerly active muscles either. In normal physiologic conditions, the feeling of muscle fatigue is present only during activity. It can be related to the mobilization of extra motor units to deliver a certain force or power. The underlying mechanism could be a disconnection of electrical and mechanical events in some muscle fibers. If an electrically activated muscle fiber lacked ATP, a weakened or an absent contraction would ensue. This situation can arise after either intensive (inhibition of glycolysis by accumulated lactate) or endurance (glycogen depleting) exercise. During beta-receptor blockade, the regulatory mechanisms adapting muscular blood flow and/or metabolic pathways to an enhancement of metabolic rate have a delayed response. In consequence, oxidative phosphorylation in some muscle fibers might be disturbed, leading to mechanical inactivity. To meet the desired strength or power output, extra motor units would have to be mobilized, this being experienced as muscle weakness or fatigue.

EXERCISE PRESCRIPTION AND TRAINABILITY DURING BETA-BLOCKER TREATMENT

Many patients on chronic beta-blocker therapy are stimulated to be physically active. In patients with ischemic heart disease, beta-blocker treatment improves exercise tolerance in a dose-dependent way. Physical activity is best performed at the moment when control of effort angina pectoris is maximal. In hypertensive patients, the exercise capacity is often impaired by beta-blockade, and the accompanying feelings of muscle fatigue may discourage such patients from participating in exercise programs. The reduction of exercise capacity depends on the degree of beta-blockade, and thus on dose and time after intake of medication. The dose should thus be kept as low as possible for optimal blood pressure control, and exercise is best performed at minimal plasma levels of the beta blocker; that is, just before the next dose is taken. Because of the risk of hypoglycemia, it is better not to exercise after several hours of fasting. If exhausting exercise is involved, beta-1 selective blockers seem preferable to nonselective blockers. Intrinsic sympathomimetic activity (ISA) does not play an important role during exercise when the level of sympathetic activity is high.

Many patients are not only physically active, but also engage in regular physical training. The question arises whether physical conditioning is impaired by beta-blocker treatment, since it has been suggested that adrenergic stimulation is an important component of physical conditioning. Fortunately, most studies have shown normal training responses during chronic beta-blocker treatment both in healthy subjects and in cardiac patients. Target exercise heart rates are shifted toward a higher percent $\dot{V}o_2$max for the same percent HRmax during chronic beta-blocker treatment, but the shift is relatively small compared to interindividual variations in this relationship. Therefore, for practical purposes, the normal relationship can be assumed during beta-blocker therapy. Nevertheless, it should be kept in mind that during beta-blocker treatment, determinations of HRmax and training heart rates have to be performed at approximately the same time after intake of the drug.

EXERCISE IN PEDIATRIC CARDIOLOGY

ROLF MOCELLIN, M.D.

In the last 20 years many authors have tried to quantify the functional ability of children with different cardiac malformations. However, the results have been by no means consistent, and it appears rather difficult to obtain an idea of the cardiovascular performance capacity of children with cardiac diseases by studying the literature.

VARYING REPORTS OF DISABILITY

There is agreement that exercise ability is diminished in the presence of a right-to-left shunt, even if the shunt is only apparent with exercise and not yet at rest. In contrast, children with a left-to-right shunt at the ventricular or atrial level or with stenotic malformations of the right or left ventricular outflow tract have as often been found to have normal test results as to be generally disabled. A more detailed hemodynamic analysis seemed to reveal that an elevation of pulmonary arterial pressure in children with ventricular septal defect was regularly associated with a decrease of cardiovascular ability, and that the extent of disability in patients with right or left ventricular outflow tract obstruction depended on the pressure gradient across the obstruction, measured at rest. These findings, though highly suggestive, have not always been confirmed.

The reasons for the striking differences of results between different investigations are manifold: In view of the great variability of aerobic power in a normal population (range 30 to 60 ml/kg/min in male adolescents), it is not surprising that discrimination between individual children with and without cardiac malformations is difficult. Even when dealing with a group of children suffering from the same cardiac malformation, discrimination from normal individuals is hampered because the heart muscle has a strong tendency to compensate for the specific defect as far as is possible. Unlike the situation of adults with coronary heart disease, the heart muscle is healthy in children, and it may overcome a mild-to-moderate pulmonary stenosis or an atrial septal defect by right ventricular hypertrophy or dilatation, re-establishing a rather normal functional ability.

METHODS OF ASSESSMENT

Patterns of ECG strain, such as ST-segmental depression, are rare and of minor importance when judging exercise reactions in patients with congenital heart disease. The direct determination of cardiovascular performance capacity through the measurement of aerobic power can generally be performed without problem in all patients who have reached at least 6 or 7 years of age. If adequate equipment is not available, indirect measurements of cardiovascular performance, such as the PWC 170 (the ergometer loading at a heart frequency of 170 beats per minute) may be employed. However, the indirect methods are rather unreliable.

THE ROLE OF EARLY SURGERY

During the last 20 years, cardiac surgery has made substantial advances, and operations at an early age have become more and more common. Accordingly, the situation concerning the exercise capacity of young cardiac patients has changed considerably. At present, corrective surgery of most hemodynamically relevant heart malformations is performed in infancy or before school age, at an age when ergometric determinations of functional ability are not yet possible, and participation in sport training is not yet a topic of discussion. This is the situation for children with a large ventricular septal defect, Fallot's tetralogy, transposition of the great arteries (including cases with additional ventricular septal defect or left ventricular outflow tract obstruction), coarctation of the aorta, large persistent ductus arteriosus, severe pulmonary stenosis with intact ventricular septum, severe aortic stenosis, and complete atrioventricular defect. Consequently, the main question posed by such patients is whether normal or approximately normal functional capacity has been achieved by the operation. If function remains subnormal, it may also be asked what kind of residual malformation is responsible.

FINDINGS IN LESS SEVERE MALFORMATIONS

Cardiac malformations which have not received surgical correction prior to school-age are mainly hemodynamically less severe malformations (for instance, a small or medium-sized ventricular septal defect, a mild-to-moderate pulmonary or aortic stenosis, an atrial septal defect, a partial anomalous pulmonary venous connection, a coarctation with sufficient collaterals, or a small persistent ductus arteriosus). Many of these children do not need an operation at all, and their functional ability is comparable with that of healthy children. Accordingly, there are no objections to their participation in sports events. In other children of this group, cardiac surgery is required. The decision to perform surgery on a child without evident complaints or symptoms is based on our knowledge of the natural history of the disease, derived from observations made when cardiac surgery was not yet available. The functional ability of these children is also within the normal range, so that there is no reason to limit their participation in school sports, either.

CONTRAINDICATIONS TO EXERCISE

One group of patients, those with aortic valve stenosis, cannot be allowed to participate in sports events because they are at risk of sudden death. The risk increases with the degree of stenosis and is imminent in cases showing ECG strain. Patients with a stenotic gradient exceeding 50 mmHg will undergo surgical correction, and their physical activity should be restricted before operation. Children with a gradient of less than 50 mmHg usually are not operated on. Despite their relatively low risk of sudden death, strenuous activities should not be encouraged; nevertheless, school sports may be allowed.

The small group of school-age patients with cyanotic heart disease who have not yet had an operation comprise patients with complex malformations; either additional pulmonary stenosis is present, or palliative banding of the pulmonary artery has been performed during infancy. Venous admixture increases with exercise, resulting in a further decrease of arterial oxygen content. Maximal oxygen intake lies in the range of 30 to 50 percent of normal. Training of the cardiovascular system is not possible for such individuals.

CHANGES OF FUNCTION AFTER SURGERY

As cardiac performance is not substantially impeded in many patients with congenital heart disease prior to surgery, operation does not necessarily bring about any direct increase in functional ability. However, prognosis concerning physical working capacity will be better, the more completely a malformation of the heart or of the great vessels has been corrected. A complete anatomic correction is possible, for example, in patients with patent ductus arteriosus, coarctation of the aorta, and atrial or ventricular septal defect, although postoperative function may be impaired by cardiac dysrhythmias following intraoperative lesions of the sinus node region or of the conducting tissue.

For patients with valvular disease, the prospects after operation are less satisfying. After valvotomy of pulmonary stenosis there may be some degree of pulmonary incompetence, although this generally has no significant influence on the patient's exercise capacity. A residual valvular pressure gradient, when combined with inadequate compliance of the right ventricle, may result in a decrease of stroke volume during exercise. When the cardiovascular performance of these children remains significantly reduced, a further operation should be considered.

After a valvotomy of an aortic stenosis, aortic insufficiency is generally present, especially if the valve was considerably malformed. It may happen that functional disability is more pronounced after operation than it was before. Moreover, valvotomy in aortic stenosis during infancy and childhood is usually a palliative measure, to be followed by valve replacement in the adult.

In patients with cyanotic congenital heart disease, considerable improvement of exercise capacity is the rule after corrective surgery. Nevertheless distinct limitations of functional ability remain in the majority of patients. In Fallot's tetralogy, the mean postoperative cardiovascular performance is about 85 percent of normal. Residual limitation of these patients is due mainly to a diminution of stroke volume. This cannot simply be attributed to persisting anomalies of the right ventricular outflow tract or to the insertion of an outflow tract patch. Pulmonary incompetence can contribute to the diminution of stroke volume, but as in isolated pulmonary stenosis, a reduced compliance of the right ventricle and residual stenosis may be more important causes of limitation. Intensive physical training might be considered as a means of restoring physical performance, but it cannot be recommended because of the remaining anatomic and functional disorders. Participation in regular school sports, however, seems justified.

Unlike children with tetralogy of Fallot (who have been extensively investigated after corrective surgery), there is little information available on the functional capacity of children after a Mustard or Senning procedure for transposition of the great arteries or after the Fontan procedure used in children with tricuspid atresia or single ventricle. This is partly due to the fact that many of the patients concerned have not yet reached an age at which precise testing is possible.

In patients who have undergone a Senning or Mustard procedure, and in whom significant tricuspid regurgitation, caval or pulmonary vein obstruction, left ventricular outflow tract obstruction, or cardiac dysrhythmias are present, normal functional ability is not to be expected. With improvement in surgical techniques, residual defects are now seen less frequently, and accordingly a better functional result may be anticipated. However, the right ventricle remains the systemic ventricle, and hemodynamic studies in such patients have shown a postoperative right ventricular ejection fraction of about 50 to 55 percent, compared to the normal value of 65 percent. Thus, normal physical performance after a Senning or Mustard procedure is generally possible only if stroke volume is maintained by a compensatory enlargement of the right ventricle.

Impaired cardiovascular performance is to be expected especially after the Fontan procedure, which is applied more and more frequently not only in patients with tricuspid atresia, but also in those with single ventricle. Even if the result of the operation is optimal, the right atrium now serving as the pumping chamber for the pulmonary circuit cannot be expected to react sufficiently to the demands of the organism in exercise. Preliminary data on the resting left ventricular ejection fraction after Fontan procedures demonstrate distinct functional limitation.

CONGENITAL HEART DISEASE AND SPORTS PARTICIPATION

With regard to the participation of patients with congenital heart disease in special sport events before or after "corrective" surgery, some basic aspects need to be presented. Cardiovascular performance is only one of the factors determining physical ability. Others include muscular strength, anaerobic capacity, and motor performance, the last being a complex term including velocity of movements, coordination ability, body balance, and hand dexterity. All of these factors vary more or less independently of each other and can be trained separately to a certain degree. All of them are usually involved in sports activities, though to a different extent and in differing combinations, depending on the kind of activity under consideration. Cardiovascular performance does not generally play a dominant role. In technical disciplines and in activities in which short-term efforts are required, the prevailing factors are not cardiovascular. This means that even if the cardiovascular capacity is diminished, rather good results can often be achieved. Cardiovascular capacity becomes important only for activities requiring endurance.

The limits of cardiovascular capacity may be estimated by measuring aerobic power and comparing results with normal values. Standardization of aerobic power in adolescents is meaningful only if body development, sex, and age are taken into consideration (Table 1).

If maximal oxygen intake is found to be reduced, this does not imply that participation in sports events is impossible. However, one should consider kinds of physical activity that are less dependent on cardiovascular capacity and are determined more by other factors such as motor skills.

INVASIVE ASSESSMENTS

When assessing cardiovascular performance postoperatively, more detailed information on cardiac output, stroke volume, and pressure gradients may be required. Such information demands at least central

TABLE 1 Absolute and Relative* Standards of Aerobic Power ($\dot{V}O_2$max) in Relation to Sex and Age

Age (years)	Boys		Girls	
	$\dot{V}O_2$ max (l/min)	$\dot{V}O_2$ max/m² (l/min/m²)	$\dot{V}O_2$ max (l/min)	$\dot{V}O_2$ max/m² (l/min/m²)
6.5	1.04	0.71	0.93	0.66
7.5	1.17	0.72	1.03	0.66
8.5	1.29	0.74	1.14	0.67
9.5	1.41	0.75	1.24	0.67
10.5	1.53	0.76	1.35	0.67
11.5	1.65	0.77	1.47	0.67
12.5	1.81	0.79	1.62	0.68
13.5	2.05	0.81	1.73	0.69
14.5	2.32	0.84	1.80	0.70
15.5	2.55	0.88	1.86	0.71
16.5	2.71	0.91	1.87	0.71
17.5	2.81	0.93	1.87	0.71

* Expressed relative to the square of stature, measured in m².

venous catheterization and arterial cannulation during exercise. One should thus consider carefully whether the information expected justifies the use of invasive methods. For meaningful interpretation, reference standards of cardiac output and stroke volume must refer to boys and girls of comparable age. Otherwise, findings such as a "low" cardiac output in relation to oxygen uptake may turn out to be misinterpretations, based on incorrect assumptions concerning the normal relationship between oxygen uptake and cardiac output in children of different ages and sex.

CONGENITAL HEART DISEASE AND TRAINING RESPONSE

In view of residual functional and anatomic disorders in many adolescents after open heart surgery (for example, after "correction" of tetralogy of Fallot, after Senning and Mustard operations in transposition of the great arteries, after a Fontan procedure for tricuspid atresia or single ventricle, as well as in complete atrioventricular defect or aortic stenosis, it is difficult to offer advice concerning physical training.

Some investigations have demonstrated significant improvements of maximum work capacity after 6 to 9 weeks of training in children following repair of tetralogy of Fallot, ventricular septal defect, aortic stenosis, and transposition of the great arteries. Training consisted in one study of jogging at heart rates of about 70 percent of maximal heart rate, performed for 30 minutes three times a week over a 9-week period. A second trial used graded interval exercise on a cycle ergometer for 6 weeks, four to six repetitions of 3- to 6-minute bouts of exercise at about 70 percent of maximal oxygen intake being performed during the final 4 weeks of training.

Interestingly, no significant increase of maximum oxygen intake was seen after training, but a higher work rate was tolerated, owing to either a signficant improvement in efficiency of performance or an upward shift of the point at which lactate production exceeded its elimination (the "anaerobic threshold").

If a higher mechanical efficiency was responsible for the increased maximum work rate following training, an improved coordination of movements would be assumed. In this manner, submaximal training could have a positive influence on exercise capacity despite the lack of any increase of aerobic power. More intensive training could perhaps result in an increase of aerobic power. However, the indications for endurance training should be considered cautiously when anatomic disorders are still present after "corrective" surgery.

ABNORMALITIES OF HEART RHYTHM AFTER SURGERY

Postoperative cardiac function may be impaired by dysrhythmias, especially if the sinus node region or the conduction tissue has been injured during the operation. Exercise may reveal rhythm disturbances not present at rest, and it may also either exacerbate or attenuate abnormalities present at rest. In cases in which sinus node function is impaired, as may happen for instance after Mustard or Senning operations or after closure of an atrial septal defect, the resting heart rate may be slowed, but a decrease of maximal heart rate is much more common, causing a considerable reduction of exercise capacity.

In children with congenital complete heart block, the ventricular rate during exercise often increases more than twofold, and an increase of stroke volume to about 150 percent of normal values may bring exercise capacity within the normal range, provided such dysrhythmias as premature ventricular contractions do not cause additional impairment. In children with acquired complete heart block, the lesion is more often located within or below the bundle of His, and the increase of ventricular rate during exercise is then often less than 10 beats per minute. In such patients, stroke volume cannot be elevated sufficiently to compensate for the low ventricular rate, and in consequence there is a considerable reduction of aerobic power.

IMMEDIATE POSTOPERATIVE CARE

It should be mentioned, finally, that the utmost caution is needed concerning physical activity in the first 3 to 4 weeks following cardiac surgery. Only gradually should the patient be allowed to participate in daily activities; participation in school sports events should be prohibited for 6 months after cardiac surgery.

EXERCISE IN THE PRIMARY PREVENTION OF ISCHEMIC HEART DISEASE

RALPH S. PAFFENBARGER, Jr., M.D., D.P.H.
ROBERT T. HYDE, M.A.

Many studies since 1950 have shown that adequate physical exercise should have real potential as an intervention regimen against ischemic heart disease (IHD). While occupational demands for strenuous physical activity have been disappearing, the more developed countries have experienced a boom in highly active recreational pursuits.

Level of habitual energy expenditure is inversely related to incidence of nonfatal and fatal IHD, and this association is at least partly independent of other influences. Various complexities of the total lifestyle picture have clouded the issues and led some observers into unwarranted skepticism. Unlike obesity, cigarette smoking, hypertension, and several other characteristics known to influence IHD risk, exercise is experienced by everyone to some degree. With so many interacting variables, precisely controlled studies of exercise are difficult to arrange and maintain, and more reliance must be placed on investigations of "natural" circumstances assessed by epidemiologic methods. Results from such studies will be described briefly.

OCCUPATIONAL PHYSICAL ACTIVITY

Hippocrates observed that a sedentary lifestyle was detrimental to health and in 1700 Bernardino Ramazzini contrasted the health hazards of tailors with those of messengers or "runners". However, IHD was not defined until 1912, and its inverse relationship to adequate vigorous exercise was not pointed out until J.N. Morris and associates, in 1953, described how physically active conductors, scrambling to collect tickets on London double-decked buses, had a much lower risk of IHD than the bus drivers who sat steering all day.

Other reports noted inverse patterns of exercise level and IHD risk between letter carriers and mail clerks, farmers and sedentary townsmen, workers on different jobs in kibbutzim in Israel, railroad track workers and clerks, and San Francisco longshoremen loading cargo or tallying it into warehouses. However, even the most persuasive studies drew attention to the problems and different ways of assessing exercise and its relationships to IHD risks.

Not all reports were positive for exercise, partly because other influences such as cigarette smoking, diet, and serum lipid levels were receiving new attention; populations differed in lifestyle, and there were wide departures in availability of data and methods of analysis. Even more important, many studies were not designed to test the exercise-IHD hypothesis, and "afterthought analyses" often were based on inadequate assessments of physical activity. Findings were negative among civil servants in Los Angeles and Chicago industrial workers, perhaps because the occupational categories lacked contrast in physical activity, or leisure-time energy output had not been evaluated. Ethnic and cultural differences apparently compounded such problems when a complex 10-year study was attempted of 16 cohorts in seven countries. If the interacting characteristics of lifestyle, such as diet, are not adequately defined and considered, the conclusions drawn from an analysis may become contradictory or confused, and in some cases, apparently inconclusive findings have been refuted in later reports. Newer methods and criteria have been developing as the various factors involved have become better understood, with refinements in data gathering instruments, study design, trend sampling, coding, data processing, evaluation, and interpretation of results.

The San Francisco Longshoremen Study. After a multiphasic screening examination in 1951, the San Francisco longshoremen were followed for 22 years. Assessments of their exercise patterns were based on actual on-the-job energy output measurements (kilojoules/week). Changes in job assignments were checked annually, and IHD mortality rates were derived from official death certificates and man-years of observation. Cargo handlers contrasted strongly with sedentary foremen and clerks. Weaklings were unlikely in either group, as union rules required all members to be cargo handlers for at least 5 years. Many did heavy work for much longer, 13 years on average. The differing IHD rates for high and low energy output jobs could not be explained by hereditary self-selection, nor by job transfers that might have accompanied premonitory symptoms.

Rates of fatal IHD among 3686 longshoremen from 1951 through 1972 were computed per 10,000 man-years of work, by age at death and job category. There were 395 IHD deaths (11%) during the follow-up, but the rate for cargohandlers who expended over 35 MJ/week at work (totalling 32 percent of the man-years of follow-up) was only about half (0.56) the rate for men in less energetic jobs. This saving effect was greatest at younger ages, but evident at all ages. Leisure-time exercise was of little importance alongside the exceptionally high occupational energy output. Shifting trends, including changes in technology, are among several reasons why the protective effect of exercise at work was seen only in the youngest two of the four 10-year cohorts born between 1877 and 1916.

High-energy workers had much lower risk of sudden death from IHD than their more sedentary fellows. Data on nonfatal IHD were lacking, but the cargo handlers may have been less likely to have an attack or better able to withstand one. The sudden death findings are of further interest, since in this comparison there is less likelihood that overt premonitory symptoms induced a change to lighter work assignments, thus discounting the issue of self-selection. Adjustment for job transfers did not appreciably alter the results of analysis for any

IHD mortality categories, sudden or delayed. Factoring out the influences of age, cigarette smoking, obesity, higher blood pressure, and prior IHD confirmed a progressive lowering of fatal IHD risk among longshoremen as energy output on the job rose from 20 to 45 MJ/week. Risk was reduced about 50 percent when energy output was twice the baseline level.

LEISURE-TIME PHYSICAL ACTIVITY

Morris and his colleagues saw that leisure-time exercise could have an important influence on IHD risk among workers whose sedentary jobs did not afford adequate energy output. A population of 17,944 middle-aged male British civil servants submitted a standard diary form logging their physical activities by 5-minute intervals for one work day and one consecutive leisure day. During 8.5 years of follow-up, there were 1138 first clinical attacks. Those who had reported vigorous leisure activity had an IHD rate of 3.1 percent versus 6.9 percent for men lacking vigorous exercise. Fatal first-attack rates of IHD for these groups were 1.1 and 2.9 percent, respectively, and for sudden deaths (unheralded by advance sick leave), 0.65 and 1.60 percent. Retirees differed likewise. Even more notably, the rise of IHD *morbidity* with age was prominent only among the nonexercising groups; there was relatively little increase among men who had reported habitual vigorous exercise.

As for occupational exercise, investigations of leisure-time physical activity and IHD risk have yielded widely varying results. In some studies, occupational differences may not have been recognized. In others, the methods of rating leisure-time exercise may not have been sufficiently refined. A number of recent studies have assessed both occupational and leisure-time physical activity.

The United States College Alumni Study. Patterns of leisure-time exercise, other lifestyle elements, and health status have been examined among 50,000 former students from Harvard University and the University of Pennsylvania in order to determine how past and contemporary physical activity relate to IHD risk. Data extending from 1900 to the present time have been obtained from physical examination and other college records on students who matriculated during the years 1916 to 1950, plus alumni responses to self-administered mail questionnaires, and terminal findings from death certificates. Subsets of the total population have been studied for personal characteristics of college days as well as for present-day exercise habits and physician-diagnosed IHD. Analysis has shown that current and continuing adequate exercise, rather than a history of youthful or hereditary vigor and athleticism, is associated inversely with risk of IHD in all age brackets studied.

Rates of first attack of IHD among 16,936 Harvard University alumni during 10 or 6 years (1962 or 1966 to 1972) were calculated per 10,000 man-years. There were 572 first attacks. Age-specific rates of IHD declined consistently with increases in energy expenditure by

stair-climbing, walking, and sports play as determined from mail questionnaires, and with increasing kJ/week in a composite physical activity index. Like trends were found for both nonfatal and fatal clinical events (angina pectoris, myocardial infarction, and, to a lesser degree, sudden death). Overall IHD risk patterns were similar in each 10-year age class from 35 through 74 years. The cardiovascular health advantage of continuing adequate exercise held good over a wide range of lifestyles and at all ages studied. The saving effect of current exercise was heightened by vigorous sports play. In summary, alumni still engaging in strenuous activities plus at least 4200 additional kJ/week of stair-climbing, walking, and other light activities had less than half (0.42) the IHD incidence of their nonathletic, most sedentary classmates.

Table 1 presents relative risks for first attack of IHD (nonfatal or fatal) by presence versus absence of each of five beneficial characteristics, adjusted for differences in age, follow-up interval, and each of the other characteristics listed. Thus, men with adequate exercise were at 67 percent of the risk for men less active; the nonsmokers were at 77 percent the risk of smokers; men who maintained their weight-for-height at modest levels had 76 percent the risk of men more obese; the normotensives had 43 percent the risk of hypertensives; and men without history of parental IHD were at 78 percent the risk of their counterparts with such history.

Whether considered positively or negatively, each of the five characteristics contributes independently to IHD risk. The impact of adverse traits is seen in Table 2. Hypertension is the most potent predictor clinically but least prevalent, while sedentary lifestyle is most prevalent and contributes the greatest percentage to IHD risk. If adverse levels of all five characteristics could be eliminated, first attacks of IHD among the alumni would be reduced by 67 percent. This compared with an 88 percent reduction of fatal IHD computed for longshoremen if they were to eliminate low activity, cigarette habit and hypertension.

TABLE 1   Relative Risks of First IHD Attack (Nonfatal or Fatal) Among 16,936 Harvard Alumni, 1962–1972, by Selected Beneficial Characteristics

Alumnus Characteristic	Relative Risk[1] of IHD, % (1 standard error)	P
Adequate exercise[2]	0.67 (0.08)	<0.001
No cigarette smoking[3]	0.77 (0.08)	0.016
Body mass control[4]	0.76 (0.08)	0.010
Normotension[5]	0.43 (0.06)	<0.001
No history of parental IHD[6]	0.78 (0.09)	0.024

[1] Risk from presence of the characteristic as compared with risk from its absence; adjusted for differences in age, follow-up interval, and each of the other characteristics listed.

[2] 8400 kJ per week expended in walking, stair-climbing, and sports play.

[3] Complete abstention.

[4] Less than 20 percent over ideal weight-for-height by 1959 Metropolitan Life Insurance Company standards.

[5] Absence of physician-diagnosed hypertension.

[6] Alumnus-reported.

TABLE 2 Clinical and Community Attributable Risks of First IHD Attack (Nonfatal or Fatal) Among 16,936 Harvard Alumni, 1962–1972, by Selected Adverse Characteristics

Alumnus Characteristic	Prevalence %	Attributable Risk[1] of IHD, % Clinical	Attributable Risk[1] of IHD, % Community
Sedentary lifestyle[2]	61	33	23
Cigarette smoking[3]	52	23	13
Obesity[4]	38	24	11
Hypertension[5]	9	57	10
History of parental IHD[6]	39	22	10

[1] Theoretical risk accounted for by presence as opposed to absence of the characteristic; adjusted for differences in age, follow-up interval, and each of the other characteristics listed.

[2] <8400 kJ per week expended in walking, stair-climbing, and sports play.

[3] Any amount.

[4] 20 percent or more over ideal mass-for-height by 1959 Metropolitan Life Insurance Company standards.

[5] Physician-diagnosed.

[6] Alumnus-reported in either or both parents.

With increasing interest in athletic energy output as a regimen for maintenance of cardiovascular health, attention has sharpened on both the benefits and the hazards of endurance exercise (Table 3), which may be defined as "sustained, rhythmic, large-muscle movement for 30 or more minutes, at three-quarters estimated maximum heart rate, four or more times weekly". Basic precautions for this exercise are: (1) avoid unaccustomed strain on an untrained system, (2) start slowly, (3) exercise prudently, and (4) taper off. As Table 3 shows, neither the benefits nor the hazards of exercise are limited to the cardiovascular system. For any average individual, the benefits are likely to be spread over nearly all body systems, while hazards might affect chiefly a weakest point, such as skeletal porosity in the elderly person. Overstress is unwise for anyone, but is especially contraindicated in the presence of known or probable cardiovascular abnormalities. Body thermal and psychologic excesses may be more subtle in onset than musculoskeletal or cardiorespiratory overstress events, but they are also very common and to be avoided.

Recent Supporting Studies. In 1975, P. Leren et al reported on IHD risk among all Oslo men aged 40 to 49 and a 7 percent random sample of men aged 20 to 39. Risk was higher for men rated highly active at work than for men with sedentary jobs but highly active in their leisure time. This finding may reflect a blue-collar versus white-collar selectivity involving other lifestyle differences, but it also points toward possible advantages of leisure-time exercise programmed and designed to suit the individual.

In Framingham, W.M. Kannel and P. Sorlie followed 1909 men and 2311 women originally without IHD. For 14 years the mortality rate, especially IHD mortality rate, was inversely related to exercise level in the men, but not the women. The largely sedentary study population was administered a simplified interview questionnaire which evaluated hours of rest and occupational

TABLE 3 Beneficial Effects and Potential Hazards of Endurance Exercise* as a Defense Against IHD†

Benefits

Enhanced physical work capacity, hemodynamic function, hematologic action, and cardiovascular fitness

Improved profiles of plasma lipid, lipoprotein, and glucose

Increased maximum breathing capacity and oxygen utilization

Improved individual lifestyles (prudent diet, cigarette abstention, body mass control, coping with stress)

Enhanced mood, thought, and psychologic behavior

Reduced physiologic precursors of cardiovascular disease (obesity, hypertension, and electrocardiographic abnormalities)

Decreased risks of atherosclerotic hypertensive, and ancillary diseases (angina pectoris, coronary insufficiency, myocardial infarction, stroke, peripheral vascular, renal, and diabetes mellitus), together with their consequences

Hazards

Increased risk of sudden death in susceptible (untrained and overstressed) individuals

Contraindicated for subjects with acute myocardial infarction, acute coronary occlusion, myocarditis, marked aortic stenosis, uncontrolled hypertension

Exercise-induced asthma and anaphylaxis

Sports anemia

Induced electrolyte and temperature imbalances

Exercise addiction and anxiety

* Sustained, rhythmic, large-muscle movement for 30 or more minutes, at three-quarters estimated maximum heart rate, four or more times weekly. (Avoid unaccustomed strain on an untrained system. Start slowly, exercise aerobically, and taper off.)

† It is recognized that exercise influences many other body systems, such as the musculoskeletal, in both beneficial and hazardous ways.

and nonoccupational pursuits rated as sedentary, light, moderate, or heavy on the basis of estimated oxygen consumption. Findings were rather indefinite, perhaps because the questionnaire or index did not identify high and low exercise groups sufficiently. They stated, "While the data fall short of either proving or disproving that an increased level of habitual exercise is beneficial, . . . the need to regain more vigorous exercise habits seems urgent for general well-being". T.R. Dawber analyzed the same data over a 24-year follow-up period, and found that exercise level was inversely related to IHD incidence in both men and women.

K. Magnus et al conducted a case-control study of first attack of IHD versus leisure-time walking, cycling, and gardening exercise levels in four residential areas of Holland from 1970 to 1974. Data were obtained by interviewing patients (or their nearest surviving kin) and 875 randomly selected IHD-free control subjects. Exercise levels were defined as *habitual* (more than 8 months/year), *seasonal* (4 to 8 months), or *occasional* (less than 4 months), and by participation in hours/week. Habitual-level activities and IHD events were significantly inverse in relationship, but seasonal or occasional activities did not predict low IHD. IHD risk did not depend on hours per week of walking, cycling, and gardening, nor did vigorous participation show any added influence. The case-fatality ratio (death within 4 weeks of IHD onset) was highest in the least active subjects, i.e., the occasional participants.

M. Karvonen et al followed two Finnish cohorts for a total of 15 years, relating IHD mortality and total mortality to exercise levels as assessed by an extensive, prestructured interview. Prevalence figures strongly related sedentary habits to atherosclerotic trends (IHD, stroke, and claudication) in men aged 50 to 69. In 1310 men, both IHD mortality and total mortality over a 5-year follow-up were inversely related to habitual exercise. However, in a subset of 838 men initially free of IHD, mortality from this cause was unrelated to exercise, although combined incidence rates of myocardial infarction and IHD death declined somewhat from the least to the most active subjects.

M.R. Garcia-Palmieri reported an 8.5-year follow-up study of 2585 rural and 6208 urban Puerto Rico men aged 45 to 65. He found a significant inverse association between exercise and risk of IHD (minus angina pectoris), as assessed by a Framingham physical activity index. Men with vigorous exercise habits had 50 percent less IHD than sedentary men. Physical activity influences were independent of other IHD predictive factors—cigarette smoking, hypertension, obesity, faster heart rate, and higher levels of serum cholesterol. When the first 2.5 years of follow-up were omitted, to avoid premonitory selection, results changed very little. At the highest activity level, nonsmokers had still less IHD, but smokers had an increased risk. Since the overall heart attack rate was only about half that on the mainland, the investigator concluded that, "The benefits from the higher activity levels in Puerto Rico probably reflect a lifetime pattern of steady activity rather than a recent increase in exercise".

P.R. Pomrehn et al studied 62,000 deaths among Iowa men aged 20 to 64. Physically active farmers had about 10 percent lower IHD mortality than nonfarmers. The farmers also had higher energy intake and slightly higher cholesterol levels and body-mass index, but were less obese by skinfold test, and their frequencies of cigarette use and alcohol consumption were more than doubled by nonfarmers. The farmers were physically active twice as often and had higher HDL-cholesterol levels than nonfarmers. They also were more fit by treadmill test. The lower IHD mortality risk of the farmers was credited to their healthier lifestyle (including less smoking). They consumed more energy because they did more physical work, but their energy output was sufficient to avoid either obesity or elevated LDL-cholesterol. This suggests that a diet matched to a vigorous exercise program is perferable to reduction of energy intake without adequate exercise.

The association of vigorous activity with low risk of sudden death from IHD was obvious among the London busmen, San Francisco longshoremen, and British civil servants, but less certain in the Harvard alumni study. However, D.S. Siscovick et al, in Seattle, found that risk of primary cardiac arrest (PCA) was less than half as great in persons who had high-intensity leisure-time activity demanding at least 60 percent of maximum oxygen uptake, as contrasted with PCA risk in persons without such exercise. The analysis included only subjects who had no record of prior morbidity and had been able to be active. Personal and exercise data were gathered by telephone interview from spouses of PCA decendents and matched controls. Exercise levels were indexed much as they were in the United States college alumni study. However, efforts to avoid possible selection or bias reduced the roster of decedents from 1250 to 163 (about 13%, a rather startling attrition). Also, the testimony of bereaved spouses might be of dubious certainty, but no special bias was found in their reports.

J.T. Salonen and associates made a longitudinal 7-year study of 7666 men and women aged 30 to 59 in East Finland. Low physical activity at work increased acute myocardial infarction, cerebral stroke, and mortality from any disease. Their analysis adjusted for differences in age, serum total cholesterol, diastolic blood pressure, height, body mass, and smoking. Low physical activity at work led to acute myocardial infarction risks of 1.5 in men and 2.4 in women relative to workers most energetic on the job. Over the first 2 years of follow-up, limited leisure activity increased risk of death, but not of acute myocardial infarction or stroke. Exercise level was estimated from the response to a single multiple-choice question. Risks of cardiovascular disease were significantly increased in individuals with low energy output. The findings for leisure-time exercise were less consistent than for occupational activity, perhaps because they were confounded by smoking or other leisure-time adversities. But since physical activity may enhance favorable serum lipids and HDL-cholesterol, the analysis probably should not have adjusted for them; adjusting for cholesterol levels could also be controlling for exercise, thus masking the measurement instead of sharpening it.

In Los Angeles, R.S. Peters et al followed 2779 healthy public safety officers for 13,317 man-years. Men aged 35 to 54 were rated into categories below or above medium values of fitness (cycle ergometer test), blood pressure, total serum cholesterol, body mass, body-mass index, lean body mass, and habitual activity. Cigarette smoking and family history of heart disease were logged as present or absent. Within an average follow-up of 5 years, 36 men had first symptomatic myocardial infarctions (5 fatal). The subjects below median fitness were at more than double the risk of IHD than men more fit, after adjustment for other influences. Men at highest risk were chiefly smokers or above median in cholesterol and blood pressure. Those less fit with any two or all three of these traits had at least six times greater risk of myocardial infarction than men more fit with the same characteristics.

D.M. Kramsch et al found that adequate physical conditioning could retard coronary (and other large-vessel) atherosclerosis in monkeys. Treadmill-exercised and sedentary adult male monkeys were compared for ischemic electrocardiographic changes, angiographic signs of coronary artery narrowing, and gross and microscopic pathologic findings. The exercised monkeys had lowered heart rates at rest and after exercise, increased heart size, a loss and regain of body mass (probably exchanging body fat for body lean), small increases in HDL-cholesterol and large decreases in total LDL- and VLDL-triglycerides, and little change in blood pressure levels. Moderate exercise also reduced coronary surface involvement and lesion size (intimal thickening), suppressed collagen accumulation, and widened lumina, in contrast to findings in sedentary animals. Retarded lesion growth in exercised monkeys was accompanied by inhibited atherosclerotic change in the aorta and other arteries.

Acknowledgments: This work was supported by the Union Carbide Corporation; the Exxon Corporation; the Mobil Foundation; the Marathon Oil Foundation, Inc.; the Phillips Petroleum Foundation, Inc.; and the Sun Company, Inc.

EXERCISE IN THE SECONDARY PREVENTION OF ISCHEMIC HEART DISEASE

VEIKKO KALLIO, M.D.

Data from a number of both uncontrolled and controlled studies indicate that physical exercise has similar effects in patients who have had myocardial infarction and in healthy individuals of the same age. Training, even at maximal intensity, is feasible in selected groups of patients, resulting in a physical working capacity that has sometimes allowed participation in marathon running. Several reports based on uncontrolled studies suggest that patients participating in physical training programs have a lower mortality than less active patients. The physical activity level before infarction is also related to prognosis, a high level of physical activity before infarction being correlated with a lower mortality rate after infarction.

In view of these interesting data, and the known effects of exercise upon such factors as hemodynamics and blood lipids, one might expect that a large controlled trial would have been undertaken in order to determine the secondary preventive value of physical training after myocardial infarction. However, such a study has not been performed. Practical difficulties include the large number of patients required, a high dropout rate and a low compliance in any training group, and a high drop-in rate among patients allocated to a control group.

In spite of the fact that we lack a definite answer to our problem, based on a sufficient number of patients and an adequately designed study, a few controlled feasibility studies and clinical trials have produced interesting data. These studies will now be briefly discussed.

SWEDISH TRIAL

A Swedish trial, started in 1968 by Sanne, Wilhelmsen, and co-workers, studied the feasibility of supervised physical training and its effects on mortality and nonfatal reinfarctions in unselected patients. A total of 313 consecutive cases less than 55 years of age were randomly allocated between a physical training and a control group, following myocardial infarction. Other details of follow-up procedure and treatment were similar for all patients. About 27 percent of those assigned to the training group had to be excluded because of cardiac contraindications or poor cooperation. The program, initiated 3 months after myocardial infarction, consisted of three half-hour training sessions per week, supervised by a physiotherapist but with a physician available. The highest training heart rate reached in patients with no evidence of residual cardiac problems averaged 144 beats per minute, 80 percent of their heart rate reserve.

Cardiac complications during training were remarkably few. One reinfarction, starting with ventricular fibrillation, was encountered in some 10,000 training sessions. The patient was successfully resuscitated and made a full recovery. The main problem was a high dropout rate from the supervised training program; only 39 percent of those who began training were still exercising at the hospital after one year, although a further 29 percent of patients continued to train at home. One year after myocardial infarction, the physical working capacity was significantly greater in the training group, but they showed no advantage of mortality or reinfarction rate.

During the next 3 years, the number of dropouts continued to increase. At 4 years, 18.2 percent of patients in the intervention group had died, compared with 22 percent in the control group. The percentages of nonfatal reinfarctions were 16 and 18, respectively. Neither of these differences was significant, although the high dropout rate from the training program may at least partly explain the negative outcome.

FINNISH OUTPATIENT TRIAL

A Finnish study was launched by Kentala almost concomitantly with the Swedish trial. This feasibility study involved 298 consecutive hospitalized male patients under 65 years of age. They were randomized to a training or a control group on admission to the hospital. At discharge, there were 81 patients in the control group and 77 in the training group. All patients were subsequently seen once a month at the hospital outpatient department. The exercise group began training 6 to 8 weeks after infarction, with 2 to 3 exercise sessions per week. The intensity of the 20-minute endurance phase was regulated to keep the heart rate about 10 beats below the maximum tolerated in the exercise test. Physical activity at home was also encouraged.

As in the Swedish trial, the dropout rate was high, particularly during the second half of the one-year training period. An attendance rate of 75 percent or more proved feasible in only a fifth of the patients. On the other hand, 11 of the 81 control patients maintained physical activity at an effective training level on their own initiative.

There were no differences in physical working capacity between training and control groups at the one-year follow-up. One recurrence of infarction occurred during training. There were, altogether, five deaths from myocardial infarction in the training group, compared with four deaths from myocardial infarction and three sudden deaths in the control group. The number of nonfatal reinfarctions was five in the training group compared with four in the control group. These differences in mortality and morbidity were not statistically significant.

FINNISH HOME-TRAINING TRIAL

The feasibility and effects of a physical exercise program based on spontaneous home training were examined in another Finnish study by Palatsi. The patients included both men and women, but excluded individuals with severe motor disorders, psychiatric problems, or severe decompensated heart failure. The training group consisted of 180 patients and the control group of 200 patients, all under 65 years of age. The exercise program began 10 weeks after infarction and continued for 12 months, with patients attending a calisthenic session in groups of 5 to 7 once a month. The 30-minute program was conducted by a physiotherapist and supervised by a physician. Training became progressively more demanding in successive months. Between supervised sessions, the patients trained at home, making notes of their personal activity. Their target was a pulse rate at least 70 percent of the maximum age-predicted value. Apart from a monthly ergometer exercise test, no special program was organized for control patients.

At one-year, 51 percent of the men and 73 percent of the women were still carrying out their exercises 6 to 7 days per week.

An insignificant trend to reduced mortality and morbidity favored the training group. During the first year, 3.5 percent of the trainers and 8 percent of controls died; the second year the mortality was 3.6 percent in the training group and 5.5 percent in the control group.

AMERICAN TRIAL

The U.S. National Exercise and Heart Disease Project (NEHDP) involved 651 men with myocardial infarction at five participating centers. The subjects covered a broad age range (30 to 64 years) and were referred for study from as early as 8 weeks to as late as 36 months after their myocardial infarction, 43 percent of them being first seen more than one year after the infarction. Patients were allocated randomly to a training or a control group. The exercise prescription called for a target heart rate that was 85 percent of the peak value achieved during a semi-annual exercise test. The program, which was held three times per week for 34 months, included games, walking, jogging, calisthenics, and swimming. The patients of the control group were re-evaluated at the same intervals as those who received training.

By the end of 2 years, 23 percent of the exercise group had dropped out, while 31 percent of control subjects were exercising regularly.

The cumulative 3-year mortality rate was 4.6 percent for the exercise group and 7.3 percent for the controls, but this difference was not significant. The 3-year rates for recurrent myocardial infarction were 5.3 percent and 7.0 percent, respectively.

Although the results from this study did not prove the case for exercise in persons with known myocardial infarction, the data are consistent with an assumption of benefit from exercise. The low mortality in the control group was not foreseen when designing the study and is partly due to the late entry of many patients into the study. It is a pity that the much larger initially anticipated number of patients could not be recruited because of financial problems.

CANADIAN TRIAL

The Ontario Exercise-Heart Collaborative Study examined the effect of high-intensity exercise on prognosis following myocardial infarction; 751 patients less than 54 years of age were recruited in seven centers 3 to 12 months after myocardial infarction. The subjects were placed on high- or low-intensity exercise by stratified random allocation. The high-intensity exercise group attended supervised sessions, usually twice weekly, carrying out the same exercise prescription on their own for a total of at least four times per week. The exercise prescription was calculated to provide walking or jogging programs requiring between 65 and 85 percent of the subjects' estimated maximal oxygen intake. The low-intensity exercise group met at least once a week for recreational activities developing a heart rate less than that observed at 50 percent of the estimated maximal oxygen intake. In addition to exercise, the participants were encouraged to stop smoking and to control obesity. Elevated serum lipid levels were also treated by the family physician. The overall dropout rate in both groups was over 45 percent which clearly exceeded the expected 35 percent.

During the 4 years of follow-up, the percentage of fatal reinfarctions in the high-intensity exercise group was 4.0 percent compared to 3.7 percent in the low-intensity exercise group. These extremely low mortality figures are similar to those encountered in the NEHDP project and, together with the high dropout rates, decreased the power of the trial to detect any differences between the two groups. The rates of nonfatal reinfarctions were 10.3 percent and 9.3 percent, respectively.

The results of the study are important, as they indicate that an aggressive exercise prescription requiring close supervision of the patients offers no advantage over a low-intensity exercise program with regard to secondary prevention.

WORLD HEALTH ORGANIZATION TRIAL

A multifactorial intervention program was adopted in a WHO coordinated study. It included physical exercise, applied in each of 24 individual centers according to the best of their knowledge. For various reasons, the morbidity and mortality data of some 3000 recruited patients could not be pooled at an international level. The study, therefore, did not answer questions about morbidity and mortality following a multifactorial intervention that included physical exercise. The results of the Finnish substudy, performed in Turku and Helsinki, have been published separately and are discussed below.

The Finnish component of the study included 375 consecutive male and female patients under 65 years of age who had been admitted to the hospital because of acute myocardial infarction. At discharge, they were randomly allocated between an intervention and a control group. The intervention included frequent contacts with an internist, optimal medical care, antismoking and dietary advice, a physical exercise program, and advice on psychosocial problems. The program started 2 weeks after discharge from the hospital. In Turku, there were three weekly exercise sessions during the first 10 weeks, and thereafter one session a week for the next 9 months. The training heart rate was determined by a maximal symptom-limited cycle ergometer test, using the formula:

Training heart rate = Resting heart rate + 60% (Maximal heart rate − Resting heart rate)

Eighty-three percent of patients participated adequately in the exercise program. The adherence rate was remarkably high, probably on account of the study design, since the period of frequent attendance lasted only 3 months. In Helsinki, patients were given structured advice on home training, the intensity being adjusted on the basis of exercise testing.

Control patients were followed up by their own doctors and were seen by the study team only once a year during the 6-year trial. We wanted to avoid too many contacts with the control patients, because of the risk of contamination with an interest in physical activity. The compliance with the intervention program was excellent. This was reflected in mean values for body mass, serum cholesterol, serum triglycerides, and systolic and diastolic blood pressure values, all of which were significantly lower in the intervention group than in control patients at the yearly follow-up. However, there was no intergroup difference of physical working capacity one year after the initial infarction.

The cumulative coronary mortality in the first 3 years of follow-up was significantly lower in the intervention group (18.6%) than in controls (29.4%, p = 0.02). This difference was mainly due to a reduction in the number of sudden deaths, the corresponding percentages being 5.8 in the intervention group and 14.4 in controls (p<0.01). The same significant trend was still observed at the 6-year follow-up. No significant difference in the number of clinically verified reinfarctions was seen between groups.

The results thus suggest that coronary mortality and, in particular, the number of sudden deaths can be reduced by a multifactorial intervention program started a few weeks after an acute myocardial infarction. The individual role of exercise or indeed any other component of the multifactorial intervention cannot be determined. The practical conclusion seems that while the best results may be expected in relatively low-risk patients, all patients should receive appropriate advice and well-organized care including physical exercise. The program should start on discharge from hospital, with most frequent attendance during the first 3 to 6 months after myocardial infarction.

The studies described have not proven that physical training has secondary preventive value after myocardial infarction. However, all but one have shown a trend in favor of this hypothesis. Physical exercise should be included in comprehensive rehabilitation and multiple risk factor intervention is a prudent approach to secondary prevention after myocardial infarction. The intensity of training does not seem a major consideration when aiming at secondary prevention. Physical activity programs are an integral part of good quality care after myocardial infarction and influence the quality of life, an aspect that should not be forgotten.

EXERCISE AND MOOD STATE

ROY J. SHEPHARD, M.D. (Lond), Ph.D.

Many middle-aged patients tell their physician that the main reason for exercising is to "feel better". Nevertheless, there have been remarkably few scientific studies examining the value of exercise in treating the mild depression and anxiety which is so commonly encountered in general practice. This chapter will offer some brief comments on the value of exercise, both in otherwise healthy patients and in those suffering a reactive depression following myocardial infarction.

THE EXERCISE "ADDICT"

There is increasing evidence that very vigorous exercise stimulates the body production of morphine-like substances, the beta-endorphins. A linkage has been suggested between this phenomenon and the "runner's high", with the further implication that regular release of endogenous morphine-like compounds creates a chemical dependence upon running. Certainly, there are some data indicating "withdrawal symptoms" when an avid runner cannot get the daily dosage of kilometers, although it is difficult to be sure whether this is a true chemical dependence or merely a sign of an obsessive personality.

The logical leap of faith is that regular running might replace the tranquilizers and pain-killers currently prescribed in such large quantities, by virtue of beta-endorphin production. Unfortunately, both the quantity and the intensity of activity needed are high (perhaps an hour of near maximal exercise per day), and an exercise prescription of this order is unlikely to be filled by a patient who is currently receiving tranquilizers or analgesics on a regular basis.

BASIS OF MOOD ELEVATION

Although the beta-endorphin mechanism can probably be ruled out in the average patient, there is nevertheless objective evidence of an improved mood in response to the type of exercise encountered in an employee fitness program. This can be demonstrated by such tests as the "profile of mood states" (POMS) and the manifest anxiety scale. Moreover, the benefit is greater in patients who initially show some anxiety or depression, perhaps in part because they can see more "reason" for involvement in the exercise program.

The optimal type of exercise probably varies with the nature of the disorder. A mildly depressed patient is generally under-aroused, and the proprioceptive stimuli from vigorous movement help to increase arousal. The social contacts and the rhythmic music of a group calisthenic session may further encourage this process. An anxious person, in contrast, is over-aroused, and the optimum pattern of exercise is then relaxing, for instance, a leisurely walk or cycle ride with a familiar and sympathetic friend.

The nature of the feedback provided by the class instructor is also important when there are psychologic disturbances. Many group exercise programs are performance-oriented, and if a class leader sets targets or assigns contracts that cannot be met, depression may be deepened or anxiety heightened. The manner of presentation should be arousing for the depressed and soothing for the anxious, but in both cases, feedback should be warm and encouraging.

APPLICATION TO "POSTCORONARY" PROGRAMS

Several studies have now shown that the average patient who reports to a coronary rehabilitation program 2 to 3 months after infarction is suffering from a moderate-to-severe depression. Although there have been some suggestions that this is an inherent part of the coronary-prone personality, or a reaction to medication, the main basis for the depression is undoubtedly an acute reaction to the cardiac episode. Many adjustments are required: income expectations must be scaled downward and occupational ambitions jettisoned; the patient must also accept more dependence upon the spouse, and in many instances normal sexual activity is modified or interrupted. It is thus hardly suprising that tests such as the Minnesota Multiphasic Personality Inventory (MMPI) show a depression score that in a third of postcoronary patients is two standard deviations greater than normal.

Studies at the Toronto Rehabilitation Center have indicated that patients falling in this severely depressed category can move as much as half of the way back to a normal personality profile over a few years of vigorous, exercise-centered rehabilitation. Part of this change may be a spontaneous recovery, but a causal relationship to the exercise rehabilitation is suggested by the fact that poor adherents to the exercise program fail to show this benefit.

Many psychologists have argued that the MMPI measures trait rather than state depression, and the change resulting from exercise is thus all the more remarkable. Application of the POMS instrument to "postcoronary" patients also brings out an abnormal mood state, although the features revealed by the POMS questionnaire are tension/anxiety, confusion, and loss of vigor, a pattern more suggestive of an anxiety state than of depression. Indeed, scores on the POMS depression scale remain normal. This reflects the less subtle wording of the POMS instrument, and emphasizes the tendency of postcoronary patients to deny both their disorder and their depression. Nevertheless, the abnormal scores of the POMS test all show substantial improvement over as little as a year of progressive training, and again there is some suggestion that this is linked to exercise compliance.

One final comment should be offered on the

dangers of symptom denial. Particularly in a "Type A", time-oriented individual, denial of symptoms may lead to a dangerous exceeding of exercise prescriptions. It is

thus important that exercise be performed initially under close supervision, so that the reactions of the patient to his or her prescription can be gauged accurately.

CORONARY BYPASS AND EXERCISE PRESCRIPTION IN ISCHEMIC HEART DISEASE

DHUN SETHNA, M.D.
JACK M. MATLOFF, M.D.
RICHARD J. GRAY, M.D.

A deconditioned state is virtually unavoidable after any major surgery, but particularly after cardiovascular surgery. Angina, dyspnea, and symptoms of lower extremity atherosclerosis often limit physical activity before operation in the patient presenting for coronary artery bypass surgery, for instance. The debilitating effects of the actual surgery, bed rest, and the metabolic demands of recuperation further depress the level of physical fitness. Decreased skeletal muscle mass, contractile strength, and efficiency are all associated with postoperative deconditioning.

Initial mobilization is frequently associated with a pronounced tachycardia and postural hypotension. This reflects a reduction of cardiac stroke volume (which may result from decreased venous return as well as poor cardiac function), hypovolemia, loss of normal vasomotor postural reflexes, and postoperative anemia. On occasion, plasma volume may be decreased more than red blood cell mass; the increase of blood viscosity, coupled with venous stasis created by bed rest, predisposes to thromboembolism.

Institution of physical training very early after coronary artery bypass surgery is not associated with increased morbidity or mortality. Rather, the duration of hospitalization is shortened, and increased functional capacity at the time of discharge results in an earlier and more complete resumption of normal activities.

INITIATION OF EXERCISE THERAPY

The patient who has undergone coronary bypass surgery with an uncomplicated preoperative and post-operative clinical course should begin activity 24 to 48 hours after surgery and occasionally while still in the cardiac surgical intensive care unit. An uncomplicated clinical course is one wherein the patient has no preoperative hemodynamic compromise or myocardial infarction. Furthermore, postoperatively there should be no significant dysrhythmia, hemodynamic instability, active

bleeding, or serious postoperative neurologic or pulmonary complication. The occurrence of an uncomplicated perioperative myocardial infarction need not alter the plan of early exercise therapy.

Most patients are extubated on the evening of surgery, or early the following day. On the first post-operative day, activity should approximate 1 to 2 met, that is, 1 to 2 times the resting metabolic rate (1 met is equivalent to an oxygen consumption of 3.5 ml/kg/min). Recommended activities include partial self-care (washing hands and face, brushing teeth), simple active and passive arm and leg movements, and active plantar and dorsiflexion of ankles several times a day. If the mediastinal chest tubes have been removed, the patient is encouraged to sit with the head of the bed raised to a 45-degree angle and with the trunk and arms supported by an overbed table. The patient should also dangle his or her legs on the side of the bed at least once on this day. Young and middle-aged otherwise healthy patients may be assisted to a bedside chair in the afternoon of the first postoperative day or may even be transferred from the intensive care unit by wheelchair to a monitored ward bed.

By the second postoperative morning, the patient is usually eating a soft diet by himself or herself, albeit quite shakily, and is assisted to a bedside chair. A bedside commode can be used at this time; indeed, the commode involves less energy expenditure and myocardial work than does the use of a bedpan. On transfer out of the intensive care unit, (usually 24 to 48 hours after surgery), some patients may walk around the room with the help of a nurse. At all times, the patient is monitored clinically and electrocardiographically, and the extent of ambulation is decreased if any of the following criteria are observed: (1) a heart rate greater than 120 beats per minute, (2) occurrence of a dysrhythmia or ST segment displacement, (3) decrease in systolic blood pressure, or (4) development of chest pain, fatigue, or dyspnea. The usual blood pressure response to exercise is an elevation of systolic pressure, and a fall of systolic pressure is evidence that cardiac output is not meeting the demands of exercise. Isometric maneuvers, which may elevate blood pressure and precipitate dysrhythmias, contribute little to cardiovascular conditioning and are strictly avoided.

PROGRESSIVE IN-HOSPITAL EXERCISE

The objective of rehabilitation after release from the intensive care unit is to develop a conditioning routine that will prepare the patient for complete self-care on discharge from the hospital. In general, low-intensity (2 to 3 met) isotonic calisthenics and exercises designated to maintain muscle tone, coordination, and joint mobility are initiated. At each stage of recovery, the level of activity chosen is one that can be performed without hazardous abnormal responses. A distinction between discomfort and pain must be appreciated by the patient, as incisional discomfort is unavoidable. Thoracic skeletal pain associated with normal postoperative convalescence can be quite remote from the sternum, involving in particular the axillary, lateral chest, dorsal and cervical spine, and shoulder areas. Rehabilitation is decreased or even discontinued temporarily if any of the criteria mentioned above are exceeded.

The patient should sit in a chair for all meals, frequently getting in and out of bed and standing up; walking (with assistance initially, as for all activity) is encouraged. Casual but routine walks with a nurse gradually supplement the calisthenics, and a walking program is initiated in the hospital corridors, wherein distance walked and pace are progressively increased. Frequent observation of vital signs determines when the pace may be increased and the distance extended. Assistance during walking is usually required for 48 hours (third to fifth postoperative day). Thereafter, the average patient should feel stable enough to walk alone or with a family member. By the sixth or seventh postoperative day, he or she should walk comfortably alone. When such a level of activity is achieved, the patient is often ready for discharge from the hospital.

PRE-DISCHARGE LOW-INTENSITY CARDIAC FUNCTION TESTING

A low-intensity treadmill test may be performed the day before hospital discharge. The test is explained in detail and an informed consent is signed. For morning tests breakfast is withheld, and for afternoon tests breakfast but not lunch is allowed, as ST or T wave changes may be associated with the postprandial state. A standard 12-lead ECG is recorded and blood pressures are obtained, ST segments, T waves, and cardiac rhythm being evaluated in the supine and standing positions, and during hyperventilation and Valsalva maneuvers. Treadmill exercise is then started at a low speed (2.7 km/h) and zero degree elevation (1.7 MET). The speed and/or the elevation are increased every 3 minutes, so that at successive stages the work rates are: 2.5, 3.4, 4.2, 5.4, and 6 to 7 METs. The speed may be held at 2.7 km/h and the elevation increased by 2 to 3 degrees per stage up to a maximum of 14 degree grade (6 to 7 METs). Alternatively, the speed may be increased at the first two stages to 4.0 km/h and 5.4 km/h respectively at zero grade; thereafter, speed is held to 5.4 km/h, but the grade is increased by 2 degrees per stage up to a maximum of 6 degrees grade (6 to 7 METs).

The test is stopped if the patient develops (1) symptoms of angina, excessive fatigue, dyspnea, or claudication, (2) a decrease in systolic blood pressure of more than 10 mmHg relative to the preceding pressure, (3) cardiac arrhythmias (significant supraventricular ectopics, salvos of 3 or more ventricular ectopic beats, Mobitz type 2 or third-degree heart block), (4) a target heart rate of 130 beats/min, or (5) the intended maximal exercise level (7 METs). Some investigators have advised continuation until other end points are reached; ST segment depression would be a relative indication for stopping the test. If a patient is receiving beta-adrenergic blocking medication, a target heart rate of 100 beats/min is often used.

A patient taking a cardioactive drug continues medication exactly as if he were at home. This is most important since one of the purposes of functional testing is to detect symptoms of cardiac decompensation or cardiac arrhythmia that might be dangerous if the same work rate were developed at home.

Low-intensity treadmill testing assesses postoperative functional capacity and allows a safe target heart rate to be determined. Each patient is instructed to measure his or her pulse before and after exercise. Should the measured pulse rate exceed the target figure, the patient is advised to decrease activity. Finally, the presence of exercise-induced arrhythmias or ischemia must be considered when making recommendations for continuing rehabilitation at home (Tab. 1).

POST-DISCHARGE PROGRAM

After discharge, the calisthenics initiated in the hospital are continued, with a progressive increase in the number of repetitions, the maximum number being attained by 4 to 6 weeks. Routine casual walking, both around the house and outside, is continued and progressively increased.

The patient is warned that swelling of the venous donor ankle may occur initially, and that this is not an indication for decreasing the level of activity. Leg elevation and occasionally elastic stockings are required to decrease ankle swelling. Muscle soreness and thoracic skeletal pain should have decreased appreciably at this stage of rehabilitation, and the patient should be able to undertake increasing amounts of exercise with better overall tolerance and less discomfort and fatigue.

If the patient encounters no shortness of breath, chest discomfort, or palpitations with this regimen, then approximately 2 weeks after surgery a program of sustained daily walking is initiated. Initially, 0.8 km is covered in 15 minutes. The distance is progressively increased, if well tolerated, to 1.6 km in 20 minutes, and then more gradually to 3.2 km in 45 minutes. By the end of 8 weeks the average, uncomplicated patient should be walking 4.8 km in one hour. Loose-fitting clothing and comfortable shoes are advised. Exercise should be avoided during extreme weather conditions (heat, cold, humidity, ozone alerts) and after meals. Fatigue is a desirable result of exercise, but exhaustion is to be avoided. The patient is instructed to stop the exercise program and consult a cardiologist if unusual discomfort

TABLE 1   Energy Cost of Common Activities

There are recommended activities at various MET levels. One MET is the resting energy expenditure (equivalent to an oxygen consumption of 3.5 ml/kg/min).

1–2 MET level

Reading
Letter writing
Playing cards and table games
Sedentary hobbies at table level
Hand sewing
Light desk work
Typing (electric)
Light dusting
Dressing
Shaving while sitting
Relaxing with immediate family
Slow walking on level at 1.6 km/h (fewer than 80 steps/min)
Exercises as prescribed by the therapists

3–4 MET level

All self-care
Work involving use of hands, standing and walking
Ironing
Use of washer and dryer with light loads
Making beds
Meal preparation
Auto driving (low-stress area)
Walking at 4.8 km/h (120 steps/min)
Exercise as prescribed by the therapists
In moderation:
   Dining out
   Religious services
   Movies
   Concerts
   Plays

2–3 MET level

Typing
Showering
Shampooing hair with assistance
Small home repairs
Playing piano
Peeling vegetables
Snack preparation
Washing small clothes by hand
Light polishing
Folding clothes
Having a few visitors in
Walking at 3.2 km/h (fewer than 100 steps/min)
Exercises as prescribed by the therapists

4–5 MET level

Mopping, cleaning windows
Vacuuming carpets
Light gardening
Carrying out garbage, using a dolly
Golf, using a cart
Bowling
Ballroom dancing
Swimming at 20 m/min
Normal social activities (e.g., entertaining, attending meetings)
Grocery shopping (avoid standing in lines and carrying
   heavy loads)
Walking at 5.6 km/h (more than 120 steps/min)
Walking up stairs slowly, pausing at each level

Remember to incorporate good body mechanics and apply energy conservation techniques with all activities. Always follow the guidelines for the home exercise program.

Source: Courtesy of Cedars-Sinai Medical Center, Los Angeles, California.

or stress occurs. Exercise is also to be avoided if the patient is ill or overly tired.

Considerable variation in exercise tolerance is seen, depending on preoperative status, sex, age, motivation, and the presence of associated disease. The exercise prescription must thus be individually tailored to clinical status and response; in general, if the duration of activity can be doubled or tripled at a given intensity without symptoms, progression to the next higher level of intensity is indicated. The response to an increased duration and frequency of activity may be monitored by the patient, based on the presence or absence of symptoms and the heart rate attained.

The eventual optimal exercise session consists of a warm-up period (10 minutes), a dynamic period during which the real training exercise is done (40 minutes), and a cooling down period (10 minutes). The warm-up period usually consists of calisthenics designed to stretch the major muscles and joints; this should always precede the dynamic interval. The dynamic interval comprises sustained walking, programmed to increase the heart rate to 70 to 85 percent of the measured maximum as determined by treadmill testing. The cool down period involves low-intensity exercise, allowing the heart rate to decrease slowly and preventing pooling of blood in the

legs; it avoids undesirable complications of abrupt stopping, such as syncope, light-headedness, nausea, or vomiting.

RETURNING TO WORK AND LIFETIME EXERCISE

Approximately 8 to 10 weeks after surgery, a submaximal (85% of predicted maximal heart rate) treadmill exercise may be performed. The results of this evaluation are used to further advise the patient regarding return to work and continuing exercise prescription. At this stage, physical function can be further enhanced by participation in individual or supervised community physical conditioning programs.

To maintain training, the exercise prescription should require (1) an intensity 70 to 80 percent of the maximum heart rate safely achieved at prior exercise stress testing, (2) a duration of 30 to 60 minutes per session, including warm-up and cooling down periods, and (3) a frequency of 3 to 4 times per week, preferably not on successive days. It is not known whether similar benefit could be obtained with a less prolonged or a less intense exercise training program. The patient is advised to work out at the same time and on the same days of the week in order to establish a routine. The level of exertion is increased only after appropriate testing, and if exercise is discontinued for 2 or more weeks, re-evaluation may be required.

Driving a car is acceptable after 6 weeks; the patient should drive on side streets for 2 weeks, and progress gradually to the main highways. A person who can walk at a speed of 4.8 km/h without difficulty or symptoms can return readily to most semi-sedentary occupations, which require an energy expenditure of 3 to 4 mets. Occupations demanding a higher energy expenditure call for more intense and prolonged training before return to work. Nevertheless, most patients can return to physically demanding work 2 months following bypass surgery, and work that requires less physical activity can be initiated whenever the patient is ready, as determined by a physician who knows the individual well.

SEXUAL ACTIVITY AFTER CORONARY ARTERY BYPASS SURGERY

Counseling regarding sexual activity is part of overall rehabilitation. It is a fair presumption that the postoperative patient has concerns about possible infarction or death during sexual activity. Such fears may be enhanced by vague statements or a total failure to discuss the topic. Myths about sudden death during sexual intercourse are widespread, and to a patient not properly informed, it may seem logical that sexual activity would stress the heart excessively.

Information on the physiologic demands of coitus after myocardial infarction indicates that work requirements during coitus are moderate, being in most instances less than the demands of daily work. Studies in which postinfarction patients wore Holter electrocardiogram (ECG) recorders during coitus with their spouses in a home setting showed that the average maximal heart rate at orgasm was 117 beats/min, with the average for 2 minutes before and 2 minutes after maximum being 97 beats/min. The maximal heart rate during work in these same patients averaged 120 beats/min. Activities inducing this heart rate included walking, climbing stairs, and doing paperwork. When exercised on a cycle ergometer within weeks of the sexual study, these same patients reproduced the peak coital heart rate at an oxygen consumption of only 15 ml/kg/min, suggesting that the energy requirements for coitus are modest.

Other studies involving the direct measurement of heart rate and blood pressure by automated devices in patients climbing two flights of stairs and during coitus in the home setting have confirmed the similarity of the double product (heart rate $\times$ blood pressure) for these two activities. Moreover, the double product during coitus remains the same regardless of the positions used by the couple. Thus, appropriate positioning should be a function of comfort rather than physiologic considerations.

Experience with postinfarction patients thus suggests that the majority of patients who have recovered from uncomplicated coronary bypass surgery should achieve an exercise capacity and an ischemic threshold that easily exceed the demands of coitus. Sexual activity can be resumed safely in the average patient who is walking distances of more than 3 km at a regular pace, without shortness of breath, palpitations, or chest pain. Since the heart rate during coitus and orgasm is usually less than 120 beats/min, exercise testing soon after coronary bypass surgery may provide information as to whether a given patient can attain a heart rate of 115 to 120 beats/min without symptoms. In suitable patients, the test is carried to a heart rate of 130 beats/min, or to an ischemic endpoint, either at the time of hospital discharge or within the next 4 weeks. Specific counseling on coital activity can then be provided. Given a good exercise capacity and no ischemic changes at a heart rate below 130 beats/min, sexual activity may be resumed in an unrestricted fashion.

The patient with severely limited exercise tolerance or a low ischemic threshold is told to avoid active participation in sexual behavior. The active role is delegated to the partner; further convalescence with retesting provides a scientific basis for determining the safety of progress from passive to active sexual involvement. If the ischemic threshold or the exercise capacity continues to be in a marginal range, the patient may be retested after taking a nitrate preparation and may be allowed to resume sexual activity with the use of this drug. Nitroglycerin taken approximately 15 minutes prior to coitus allows coital activity without pain or ECG evidence of ischemia.

Participation in an exercise training program has clinical and physiologic value as regards sexual activity. Patients who engage successfully in an exercise training program report fewer symptoms and have an increased coital frequency. Achievement of sexual gratification postoperatively often parallels the achievement of independence in regard to work. Since the goal of coronary bypass surgery is to allow a return to normal life, appropriate guidance in relation to physical activity is an important part of overall therapy.

Thoracic skeletal pain may be a major symptom experienced by the post-bypass patient on resumption of sexual activity. While the double product achieved during coitus is the same regardless of position, weight-bearing by the sternum should be avoided. On the average, it takes up to 12 weeks for good osseous healing of the sternum.

EXERCISE IN THE CONTROL OF HYPERTENSION

HEIKKI A. SALMI, M.D.

Physical exercise is often considered as a possible nonpharmacologic treatment modality in hypertension. Other possibilities include the reduction of excess body mass, restriction of salt intake, and avoidance or reduction of psychosocial stress. The long-term results of "weight reduction" programs are poor, even if the immediate results are promising. Limitation of sodium ingestion is also difficult under urban living conditions, where a major part of the diet is industrially produced. The reduction of psychosocial stress often remains an unrealistic wish, because in practice the patient is unable to change his or her way of life. Commitments to the working community, career, and family are stronger than the doctor's orders to relieve the burden of a hectic life style. Thus, physical exercise is often a good alternative therapy, although it is not universally applicable. Physical exercise can also be used as an adjunct to "weight reduction" programs.

The most crucial question the clinician must answer is: Does my patient need drug therapy for an elevated blood pressure? The modern concept is that blood pressure levels are distributed in a continuous fashion across the community. Hence, there is no clear-cut threshold between normotension and hypertension; high blood pressure is more truly a risk factor than a disease. In practice, there is a broad gray area, where we do not know whether we should start drug treatment and the patient does not know whether it is acceptable. In deciding whether to use drugs in treating a patient with mild hypertension, there still are no strict rules, although the newest epidemiologic studies favor a more active pharmaceutical treatment than was previously accepted.

Many patients today have a tablet resentment syndrome, and immediate commencement of drug treatment is not the best solution, since many patients will not comply with therapy. Even if drug treatment is the therapy of choice according to our criteria, the patients concerned need a "brain wash" period to be psychologically prepared and motivated to accept continuous drug therapy for what may be a symptom-free long-term disease. A similar reasoning applies to the doctor, who is not always quite sure whether continuous drug treatment should be initiated. The response to this dilemma is a nonpharmacologic treatment, which in many instances, can take the form of physical exercise. The aspect of active participation is important for many patients whose attitude toward life is aggressive. They are not content with passive observation of blood pressure values, but insist on doing something themselves to correct the situation. This type of personality is common in Western societies. Active physical exercise provides a suitable outlet for such individuals to achieve a feeling that they have done all they can to avoid the feared drug treatment. The psychologic motivation to start pharma-

ceutical treatment is then in place and when the moment the doctor already knew in the beginning has come: initiation of drug therapy.

Physical exercise can also be used as an adjunct to drug therapy. However, this can create a new set of problems, because not all hypotensive drugs are suited for use with physical exertion.

THE PHYSIOLOGIC BASE

Most investigators agree that normal blood pressure is not reduced as a result of physical exercise. However, the practicing clinician is more interested in results with hypertensive persons.

The classification of hypertension is as follows: (1) the initial phase of hypertensive disease—latent, marginal, labile, or borderline hypertension, and (2) the later phase of hypertensive disease—fixed or established hypertension. According to this concept, the typical characteristic of (1) is a hyperkinetic circulation, while that of (2) is an increased peripheral resistance. The validity of this hemodynamic concept has recently been challenged. For practical purposes it might possibly be more correct to speak about mild and severe hypertensive disease, without any consideration of differences in hemodynamics.

MILD HYPERTENSION

Physical exercise increases both systolic and diastolic blood pressures during activity. The increase depends on the intensity of exercise and is usually greater in hypertensive persons than in normotensive individuals. The hypertensive reaction to any given absolute intensity of exercise is decreased by training. The clinician is interested in the effects of training on the blood pressure at rest because he employs physical training as a treatment modality instead of, or in addition to, drugs.

The blood pressure lowering effect seems most clear-cut in the initial labile phase of hypertensive disease. The hyperkinetic stage of hemodynamics, which is peculiar to the initial phase of hypertensive disease, seems to react relatively well to physical exercise. The predominant hemodynamic features are increased heart rate and increased cardiac output at rest. Logically, the treatment of choice would lower both heart rate and cardiac output as, for example, through a reduction of sympathetic tone and/or an increase of vagal tone. Since decrease of resting heart rate and of cardiac output are generally observed with the physical training of healthy individuals, physical conditioning might be expected to benefit subjects with early latent hypertension.

A summary of experimental studies and examples of the dosage of exercise adopted in labile hypertension are given in Table 1.

FIXED HYPERTENSION

The results in more advanced hypertensive disease are much worse or nonexistent. At this stage, a

TABLE 1 Physical training in mild hypertension — Some experimental results from the world literature

Subjects	Training description	Changes in hemodynamics	Changes in physical fitness
2 men (30-39 yrs) (+ 6 men with essential hypertension	1 hour *tiw* for 28 weeks — muscle flexibility, running, ball games	SAP, DAP decreased at rest, and during submax. exercise	$\dot{V}O_2$ ma increased from 2.1 to 2.9 1/min (or 41 ml/kg min)
37 men (+ 128 normotensive men)	3 h/wk — calisthenics, jogging volleyball, 10-15 min × 7/wk calisthenics at home 24 wks	SAP, DAP decreased at rest, during submax. exercise	PWC_{150} increased 18% (16% in normotensives)
5 men (26-38 yrs)	1 hour *tiw* for 6 weeks — cycle ergometer, peak HR 150-160 /min	Mean BP, HR, CO decreased at rest and during submax. exercise, a-v diff., total peripheral resist. unchanged at rest or during exercise	
7 men (23 yrs) (35 older healthy men, 5 older men with essential hypertension)	4-5 h/wk, 8-12 wks — calisthenics, swimming, running, games	SAP, DAP, HR unchanged at rest or during exercise	Initial $\dot{V}O_2$ max 36.3 ml/kg min, increased 33% (15% increase in normot., 8% increase in hypert., initial $\dot{V}O_2$ max lower)
27 obese women (37 yrs)	55 min *tiw* for 24 wks — jogging, calisthenics, cycle ergometer HR max minus 10-15 bpm	BP decreased at rest and during submax. exercise	HR decreased during submaximal work
88 patients	30 min daily for 28 days ergometer	SAP + DAP decreased in 42 percent of patients	
25 patients borderline hypertensive + 34 normotensives	50 min/*tiw* for 4 mos. — ergometer		$\dot{V}O_2$ increased significantly in trained hypertensives and normotensives

*Age either mean or range. Abbreviations: h = hour; wk = week; SAP = systolic arterial blood pressure: DAP = diastolic arterial blood pressure: BP = blood pressure; CO = cardiac coutput; $\dot{V}O_2$ max = maximal oxygen intake; PWC = physical working capacity at certain heart rate: HR: (bpm) = heart rate (beats/min): diff. = arteriovenous difference in blood oxygen concentration: total peripheral resist. = total peripheral resistance.

normokinetic resting circulation is typical. The most important aspect of pathophysiology is a permanently increased peripheral vascular resistance, due to structural vascular narrowing. Physical exercise decreases the peripheral resistance, but in practice its effect is not great enough to achieve a clinical response. Pooling detailed hemodynamic findings from several studies indicates that, if anything, the blood pressure at rest tends to be somewhat higher after training. Considering the theoretical possibilities for induction of a lasting blood pressure reduction, it also seems rather improbable that physical conditioning alone could induce hemodynamic changes of a magnitude that would lower the systemic blood pressure substantially. The results in the established phase of hypertensive disease are thus either negative or indeterminate.

A WHO expert group considered the effect of physical training alone to be of too little value to deserve further studies.

A summary of the experimental studies and examples of the dosage of exercise adopted in fixed hypertension are given in Table 2.

In general, it can be stated that physical exercise is less effective than antihypertensive drug treatment. However, physical exercise has indirect value as an adjuvant in the treatment of obesity; hypertension is strongly correlated with obesity.

HYPOTHESES ON THE MECHANISM OF ACTION OF EXERCISE

Psychic Relaxation. The mental relaxation induced by physical exercise is given as a possible explanation of any decrease in systemic pressure. The concept is diffuse, and research using the methods of biologically oriented medicine is difficult. The mechanism would be analogous to yoga, meditation, autogenic training, and psychotherapy, all of which have been tried in the treatment of arterial hypertension. Quantification and measurement are difficult not least because language and concepts differ from those conventionally used in exact sciences.

Lowering of Adrenergic Tone. The hemodynamic effects of endurance training correspond closely to the alterations achieved by sustained administration of beta-adrenoceptor blocking drugs. Very probably, the hemodynamic changes induced by physical exercise indicate a lowered adrenergic tone, that is to say, a physiologic beta-blockade. Thus, physical exercise causes an adaptation in both the central and peripheral sympathetic nervous systems.

A second typical characteristic of the labile hyperkinetic phase of hypertension is parasympathetic underactivity. Activation of vagal tone is a plausible explanation.

TABLE 2   Physical Training in Fixed Hypertension — Some Experimental Results from the World Literature*

Subjects	Training description	Changes in Hemodynamics	Changes in Physical Fitness
4 persons	35 min *tiw* — treadmill, HR >150 beats/min	BP unchanged at rest or during exercise	Submax. $\dot{V}O_2$ decreased
23 men (35–61 yrs) (+ 22 normotensive men)	45–55 min *biw* for 24 wks — walking-jogging HR: resting HR + 60–70% (max.-resting HR)	BP decreased at rest (DAP decreased in normotens.)	
10 men (48 yrs) WHO stage II	30 min × 5/wk for 4 wks — cycle ergometer HR: 120–140 beats/ min (=70% aerobic capac.)	BP at rest unchanged, BP during submax. exercise decreased; total peripheral resist. increased at rest	PWC increased 20% submax. $\dot{V}O_2$, HR decreased
10 men and women. WHO stage II, 6 training (44 yrs) 4 sedentary (47 yrs)	60 min *tiw* for 12 wks — calisthenics, walking-jogging, cycle ergometer 60–70% /$\dot{V}O_2$ max	BP unchanged (training, sedentary) BP unchanged during exerc.; a-v differ. increased during submax. exercise (training); total peripheral resist. increased at rest (training)	VO_2 max increased 13% in the training, 3% in the sedentary
30 women (30–69 yrs), WHO stage II	30 min *tiw* for 52 (–120) wks (after first 12 wks, 12 wks of detraining) — calisthenics, walking-jogging, cycle ergometer; HR 50% max HR (finally 75–85% during the last 52 wks)	BP decreased at rest, during submax. exercise	VO_2 max increased 26% (after 76 wks)

* For abbreviations, see Table 1

Peripheral Vasodilation.   There are experimental results indicating that the vasodilating effect of physical exercise results in a reduction of blood pressure. As stated above, the clinical effect in established hypertension is poor or nil. The reason for failure could be that organic alterations in the vasculature have occurred at this stage of the disease.

Altered Receptor Function.   As a result of physical exertion, baro/vascular/volume receptors might find a new level of function. The blood pressure regulating system in toto tries to find a new level, which it then seeks to maintain.

Improvement of neuromuscular relaxation.   This hypothesis is offered as a plausible explanation. The concept is unclear and diffuse and might perhaps be considered as a part of reduction of sympathetic overactivity.

Loss of Water and Electrolytes.   The idea has been advanced that prolonged strenuous exercise might cause fluid and electrolyte loss, establishing a chronic low-grade volume depletion corresponding to treatment with diuretics. It seems illogical, since there is substantial experimental evidence that training increases the circulating plasma volume.

Insulin-Sodium Reabsorption Blockade Mechanism. Physical exercise induces a decrease of plasma insulin levels, leading to a diminished tubular sodium reabsorption. Physical training results in a decrease in both fasting and stimulated plasma insulin concentrations, with an increase in the sensitivity of peripheral tissues to insulin action. It is not well understood how endurance training affects the action of insulin on the renal tubules, but it is possible that lower plasma insulin concentrations after

physical conditioning may diminish sodium retention and consequently reduce blood pressure. Frequent training sessions decrease both plasma insulin and glucose. They also increase blood levels of fatty acids, ketone bodies, and glucagon. The effect of repeated bouts of exercise is a decreased sodium retention and a fall in blood pressure.

Decreased Catecholamine Response.   Both plasma norepinephrine and epinephrine increase during exercise. Epinephrine secretion from the adrenal gland reflects blood glucose concentration. The plasma responses of catecholamines are lower in physically trained individuals than in the untrained. The result is a decrease in peripheral vascular resistance both at rest and during submaximal exercise. The catecholamine hypothesis is closely connected to theories of a lowered activation of the sympathetic nervous system and possibly the effective mechanism is the general theory of a decreased peripheral vascular resistance, already discussed.

Risks.   When prescribing exercise as a form of treatment, the physician must keep in mind that advantages and drawbacks have to be weighed in the same basic way as when prescribing drugs. In general, exercise is relatively harmless and free of side effects, and the physician should not induce unnecessary anxiety in the patient. However, the risk of a cardiovascular disaster should not be ignored. Patients with high initial blood pressure readings and cardiovascular complications are at particular risk. A sudden large rise of blood pressure may cause a vascular catastrophe or cardiac dysrhythmia, and it may precipitate angina or induce pulmonary edema due to the sudden rise of left ventricular end-diastolic pressure. Most antihypertensive drugs are incapable of preventing the transient rapid rise of blood pressure associated with isometric exercise. Isometric activities may induce very sharp and high transient peaks of blood pressure. Dynamic isotonic training increases blood pressure much less during physical activity.

Type of Exercise. Dynamic exercise (walking, jogging, cross-country skiing, biking, or rowing) is to be preferred to static isometric exercise (weight lifting, body building, wrestling). It is generally believed that the desired antihypertensive effect is achieved by dynamic but not by isometric exercise. In addition, isometric exercise can be harmful; in labile hypertension, static exercise increases the heart rate without altering peripheral resistance. On the contrary, in established hypertension the heart rate remains unchanged, while peripheral resistance increases strongly.

PHYSICAL EXERCISE IN PATIENTS RECEIVING ANTIHYPERTENSIVE DRUGS

Beta-blocking agents are the most common first antihypertensive drugs to be used in treating a young or middle-aged patient. Beta-blockade is a logical approach, especially in the initial labile and hyperkinetic phase of hypertension. The physical working capacity is reduced by the beta-blocking agent because it diminishes (1) the positive inotropic action of exercise upon the heart, (2) heart rate, (3) cardiac output, and (4) contractility of the heart muscle. Stroke volume is somewhat increased, but the heart rate is so markedly reduced that the end result is a decline of cardiac output. An increase of arteriovenous oxygen difference alleviates the situation to some extent. In addition to these central hemodynamic side effects, peripheral side effects are encountered: muscular weakness in the legs and a feeling of coldness in the digits. Several hypotheses on the pathomechanism of these phenomena have been proposed, both hemodynamic and metabolic.

Theoretically, beta-blockers with ISA (intrinsic sympathomimetic activity) and/or specific beta 1-blocking properties (cardioselective) are less harmful because peripheral hemodynamic and metabolic effects are milder.

Unfortunately, the degree of selectivity for the cardiac, or beta 1, receptor is insufficient to avoid a substantial degree of peripheral beta-blockade when higher doses are used. In addition, the central cardiac effect may be so strong that problems arise when an athlete uses a cardioselective beta-adrenergic blocking drug, despite the theoretical advantages of selectivity. The practical solution is to combine a beta-blocking agent with a diuretic and/or a vasodilator, thus reducing the dose of beta-blocker.

Diuretics are a suitable group of antihypertensive drugs to prescribe for athletes, if one keeps in mind their general side effects (e.g., hypokalemia). The reduction of circulating plasma volume is not harmful because endurance exercise will tend to restore plasma volume.

Peripheral vasodilators and alpha-receptor antagonists (hydralazine, dihydralazine, prazosin, minoxidil) are also suitable. Centrally acting alpha-agonists such as methyldopa and clonidine are well tolerated by athletes, but the general side effects must be kept in mind. Angiotensin converting-enzyme-inhibitors (captopril) are suited for use with physical exercise.

The norepinephrine-depleting agent, reserpine, does not interfere directly with physical exercise, but its general side effects and limited effectiveness have diminished its clinical use. Ganglion-blocking agents (for instance, guanethidine, bethanidine, debrisoquine, guanoxan) are the least acceptable group of antihypertensive medicines because of marked orthostatic side effects. Unpleasant and dangerous orthostatism is severely aggravated by physical stress. High ambient temperatures aggravate the situation, and a sudden circulatory collapse may result. A decrease of cerebral and cardiac perfusion and an increased risk of stroke and myocardial infarction have been demonstrated when physical exercise has been combined with use of these drugs.

PRACTICAL RECOMMENDATIONS

Evidence concerning the effect of physical exercise on blood pressure is far from unequivocal. Consequently, the patient cannot be given any firm promises as to the effectiveness of such treatment. In general, it seems less effective than drug therapy. However, many patients who, according to present criteria, have to be treated with hypotensive drugs need a "brain wash" period of psychological preparation for pharmacologic treatment. Because these patients anticipate that taking pills every day will cause a decline in the quality of their life, they try to find an alternative approach. Individuals with an active type of personality in particular, insist on doing something to resolve the problem themselves. Physical training is an active and aggressive approach suited to the needs of such patients.

Borderline and mild hypertensives benefit most from physical exercise, and this treatment is risk-free in them. The results in more advanced hypertensive disease are poor. The risks of cardiovascular disaster should not be ignored. Patients with more severe and long-lasting hypertension complicated with cardiovascular damage are vulnerable to cardiovascular disaster.

Physical exercise is also a useful adjunct in an obesity treatment program, hypertension being closely correlated with obesity. However, the decrease in blood pressure shown by mild hypertensives after physical training is independent of changes in body mass. On the other hand, several studies have shown large decreases of blood pressure when body mass is reduced by dieting without salt restriction.

Choice of the type of physical exercise can in general be left to the patient. However, dynamic isotonic training should be recommended. It must be stressed that isometric static exercise has no effect upon resting blood pressure and can be hazardous. It is useless and may even be harmful to prescribe physical training if the patient does not like it or does not have opportunity to carry it out. The "skipping" of a prescribed program induces anxiety. If the patient is allowed to choose the type of physical activity, adherence is better and there are less likely to be attacks of "bad conscience" when the program is neglected.

Available scientific information is insufficient to suggest an appropriate amount of exercise. Published training programs are too varied to give a firm scientific base to any recommendations (see Tables 1 and 2). One has to rely on generally accepted principles of exercise prescription.

The patient characteristics to be considered include age, primary physical condition, possible concomitant diseases, and possible end-organ damage caused by hypertension.

Exercise should be dynamic, loading large groups of muscles. Daily bouts of 10 minutes training at 70 percent of maximal oxygen intake induce measurable training effects over a few weeks. If the intensity is diminished, the duration of the training session must be prolonged. Most recent studies have shown that low-intensity activities such as walking can bring about considerable improvement of physical condition if a person is originally in poor physical shape. In practice, the best advice seems to undertake from half to one hour of training at a pulse rate of 70 percent of the age-predicted maximum two to three times per week.

Considering existing evidence on the risks of physical activity in relation to its intensity, it should be emphasized that "it is not the distance, but rather the speed that kills". An appropriate recommendation for the public at large is "walk for your health" rather than "run for your life".

SICKLE CELL ANEMIA AND EXERCISE

WILLIAM B. STRONG, M.D.

Sickle cell anemia was first described by Herrick in 1910. The gene frequency is approximately 8 percent in American blacks, with an autosomal pattern of inheritance. The disease, therefore, affects a large number of citizens of North America and is responsible for a significant number of lost school and work days as well as an extremely unfortunate derangement of health and lifestyle.

There is already a plethora of material devoted to the basic physiological disturbances, diagnosis, and treatment of patients with sickle cell disease (and trait). The purpose of the present chapter is to review the results of exercise testing in sickle cell patients, especially with regard to pediatric patients.

PHYSIOLOGY AND CLINICAL MANIFESTATIONS

Sickle cell disease is a clinical manifestation secondary to the substitution of valine in the number 6 position of the beta chain of hemoglobin. A variety of clinical effects arise from the sequestration and destruction of the affected erythrocytes.

The first and most important clinical manifestation is anemia which leads to a sustained increase in cardiac output when the hemoglobin is less than 8 g/dl, a typical figure encountered in sickle cell anemia. There is usually an elevation of stroke volume, but resting heart rate is either normal or only mildly elevated relative to age matched controls.

Although oxygen carrying capacity is reduced, there is not the decreased blood viscosity commonly seen in non-sickle cell anemias. However, there is a rightward shift of the oxyhemoglobin dissociation curve secondary to an increase of 2,3-DPG concentration; this serves to decrease the binding of O_2 and increases oxygen delivery at the tissue level.

Much attention has been paid to the possibility that the increased alveolar-arterial oxygen tension gradient found in sickle cell patients is due to ventilation/perfusion abnormalities secondary to erythrocyte sludging. Pulmonary hypertension has been found in only a small percentage of patients, but the majority show some cardiomegaly.

A search for a cardiomyopathy which would be characteristic of sickle cell disease has been singularly unrewarding. There has been no consistent microscopic evidence of ischemic myocardial injury on necropsy. Indeed, the primary causes of death in sickle cell patients are infection in children and renal failure in adults; at post-mortem, there is no evidence of arteritis or coronary thrombosis. Possibly, the high rate of flow induced by anemia moves the erythrocytes through the heart before sludging can occur.

The cardiovascular features of sickle cell patients are generally those of any long-standing anemia, but they appear earlier in sickle cell disease and are seen at higher levels of hemoglobin (8–10 g/dl) than in other forms of chronic anemia (7 g/dl). The physical examination almost always shows a hyperdynamic precordium and a nonspecific ejection murmur that is loudest at the upper left sternal border. There is frequently a third heart sound and accentuation of S_2. There is persistent expiratory splitting of S_2. This "fixed" splitting of S_2 and the increased pulmonary flow seen on x-ray examination has frequently led physicians to the incorrect diagnosis of atrial septal defect. The presence of hepatosplenomegaly is variable, depending on the degree of pulmonary congestion and whether or not the spleen has infarcted.

Routine ECG shows a pattern of nonspecific ventricular enlargement. A chest film may show infiltrates, scarring or atelectasis, and almost always cardiomegaly, with an increased pulmonary flow and an enlarged main pulmonary artery segment.

EXERCISE TESTING

The role of exercise testing in a clinical setting has been continuously expanding since the early testing of adults in the 1940s. Exercise testing has been quite helpful in demonstrating cardiovascular abnormalities in sickle cell patients. Nuclear imaging and echocardiography have both helped to delineate hemodynamic abnormalities in sickle cell patients.

The earliest exercise testing primarily used electrocardiography. The basic finding was, that with increasing levels of exercise, there was a gradual shift of the mean QRS vector to the right. Additionally, T-wave duration decreased, while T-wave amplitude initially decreased but then increased as maximal work rates were reached.

Subsequent work by Alpert, comparing 47 patients with sickle cell anemia and 170 healthy blacks, showed the patients to have higher resting heart rates than the controls. What is more, 15 percent of the sickle cell patients had definitely ischemic responses to exercise, with a lower maximum heart rate response. Another 34 percent of the sickle cell patients had equivocally ischemic responses to exercise, although their maximum heart rates were consistent with the control group. Thus, almost one-half of the sickle cell group had either definite or equivocal ischemic changes, while none of the control group had ischemic changes and only 2 percent had equivocal changes. The increase of resting heart rate in pediatric sickle cell patients is in contrast with findings in other forms of anemia, in which the resting heart rate is not significantly increased. It also contrasts with the normal heart rates seen by Miller in adult sickle cell patients.

Alpert further demonstrated that patients with sickle cell anemia had a decreased blood pressure response at maximal voluntary effort and a marked reduction of maximal work capacity when compared to controls. The ischemic group had the lowest maximal work capacity (and the lowest hemoglobin readings); the male ischemic group had a lower blood pressure response to exercise than did the female ischemic group.

The explanation for the ischemic response, the decreased rise of blood pressure, and the reduced working capacity probably lies in a limitation of oxygen transport to the myocardium. The already tenuous oxygen supply is taxed beyond the patient's ability to compensate during exercise. D.M. Miller has shown that by using a partial exchange transfusion, thereby increasing the oxygen carrying capacity of the blood (although not the hemoglobin level), maximal work levels were reached with a higher anaerobic threshold.

The echocardiogram is a tool which has become increasingly valuable. Gerry showed that although sickle cell patients had increased LV mass, LV systolic index, LV diastolic index, and stroke volume index, they did not demonstrate any significant differences in circumferential shortening, ejection fraction, or systolic time intervals. Rees studied children who had complaints of exertional dyspnea, showing a definite decrease in ejection fraction and shortening, with an increase in cardiac index. Balfour and Covitz used digitized echocardiography to show that ischemic sickle cell patients had a decreased rate of left ventricular filling. Arensman employed the same type of apparatus to demonstrate that sickle cell patients had a delay in attaining maximal free LV wall and septal thickness during systole. They also showed a delay in LV wall and septal thinning during diastole, leading to a decreased rate of LV filling. The patients with the most significant diastolic thinning were the ones who had the highest incidence of exercise intolerance and ischemic changes during stress testing.

Alpert performed exercise ergometry on 48 children with sickle cell trait. Lower values were shown for maximal heart rate and work rate, but blood pressure changes were normal. None of the patients had definite ischemic responses, but 8.3 percent had equivocal changes.

The exercise responses of patients with sickle cell disease apparently differ with age. It may be that those members of the pediatric group who develop significant cardiac dysfunction do not survive to adulthood. The role of exercise testing in management is increasing in importance, especially as a means of identifying candidates for partial exchange transfusions. Efforts are focused upon patients with ischemic exercise responses, and even younger patients with abnormal digitized echocardiographic measurements. Those patients who show equivocal responses can be followed to find out whether or not they progress to definite ischemia.

It seems likely that the role of exercise testing in assessing patients with cardiovascular dysfunction will continue to expand. Only one of my sickle cell patients, when exercised to maximum voluntary effort, has experienced a mild post-exercise crisis. Thus, I do not restrict youths with sickle cell disease from doing whatever they can. Realistic exercise prescriptions can be developed by exercise testing, although more research is needed to determine to what degree patients with sickle cell anemia can benefit from an increase of physical activity.

BLOOD DOPING AND PERFORMANCE

BJÖRN T. EKBLOM, M.D.

PHYSIOLOGIC BACKGROUND

Physical performance depends on many factors of which energy liberation, neuromuscular function, and psychologic factors are the most important. During heavy muscular work involving large muscle groups (tasks such as cross-country skiing or uphill running), maximal aerobic power is closely related to performance. But oxygen transport is also of importance in many other individual and team sports. In endurance events, local muscular factors such as glycogen content, muscle fiber distribution, or capillary density may also determine how long an individual can continue at a certain speed.

Maximal aerobic power is limited mainly by the product of cardiac output times arterial oxygen content. Maximal aerobic power is reduced after bloodletting and after exposure to altitude or carbon monoxide. Evidently, in such situations maximal cardiac output cannot be increased sufficiently to compensate for the reduced oxygen content of the arterial blood.

A few years ago the question was raised whether increasing the oxygen content of the arterial blood through an augmentation of hemoglobin concentration would increase maximal aerobic power and thus enhance physical performance. Alternatively, it was suggested that the increased viscosity, which would probably follow the increase of hemoglobin concentration, would reduce maximal cardiac output. Furthermore, doubts were expressed whether the peripheral muscles could increase their aerobic energy liberation and transfer if maximal aerobic power was increased. Studies were conducted in our laboratory to answer these problems. Well-trained physical education students with a maximal aerobic power between 50 and 65 ml/kg/min were used to ensure that repetition of the maximal exercise tests did not increase maximal aerobic power and performance.

After initial baseline tests, 800 or 1200 ml of whole blood was withdrawn and stored in a blood bank. Hemoglobin concentration fell as expected, with a parallel reduction of maximal aerobic power and physical performance. After 30 to 35 days, hemoglobin concentration was restored through normal erythropoiesis and maximal aerobic power and performance returned close to values obtained before the blood withdrawal.

At this point, the subjects were reinfused with their own red blood cells and tested again on the following day. Hemoglobin concentration and blood volume were increased, while the maximal cardiac output and the red cell 2–3 diphosphoglycerate were unchanged relative to either prebleeding or prereinfusion values. Maximal aerobic power and physical performance (the latter measured as the time to exhaustion at a standard maximal treadmill load) increased in all of the subjects tested.

The average increase of maximal aerobic power for the first 25 subjects tested in our laboratory following this procedure was close to 10 percent. Practical tests, such as work time on a cross-country track, showed a parallel improvement of performance, with a 10 to 15 percent reduction of times for a given distance. The enhanced maximal aerobic power and physical performance persisted from a few up to 14–18 days. The reason for interindividual discrepancies in this response is not known.

The magnitude of the increase in maximal aerobic power and physical performance cannot be applied directly to elite athletes, since so many factors are involved in high-level sports. But there is no doubt that the procedure described above will increase maximal aerobic power and improve physical performance even in a top-trained athlete, although the increase may be somewhat less in such individuals.

Thus the theory that an increase in the oxygen content of the arterial blood would increase maximal aerobic power and improve physical performance is valid. Our studies also showed some increase of blood viscosity due to the increased hemoglobin concentration, but this did not affect the cardiac "afterload," so that the maximal cardiac output remained unchanged. Furthermore, the working muscles were able to consume the increased delivery of oxygen "offered" by the arterial circulation. Some argue that the "overnight" improvement in performance is psychologic, which can be ruled out by the type of testing used; others believe that the increase of maximal aerobic power and performance is the result of repeated testing. The latter hypothesis can be ruled out by the fact that we used well-trained subjects who normally trained 4 to 6 days per week. Furthermore, a comparable effect has been seen in other studies using approximately the same methods and procedures.

So far, no studies have been reported on the effect of increasing the oxygen content of arterial blood upon the performance of physical exercise involving small muscle groups. Nor have there been any studies about possible effects on mental performance during physical exercise or upon performance in team sports.

It should be stressed that our experiments were never intended to be used in sports, either by us or by any other parties. The term "blood doping" for the increase of hemoglobin concentration induced by autoinfusion was introduced by the mass media. Some athletes now report using blood doping in sport events even at the Olympic level, a development which I certainly regret. As far as I know, no Swedish athletes have ever used this method in any sport event.

ETHICS

The transfusion of red blood cells (blood doping) to an athlete in connection with any competition is a violation of the rules of The International Olympic Committee. These state:

"Doping is defined as the administration or use of substances in any form alien to the body or of physiological substances in abnormal amounts and with abnormal methods by healthy persons with the exclusive aim of attaining an artificial and unfair increase in performance in sports."

In the case of blood doping, the substance—although the individual's own blood—is given by an abnormal means and often in an abnormal amount with the aim of increasing physical performance. Therefore there is no doubt that *this procedure must be regarded as doping*.

RISKS

Any medical treatment or physiologic procedure that involves venipuncture has some hazard for health.

This applies also to blood letting and subsequent reinfusion of one's own blood. Risks include allergic reactions and infections, although no side effects have been reported in any studies in which this method has been used to date.

DETECTION

So far, there is no practical method available to detect the use of blood doping. However, this does not necessarily imply that in the future methods may not be developed, especially if athletes will accept venipuncture as a part of the doping tests to which they must submit.

EXERCISE-INDUCED BRONCHIAL OBSTRUCTION

HERMAN J. NEIJENS, M.D., Ph.D.
ERIC J. DUIVERMAN, M.D.
KAREL F. KERREBIJN, M.D., Ph.D.

Asthmatic subjects may develop a bronchial obstructive reaction after exercise. This is usually called exercise-induced bronchial obstruction (EIB) or exercise-induced asthma.

The phenomenon occurs almost exclusively in asthmatic subjects. The prevalence of EIB seems relatively high in children with asthma as compared to adult patients. Our clinical impression is that EIB gives rise to an important part of the symptoms experienced by asthmatic children, especially around puberty. Many of such children are limited in both their daily activities and sports by the occurrence of EIB.

FORMS OF EIB

EIB follows various types of exercise, although running or cycling is generally the relevant activity in practice. Typically, a short period (5 to 8 minutes) of strenuous exercise results in shortness of breath, but the phenomenon may also become manifest after a longer period of exercise, depending on the intensity of work and the sensitivity of the patient. The symptom of dyspnea, regardless of severity, is usually most marked during the first 10 minutes after exercise, decreasing over the next 15 to 45 minutes. In contrast to the early reaction immediately after exercise, a delayed bronchial obstruc-

tive reaction has been observed recently; the latter is similar to delayed reactions in antigen-induced bronchial obstruction. The late type of reaction occurs 4 to 24 hours after exercise. Prolonged early reactions are also found occasionally. Delayed reactions are observed particularly in children, and they have clinical implications. An apparent spontaneous nocturnal exacerbation of asthma may be related to a bout of exercise that was undertaken several hours earlier.

The occurrence of EIB can often be determined from the history. It may also be ascertained by an exercise test in the laboratory or in a natural setting. A variety of factors influence the degree of bronchial obstruction after exercise (see causes). In the laboratory, the test exercise can be performed on a treadmill or a cycle ergometer; the heart rate should be brought to at least 90 percent of the age-related maximal value. The corresponding work rate is maintained for 6 to 8 minutes. The degree of bronchial obstruction is usually expressed as the difference in lung function before and after exercise. If the same exercise test is repeated within a couple of hours, the degree of bronchial obstruction after the second test is generally much lower or even nil when compared to that observed in the first test. The ability to induce the same amount of bronchial obstruction reappears after 2 hours, and it is nearly always fully restored within 4 hours. In essence, there is a refractory period of about 2 hours.

The severity of EIB varies greatly, both between patients and in the same patient at different times. An occasional patient develops serious, prolonged, and potentially life-threatening attacks of dyspnea, stridor, erythema, itching of the skin, angioedema, gastrointestinal colic, and headache. Such attacks are described as exercise-induced anaphylaxis. Exercise-induced anaphylaxis may occur only once in a life-time, but in some patients it recurs repeatedly.

EIB has to be distinguished from the post-exercise tachypnea seen in patients with restrictive pulmonary diseases. These latter abnormalities are important to recognize because such patients are at risk of hypoxia.

CAUSES OF EIB

A number of factors affect the response to exercise.

Amount of Metabolic Stress

Postexercise bronchial obstruction sharply increases with both the duration and the intensity of exercise. A plateau of response is reached between 60 and 85 percent of the maximal working capacity.

Type of Exercise

Free-range running reportedly causes more bronchial obstruction than the same intensity of treadmill running. Cycling induces a smaller drop in lung function than running, while walking and swimming are even less effective methods of revealing postexercise EIB. Sports such as swimming and rowing a kayak, which use primarily the arms, seem less likely to induce bronchial obstruction.

These differences in response were originally thought to reflect differences in the characteristics of the predominant muscle groups used for the various types of exercise. However, doubt about this explanation has been raised by several more recent studies. If the several types of exercise are carefully matched in terms of oxygen consumption, the differences in EIB disappear. A linear relationship exists between oxygen consumption and the muscle volume that is activated. Differences of EIB between the several kinds of sport and between persons of differing age and sex diminish markedly if a correction is applied for the muscle mass that is involved.

Temperature and Humidity of Inhaled Air

EIB is more severe if the air is dry than if it is humidified. Clinical observations on the importance of humidification have been confirmed in a climatic chamber, where exercise at a high relative humidity (90%) gave rise to a much smaller bronchial response than exercise at a low relative humidity (25%).

Nasal breathing virtually abolishes postexercise bronchial obstruction. This is due to the humidifying and heating capacity of the nose. An excellent relationship has been demonstrated between the temperature and the humidity of inspired air and the degree of bronchoconstriction that develops after exercise.

One study compared the importance of temperature and humidity. Heating the air from room to body temperature in itself had no marked effect upon the bronchial response. However, when the humidity was also increased, the degree of bronchial obstruction was diminished, and the changes of lung function were completely averted by inhaling fully saturated air at room temperature. It thus seems that the humidity of the inhaled air is more important than its temperature; temperature has a role mainly because a decrease of temperature leads to a diminution of water content.

By the time inspired air approaches the alveoli, it has become fully saturated with water vapor at body temperature. Heat and water vapor move from the bronchial mucosa to the incoming air, as a function of temperature and vapor pressure gradients and the geometry of the exchanging surface. Heating occurs by both conduction and convection. As the air is warmed, its capacity to hold water increases, and humidification occurs by evaporation from the surface of the airway mucosa.

The net effect is mucosal cooling and drying. This depends on (1) the temperature and water content of inspired air, (2) the intensity of ventilation, and (3) the duration of exposure. A combination of high levels of ventilation with relatively cold air surpasses the warming and humidifying capacity of the upper airways, challenging the deeper airways with cooling and drying. The decrease in temperature of the intrathoracic airways is confirmed by measurements made in the retrotracheal part of the esophagus; the extent of changes reflects the minute ventilation and is inversely related to the inspired temperature and water content. When inspiring air at $-17°C$ with moderate hyperventilation, a mean temperature of $20°C$ has been found in the trachea, and $27°C$ deep in the right lower lobe of the lung. This indicates that very cold air is needed to drop the temperature of the intrathoracic airways in the case of modest hyperventilation. However, with the more pronounced hyperventilation of heavy exercise, less cold and dry environmental air can induce a bronchial reaction; critical values are a temperature of less than $20°C$, and a water content below 30 mg/L.

Mechanisms of Bronchial Obstruction

Bronchial reactivity is a characteristic of asthma which can be quantified by testing the response of the bronchi to a standardized stimulus; for example, examining changes of lung function after the inhalation of histamine or metacholine. The degree of bronchial obstruction after exercise and the extent of the reaction after inhaled histamine appear to be related. This suggests that similar mechanisms are involved in the two reactions.

Since the severity of asthma is related to bronchial reactivity, which in turn is related to EIB, the complaints caused by EIB are more intense among those with severe asthma. Considerable variation in the severity of EIB may occur over the year, corresponding to seasonal remissions and exacerbations of asthmatic symptoms. The variation of EIB probably reflects changes in airway reactivity to histamine or metacholine. The presence of a viral respiratory tract infection or a recent vaccination against influenza can increase the severity of EIB. Indeed, any factor that increases the reactivity of the respiratory tree accentuates the response to exercise. The biologic significance of EIB may be a protection of the lung against excessive heat and water loss. An increase in airway resistance decreases ventilation and hence thermal demands. Why asthmatics respond more intensely than healthy individuals is not completely known, but it may represent no more than the heightened airway reactivity of asthma. Parts of the bronchial mechanism contributing to an exaggerated bronchial reaction include the status of the mucosa (increased permeability or sensitivity to physical chemical changes), the parasympathetic nervous system, the mast cells (more ready release of histamine), and possibly other factors. Information about such disturbances is important to a rational plan for the prevention of EIB.

PREVENTION AND TREATMENT
General Advice

The following actions are currently recommended to combat EIB. Based on the information about airway drying and cooling, the patient is advised to inspire through the nose. If the nose is seriously obstructed, reasons for this disturbance should be examined. Mucosal swelling can often be treated with drugs, whereas anatomic abnormalities such as deviations of the septum or polyps may require surgical correction. Gymnasiums should provide an atmosphere with optimal temperature and humidity.

One can further advise an asthmatic patient to increase running speed gradually. In this manner, pronounced bronchial obstruction is avoided and a refractory situation is created (in effect "running through one's asthma").

Certain sports are more acceptable than others. Swimming, wrestling, sprinting, and team sports in which running is of short duration are usually well tolerated. Cold-weather sports, however, are often more difficult for asthmatics than for healthy children. Downhill skiing is often well tolerated, and the same is true of activities in warm and moist air (particularly indoor swimming).

Prophylaxis

Proper medication, taken prior to exercise, allows most asthmatic children to participate in nearly all sporting events. A number of drugs are effective. Their potency in a given individual can be tested by measuring the exercise reaction with and without administration of a given agent. Atropine and related parasympathetic blocking agents may protect against EIB if administered by aerosol. Results vary from no effect to partial protection. Better protection is usually seen after inhalation of disodium cromoglycate (Lomudal). Beta-sympathetic agonists are highly effective in most patients when given by aerosol, but oral preparations have variable and less pronounced effects.

Xanthine derivatives, such as aminophylline and theophylline, also offer protection, but for a reasonable result a serum level of at least 10 g/L is needed. Calcium blockers have only a slight protective effect. However, future developments may yield more specific calcium blockers for the bronchi. Oral or inhaled corticosteroids have little immediate value against EIB.

Adequate protection sometimes requires careful titration of optimal dosage for an individual drug or a combination of drugs.

The therapeutic effectiveness of drugs in EIB can be summarized as follows: usually, beta-sympathetic agonists are the most effective, while parasympathetic antagonists are the least effective. Disodium cromoglycate has an intermediate effect and is of sufficient potency for the majority of patients. Since disodium cromoglycate is still without observed side effects after 15 years of experience, it is an important drug for the prevention of bronchial reactions during sports. Many asthmatic children with EIB can participate in sports if they take disodium cromoglycate before a game; the dose may need to be repeated after one or more hours. If disodium cromoglycate does not offer sufficient protection, the inhalation of a beta-sympathetic agonist may be considered, but too frequent use (an arbitrary ceiling of more than 2 puffs per 4 hour) may result in complications, such as tremor or tachycardia.

A well-adjusted plan of treatment is, for many asthmatic patients, essential to the performance of daily activities, sports participation, and maintenance of physical condition.

VALUE OF EXERCISE IN ASTHMA

Exercise can benefit most children, including those with EIB. Before starting a training program, one must identify those children with other lung diseases and disturbances through a careful clinical examination and appropriate exercise tests.

Physical training should be individually tailored, to allow children to realize their potential irrespective of initial physical conditions. The effect of training upon asthmatics is mainly confined to an improvement of fitness. Variables such as ventilatory muscle performance and circulatory adaptations to effort may be improved with training. Psychologic encouragement probably also makes an important contribution to the subjective gains often reported after training. Sports participation improves general well-being as well as fitness, with good effects upon an asthmatic subject. Exercise tolerance may be increased because of a lesser hyperpnoea at any given level of oxygen consumption in a fit person compared to someone who is unfit. In consequence, low levels of physical activity can be performed without respiratory distress, and less medication may be needed to control EIB. On the other hand, there are no important changes of lung function or liability to EIB. Nevertheless, the patient can avoid EIB and undertake a training program by following the regimen described in the previous paragraphs.

EXERCISE IN CYSTIC FIBROSIS

GERARD J. CANNY, M.B., F.R.C.P.(C)
ROBERT K. GRISDALE, B.A.
JACQUES E. MARCOTTE, M.D., F.R.C.P.(C)
HENRY LEVISON, M.D., F.R.C.P.(C)

Although cystic fibrosis is a multisystem disease, most of the morbidity and almost all of the mortality are attributed to progressive lung disease. Pulmonary disability in cystic fibrosis results from bronchial obstruction, which is initially confined to small airways, but involves progressively larger airways as the disease advances. This airway obstruction arises from blockage by mucopurulent secretions and thickening of the airway walls as a result of squamous metaplasia, glandular hypertrophy, and eventually bronchiectasis. Mismatch between alveolar ventilation ($\dot{V}_A$) and perfusion ($\dot{Q}$) occurs and results in abnormal gas exchange. Thus, early in the course of the disease, mild hypoxemia and a widening of the alveolar-arterial oxygen difference may occur in the absence of other abnormalities of pulmonary function. Advanced disease is characterized by chronic airflow limitation, severe hypoxemia, pulmonary hypertension, and cor pulmonale.

Progression of lung disease in cystic fibrosis often results in a reduced capacity for physical activity, and this in turn can affect patients' life style, self-esteem, and employment opportunities. In recent years, research from several laboratories has increased our understanding of the physiologic mechanisms for effort intolerance in cystic fibrosis. This information has provided a scientific basis for the management of patients through exercise prescription, vocational counseling, and evaluation of treatment.

EXERCISE LIMITATIONS IN CYSTIC FIBROSIS

Several investigators have shown that cystic fibrosis patients retain a remarkable ability to exercise in spite of significant degrees of lung disease. In general, however, exercise tolerance correlates with clinical status and abnormalities of lung function. The severity of airway obstruction is thought to play a major role in limiting exercise tolerance in the disease. Airway obstruction limits ventilatory capacity. In addition, ventilatory requirements are increased in cystic fibrosis as a result of enlarged physiologic dead space and hypoxemia. During exercise, therefore, patients with cystic fibrosis tend to maintain a high minute ventilation ($\dot{V}_E$), as compared to normal subjects, resulting in a high ventilatory equivalent for oxygen ($\dot{V}_E/\dot{V}_{O_2}$). The ventilation at maximal exercise, particularly in more disabled patients, may approach or exceed the estimated maximum voluntary ventilation (MVV), indicating that a ventilatory limit has been reached. By contrast, normal subjects reach maximal exercise with a considerable ventilatory reserve ($\dot{V}_E$ at maximum work level is seldom greater than 70 percent MVV).

The ability of some patients with cystic fibrosis to achieve levels of ventilation in excess of MVV during exercise reflects a form of bronchial lability, unique to the disease. Several studies have shown that patients with cystic fibrosis may experience dramatic increases in peak flow rates during exercise and only minimal bronchoconstriction following exercise. This bronchial lability is due mainly to flow transients which result in higher peak flow rates.

Major alterations in arterial blood gases from resting levels are not generally seen during exercise in cystic fibrosis. The majority of patients are able to maintain arterial oxygen pressures (PaO_2) during exercise as a result of an improvement in $\dot{V}_A/\dot{Q}$ distribution which reduces venous admixture ($\dot{Q}va/\dot{Q}t$). Similarly, the increased minute ventilation seen during exercise allows these patients to compensate for increased dead space, thus maintaining adequate alveolar ventilation and preventing CO_2 retention. In patients with advanced lung disease, however, these compensatory mechanisms may not be adequate. Significant venous admixture may persist, and alveolar hypoventilation may develop during exercise, resulting in arterial oxygen desaturation and CO_2 retention. Unfortunately, patients who develop blood gas abnormalities during exercise cannot be identified from resting pulmonary function tests. Exercise testing should, therefore, be mandatory for patients with advanced lung disease before commencing a reconditioning program.

Respiratory muscle fatigue may also contribute to exercise limitation in cystic fibrosis. A number of factors compromise inspiratory muscle function, particularly that of the diaphragm, as the disease progresses. As a result of chronic hyperinflation, the inspiratory muscles are shortened and forced to operate on an inefficient portion of their length-tension curve. Extreme hyperinflation of the lungs also increases the radius of curvature of the diaphragm and curtails its ability to generate inspiratory pressure. In addition, the reduction in lung compliance that accompanies air trapping substantially increases the work of breathing through its detrimental effect on the pressure/volume relationship of the lung. Hypoxemia and malnutrition, common features of cystic fibrosis, can also have a deleterious effect on diaphragmatic strength and endurance. During exercise, therefore, when ventilatory requirements are particularly high, the impaired status of the inspiratory muscles may contribute, in varying degrees, to exercise limitation. Although diaphragmatic fatigue is not implicated in exercise limitation in normal subjects, one study has shown electromyographic patterns suggestive of fatigue in the inspiratory muscles of patients with cystic fibrosis while they are performing exhausting work.

In contrast, cardiovascular factors appear to play a relatively minor role in limiting exercise tolerance in cystic fibrosis. Cardiac output, at rest and during exercise, remains normal until the preterminal stage of the disease, when right ventricular failure commonly occurs. Although patients with advanced lung disease tend to have higher heart rates than normal patients at comparable work loads, they invariably fail to achieve predicted peak heart rates, suggesting that exercise is interrupted before the cardiovascular system becomes maximally stressed. The increase of cardiac output during exercise in patients with advanced disease is generated primarily by an increase of heart rate rather than an increase of stroke volume. This impaired cardiac response to exercise in patients with advanced disease has been confirmed by radionuclide techniques. The right ventricular ejection fraction either may fail to show an appropriate increase or may even decrease on exercise, presumably owing to increased afterload on the right ventricle. Similarly, left ventricular dysfunction during exercise has been demonstrated by these techniques in a minority of patients. The cause of the impaired left ventricular function is controversial. The most likely factors are (1) an increased afterload on the left ventricle as a result of abnormal swings in intrapleural pressure during exercise, and (2) impaired filling and emptying of the left ventricle due to compression by an enlarged right ventricle.

In conclusion, exercise tolerance in cystic fibrosis, although practically normal in mildly affected patients, becomes progressively more limited as the disease advances. Although abnormalities of cardiac function are seen in some patients during exercise, the major mechanisms responsible for exercise intolerance are related to the underlying pulmonary pathophysiology and include mechanical factors, ventilatory inefficiency, gas exchange abnormalities, and possibly fatigue of the respiratory muscles.

PHYSICAL REHABILITATION IN CYSTIC FIBROSIS

Respiratory Muscle Training

Since cystic fibrosis increases the work of breathing while diminishing the effectiveness of the respiratory muscles to perform work, it is conceivable that ventilatory muscle training could improve exercise tolerance in the disease. Previous work from our laboratory has shown that specific ventilatory muscle endurance training (maximal normocapnic hyperventilation for 25 minutes per day, 5 days per week) does increase maximum sustained ventilatory capacity (MSVC), thus allowing an increase in the minute ventilation potentially available during exercise. Similarly, inspiratory muscle training using a resistive load (15 minutes twice daily) improves both ventilatory muscle strength and endurance in the disease. It is possible that the improved respiratory muscle function achieved by the above techniques may, in some patients, delay the onset of inspiratory muscle fatigue and thus improve exercise tolerance. Furthermore, the improved respiratory muscle function should in turn help patients to cope with the added respiratory load during an acute exacerbation of their lung disease.

Specific ventilatory muscle training programs are rather tedious, and deconditioning occurs rapidly when training is discontinued. Fortunately, respiratory muscle function can be improved equally well by conventional physical training. Two independent studies have shown that programs consisting of swimming/canoeing and running enhance respiratory muscle endurance in patients with cystic fibrosis. Participation in appropriate exercise programs appears therefore to be a more practical way of maintaining ventilatory muscle endurance in patients with cystic fibrosis.

Aerobic Exercise Training

Physical training programs are widely used for rehabilitation of adult patients with chronic lung diseases. Although the exercise tolerance of these patients can be extended by training regimens, little agreement exists as to the mechanisms responsible for this improvement. Pulmonary function tests and arterial blood gases remain essentially unaltered with training. Likewise, a training bradycardia has not been consistently observed in the studies reported to date. Some investigators have noted a reduction in ventilatory requirements at equivalent work loads after training, but this change is most likely due to improved neuromuscular coordination. Much of the improvement in exercise tolerance after training is undoubtedly due to subjective factors, such as increased confidence, motivation, and tolerance to the sensation of dyspnea on the part of the patient. However, this should not detract from the potential value of exercise programs in rehabilitating patients with chronic lung diseases.

Although medical personnel have intuitively recommended that patients with cystic fibrosis lead active lives, the physiologic effects of exercise programs on the course of the disease have only recently been examined. One controlled trial demonstrated the benefits of an intensive running program. After 3 months of training, the exercise group had significantly increased exercise tolerance and peak oxygen consumption, while a training bradycardia indicated increased cardiovascular fitness. No improvement in lung function, however, was observed after training. Exercise has also been shown to increase mucus clearance in the disease, but no data exist as to whether a training program can replace conventional chest physiotherapy in the form of postural drainage with percussion and vibration.

Implementation of Training

In patients with cystic fibrosis, long-term training programs obviously need to be tailored to the individual's physical capability and should take into account the degree of respiratory disability as assessed clinically, through pulmonary function tests, and by graded exercise testing if necessary. Patients with mild-to-moderate lung disease should be encouraged to participate in aerobic endurance exercises which will promote and maintain cardiovascular fitness. Suitable examples include swimming, jogging, cycling, and cross-country skiing. Patients should exercise at least 20 to 30 minutes a day, 3 to 5 days a week. Activities requiring effort against resistance, e.g., weight-lifting, while doing little to improve cardiovascular fitness, should not be discouraged, but rather included in a combined cardiovascular and strength training regimen.

Debilitated patients with advanced lung disease require an individualized exercise program. Ideally, the exercise prescription for such patients should be based on the findings of a progressive exercise test. In this way the patient's exercise tolerance (Wmax) and maximal attainable heart rate can be determined. In addition, by monitoring transcutaneous oxygen saturation during the test, patients who desaturate during exercise can be identified. Graded treadmill walking or bicycle ergometer exercise is usually preferred in the initial stage of rehabilitation. The exercise program should begin with a low-intensity exercise, and as exercise tolerance improves, the training level can be gradually increased toward a target intensity at which 70 to 80 percent of maximal heart rate, as determined by initial testing, can be maintained for a 20 to 30 minute exercise session. Each training session should be divided into a warm-up period of 5 to 10 minutes, at least 15 minutes of continuous exercise, and then a 5 to 10 minute cool-down period. Patients should exercise at least 3 to 5 times weekly with no more than 2 days between workouts. As soon as a satisfactory level of cardiovascular fitness is attained, the program should be adapted to include less formalized activities for continued use at home. It should be emphasized that fitness rapidly deteriorates when exercise is stopped. Thus, maintenance of fitness requires a life-time commitment to an exercise program.

ADJUNCTS TO REHABILITATION

Supplemental Oxygen During Exercise

In adult patients with chronic obstructive pulmonary disease, supplemental oxygen therapy during exercise can improve exercise endurance at submaximal work loads. The role of oxygen therapy during exercise in cystic fibrosis has not been studied, and no guidelines exist as to when oxygen should be used. Supplementary oxygen during exercise should certainly be considered for patients with severe hypoxemia at rest or for patients who develop marked arterial oxygen desaturation on exercise.

Possible explanations for improved exercise endurance while breathing supplementary oxygen in patients with chronic lung diseases include a reduction in the ventilatory cost of exercise, improved respiratory muscle endurance, and possible relief of pulmonary hypertension.

Pharmacologic Intervention

Oral theophylline improves effort tolerance in chronic obstructive lung disease. This improvement may, to a large extent, reflect the direct effect of the drug on diaphragmatic contractility, rendering it less susceptible to fatigue. Digoxin, on the other hand, does not increase the maximum exercise capability of patients with cystic fibrosis. The effect of pulmonary hypotensive agents on exercise tolerance in cystic fibrosis has not been delineated.

Assisted Ventilation

Recent work in adult patients with chronic obstructive pulmonary disease has shown that some patients with advanced disease develop respiratory muscle atrophy, leading to fatigue and chronic hypercapnia. As the respiratory muscles of these patients are already overburdened, even at rest, exercise rehabilitation is unlikely to be successful and may cause further damage to the muscle fibers. Resting the respiratory muscles of such patients by nocturnal negative pressure ventilation can improve respiratory muscle function, and this seems preferable to aggressive exercise training. It remains to be determined whether patients with advanced cystic fibrosis will respond to such resting programs, and if so, whether rest vis-a-vis exercise training is the more appropriate form of treatment for a given patient.

IMPACT ON PROGNOSIS

The majority of cystic fibrosis patients can be expected to benefit from an exercise program in terms of increased exercise tolerance and ventilatory muscle endurance. The increased exercise tolerance should in turn help patients to cope with the activities of daily living and thus improve self-esteem and general well-being. Exercise training will not improve pulmonary function. However, the unrelenting pulmonary deterioration which characterizes the disease may be attenuated by exercise training. If this speculation proves correct, continued participation in exercise programs should improve the long-term prognosis for patients with cystic fibrosis.

EXERCISE IN CHRONIC OBSTRUCTIVE LUNG DISEASE

ANTHONY S. REBUCK, M.D., M.B., B.S.,
F.A.C.P., F.C.C.P., F.R.C.P.(C)
ANTHONY D. D'URZO, B.P.H.E.
KENNETH R. CHAPMAN, M.D., M.Sc.,
F.R.C.P.(C), F.C.C.P.

MECHANISMS OF DYSPNEA

The act of breathing comprises a series of rhythmic "voluntary" muscular contractions that are maintained through sleep and unconsciousness. It requires only a minor shift in attention for a person to become aware of his breathing and of its rate and depth. When the awareness of breathing becomes excessive or the act uncomfortable, one is said to be dyspneic. Dyspnea can be induced in several ways, but the unifying feature is the force generated by the respiratory muscles. The relationship between this force and the resultant volume change depends upon the elastic and resistive properties of the respiratory system, more force being required when the mechanical properties are disrupted by disease. Dyspnea can arise when an increased force evokes a conscious response, when the respiratory muscles are weakened or fatigued, or when a subject with a healthy ventilatory pump is stimulated to increase the rate or depth of breathing. Quantitatively, the most demanding of these stimuli is exercise, but the manner in which it is perceived is influenced not only by the intensity of exercise, but also by the psychophysical discrimination of the subject.

The sensory impression of dyspnea depends upon the relationship between the stimuli generated by exercise and the evoked conscious response. Before experiencing dyspnea, one must *detect* a stimulus. One must then *discriminate* the altered physiology from the normal stable condition, and *recognize* the sensation for what it is, before embarking on the process of *scaling* its intensity. The basic respiratory sensations perceived by the exercising subject derive from vagally mediated stretch receptors, joint receptors, and muscle spindles in the chest. The relationship between subjective sensation and the volume changes induced by both inspiratory and expiratory muscles is best described by a power function. However, force or effort provides an important input to the perception of volume change in the respiratory system; as respiratory muscles fatigue, the sense of effort continues to increase.

Patients with airflow obstruction complain of breathlessness on exertion and have a limited exercise capacity. An important distinction must be drawn between the exercising asthmatic and the patient with chronic airway obstruction. The flow limitation of the asthmatic changes as a result of the exercise itself. Expiratory flow rates usually increase during the first few minutes of exercise, but as exercise continues, respiratory function begins to deteriorate. Soon after quitting, the asthmatic usually experiences a transient, self-limited increase of bronchoconstriction. By contrast, in chronic obstructive lung disease (COPD), the abnormalities of lung mechanics prevent ventilation from meeting the metabolic demands of work. Even though airway obstruction does not develop during exercise in these patients, flow limitation does increase.

During exercise, patients with chronic airflow obstruction are more dyspneic than normal subjects at comparable levels of ventilation. The maximum levels of ventilation are determined by the maximal force the patient can maintain without fatigue and by the impedance of the respiratory system. As the force required of the inspiratory muscles is directly related to impedance, impedance must determine much of the respiratory distress during exercise. In "loaded breathing" studies, healthy subjects have been asked to exercise while breathing through narrow tubes or resistances in order to simulate the impedance experienced by patients. The resultant impaired exercise performance adds weight to the argument that the reduction of ventilatory capacity dominates the reduction in maximum power output.

Even though mechanical loads accurately mimic the ventilatory patterns seen in patients, they fail to explain the differences in respiratory distress reported by some patients at comparable levels of airway obstruction. Some patients ("fighters" or pink-puffers) complain of more dyspnea than others ("nonfighters" or blue-bloaters). With the current popularity for personality testing as an adjunct to physiologic measurement, and of psychophysics for quantifying input and output variables, it is tempting to offer a behavioral explanation for the differences between fighters and nonfighters. However, a difference of pathologic process is more likely. Type A, the fighters, have large lungs, a loss of lung elastic recoil, a reduced surface area for gas exchange and, until late in the disease, adequate alveolar ventilation at rest. Hence, a normal arterial Pco_2 is characteristic of dyspneic patients with emphysema. By contrast, type B, the chronic bronchitic nonfighters, have smaller lungs, much of which are composed of well-perfused but poorly ventilated "slow spaces". Resting hypercapnia, hypoxemia, and cardiac failure are frequent in such patients. The emphysematous patient with an $FEV_{1.0}$ equal to that of a chronic bronchitic will invariably experience more exercise dyspnea than the latter. Such a person has, or is likely to have, a higher alveolar ventilation, a lower arterial Pco_2, and little or no change of venous admixture during exercise. The bronchitic, on the other hand, is likely to improve gas exchange, increases in tidal volume reducing regional inequalities of alveolar ventilation. As airway obstruction becomes more severe, end-expiratory lung volume increases. Inspiratory muscle length then inevitably shortens, forcing the muscles to work at a mechanical disadvantage, so that for a given impedance, it becomes likely that the sense of effort would increase.

From these arguments, the term "chronic airway obstruction" is inadequate to describe the various subtypes of respiratory disorder covered by this blanket term. In order to understand the exercise limitation and resultant dyspnea, it is necessary to go beyond a simple measure of airway resistance or resting expiratory flow rates. Dyspnea during exercise results from a quantitative disturbance of the sense of respiratory load. In order to appreciate the differences experienced among asthmatics, bronchitics, and emphysematous patients, it is necessary to record the effect of exercise on their respiratory impedance, and to quantify the impedance in terms of the lung volume changes that accompany it.

INITIAL EFFORT TOLERANCE

Shortness of breath and effort intolerance are major symptoms in patients with COPD, regardless of whether they are classified as type A (emphysematous) or type B (bronchitic). In the latter, exercise capacity is limited primarily by an inability to increase ventilation in proportion to metabolic demands; the absence of an adequate ventilatory reserve is plain, since maximal exercise ventilation frequently attains the maximal voluntary ventilation (MVV) achieved at rest. By contrast, the ventilatory response to heavy exercise seen in healthy subjects (usually between 60 and 80% of MVV), exceeds any increase of oxygen consumption ($\dot{V}_{O_2}$), carbon dioxide output ($\dot{V}_{CO_2}$), or pulmonary blood flow ($\dot{Q}$). This ensures maintenance of arterial oxygen tension, PaO_2, acid-base homeostasis, pH, and efficient oxygen delivery to the working muscles.

Reductions of maximal exercise power output and $\dot{V}_{O_2}$ in patients with chronic airflow limitation are related to reductions in resting $FEV_{1.0}$. The relationship becomes closer if age and pulmonary carbon monoxide diffusing capacity (Dco) are also considered. The close relationship between maximal exercise ventilation and $FEV_{1.0}$ at rest provides further support for the contention that an impaired ventilatory pump limits exercise capacity in COPD.

When considering the relative impact of airflow obstruction and other physiologic abnormalities upon exercise ventilation, useful information may be obtained by evaluating the exercise-induced changes of ventilation ($\dot{V}_E$), tidal volume (V_T), breathing frequency (f), and the timing of breathing (inspiratory versus total time, Ti and Ttot). The mechanical properties of the respiratory system dictate that adaptations must operate within the constraints set by the total lung capacity, the pressure/volume characteristics of the respiratory system, and the flow/volume loop for inspiration and expiration. A common finding in COPD patients is an elevated FRC, which results from a loss of elastic recoil and increased expiratory airflow resistance. Thus, during expiration the maximal expiratory limb of the flow volume curve is reached even at rest. During exercise, increases in minute ventilation are usually accompanied by increases of end-expiratory volume, tidal volume, and inspiratory flow; expiratory flow cannot exceed the expiratory limb of the flow-volume loop. Thus Ti/Ttot may fall to 0.3 or less compared to normal values of 0.4 to 0.5, as a functional adaptation to expiratory flow limitation. However, this adaptation becomes self-limiting if increases in lung volume alter the force-length relationship of the inspira-

tory muscles, causing them to work less efficiently. Furthermore, changes in volume and flow necessitate high force development by the inspiratory muscles, and respiratory muscle fatigue may limit further increases in ventilation.

In comparison to healthy subjects, patients with chronic airflow limitation must perform more respiratory work at comparable submaximal work loads. The energy requirement may amount to as much as 20 to 30 percent more oxygen at a given power output, a substantial increase for subjects whose maximum oxygen intake may be limited to 1 L/min or less. If total ventilatory changes at a given work rate are considered, it is not uncommon to find that some patients hyperventilate (type A), whereas others hypoventilate (type B). Ventilatory changes during exercise can be examined in terms of gas exchange efficiency, through measurements of $\dot{V}_E/\dot{V}_{O_2}$, $\dot{V}_E/\dot{V}_{CO_2}$, $PaCO_2$, V_D/V_T ratio and venous admixture.

A distinguishing feature among patients with COPD is the elevated ventilatory equivalent for both oxygen and carbon dioxide ($\dot{V}_E/\dot{V}_{O_2}$ and $\dot{V}_E/\dot{V}_{CO_2}$) during exercise. This reflects a rather inefficient ventilatory pump, since the added ventilation does not take part in gas exchange. There seems to be no association between the severity of obstruction and progressive increases in $\dot{V}_E/\dot{V}_{CO_2}$. This is not surprising, since abnormalities of ventilation-perfusion-diffusion relationships may also impair the efficiency of gas exchange in these patients. During exercise, $PaCO_2$ usually increases, and arterial oxygen tension (PaO_2) may drop below resting values. The ratio of dead space to tidal volume (V_D/V_T) may worsen or remain unchanged. Thus, abnormalities are relatively greater during exercise than at rest. Venous admixture may improve with exercise, reflecting changes in ventilation-perfusion distributions.

The severity of dyspnea is to some extent related to pulmonary gas exchange impairment, since poor gas exchange increases the ventilation required to maintain homeostasis at a given metabolic demand. The increased respiratory work encroaches upon a limited ventilatory reserve, causing the patient to terminate exercise because of breathlessness.

In COPD, the cardiac output response to exercise may be normal or even increased. However, large intrathoracic pressure swings can cause changes in left ventricular transmural pressure and thus afterload to the left ventricle; a reduced cardiac ejection fraction then results in a limited cardiac output response. Although these patients may exhibit mild-to-moderate degrees of arterial hypoxemia at rest and during exercise, oxygen delivery to exercising muscle is usually maintained. This accounts for the commonly observed lack of correlation between the severity of hypoxemia and reduction in maximal power output.

The major factor that limits exercise in COPD lies in the abnormal mechanical characteristics of the respiratory system. This abnormality is aggravated by increased ventilatory requirements, secondary to ventilation/perfusion mismatching and any vein-to-artery shunting.

The combined effects of these mechanical and physiologic abnormalities become manifest as the sensation of dyspnea.

EXERCISE PROGRAMS

Twenty years ago, clinical dogma dictated that patients with COPD were best treated with rest and avoidance of stress; suggestions that exercise programs could play a useful role in the "reconditioning" of such patients were viewed with skepticism. Attitudes have changed dramatically as numerous investigations have demonstrated improvements in exercise tolerance and well-being following appropriate exercise therapy. Although the physiologic mechanisms responsible for these improvements remain unclear, exercise conditioning has become an established part of rehabilitation programs for patients with chronic airflow obstruction.

PROPOSED BENEFITS

A major difficulty in evaluating studies of exercise reconditioning in COPD is the inadequate characterization of patients. In addition to classification as emphysematous or bronchitic, patients may differ with respect to the presence or absence of coexisting cardiovascular disease, duration of illness, nutritional status, bronchial hyperreactivity, and previous athletic experience and conditioning. Evaluation of data is also made difficult by the lack of standardized protocols among laboratories for testing and training patients.

It is generally agreed that exercise conditioning produces no improvement of pulmonary mechanics and probably does not alter the rate of decline in lung function. Effects on mucociliary clearance and other lung defense mechanisms are unknown, but are probably minimal. Nonetheless, exercise conditioning allows COPD patients to exercise at similar work rates with a lower heart rate, respiratory rate, minute ventilation, and CO_2 output than before conditioning. Whether single-level or incremental tests are used, exercise tolerance is improved following training. Cardiac function does not improve, probably because symptoms limit the conditioning exercise to work rates well below those necessary to produce cardiovascular training. Much of the improvement in exercise tolerance is task-specific, suggesting that patients improve the skills with which they perform these tasks. Increased oxygen extraction by exercising muscles has also been postulated as a reason for improvement, but it is again unlikely that patients with COPD achieve work loads high enough to alter the metabolic function of skeletal muscles. Several studies have failed to show any changes in the skeletal muscle enzymes that deliver ATP to the myofibrils. Psychologic factors may play a significant role; the response to both exercise and rehabilitation programs is to some extent a function of patients' premorbid personalities and coping mechanisms. The success of exercise therapy has been better correlated with psychiatric data and improvement

in symptom scores than with changes in any physiologic data. It has also been postulated that training "desensitizes" patients to the dyspnea of exercise. Whether such "desensitization" is purely psychologic and a consequence of greater confidence or results from physiologic changes is unknown. In this respect, attention must be directed to the possible importance of the respiratory muscles; they play a major role in the perception of dyspnea, with muscle fatigue augmenting the sensations produced by resistive and elastic loads. Inspiratory muscle training alone can improve exercise tolerance in COPD patients, giving rise to speculation that resistance to fatigue and/or altered perception of dyspnea may underline much of the improvement with exercise conditioning. There is as yet no evidence that exercise programs alone alter long-term prognosis, although comprehensive rehabilitation programs which incorporate exercise training may improve the level of function and decrease the number of hospitalizations for COPD patients.

MEDICAL THERAPY

Exercise training is begun when patients are clinically stable or have largely recovered from any acute exacerbations of their disease. The benefits of exercise training are lost following acute illness, and patients must be re-evaluated thoroughly following intercurrent illness before exercise programs can be resumed. The ventilatory limitation to exercise in COPD dictates that pulmonary mechanics should be optimized with available medical therapy. Clearly, the most important first step of treatment is smoking cessation. Beta-2 selective agonists (for example, fenoterol, salbutamol, terbutaline) are useful bronchodilators, best administered by the aerosol route to minimize side effects. If patients are unable to use conventional metered-dose inhalers, compressors for nebulization of medication should be considered. Beta-2 agonists may to some extent be replaced by newer anticholinergic agents such as ipratropium bromide; these are effective bronchodilators in COPD, and are free of significant cardiovascular and other systemic side effects. Theophylline, in a sustained-release formulation administered twice daily, is a useful adjunct to aerosolized bronchodilators. Objective measures of improvement should be sought to determine the most effective bronchodilator regimen for each patient. Beta-2 agonists and theophylline, in addition to their bronchodilating properties, may improve mucociliary clearance and stimulate ventilation, while theophylline may also help prevent respiratory muscle fatigue. Thus, the absence of major changes in pulmonary function should not discourage use of these medications if the patient reports significant subjective improvement. The role of corticosteroids in stable COPD is not well established, and in view of potential serious side effects, they should not be prescribed in the absence of objective improvement in pulmonary function. To reduce the incidence of intercurrent infections, polyvalent pneumococcal vaccination should be administered once, and influenza vaccination should be given annually in the fall. Reliable patients may be given a supply of a broad-spectrum oral antibiotic for prompt use at the onset of any exacerbation of their condition. A discussion of continuous or nocturnal low-flow oxygen therapy is beyond the scope of this chapter, but such measures should be considered in patients with resting arterial hypoxemia, repeated and severe nocturnal oxygen desaturation, and polycythaemia. The role of supplemental oxygen during exercise is considered under *Adjuncts*.

TESTING PROTOCOLS

There is no consensus with respect to the best exercise testing protocol for COPD patients. A useful approach is initial evaluation by progressive testing, supplemented by steady state tests for serial assessment. Incremental tests to a symptom-limited maximum offer information as to the choice of initial work load for training and may identify significant cardiac or peripheral vascular disease (which might modify the training program). Initial assessment must include electrocardiographic monitoring to detect significant cardiac dysrhythmias or ECG signs of ischemic heart disease, both common complicating factors in this population. Arterial oxygen saturation should be monitored continuously by oximeter to identify patients who desaturate with exercise and who thus require supplemental oxygen. Exercise at a constant submaximal work rate allows the determination of endurance time, a useful measurement for serial testing during and after training. A practical approach to serial evaluation is the 12-minute walk, in which the patient is instructed to cover as much distance within 12 minutes as he is able, walking at his own pace and pausing as necessary. The test may be conducted in hospital or clinic corridors, monitored by paramedical personnel or by the patient himself. The results of the test are a comprehensible yardstick for patients, offering incentive as well as a means for serial self-testing beyond the period of training.

TRAINING PROTOCOLS

The methods and duration of training are not uniform among laboratories, but the following general principles are offered. Given that improvement with exercise training is to some extent task-specific, it is most helpful to the patient if treadmill exercise is used. Not only is walking an important activity of daily living, but a walking program may be prescribed to maintain gains following the completion of the formal training program. One small advantage of cycle ergometer exercise is the availability of relatively inexpensive stationary cycles for home use in inclement weather. Alternate forms of exercise such as swimming have not been evaluated extensively, but may be useful for select patients who have disorders of weight-bearing joints or other complications which prevent walking or cycling.

A reasonable goal for most patients with moderate-to-severe COPD is to exercise at or near the symptom-limited maximal work rate for 20 to 30 minutes per session. This may be achieved for most patients by initial training periods of between 10 and 20 minutes at a very low work rate, increasing the work rate and duration during thrice-weekly sessions. The most marked improvements occur during the first 2 to 3 weeks of a training program, but the total program length has varied among studies from 2 months to 2 years. A realistic program is of 1 to 2 months' duration, followed by a home prescription to maintain "conditioning". Re-evaluation should be performed at regular intervals (3 to 6 months), using either formal steady-state protocols or the 12-minute walk test.

ADJUNCTS
Breathing Retraining

Pursed-lip breathing is adopted spontaneously by many emphysematous patients and has been taught widely as part of pulmonary rehabilitation programs. This pattern of breathing may reduce the sensation of dyspnea by preventing airway collapse and decreasing respiratory rate and work of breathing. Such teaching is often combined with attempts to assist diaphragmatic function with learned patterns of abdominal breathing. The abdominal muscles are stiffened during expiration to push abdominal contents upward; during inspiration the abdominal muscles are relaxed and the abdominal contents fall, assisting the diaphragmatic descent. Such breathing maneuvers appear to have no training effect on diaphragmatic strength or endurance and are not continued unconsciously by patients. Such teaching therefore offers a conscious pattern of behavior that may provide mild relief during episodes of dyspnea and during exercise. These subjective benefits, while minimal, are available at little cost or side effect and may reasonably be incorporated in exercise programs.

Nutrition

Although there is good evidence that starvation accelerates the development of emphysema in animal models, the role of nutrition and dietary manipulation in humans is unclear. Further investigations of the metabolic consequences of COPD and the benefits and side effects of dietary alteration will be required before specific recommendations can be made.

Drugs

In addition to bronchodilating drugs, pharmacologic interventions in COPD may include attempts to improve exercise function with inotropes, such as digoxin, or afterload-reducing agents, such as hydralazine. Preliminary studies suggest that there is little benefit from such agents in patients without significant coexisting left ventricular dysfunction. Right ventricular function alone appears to be unaltered or altered unpredictably by digoxin or vasodilators in the majority of COPD patients. At present such therapy cannot be advised for routine use, but further investigations might identify a subset of patients who would benefit. Opiates, benzodiazepines, and alcohol have provided relief of dyspnea in acute administration studies, but their long-term role has not been defined.

Oxygen

Oxygen administration during exercise relieves dyspnea and improves exercise tolerance in many patients at the expense of transient increases in arterial CO_2. Although some benefit has been reported with oxygen administration preceding exercise, it is most appropriately administered by face mask or nasal prongs during exercise. Although patients who are hypoxemic at rest or during exercise are most likely to benefit, some normoxic patients appear to improve as well.

Inspiratory Muscle Training

It is becoming increasingly clear that respiratory muscle dysfunction and fatigue play a major role in the pathophysiology and symptomatology of COPD. Specific conditioning programs for the respiratory muscles have been investigated as potentially useful forms of treatment. Periods of isocapnic hyperpnea improve respiratory muscle endurance and increase exercise tolerance. Added inspiratory resistive loads have also been used to train respiratory muscles, and in one study, such inspiratory muscle training alone produced greater improvement in exercise tolerance than a conventional exercise program. At present, the duration of the training effect is unknown, and the most effective conditioning schedule has not been established. Some studies have used EMG criteria of respiratory muscle fatigue to guide training, a technology that is not routinely available in most exercise facilities. It is uncertain which patients will benefit most from such training, and a risk exists that some patients may develop respiratory muscle fatigue with such manipulations. While this treatment modality appears promising, it cannot be recommended routinely at this time.

EXERCISE IN THE TREATMENT OF DIABETES MELLITUS

GÖRAN A. L. HOLM, M.D.
MARCIN J. KROTKIEWSKI, M.D.

Physical exercise has been described as a means of treating diabetes mellitus from ancient times. After the discovery of insulin, Joslin introduced his famous triad (exercise-diet-insulin) as the so-called cornerstones of diabetic treatment. Joslin's triad is found in almost all textbooks on diabetes. However, scientific evidence for the beneficial effects of physical exercise in diabetes has been scarce. Indeed, reports during the last few years have shown that exercise is no universal remedy for diabetes. The effect of exercise varies from one group of patients to another, and in some cases it may even cause adverse effects.

It is particularly important that the young patient with type 1 diabetes requiring insulin treatment should understand the effects of physical exercise and know whether he or she can participate in games or sports without restriction.

The incidence of type 2 diabetes has apparently increased with improved living standards, and adult diabetes is nowadays a frequent disease in the western world. Obesity with insulin resistance seems to be a contributing factor in the development of this type of diabetes. A second important issue is thus whether physical exercise can improve glucose tolerance or even prevent the appearance of diabetes in older individuals. Finally, it is well known that diabetes is associated with an increased risk of cardiovascular disease. Insulin resistance, hypertension, and an abnormal lipid profile can all contribute to macrovascular disease. Does physical exercise have a beneficial effect on these so-called risk factors? Each of these three questions will be discussed in this chapter.

TYPE 1 DIABETES

There are only a few reports suggesting that glucose tolerance is improved after physical training in patients with type 1 diabetes. It is often very difficult to draw definite conclusions as to which factor was the more important in these studies—insulin, diet, or exercise. In one group of patients with type 1 diabetes but no complications, we could not see any evidence of improved metabolic control in blood glucose, urinary glucose, or glucosylated hemoglobin after completing 3 months of physical training. Neither did the required dosage of insulin change. However, the initial metabolic control of this group was suboptimal, and it is possible that a different result might have been obtained if the metabolic control had been better from the beginning, for example, if the patients had been treated with a continuous insulin infusion system. In such a study, it would also have been easier to follow changes in insulin requirements.

Type 1 diabetics nevertheless show an increased sensitivity to insulin after physical exercise, if this is measured with the euglycemic insulin clamp method. Not only does glucose disposal increase, but insulin clearance is also augmented. In vitro studies on adipose tissue do not show any changes in the number of insulin receptors or their insulin-binding capacity, so that the increased insulin sensitivity as measured by the clamp method seems dependent on postreceptor mechanisms. However, most of the glucose is taken up by muscles. Change or lack of change in adipose tissue therefore cannot necessarily be extrapolated to the status of the muscles.

There are no conclusive studies suggesting that physical exercise per se can improve metabolic control in type 1 diabetes. On the other hand, metabolic control has great importance for the performance of physical exercise. If metabolic control is poor, the muscle glycogen depots are depleted, contributing to an impaired work capacity. On the other hand, if metabolic control is good, there is no difference of glycogen storage or work capacity between the diabetic and a normal subject. If diabetes is poorly controlled, the metabolic status may deteriorate even further with the increase of plasma glucose, free fatty acids, and ketone bodies that develop during exercise. This deterioration most likely reflects insulin deficiency, with a decreased glucose uptake by the working muscle. Other studies have shown that the poorly controlled diabetic patient has higher plasma levels of anti-insulin hormones such as growth hormone, corticosteroids, and catecholamines. Such abnormalities are accentuated even further during physical activity, worsening metabolic control and possibly contributing to the development of microangiopathy. Moreover, if metabolic control is improved, for instance, by use of a portable insulin infusion pump, these hormone levels are normalized both in the basal state and during exercise.

Episodes of hypoglycemia after exercise are a common problem for the patient with type 1 diabetes. Only a couple of years after the discovery of insulin, Lawrence described young diabetic tennis players who experienced hypoglycemic symptoms following tennis matches. Such episodes appear in patients whose diabetes is normally well controlled by insulin; the difficulty seems an inappropriate regulation of insulin. Normally, physical exercise leads to an inhibition of insulin release, and plasma insulin levels decrease. A low concentration of plasma insulin favors the mobilization of substrates for the working muscle. Specifically, low plasma insulin levels reduce the inhibition of lipolysis, with an increased liberation of free fatty acids and glycerol, plus an increase of glycogenesis and glycogenolysis in the liver with an increased hepatic output of glucose. In patients with type 1 diabetes who receive exogenous insulin, these physiologic control mechanisms no longer operate normally. The insulin concentration is not reduced during work, but may actually increase on account of an increased absorption of exogenous insulin from subcutaneous depots. The mobilization of necessary substrates for the

working muscle is thereby inhibited, resulting in attacks of hypoglycemia. Another factor contributing to hypoglycemia is that exercise per se has an insulin-like effect, increasing the uptake of glucose by the working muscle. The severity of the hypoglycemic reaction in insulin-treated patients depends on the dosage of insulin, the time of maximal effect of the insulin given, and the site where the insulin has been injected. To vary these factors is quite difficult. Therefore, the best advice to offer the diabetic patient who is performing physical exercise is to eat more carbohydrates before work. The insulin dosage may also need to be reduced if more regular physical exercise is planned.

Muscle adaptations to physical exercise are normal in type 1 diabetics with respect to strength, performance, and fiber-type distribution. However, the capillary density does not increase as much in the diabetic patient as in normal individuals of the same body mass who undertake training for the same period. It is unclear as yet whether this is an effect of abnormal metabolic control or whether it depends on some other mechanism. The basal membrane of the muscle capillaries is thickened in diabetic patients. Some studies have shown that physical training reduces basal membrane thickness in type 1 diabetes, but this again may be an effect of improved metabolic control on account of an optimalization of insulin and dietary regimen.

TYPE 2 DIABETES

Type 2 diabetes must be considered as a social disease. The increasing incidence of type 2 diabetes is most likely due to a decrease of physical activity and a change of dietary habits in western society. The majority of type 2 patients are overweight. Insulin resistance is a dominant characteristic. Insulin resistance does not seem to depend on changes in the number of insulin receptors or on changes in their insulin-binding capacity, but is rather an expression of postreceptor defects. However, it is not possible to study these variables in human muscle tissue—the important target organ of physical exercise. It is well known that physical training reduces both insulin resistance and plasma insulin levels in hyperinsulinemic subjects. The reduction of insulin levels reflects partly a reduced secretion of insulin and partly an increased insulin turnover. How does physical exercise modify insulin sensitivity and glucose homeostasis in type 2 diabetics?

We investigated the effects of physical training in a large group of patients with type 2 diabetes. The patients were either on sulfonylurea therapy or on a dietary regimen alone. Most of these patients were mildly obese. They exercised for one hour, three times a week for 3 months. In a minority, there was no improvement of glucose homeostasis. Closer analysis showed that in this subgroup there were no cardiovascular responses to physical training, and no increase of insulin sensitivity as measured by the euglycemic insulin clamp technique. It is thus likely that the lack of metabolic response was due to inadequate activity during the training sessions. A further factor may have been a poor initial metabolic control, although no differences could be seen in this respect relative to the remaining subjects. The group in which glucose tolerance did improve was subdivided further into a high-insulin-producing and a low-insulin-producing class on the basis of plasma levels of C-peptide. The connecting (C—)peptide and insulin are secreted from the beta-cell in equimolar amounts, but only the insulin is taken up by the liver. Plasma concentrations of C-peptide have therefore been considered as providing an estimate of insulin secretion. Comparison between plasma levels of C-peptide and insulin also yields an estimate of insulin uptake by the liver. Plasma insulin levels were increased in both subclasses, but insulin levels fell only in the subclass with a high insulin production. The subclass with a low insulin production showed an increase in insulin release as gauged from C-peptides, but no change in plasma insulin levels. This shows the important role of the liver in insulin homeostasis during physical exercise. Regarding glucose homeostasis, clamp measurements suggested that the subclass with low insulin production was less insulin-resistant and showed a more pronounced improvement of glucose tolerance with exercise than did the subclass with a high rate of insulin production.

Physical exercise led to local adaptations in the muscles, particularly an increase in the activity of several oxidative enzymes. Changes of enzyme activity developed in parallel with an increased capillarization of the active muscles. The increased capillarization and the shortened diffusion distance were correlated with the increase in insulin sensitivity. The study therefore shows that a number of variables must be taken into account when interpreting changes in glucose and insulin homeostasis after the physical training of type 2 diabetics. The exercise must be of sufficient intensity and duration to induce adaptive changes in both the circulation and the muscles before an improvement of glucose homeostasis can occur. Possibly, the training response is less if the initial metabolic control is poor. Moreover, the degree of insulin resistance seems to influence the impact of training on glucose homeostasis.

OTHER FACTORS ASSOCIATED WITH DIABETES

Today, it is beyond reasonable doubt that good metabolic control can prevent the development of microangiopathy in patients with diabetes mellitus. The incidence of cardiovascular disease nevertheless remains high in diabetes. Both experimental and large population studies have shown that the development of arteriosclerosis is associated with insulin resistance and hyperinsulinemia. It is therefore important to normalize both insulin sensitivity and plasma insulin levels in the treatment of diabetes. As already mentioned, physical exercise is beneficial in this regard.

Insulin resistance and hyperinsulinemia can be considered as central metabolic derangements, associated with dyslipoproteinemia and high blood pressure. In diabetes mellitus, plasma triglycerides are elevated, and at the same time there is a decrease of HDL-cholesterol. Low plasma levels of HDL-cholesterol are in turn linked with cardiovascular disease. Physical exercise reduces triglyceride levels and increases HDL-cholesterol, therefore reducing the risk of atherosclerosis in diabetes. A moderate increase of blood pressure can also be corrected by regular physical exercises.

Thus, a number of so-called risk factors associated with diabetes can be affected beneficially by an exercise program. However, the question arises whether one can prevent the appearance of type 2 diabetes by exercise. Since obesity and insulin resistance contribute to the development of diabetes, it should be obvious that a program of reduction of body mass and increased physical activity reduces the risk of diabetes. Since it is often difficult to change established patterns of life style, one should first begin with some form of risk-group evaluation. Recent findings suggest that individuals with moderate abdominal obesity are particularly prone to increased insulin resistance, reduced glucose tolerance, and an increased risk of diabetes and cardiovascular disease. This group, commonly middle-aged men, should therefore be the specific target of diet information and exercise programs.

PRACTICAL CONSIDERATIONS

Despite its value, physical exercise should not be seen as a universal treatment for diabetes mellitus. Physical training should be prescribed against clear indications, in the same way as any other medical therapy is prescribed.

Type 2 diabetes with obesity and insulin resistance forms the largest group in which exercise and a "weight-reducing" diet regimen should be the first choice in therapy. The patient should be given adequate information about the beneficial effects of exercise, and then an individualized program of daily training should be prescribed. In some cases, training may begin in a group, under the supervision of, for instance, a physiotherapist. However, in the long run it is important to try to make exercise an essential component of the patient's life style. The diabetic patient usually has a poor physical work capacity, and training should therefore start at a low intensity.

Since cardiovascular disease is common in diabetes, and may not have presenting symptoms, a stress test should be performed along with a routine check of the cardiovascular system before the patient is given advice on training.

In patients with type 1 diabetes, the physician should first try to optimize metabolic regulation with multiple doses of insulin, diet, and counseling. Once the patient has established good control, and assuming that there are no late complications, no limitations need be placed upon participation in physical training or sports activities. A number of type 1 diabetics currently peform sports at the elite level.

Patients with serious microangiopathy should be dissuaded from heavy physical activity. There have been cases in which patients with serious retinopathy have had hemorrhage induced by physical activity, and there have even been cases with nephropathy that have progressed to sudden renal failure. Patients with neuropathy and a loss of sensitivity are at an increased risk of foot injury when jogging. Many patients are treated by beta-blocking agents. A selective beta 1-blocking agent should always be chosen. Possible hypoglycemic reactions after physical activity are prolonged by nonselective beta-blocking agents.

EXERCISE AND RHEUMATOID ARTHRITIS

BJÖRN T. EKBLOM, M.D.

Rheumatoid arthritis (RA) is a chronic disease, still largely of unknown origin. According to the American Rheumatoid Association (ARA), the main criteria of RA are: morning stiffness, tenderness or pain on motion, history or observation of joint swelling, subcutaneous nodules, some positive laboratory blood tests, and some radiographic and histologic changes in affected joints.

RA usually has a gradual onset, with pain, swelling, and stiffness of small peripheral joints. The disease begins most commonly between the ages of 25 and 60 years. There is a female preponderance of 3:1.

Progression is slow, with periods of exacerbation and remission. The inflammatory process involves the joints, leading to a gradual destruction of the joint surface, and also affecting the surrounding joint capsule and ligaments. Furthermore, tendons and skeletal muscles can become affected. Since the disease is systemic, symptoms from the cardiovascular (pericarditis, peripheral arteritis), pulmonary (pleuritis, fibrosis), and nervous (neuropathy, neuritis) systems are also very common.

All of these various changes affect the RA patient's ability to undertake physical exercise. The patient's general functional capacity and physical performance are often categorized as proposed by the ARA:

1. Complete ability to carry out all usual duties.
2. Adequate ability to carry out normal activities despite some handicap, discomfort, or limitation of motion.
3. Limited ability to carry out usual occupation or self-care.
4. Incapacitated, largely or totally.

PHYSICAL PERFORMANCE IN PATIENTS WITH RA

Since RA is a disease involving different parts of the body, the activity of the disease influences the patient's physical performance. During exacerbations physical performance is low, and the patient cannot carry out intense physical exercise. During remissions, the physical performance is less affected since pain is reduced with a corresponding lessening of muscular and physiologic fatigue.

A patient in functional class I may perform any type of physical exercise, since the disease involvement has not yet had any major impact upon the ability to exercise. Exceptions in some cases include hard physical exercise, running, and individual racquet sports, which put a hard "eccentric" stress on the knees and feet. Especial care is needed if there are active processes in these joints. In almost all cases, bicycle or cycle ergometer exercise remains possible.

Patients in RA functional class II and a few patients in functional class III can perform most types of physical exercise—especially bicycling and walking, but sometimes even jogging—during low-activity phases of the disease. During high-activity phases, these patients can only exercise in a "no load" or very low load condition (for example, a cycle ergometer setting of 25 watt), owing to the inflammatory process in the joints, muscles, and tendons. The ability to exercise is recovered fairly soon after the most acute phase of the disease, and it is possible to exercise a patient even though signs of active engagement of the joints have not fully disappeared.

Although a few patients in functional class III can perform walking, jogging, and similar types of exercise, most patients in this functional category can swim and exercise on a bicycle, provided the type of exercise, its intensity, and the range of movements are modified on the basis of the patient's anatomic-pathologic condition. In this functional class, polyneuritis and peripheral arteritis are common and may again modify the ability to exercise.

By definition, most patients in functional class IV are not able to carry out complicated movements. However, quite a few patients in this category can perform some physical activity, for example, while suspended in water, or exercising "free" without preset levels of intensity or frequency.

GENERAL ASPECTS OF PHYSICAL TRAINING FOR RA PATIENTS

When prescribing physical training for patients with RA, the stage and activity of the disease must be considered. During exacerbations, low-intensity exercise

—"no-load" pedalling of a cycle ergometer or swimming in warm water—can be performed. Mobility training to avoid contractures is recommended. After such a period, most patients of functional class I and II and quite a few in class III can perform walking and bicycle training to develop cardiovascular fitness and even increase muscle strength and endurance. It is important that the training session begin with a long "warm-up" (10 to 15 minutes at a fairly low intensity). Thereafter, RA patients may perform interval or continuous higher-intensity training.

If the initial few weeks of physical training is carried out carefully, most patients can continue with their daily training. In long-term follow-up studies (up to 8 years), 80 to 85 percent of patients who initially started physical training continue to do so regularly on their own. However, it is our experience that if a patient is inactivated by an exacerbation, it is important that these patients return to group training for a few weeks before taking up individual training again.

Swimming, rowing, and bicycling are in many respects good modes of exercise in RA, since the body mass does not load the joints of the lower extremities. That is part of the reason why low-intensity swimming, rowing, and bicycling are recommended for periods of exacerbation of the disease. To recommend total bed rest is not only unnecessary for most patients, but may also increase the risk of developing contractures and immobility.

EFFECTS OF TRAINING IN PATIENTS WITH RA

As mentioned earlier, the RA patient generally has a low physical working capacity. Thus, there are improvements in both subjective indices of performance and physiologic variables even after a fairly short period of time and a moderate amount of physical training.

The effects of physical performance and related physiologic, medical, and social/psychosocial factors are very evident in individual cases. In a study in Stockholm, 6 weeks of physical rehabilitation ("training") increased walking performance on level ground by 14 percent, and walking up stairs by 25 percent while bench-stepping (highest possible) increased 15 to 20 percent in a group of 23 RA patients. The training of this group comprised cycle exercise and muscle strength training once a day, 5 days a week, plus standard physiotherapy. The maximal oxygen uptake increased from 1.22 to 1.47 L/min. Dynamic and isometric muscle strength improved by 23 to 73 percent. Although there is muscular hypotrophy in RA—mainly a selective fast-twitch (type II) hypotrophy—this type of physical training increases muscle fiber area as evaluated by muscle biopsy.

Both "central" and "local" ratings of perceived fatigue are markedly reduced by short-term physical training. This implies that patients can perform a given work task with a lesser sense of exertion and also that they can elect to work at a higher intensity. This improved effort tolerance is confirmed when patients are questioned about their performance of daily activities after a period of physical training.

Long-term physical training restores physiologic variables toward or above the normal range for the corresponding age group. There are also other positive clinical, psychologic, and sociologic effects. Over an average observation period of 5.5 years, patients from a training group (n=23) had a total hospital stay averaging 16.4 days compared to 35.6 days in an equally large control group (p<0.05). In comparison with the control group, trained patients had arrested their disease progress, radiographs proving that the speed of destruction of joint cartilage and bone had been significantly reduced. Clinical examination confirmed a better joint state, and the patients reported a significantly better functional capacity in their daily activities. Trained patients also took significantly less sick leave and sick pension, staying in hospital less than half as many days as the controls.

It is obvious that training is one of the few means by which the patient can influence clinical outcome. There are many indications that an increase of physical activity also has beneficial psychologic consequences for the whole rehabilitation process. For instance, a feeling of social isolation was reported almost twice as often in controls (36%) as in the trained patients (20%).

Finally, it is important to note that in our training study all patients wished to take part in some form of training in the future.

EXERCISE FOR THE DISABLED: THE PARAPLEGIC

ROY J. SHEPHARD, M.D. (Lond), Ph.D.

The Special Olympics now offer the disabled patient the opportunity to compete against other individuals suffering a similar degree of disability; moreover, such events have been very successful both in boosting morale and in providing a stimulus to the maximizing of residual function. This chapter will offer comment on the specific problems of the paraplegic, with reference to methods of testing and training, functional classification, and sports involvement.

TESTING AND TRAINING

Arm Ergometry. Aerobic power can be assessed by either a forearm-crank ergometer or some arrangement using the wheelchair. The great advantage of a forearm crank is that conditions are held constant from one patient to another, but there is also the disadvantage that the muscles used in operating the crank are not identical with those used in propelling a wheelchair. Because the muscles involved are small, the rate of rotation (80 rpm) is higher than for normal cycle ergometry. In other respects, the protocol is much as for cycle ergometer measurements of aerobic power, although it may be difficult to demonstrate a plateau of oxygen consumption. In the field, submaximal tests can be carried out, but attempts to extrapolate findings to a predicted maximum suffer from the same problems as seen in normal subjects—a large inter-individual variation of maximal heart rate and a correspondingly large error (10 to 15%) in the predicted maximal oxygen intake. Submaximal scores may give some guidance as to the progression of training, but are of little value in advising an individual patient concerning current fitness status.

Wheelchair Tests. The simplest type of test is analogous to Cooper's 12-minute run: the distance covered in a wheelchair is measured over a 12-minute period. If conditions are carefully standardized, this may provide some indication of condition, but scores are very susceptible to the nature of the ground surface, the mass of the wheelchair, and the skill of the operator.

A second option is to ask the patient to propel a wheelchair up a special wide treadmill. This has the advantage of being a relatively "real life" task, testing the muscles important to daily performance, but scores are again influenced by wheelchair design and the experience of the user. The third possibility is to attach wheelchair rims to the drive of an ergometer.

Muscle Strength. When measuring muscle strength, the choice is again between a well-standardized laboratory method and something that has greater realism. To date, most people have opted for isometric

dynamometer and tensiometer measurements, although some have added Cybex II isokinetic measurements on the main groups of arm muscles. There seems to be a fairly close relationship between isometric and isokinetic scores, with both having an important influence upon aerobic power and endurance performance.

Body Fat. The average wheelchair patient gets inadequate exercise and thus tends to accumulate body fat, the problem becoming particularly acute if a motorized wheelchair has been provided. Skinfolds can be measured as in a normal individual, but it is not possible to predict body fat or lean mass using standard equations, since there is generally wasting (or absence) of the lower part of the body.

Potential Condition. Well-trained wheelchair athletes are capable of developing a remarkable aerobic power (3.5 to 4.0 L/min, much more than is found in a sedentary young adult). Equally, there is tremendous muscle hypertrophy, individual muscle fibres being up to three times larger than in a normal person. In women, there seems as yet relatively little selection of wheelchair competitors, and maximum scores are no higher than would be produced by moderate training. However, male competitors probably reflect not only the potential training response of the average individual, but also some selection of the well-endowed.

Training Program. To date there have been few systematic studies of training in wheelchair patients, but current indications are that intensity (relative to the individual's maximum), frequency, and duration of conditioning all influence the training response. Not only is aerobic power increased, but there are also gains of muscle strength, particularly at high speeds of movement (e.g., 180° per second). Moreover, the increments of muscle strength seem important in enabling the well-trained individual to sustain a large stroke volume and cardiac output at high work rates. In general, the optimal prescription seems, as in a normal patient, 30 minutes of exercise at 60 to 70 percent of maximal oxygen intake, performed three to four times per week.

FUNCTIONAL CLASSIFICATION

There has been a great deal of debate over the past few years on the optimal method of classifying the paraplegic patient. However, the most widely used scheme is still that developed by the International Stoke Mandeville Games Federation:

Ia. Complete or incomplete quadriplegia resulting from cervical lesions, involving both hands, with weakness of the triceps and with severe weakness of trunk and lower extremities interfering with sitting balance and ability to walk.

Ib. Complete or incomplete quadriplegia resulting from cervical lesions involving both hands with normal or good triceps and with generalized weakness of trunk and lower extremities interfering significantly with sitting balance and ability to walk.

Ic. Complete or incomplete quadriplegia resulting from cervical lesions with normal or good triceps and normal or good finger flexors and extensors, but with generalized weakness of trunk and lower extremities interfering significantly with sitting balance and ability to walk.

II. Complete or incomplete paraplegia T1 to T5 or comparable, with poor or nonexistent abdominal muscle strength and no useful sitting balance.

III. Complete or incomplete paraplegia T5 to T10 or comparable, with upper abdominal and spinal extensor muscle control allowing poor sitting balance.

IV. Complete or incomplete paraplegia T10 to L2 or comparable, with weak or nonexistent quadriceps strength and limited gluteal control.

V. Complete or incomplete paraplegia (lesion below L2 or comparable) with good or fair quadriceps control.

The advantage of the ISMGF schema is that it combines information on the anatomic level of the lesion with an assessment of the quality and quantity of functioning musculature. In well-trained athletes, there seems to be a good correlation between forearm power output and ISMGF classification, but in less well-trained individuals, there is relatively little difference of score between class II and class V lesions, at least on laboratory tests. Moreover, there is little difference of condition between mobile, sedentary, and incapacitated wheelchair patients, suggesting that average use of a wheelchair by a city dweller provides an insufficient stimulus to maintain either cardiorespiratory or muscle function.

SPORTS INVOLVEMENT OF THE DISABLED

Sir Ludwig Guttmann introduced archery as a therapeutic measure for paraplegic war veterans in 1948, and the first international competition was held in 1950. By 1960, the growth in number of participants was so large that the games were moved from Stoke Mandeville

to Rome. Subsequently, the country hosting the Olympics has generally staged a Paraplegic Games, although in 1980 Russia claimed "they had no disabled," and so a competition for some 2500 competitors was held at the Dutch National Sports Center, near Arnhem.

The ISMGF promotes the basic principle that both in recreation and in competition, minimal rule changes should be made to allow the various categories of disabled individual to participate with a good chance of success in their respective classes. Wheelchair races range from 40 to 1500 meters, and unofficial marathon events have clocked times under 2 hours. Field events include all the usual throwing competitions (discus, shot-put, and javelin) performed from an anchored chair. Other individual sports include swimming, table tennis, fencing, weight-lifting, archery, rifle-shooting, bowling, and snooker. Wheelchair basketball is the most popular of the team sports. Possibilities for the winter season include downhill sledding in a "pulk" and ice hockey performed from a sled.

Recreational pursuits open to the disabled include riding, sailing, gliding, and five-pin bowling.

Disabled athletes who train for major competitions seem no more liable to injury than their able-bodied counterparts. Medical staff must be prepared to treat the usual problems of international competition— sleeplessness, exhaustion, dehydration, sunburn, gastroenteritis, minor respiratory infections, and sprains, rather than any specific problems attributable to the disability.

Participation in sport often plays an important role in promoting social reintegration following traumatic paraplegia. Some authors have found that the sports participant develops arm strength twice as fast as the person receiving traditional bedside rehabilitation. Likewise, more of the sports participants return to the labor force; they also have a lower rate of absenteeism and earn a greater wage than their sedentary counterparts. Physiologic gains are even more remarkable, and the top competitors develop a greater aerobic power and more muscle strength than their able-bodied contemporaries. Physicians should thus offer every encouragement to the sports participation of the paraplegic.

EXERCISE AND SENSORY DISABILITY

GRAHAM R. WARD, Ph.D.

Opportunities previously unavailable to the disabled now abound in education, sport, and exercise programs. Many countries have extended the level of such opportunities until they almost match those availa-

ble to the nondisabled. From a very slow beginning with little chance to excel, the deaf, blind, and other individuals with sensory problems are now openly encouraged to take part in safe, well organized school physical education programs, general exercise, and sporting activities.

In many countries, these individuals can join special associations or clubs that are affiliated to a World Sporting Body. The deaf, the blind, and other disabled groups have organizations that arrange local, regional, national, and international championship class sport competitions. Examples include the International Blind Sports Association (I.B.S.A.) and the International Committee of Silent Sports.

CHILD DEVELOPMENT

During early childhood, the child with a disability such as blindness or deafness is often hampered by lack of opportunity to take part in physical activity. The play model with other children is often either unavailable or avoided because in the main, neither parents nor potential playmates know how to communicate well with such individuals. Fortunately, over the past two decades many countries have made good progress in the way disabled children are screened and diagnosed early in their development. Earlier detection and diagnosis have led to greater understanding on the part of both parent and child. A greater number of children are being medically screened and diagnosed early, owing in part to a growing public awareness and in part to a better educational system. More and more qualified people are now dealing with the disabled, and they are aware of the early signs of disability. The sooner a child is treated, the earlier appropriate exercise opportunities can be made available. This in turn usually leads to the development of better exercise skills, with apparent benefit to other body developmental patterns. Children who are born with major hearing and sight defects often lack the basic skills that nondisabled children possess when they attempt exercise. However, if disease develops somewhat later, there is better progress in exercise because coordination patterning is more sound. Most children with poor communication skills are accommodated at schools and medical treatment centers specializing in this type of education.

Perhaps this is not always the best route to take. However, experts in lip reading, sign language, sight boards, and braille are employed at these centers, and a combination of close teacher contact, small classes, and good equipment and personnel allow the children to learn faster than at normal schools.

A recent trend has been to send disabled children to regular schools where they can be integrated with nondisabled or nonhandicapped children. In many cases, the less severely disabled children respond well to this type of learning and, in turn, develop good exercise patterns which help them in sporting activities during later life. However, many children with multiple handicaps or gross disabilities do not fare as well in their overall development if integrated. Accordingly, opportunities for both classroom instruction and exercise are still available to them at special centers. Many of these children have extreme difficulty with basic physical education, and few seem to develop sufficiently to allow them to take part in sporting or competitive activities as adults.

PHYSICAL EDUCATION

Many present-day schools offer some form of physical education for the disabled. Most classes are taught in a very similar manner to the nondisabled. The better programs include the same components of exercise offered in regular school activity with certain changes made in the use of the equipment. Most classes incorporate warm-up exercises for at least 15 minutes, including strength and aerobic components. Thereafter, they teach a skill of some type, followed by a game that includes the skill taught earlier. The class should always finish with a cool-down period. There should be lots of fun and music if appropriate. Specialized equipment may include electronic beeper balls, balls with bells inside, and other specialized audio or visual items. All can be used successfully if they are safe, colorful, and easily handled. Balls or bats may be made of sponge, plastic, foam plastic, and, in some cases, vinyl or leather (which last longer under heavy use). Other equipment is usually standard physical education apparatus.

SPORT AND EXERCISE OPPORTUNITIES

There have been sport and exercise opportunities for the blind, hearing impaired, and others with sensory disabilities for many years. Recently, opportunities to excel have grown considerably, and participation in sport and exercise has now become a normal occurrence rather than a special event.

History: Competitive sport for the blind dates back to the late 1940s, but some competitions for the deaf were held as early as the 1920s. Exercise and sports activities were usually developed from the rehabilitation process. Some evolved through schools, while others for adults were developed in hospitals after world or local wars and border disputes.

Large-scale competitive sport events are recent departure from the "old style" field, gala, or picnic day.

Classification: In all sporting events, a specific classification system has been developed for each disability group. Many athletes competing in blind or deaf sports are designated legally blind or deaf, but they are not necessarily totally blind or deaf. Nevertheless, all competitors must be tested by an ophthalmologist, an audiologist, or other specialist prior to taking part in an organized competition. This medical intervention helps to keep the competitions fair, ensuring that participants only compete alongside fellow athletes with either the same or a very similar degree of disability.

Example: Blind Classification. Set out below is one example of a classification system which is used to allow athletes to compete on an equal basis:

B1: No light perception at all in either eye up to light perception; inability to recognize objects or contours in any direction and at any distance.
B2: Ability to recognize objects or contours up to visual acuity of 2/60 and/or a limitation of field of vision of 5 degrees.
B3: Has 2/60 to 6/60 vision and/or field of vision between 5 and 20 degrees.

Recently, some events have been allowed where athletes with various disabilities have competed against one another on a functional rather than a disability basis. This interesting approach may develop more quickly with some disabilities than with others; it allows a blind athlete to compete alongside a deaf athlete or with athletes from the Cerebral Palsy, Amputee, or Wheelchair Federations.

In my opinion, this system will be neither feasible nor fair for all sporting events and all disabilities. However, it has worked in certain events with selective disabilities. The sport event list for this classification system may be its major limiting factor.

Rules: Most of the rules followed in disabled sport are the same or very similar to those for nondisabled sport. International rules and regulations for specific events such as Track and Field and Swimming are identical, with a few very minor exceptions. When rules are changed, safety, fairness, and availability of equipment are the usual reasons.

Equipment for Competition: The equipment used is rarely changed, although sometimes it is adapted from that used by International nondisabled sport groups. There are exceptions to this, especially in the case of local or regional competitions where additional competitive events not listed in the International rule books may be acceptable. This allows for the development of ethnic events and/or local athletes.

Special guide rails and guide wires may be used during blind events especially in sprint competitions. At the International level, such aids are rarely seen; the training techniques employed and the innovations adopted by coaches and teachers have almost eliminated specialty items such as stationary guide supports. During 100-meter track and swimming sprints, the fully blind are directed by following the sound of a coach's voice. During 200- and 400-meter sprints, middle- and long-distance running, the totally blind usually employ a guide runner for both training and competition. In most running competitions, the guide is tethered to the athlete by a short cloth or rope, but in training this is not necessary. In my opinion, to teach the athlete to run freely with the guide at the side does not impede racing ability as much as tethering the athlete. The guide should act as the eyes but not as the exercise machine. This decision should, of course, be left to the athlete. The guide runner should be a better athlete than the disabled person, since otherwise the disabled individual will be hindered during competition. During some events in certain countries, a blind athlete must carry a white cane. This is an unusual rule, and it impairs athletic excellence.

Electronic head sets and hearing aids have also been used in competitions for the deaf and blind. Such aids to training and competition have considerable merit. However, using such equipment to help the athlete with tactics may be unfair in competition. Innovative approaches such as a colored light system to signal the beginning of races for the deaf probably would eliminate the old handkerchief or flag drop.

Competitive Site: The competitive site must be well prepared and maintained to a high standard. All holes should be filled, paths and roads should be smooth, and all sites should be easily accessible and safe to traverse.

Running tracks, swimming pools, and other areas for competitions must be up to international caliber. The metal curb on the inner lane of the running track should be removed when the blind are competing, but very small plastic pylons or, better still, small discs should be substituted to designate the inner parameter. This is important for safety reasons. Most other competition sites should be prepared as for normal top quality competition.

The housing for the athletes should be safe and of good quality. Usually, very few changes are needed. It is desirable but not essential to house all blind or deaf athletes on the ground floor. For all disabled athletes, there should be good safety features such as well marked exits, with audio and visual emergency warning devices. Adequate arrangements should be made for guide dogs, including provision of food and exercise areas for the animals.

The normal medical back-up of doctors, physiotherapists, athletic trainers, and medical supplies must be available at all times at the games site. Often this feature is overlooked.

TRAINING

Individuals born with a sensory disability are often at a disadvantage in the level of cardiovascular fitness they can attain, owing to a lack of early childhood development. Scant research suggest these children have a subnormal maximum oxygen intake and fail to develop the normal working heart rate. This reflects a lack of training and general exercise opportunities, since when the child is trained for a few months, heart rate responses become similar to those of other athletes of the same age. Muscle fatigue is also a major limiting factor, regardless of the exercise modality used. Recent data from Toronto suggest that after 16 weeks of vigorous physical training, blind teenagers (13 to 18 years) attain fitness levels approaching those of the normal, trained teenager. Previous research done in Winnipeg in 1971 showed that the physical working capacity of deaf children (8 to 17 years) was similar to that of normal children, but was superior to that of the blind.

Arousal in deaf children, and overprotection by parents of blind children are important early obstacles to overcome if athletes are to be developed from these groups. However, once motivated and trained, such patients are able to reach normal or even above-average physical working capacities.

Until recently, most deaf, blind and other sensory disabled children were so unprepared that they could not hope to take part in sport competition. With sensible preparation covering the basic elements of training, many aspiring athletes now attempt training for high-level competition with good success. In fact, some performances in various sports are exceedingly good when compared to normal athletes.

Basic components for adequate athletic training are set out below. All elements will be included in a good training system:

1. Prolonged or continuous aerobic work.
2. Repetition work.⎤
3. Intermittent work.⎥──► aerobic or anaerobic
4. Interval work.⎦
5. Strength and circuit training.
6. Competitive aspects.

The classification covers the three major components that build up endurance, strength, and speed. If an athlete does not include training from each section, it is possible to miss that overall development which is important in the making of a top level athlete. The duration of training is of extreme importance, but depends upon the type of event for which the child is being prepared. Another important consideration is the intensity and frequency of effort relative to the endurance of the athlete. Regardless of the sport, training of the disabled athlete must be based upon sound first principles, good planning, and a sensible approach.

EFFORT TOLERANCE IN SCOLIOSIS

HANS STOBOY, M.D.

RESPIRATORY PROBLEMS

The most important clinical symptom of decreased effort tolerance in severe scoliosis is dyspnea. This is observed not only during exercise, but even at rest. The breathing pattern is marked by a small tidal volume and an increased respiratory rate. There is thus a large deadspace ventilation/minute volume ratio and a diminished alveolar ventilation. These findings become pronounced in patients with a Cobb-angle (lateral deviation of the spine) larger than 70°.

Owing to stiffness of the thoracic cage, the compliance of the respiratory system is smaller than normal, decreasing as Cobb-angle increases. This reflects a reduced chest compliance. The pressure/volume curve has a shallow slope and a diminished linear portion over mid lung volumes (30 to 40% of total lung capacity compared to 75% in normal subjects). Compliance drops to 0.04 to 0.07 L/cm H_2O, from the normal 0.2 cm H_2O. The overall compliance of the respiratory system in severe scoliosis is thus reduced from 0.1 L/cm H_2O to approximately 0.07 L/cm H_2O.

EDITOR'S NOTE

Minor deformities of the spine may spoil the appearance of an athlete, detracting from scores where appearance is a feature of judging, but otherwise have little importance in sports medicine.

Major scoliotic deformities impair balance, throw uneven strain upon other body joints, and in severe cases may impair cardiorespiratory performance, with a limitation of working capacity. In a sample of 542 children aged 6 to 12 years, we noted some degree of spinal deformity in five. The muscular strength was 96 percent of the anticipated figure in these children, but maximal oxygen intake was only 87 percent of normal. Stoboy examined older youth (13 to 20 years) with much more serious deformities (average 66-degree angulation of the spine) and their maximal oxygen transport was only 79 percent of normal. However, after a combination of surgical treatment (Harrington rod) and endurance training (cycling, supplemented by swimming after removal of the cast), aerobic power was increased to a normal level.

Others have noted improvements or aerobic power in severely deformed children after training, even in the absence of surgical treatment.

The work of breathing is greatly increased, varying as the square of tidal volume. If a patient changes from a typical tidal volume of 250 ml to a normal tidal volume of 500 ml, a 20-fold increase of breathing work can be expected.

If the deformity exceeds 70°, pulmonary hypertension precedes right heart failure in many adult patients. The increased pulmonary vascular resistance appears to be due to a combination of pulmonary vasoconstriction and vascular changes such as medial proliferation.

Lung volumes and capacities are diminished. The best-documented negative correlation relates vital capacity to Cobb-angle; at an angle of 100°, the VC is reduced by approximately 50 percent. Despite these various restrictions of pulmonary function, Haber and associates have suggested that the low aerobic power of the scoliotic patient is due exclusively to sedentary life habits. General detraining occurs because children with severe scoliosis are reluctant to take part in physical activities. But impairment of ventilation is also an important factor limiting physical performance in advanced and severe scoliosis.

EFFORT TOLERANCE

Effort tolerance depends mainly on the extent of scoliosis. Most patients with minor scoliosis (Cobb-angle smaller than 30°) have no functional restrictions. However, patients with moderate (Cobb-angle $\overline{X} = 50$ to 70°) or severe scoliosis (Cobb-angle more than 70°) show a definite decrease in pulmonary and/or cardiovascular function.

Issues in assessing effort tolerance include:

1. Which of the variables characterizing physical fitness are diminished relative to healthy subjects?
2. Does surgical correction of scoliosis and a strict regimen of rehabilitation improve function or does ventilation remain at presurgical values?
3. Do differences exist between moderate and severe scoliosis?
4. Is the limitation of physical work capacity due to morphologic and functional changes of ventilation or to detraining?
5. Is any information available concerning benefit from rehabilitation?

In moderate and severe scoliosis (Cobb-angle 39 to 102°; n = 62), the VC is decreased to 60 to 80 percent of reference values. According to Meister, a loss of VC is seen at Cobb-angles > 50°, with a drop to 50 percent of reference values at Cobb-angles > 100°. The decreases of one-second forced expiratory volume, (FEV_1) match the loss of forced vital capacity (FVC). The maximum voluntary ventilation (MVV) is sometimes said to be less restricted than VC in severe scoliosis, but we have seen a diminution to approximately 40 to 50 percent of normal values.

Maximal work rates (100 to 120 watt) are diminished by 30 to 40 percent relative to reference values. The resting heart rate of a moderate or severely scoliotic patient is 102 to 105/min, and a maximal heart rate of 185 to 200/min is reached at relatively low work loads.

The resting respiratory minute volume ($\dot{V}E$) is increased by 30 to 40 percent compared to reference values. The breathing frequency (f_R) is high (21/min), and the tidal volume (V_T) is small. The increase of f_R becomes more marked as compliance decreases. It represents an attempt to avoid an increased O_2 consumption by the respiratory muscles. This pattern of ventilation is nevertheless inefficient, leading to a diminished alveolar ventilation and an enlarged dead space (V_D) ventilation /min, with a V_D/V_T ratio of 0.40 to 0.45 compared to 0.35 in healthy subjects.

During maximum work, f_R reaches 35 to 40/min, but V_E is limited to 51 L/min. In submaximal work (1.35 W/kg), the ventilation remains inefficient, with a small V_T, an increased work of breathing (small and shallow compliance), and a respiratory O_2 consumption four to ten times larger than normal. The breaking point of V_E or work rate.

The ventilatory equivalent ($\dot{V}EO_2$; normally 28 ml/L O_2) is raised to at least 33 to 35, emphasizing the inefficient pattern of ventilation.

During submaximal ergometric exercise,the most severely scoliotic patients (120 to 160°) show a larger O_2 consumption than less restricted individuals. However, at maximal work loads, the patients with severe scoliosis show a significantly smaller O_2 uptake (1400 ml/min) than those who are less disabled (1600 ml/min). $\dot{V}O_2$ max values are about 40 percent less than reference values. The maximal O_2 uptake/kg of body mass is 30 to 32 ml/kg/min, larger than reported in some earlier studies of scoliotic children (11 to 25 ml/kg/min), but very low when compared to the figures of 40 to 55 ml/kg/min anticipated in healthy subjects.

In moderate scoliosis, the resting arterial oxygen pressure (PaO_2) is scarcely diminished. When the restriction of VC is < 60 percent, the PaO_2 increases during light exercise, but if the VC is restricted by more than 60 percent, arterial hypoxemia develops. According to Meister, hypoxemia during physical exercise is one of the most important signs of respiratory insufficiency. Nineteen patients in one study that we conducted, showed a rise of PaO_2 during maximal work, from 75 torr to 93 torr; this suggests the exercise brought about an improvement of the ventilation-perfusion ratio. Other patients showed a decrease of PaO_2 during exercise, reflecting increased venous admixture. Hypercapnia is a very rare finding in scoliosis, and is only seen with extreme restrictions of VC (< 30%).

In moderate or severe scoliosis, most of the functional and effort criteria are worse than reference values for healthy subjects or at best lie at the lower limit of the normal range.

RESPONSE TO SURGICAL TREATMENT

Most authors maintain that corrective surgery does not appreciably improve lung function, although published papers lack information concerning rehabilitation regimens, which play a major role in the successful treatment of scoliosis. In our study, all patients (n = 62) underwent endurance training and spinal mobilization therapy for several weeks prior to surgery. They remained under clinical observation for a period of 14 months. A strict regimen of casts and braces was maintained, supplemented by breathing therapy as well as strength and endurance training.

Lind and Bjüre assessed lung volumes for 5 years following surgery. They found significant increases in both static and dynamic lung volumes. Meister also noted a significant (20 to 25%) improvement of lung volumes over a 4 to 5-year follow-up. Gains were accompanied by an increase of PaO_2, especially during physical exercise, and a diminution of $\dot{V}EO_2$, with an enhanced ventilation-perfusion ratio.

In our study, patients with moderate scoliosis (Cobb-angle < 70°; n = 47) showed an improvement in nearly all variables, including an improved effort tolerance after spinal surgery and rehabilitation. Maximal benefit developed over the first 2 years, usually corresponding with the completion of body growth.

Several authors have seen significant increases of VC and FEV_1, with a return of MVV toward the normal range. Shneerson and Edgar did not find any changes after spinal fusion, but this may be due to a small sample (n = 10), a short period of observation (17 to 21 months), and a different rehabilitation regimen.

We saw a decrease of resting f_R, $\dot{V}EO_2$ and f_H until the end of the second year, an observation suggesting improved alveolar ventilation and enhanced cardiac function. $\dot{V}Emax$, $\dot{V}O_2max$ and O_2 pulse also rose until the end of the second year, confirming the enhancement of effort tolerance by spinal fusion and strict rehabilitation.

In patients with severe scoliosis, the increase of VC was proportionately the same. However, the postoperative f_R, f_H, $\dot{V}Emax$, $\dot{V}O_2max$, and O_2 pulse remained unchanged. Nevertheless, a decrease of $\dot{V}EO_2$ in this group, especially at maximal work load, indicated an improvement of alveolar ventilation during exercise.

We avoided using $\dot{V}O_2max$ per kg of body mass to assess changes of fitness, because an increase of body mass occurred following surgery (4 kg and 9 kg in two years for moderate and severe cases respectively). Subsequently, body mass remained constant (55 kg).

ROLE OF EXERCISE IN TREATMENT OF SCOLIOSIS

Haber et al stated categorically that "a reduced aerobic capacity is not the consequence of scoliosis in most patients, but the consequence of keeping the patients away from school sports and other sport activities." However, this seems only a partial explanation of the reduced effort tolerance. Certainly, children with severe scoliosis do not participate in physical exercise as they should, owing to their unattractive appearance, their exercise dyspnea, and the influence of an overprotective family and/or family physician. On the other hand, Schneerson argues that reduced ventilation and/or dyspnea are the factors limiting physical fitness. These divergent opinions reflect differing observation periods, treatments, rehabilitation regimens, degrees of scoliosis, ages, and other unpredictable influences.

We discriminate between the two patient groups (Cobb-angle $< 70°$ and $> 70°$). Both groups underwent the same treatment for one year after spinal surgery; in moderate scoliosis, most functional criteria approached the normal range postoperatively, but most values in severely scoliotic patients remained at their presurgical value after operation, although operation did prevent the deterioration of ventilation which is usually seen in untreated severe scoliosis.

Additional physical training is recommended by some authors to retard the progress of spinal curvature and to improve pulmonary function and physical working capacity. It can be assumed from the decrease of $\dot{V}EO_2$ and increase of PaO_2 that alveolar ventilation is improved during physical performance. Sünram et al and Götze et al both reported positive changes of $\dot{V}O_2max$, O_2 pulse and $\dot{V}EO_2$ after only 4 weeks of heavy training, but as far as we know, these patients have never been retested.

Bjüre et al showed an increase in $\dot{V}O_2max$ and a decrease of submaximal heart rate after 3 months of training in most of their patients. However, there was no correlation between the increase of $\dot{V}O_2max$ and gains of VC. Some patients with large curvatures did not improve with training. Approximately the same results were found in our studies. Comparing patients with moderate and severe scoliosis, the Cobb-angle could not clearly differentiate a group of patients who would benefit most from training. It may be that patients with a severe limitation of $\dot{V}O_2max$ cannot be improved by moderate training, owing to persistently hypoventilated and/or underperfused areas of lung; in general the less trainable patients are those with extremely severe scoliosis, but the issue has not been completely resolved, and additional research is required to test the correlation between the degree of ventilatory restriction and the response to physical training.

FEMALES AND PHYSICAL ACTIVITY

JANET E. HALL, M.Sc., M.D., F.R.C.P.(C)

Over the past decade, the participation of women in physical activity has increased dramatically. Women of all ages are exercising, and increasing numbers are training intensively for endurance events. This has raised a unique set of issues, many of which relate to reproductive endocrine function. Puberty may be delayed in girls involved in intensive training programs. Menstrual cycle changes have been increasingly reported and include shortened luteal phases, oligomenorrhea, amenorrhea, and anovulation. These raise concerns about future infertility and accelerated osteoporosis. In addition, many women are anxious to exercise during pregnancy, and issues of teratogenesis, fetal growth retardation, and birth complications must be addressed.

Other issues such as anemia and nutrition are important, but this chapter will deal mainly with areas related to reproductive endocrinology. After briefly reviewing the known hormonal events and the possible sites at which exercise may exert an influence on reproductive hormonal control, the aforementioned issues will be addressed in terms of therapeutic approaches.

REPRODUCTIVE MECHANISMS

Normal reproductive function in women involves a complex interplay of hypothalamic, pituitary, and ovarian factors. The hypothalamus plays a key role in coordinating and integrating signals from the central nervous system (stress, body mass, and environmental cues), with feedback from the ovary via estrogen and progesterone. Gonadotropin-releasing hormone (GnRH) is secreted in a pulsatile fashion from neurons in the arcuate nucleus of the hypothalamus into the portal circulation, which supplies the anterior pituitary. In the pituitary, luteinizing hormone (LH) and follicle-stimulating hormone (FSH) are synthesized and secreted in response to this single releasing hormone. LH and FSH are not controlled in parallel, however. The amounts and proportions of LH and FSH released are influenced separately by feedback of the ovarian steroids and possibly by the frequency and amplitude of GnRH pulsations.

Several neurotransmitters are thought to be important in modulating the basic program of GnRH pulses from the hypothalamus. Norepinephrine has a stimulatory effect on GnRH release and LH pulsations, whereas dopamine inhibits both GnRH and prolactin. Endorphins (endogenous opiate peptides) may play a role in gonadotropin secretion through direct inhibition of GnRH or possibly via their known effect of increasing prolactin, which would then inhibit dopamine and GnRH. Catechol-estrogens are structurally similar to the neurotransmitters, and their potential role in GnRH modulation is currently being investigated.

As mentioned, the ovarian steroids exert extremely important influences at the level of both the pituitary and the hypothalamus. At the pituitary, low levels of estrogen have a negative effect. With exposure to higher estrogen levels, however, there is a positive feedback effect which is facilitated by the presence of progesterone and is largely responsible for the pre-ovulatory LH surge. Estrogens also have a positive feedback effect on the frequency of GnRH from the hypothalamus. In man, the frequency of LH pulsations decreases in the luteal phase in a pattern that correlates with the duration of progesterone exposure. In animals, endorphin levels are higher in the luteal phase and are increased by estrogen and progesterone. This also may be an important mechanism in the decreased frequency of LH pulses seen in the luteal phase in women.

Prior to puberty, the reproductive axis is characterized by low levels of gonadotropins and ovarian steroids. It has long been postulated that at this time, the hypothalamus is extremely sensitive to negative feedback by the low levels of circulating sex steroids and that this super-sensitivity is lost at puberty. Recent evidence had questioned any negative feedback role of these steroids prior to puberty. Whatever the mechanism, puberty is characterized by the emergence of gonadotropin, and by inference, GnRH pulsations. This is initially manifested by LH surges, which occur only with sleep, and eventually by a pattern of LH pulsations which occur approximately every hour. Reproductive maturity is characterized by monthly ovulatory cycles. In the follicular phase, the dominant follicle emerges under the stimulation of FSH and estrogen production increases. Ovulation is preceded by an obligatory LH surge and is followed by luteinization of the follicle, with production of estrogen and progesterone in the luteal phase. Finally, as the corpus luteum ages, if conception does not occur, steroid production declines and the endometrium, which has been prepared for implantation, is shed. At about 40 years of age, the frequency of ovulatory cycles decreases in association with a diminishing number of follicles. Over the next decade, estrogen levels decrease and the menopause ensues. At this time, low levels of ovarian steroids are accompanied by high gonadotropin levels.

Influence of Exercise

Alterations in certain reproductive hormones occur with exercise and training. We initially observed acute increases in estradiol and progesterone with exercise in the luteal phase and estradiol in the follicular phase, and these observations have been confirmed by others. The work of HA Keizer suggests that these changes result from a decreased clearance of the ovarian steroids during and after exercise. Data on the gonadotropins are less consistent, and interpretation is compounded by the pulsatile nature of their secretion. It is clear that accurate characterization of the acute gonadotropin response to exercise will require careful analysis of LH and FSH pulsations with more frequent sampling and longer follow-up than has been used to date. Prolactin has also been shown to increase in response to exercise, an effect that is more pronounced in trained women. Likewise, endorphin levels are higher with exercise and appear in some studies to be augmented by training.

There are several sites at which these changes may act to alter reproductive cycle endocrine function. Elevated ovarian steroids may have an inhibitory effect at the level of the pituitary. In animals, prolactin increases the sensitivity of the pituitary to this effect. In addition, prolactin elevations may exert their effect at the hypothalamus by inhibiting dopamine and, thus, GnRH. Endorphins are increased by the ovarian steroids and by exercise and may inhibit GnRH either directly or via an increased prolactin, as above. Changes in the frequency and amplitude of GnRH pulses may alter LH and FSH production both absolutely and in relation to each other. These changes, in turn, may affect the orderly process of follicular maturation and result in either shortened luteal phases or anovulatory cycles.

An alteration of GnRH pulsations may explain the abnormally low FSH/LH ratio in the follicular phase which has been found in swimmers with shortened luteal phases. Further support for a primary hypothalamic defect comes from studies in amenorrheic runners, showing a decrease in the frequency of LH pulses in some with a normal or supersensitive LH response to exogenous GnRH, the latter suggesting that the pituitary is sensitive to whatever GnRH input it receives.

Other factors thought to be important are an excessive energy demand relative to food intake and body reserves of fat. Some authors have argued that peripheral fat provides a major site for conversion of androgens to estrogens and that estrogens drop below the critical level needed to sustain the menstrual cycle if body fat is less than some arbitrary figure variously set at 12 to 20 percent of body mass. The high core temperature associated with distance running may influence hypothalamic GnRH control and may also depress ovarian steroid secretion. Finally, the impact of anxiety upon menstrual function is well documented, and top-level athletic competitors may well face greater psychological pressures than women with other careers.

MENSTRUAL CYCLE DISTURBANCES

Delayed Menarche

Menarche, the onset of menstrual periods, is one of the final stages of pubertal development, occurring some 2 years after the beginning of breast development and pubic and axillary hair growth. Regular ovulatory menstrual cycles may take 1 to 3 years to become established.

However, the onset of menses is a point that is more amenable to retrospective analysis than other aspects of pubertal development and has been used in a number of studies comparing athletes and ballet dancers with nonexercising females.

Olympic volleyball players were found to have a later age of menarche than high school and college athletes, who in turn had a later menarche than nonathletes. Later menarche was also reported in a group of adult women running more than 48 km a week compared with nonrunning controls. Bearing in mind that international competitors are selected for characteristics that differ by 3 to 4 standard deviations from the mean, one should expect such selection to have an impact upon the age of menarche. Those with late menarche tend to remain petite in their early teen years, so at this stage may have particular success as gymnasts or ballet dancers. However, late maturation also encourages a large adult height, so that in their later teens, later maturers may have a body build well adapted to volleyball or basketball. Nevertheless, there is evidence that some factor related to competitive training may cause a later menarche. Frisch studied swimmers and runners and found a delayed menarche of 5 months per year of premenarche training, but those who began training after menarche had a menarchal age comparable to that of controls. Warren followed young ballet dancers for 4 years and documented a mean menarchal age of 15.4 years compared with 12.5 years in an age-matched control group. More significantly, progression of sexual development and onset of menses occurred during periods of forced rest, even when body composition was unchanged. There was a significant catch-up effect in pubertal progress at these times.

Studies of Olympic athletes indicate that delayed menarche is more common in gymnasts and runners than in swimmers. Those groups most affected, such as ballet dancers, are relatively lean and there have been suggestions that a critical amount of body fat is required before menarche begins. Numerous studies have failed to support the idea that leanness is the only variable responsible for delayed menarche. However, it does seem to play an important role. In Warren's study, leaner dancers were relatively more affected by alterations in energy expenditures than were their heavier peers. A population study of girls in Holland also supports a synergism between thinness and intense sports activity in delaying menarche.

Altered Menstrual Cycles

Although most women can exercise without menstrual changes, there is an increased prevalence of amenorrhea and oligomenorrhea among athletes and dancers. The figures quoted range from 3.4 percent, as in the general population, to 51 percent, depending on the group being studied and the definition of terms. Shortened luteal phases have been documented in swimmers and marathon runners. If cycle length alone were used as the basis for normalcy, many of these subjects would have been classed as normally menstruating, indicating that the prevalence of menstrual cycle changes may well be higher than the current estimates.

Longitudinal studies have documented a variability in types of menstrual cycles, so that a given woman with a normal pretraining cycle may go on to initially develop a shortened luteal phase followed by anovulation and/or amenorrhea with further training. This suggests that the short luteal phase, oligomenorrhea, and amenorrhea observed with training are part of a continuum.

Factors most often associated with alterations in menstrual function are training intensity, relative leanness, and variables relating to reproductive immaturity. Although training intensity, particularly in terms of stress, is difficult to quantify, a positive correlation between weekly mileage and the prevalence of secondary amenorrhea has been shown. Dancers and athletes frequently report changes in menstrual cycles related to alterations in training schedules. Even among athletes who train at a high intensity, amenorrhea is more common in activities that promote or require a low percentage of body fat. In many groups of runners and dancers, there is an increased reporting of amenorrhea in leaner participants, and acute changes of body mass with no alteration in training intensity have also been found to influence menstrual regularity. Thus, the potential synergism of exercise intensity and leanness noted for menarche would also appear to be operative here. Menstrual irregularities are more frequently found in athletes who experience a later menarche, in younger athletes and dancers, and in those with a history of irregular cycles prior to training. Such women may have a relatively fragile reproductive endocrine axis.

Of particular importance, longitudinal studies have now shown a return of normal menstrual function both in women who continue to train but gain mass and in those who decrease training intensity while maintaining a low body fat.

Therapeutic Approach

Any woman who presents with concerns relating to reproductive function must be seriously evaluated with her own needs in mind. As with delayed menarche, reports of the reversibility of exercise-related menstrual cycle changes are extremely encouraging for women with concerns about current or future infertility. In our enthusiasm, however, it must be remembered that exercising women are susceptible to the same problems as other women presenting with infertility or menstrual problems. Whether dealing with primary amenorrhea (delayed menarche) or secondary amenorrhea, the first responsibility of the physician is to ensure that this is related to sports participation and not to some pathology which has been overlooked. The diagnosis and treatment of other pathologies follows the general principles found in standard texts and will not be repeated here. In the exercising female, a combination of hard training and insufficient energy intake may be a factor. The possibility that legal or illegal medication is involved must also be kept in mind; examples include the therapeutic use of cortisone preparations in the treatment of musculoskeletal problems and use of anabolic steroids.

The average age of menarche in North America is 12.5 to 13 years. In dancers and athletes, this may be delayed to 15 years. It is now encouraging that following a period of relative inactivity and/or a significant weight gain, pubertal progression occurs, indicating that these effects are reversible. However, when menarche is delayed beyond 10 to 12 years in the absence of breast and pubic hair development, or beyond 16 years in their presence, medical advice should be sought. Initial evaluation should include an exercise and growth history as well as a careful family history with particular reference to pubertal development. Growth and pubertal development charts should be started and gonadotropins measured. Gain of body mass or a decrease in physical activity for several months may be suggested. This will usually be sufficient to produce pubertal progression or menstruation if there is any concern on the part of the patient, her parents or the physician. Further evaluation depends on the individual circumstances and responses to these simple maneuvers.

Evaluation of the woman with secondary amenorrhea or infertility should begin with a careful menstrual history, including age at menarche, evidence for the establishment of regular ovulatory cycles, and past pregnancies, all of which may provide clues to the maturity of the reproductive endocrine axis. It is important to inquire about contraception and about symptoms that may suggest estrogen deficiency such as painful intercourse, lack of vaginal secretions, or frequent urethritis. Questions relating to abnormal hair growth, galactorrhea, or symptoms of hypo- or hyperthyroidism should be included. A detailed exercise and weight history may provide clues to reversibility of any cycle abnormalities and should allow the practitioner to identify those in whom physical activity is part of an anorexia nervosa syndrome. Following a thorough physical examination, which should include a pelvic examination, investigations should begin with a pregnancy test in any sexually active woman, a prolactin level, and, if the woman has menstrual cycles, documentation of the basal body temperature for one month. Further hormonal evaluation may include estradiol levels, gonadotropins, and, if clinically indicated, thyroid function and androgen status.

Hypothalamic amenorrhea may be associated with low or normal estrogen levels, and this can usually be assessed clinically. Although some authors advocate the use of oral contraceptives or replacement estrogen and progestogen, their use is controversial. Oral contraceptives carry an increased risk of cerebrovascular accident, especially in patients who smoke or have a history of migraine headache. The risk of thromboembolic complications is related to estrogen dose and becomes less significant with current low-dose contraceptives. An increased risk of myocardial infarction is associated with the use of high-dose oral contraceptive medication, but information regarding the effects of currently used low-dose preparations is still awaited. A suspected association between the use of oral contraceptives and endometrial or breast malignant tumors has yet to be substantiated. In the woman under 30 who does not smoke, have hypertension or a history of migraine, oral contraceptives can be considered.

One of the practical problems arising from low estrogen levels is atrophy of the genitourinary mucosa; this leads to painful intercourse and urethritis. It can be treated with estrogen cream, applied locally several times per week, or with oral estrogens and intermittent progesterone. The last medication is an important component of therapy because of the increased risk of endometrial hyperplasia with unopposed estrogens. The other major side effect of low estrogen levels is osteoporosis (to be discussed).

The woman who presents with infrequent periods, particularly if there is heavy bleeding or prolonged spotting, may have adequate estrogen but inadequate progesterone from chronic anovulation, a situation which predisposes her to endometrial hyperplasia and adenocarcinoma of the endometrium. In this group, progesterone in the form of Provera, 5 to 10 mg for 10 days of each month, *should* be used.

If pregnancy is desired, ovulation or normalization of a shortened luteal phase can usually be achieved by modifying training schedules for several months without completely discontinuing training. In lean women, a small gain of body mass may be all that is required for the return of normal cycles. Treatment beyond this for the anovulatory woman requiring pregnancy may require ovulation inducing drugs and should be managed by physicians with particular expertise in this area. Causes of infertility other than anovulation must be considered when applicable.

For the woman who does not wish to become pregnant, contraception is important even in the absence of regular cycles. In fact, menstrual irregularity may increase the risk of unplanned conception. Barrier methods are often more acceptable to the athlete, but the birth control pill is an alternative, taking into account the foregoing comments. Two studies have now shown a decrease in muscle endurance in oral contraceptive users, and a decrease of maximum oxygen intake while taking oral contraceptives has also been observed in subjects who acted as their own controls.

OSTEOPOROSIS

Bone mass decreases in both men and women with aging, beginning at age 30 to 35 in women and about age 50 in men. In women, the loss occurs two to three times faster than in men. Around the menopause, there is a period of 5 years in which bone loss is accelerated even further. Decreased bone mass increases the risk of skeletal fractures, including hip, radial, and vertebral fractures.

Bed rest exacerbates the demineralization of bone. Conversely, exercise increases both total and local bone mass in both young people and the elderly. Even elderly postmenopausal women can increase their bone mineral content in response to exercise.

Adequate dietary calcium is essential to prevent bone resorption, as serum calcium is regulated within fine limits. Most women have a slightly negative calcium balance, and this doubles after the menopause owing to a diminished absorption of dietary calcium. Recent studies have shown an alarming deficit of calcium intake in both ballet dancers and athletes. The recommended calcium intake is 1 gram per day for premenopausal women and 1.5 grams per day for postmenopausal women, the latter being equivalent to 4 to 5 glasses of milk per day.

Estrogen is important in controlling bone resorption, and decreases blood levels of estrogen are presumably responsible for the accelerated bone loss after the menopause. In oophorectomized women, Cann has shown that bone loss stabilized after 24 months when subjects were given Premarin (conjugated estrogens), 0.6 mg/day, whereas controls continued to lose bone at 36 months. Patients with amenorrhea secondary to hyperprolactinemia have a decrease in bone mineral content, but it was expected that the protective effects of exercise would counterbalance any effects of decreased estrogen on bone in athletes with amenorrhea. Recent studies, however, have revealed decreases of vertebral density in amenorrheic runners, although dietary deficiencies may have been a contributing factor. Preliminary studies have suggested that in sports involving the upper body, the decrease in vertebral bone density is not as apparent.

Therapeutic Approach

Recommendations for the prevention of early osteoporosis in women include the building of a strong bone mass before the age of 30 and continued exercise thereafter. An adequate calcium intake is also vital. Recommendations for amenorrheic athletes and those with shortened luteal phases are controversial. Some physicians advocate estrogen replacement, particularly for those with stress fractures. In young women with no contraindications, oral contraceptives can be used. Otherwise, low-dose estrogens in the form of premarin or the newer estradiol preparations are suggested. These must be used in combination with progesterone as Provera, 5–10 mg for 10 days per month, to guard against endometrial hyperplasia. However, the use of estrogen is not universally accepted, and careful attention to dietary calcium intake may well prove sufficient to prevent accelerated osteoporosis. The information we have to date is not complete regarding this issue.

PREGNANCY

Information about the effects of exercise during pregnancy on maternal and fetal well-being is currently incomplete. Studies in developing countries and in the lower socioeconomic strata of industrialized countries suggest that women who work until term, particularly if this involves standing, have smaller babies and may have an increased incidence of stillbirths. An increase in perinatal mortality and a probable decrease of birth weight has also been described in rats trained at 80 to 88 percent of $\dot{V}O_2$ max during pregnancy. Such studies raise concerns about the adequacy of uterine blood flow during exercise and potential hypoxic effects on the fetus. Direct measurements cannot be made in humans, and animal studies are far from conclusive. Fetal hypoxia and a decrease in uterine blood flow have been documented in pregnant ewes during moderately severe and exhausting exercise, although such changes have not always been found. In the only human study labelled saline was injected into uterine and skeletal muscle. The authors demonstrated a decrease in uterine blood flow when women performed moderate exercise during the third trimester; an effect was more pronounced in preeclamptic subjects.

Fetal heart rate monitoring has been used to assess the fetal response to maternal exercise. Both bradycardia and tachycardia can reflect fetal distress. Varying exercise intensities have been used, although none have been maximal or exhausting. The usual fetal heart rate response is a mild increase, but transient initial decelerations were noted by Dale and associates. A small percentage of women in two additional studies have been shown more profound changes during exercise testing. In one of these reports, there was a high correlation with subsequent fetal distress during labor.

In one study of birth "weight", length of labor, or complications no adverse effects were noted in women who continued to jog throughout pregnancy. Another group trained women at 65 to 70 percent of maximum oxygen intake throughout the second and third trimesters; they found a trend toward increasing birth "weights" in the exercised group.

Therapeutic Approach

In general, recommendations for training during pregnancy should be individualized. Common sense is the key. Pregnancy is not the time to begin a new sport or conditioning program. In the absence of complications or significant risk factors, such as twins or hypertension, women can continue their usual activity throughout the first and second trimesters, but should expect a gradual decrease in performance, especially in the second trimester. Sports in which trauma is possible should be avoided, as should activities in which body temperature increases by more than 1°C (for instance, running and racquet sports). During the final trimester, individuals vary considerably in their exercise tolerance, but further decreases of activity are to be advised, and in some cases, exercise may need to be restricted. If training is continued at this time, it should be done only under close physician supervision, and exercise testing with fetal heart rate monitoring is recommended.

ATHLETES WITH MENSTRUAL IRREGULARITIES

DONALD W. KILLINGER, M.D., Ph.D., F.R.C.P.(C)

Menstrual problems occurring in athletes include primary amenorrhea, secondary amenorrhea, oligomenorrhea and normal menstrual cycles with a short luteal phase. These problems are relatively common in athletes, particularly those involved in world-class competition. As has been described in a previous chapter, one of the major factors involved in these menstrual problems appears to be a diminished ratio of fat to lean body mass. It has been noted, however, that individuals with normal body mass can also develop menstrual problems during strenuous exercise, and hyperprolactinemia has been recorded in some of these patients. There is also recent interest in the possible role of endorphins as a factor interfering with normal menstrual activity. It is probable that the main site of action of these opioid peptides is in the control of prolactin secretion through the hypothalamus rather than by direct inhibition of gonadotrophin secretion at the level of the pituitary. These endorphins may interfere with the dopaminergic inhibitory activity of the hypothalamus in diminishing prolactin secretion. By this mechanism, endogenous opioids can result in an increase in prolactin release and thereby affect menstrual activity.

The vast majority of athletes with menstrual irregularities do not require treatment, and the problem will disappear with a change in physical and emotional routine. There can, however, coexist any of the usual mechanisms resulting in either primary amenorrhea or other menstrual irregularities; these must be investigated prior to reassuring the patient that no intervention is required.

COMMON CAUSES OF MENSTRUAL IRREGULARITIES

The common causes of menstrual irregularities in healthy athletes include hyperprolactinemia, polycystic ovarian disease, adrenal virilism, nonfunctioning pituitary adenoma, and anabolic steroids. If a female athlete has not reached the menarche by age 16 or if secondary amenorrhea or menstrual irregularities occur at any other time, investigation should be carried out to be sure that no other underlying cause is present. Hyperprolactinemia can occur as a result of a prolactin-secreting pituitary tumor, drugs that alter dopamine release or action, or both physical and emotional stress. If the hyperprolactinemia begins at an early age, primary amenorrhea may occur. Slight elevations in prolactin levels can permit normal menstrual periods with interference in luteal function; more serious elevations can result in oligomenorrhea or secondary amenorrhea.

Polycystic ovarian disease is a common cause of secondary amenorrhea and oligomenorrhea but is rarely associated with primary amenorrhea. The major clinical features of this syndrome are obesity, hirsutism, and menstrual irregularities. Particularly in the athletic female, obesity may not be present, and this problem could go unrecognized. Adrenal virilism associated with increased adrenal androgen production can be due to the late appearance of a mild form of congenital adrenal hyperplasia due to a 21-hydroxylase deficiency. Most patients with increased adrenal androgen production do not, however, have an identifiable enzyme defect, and the etiology is unknown. The clinical features are similar to those seen in polycystic ovarian disease. A nonfunctioning pituitary adenoma may result in amenorrhea in an otherwise healthy female and must be ruled out before reassurance can be given. It should be recalled that many of the female patients who are involved in serious international athletics may be taking anabolic steroids; use of these drugs can result in menstrual irregularities.

INVESTIGATION

The minimal investigation required to rule out the problems described includes the following. A detailed drug history to determine the potential use of anabolic steroids or the use of other drugs that could increase serum prolactin levels. This drug history should include use of the birth control pill. Serum prolactin levels should be measured during basal conditions such as a morning sample. If possible, additional determinations at different phases of the menstrual cycle would be very useful; a plasma prolactin level after exercise may be helpful to detect transient hyperprolactinemia. A skull film is important to detect a pituitary tumor and would also be potentially useful in detecting a cranial pharyngioma in patients with primary amenorrhea. While a skull film does not provide as much information as a CT scan, in situations in which there is no other evidence to suggest a pituitary tumor, this relatively simple procedure should be adequate.

The measurement of testosterone, androstenedione and dehydroepiandrosterone sulphate will provide information regarding excessive androgen production of both ovarian and adrenal origin. An increase in the plasma level of dehydroepiandrosterone sulphate suggests an adrenal source of excess androgen production, while an elevated level of testosterone is more likely to be of ovarian origin. Plasma luteinizing hormone (LH) and follicle stimulating hormone (FSH) should be measured to rule out primary ovarian failure in patients with either primary or secondary amenorrhea. An abnormal LH to FSH ratio would support a diagnosis of polycystic ovarian disease.

If this investigation shows any specific abnormalities, appropriate treatment is indicated. If, however, all of this investigation is normal and the patient is otherwise healthy, continued observation is appropriate as long as the patient continues to indulge in excessive physical activity. Repeat studies, particularly of prolactin levels, should be carried out at regular intervals to be sure that there are no abnormalities in this area. There is some debate as to whether specific therapy particularly with estrogen replacement is indicated in patients with amenorrhea. It is unlikely that amenorrhea persisting over a period of a few years will contribute substantially to long-standing osteoporosis, so concerns in this area are largely unfounded. Attempts to obtain withdrawal bleeding using 10 mg of Provera daily for 5 days will help to determine whether reasonable estrogen levels are present; if withdrawal bleeding occurs, this treatment could be instituted every 3 months if spontaneous menses do not return.

Most patients with menstrual irregularities associated with exercise recover spontaneously, and reassurance is the most useful therapeutic tool available. In order to provide this reassurance then, an adequate, thoughtful investigation is required to rule out any potentially serious underlying disorder. If this can be done, then the patient can be followed at regular intervals as long as the activities persist.

EXERCISE AND PREGNANCY

EDWIN DALE, Ph.D.
LEWIS G. MAHARAM, B.A.

The question of participation in an exercise program during pregnancy is one that can only be answered after complete and thorough discussion between the prospective parent(s) and the attending obstetrician or nurse midwife. Differing viewpoints concerning the appropriateness of exercise during pregnancy must be recognized. In years past, pregnancy was considered a state of disability that would confine the woman and her activities. Today, with our emphasis on physical fitness, the suggestion is made that if exercise is good for the nonpregnant woman, then perhaps it may be extended to and be equally good for the pregnant one. Additionally, the extrapolation might be made that if exercise promotes health, then perhaps exercise during pregnancy might assure a healthy fetus.

This chapter presents some practical recommendations for the woman who wishes to be involved in some type of exercise/fitness program during her pregnancy.

We shall review the physiologic impact of pregnancy upon the mother and the exacerbation of these effects when exercise is undertaken. Emphasis is placed upon features which are both general to the overall pregnancy and specific to the particular trimester. Attention will be focused on returning to or beginning exercise in the postpartum period and the effects of exercise during pregnancy upon fetal development, labor, delivery, and subsequent child development.

EFFECTS ON MOTHER

Pregnancy represents an altered physiologic state. Briefly, cardiac output is increased by 30 to 50 percent over the nonpregnant resting state. The greatest increment occurs during the first trimester, when uterine blood flow is slightly increased and before placental vascular flow has begun. The maximal maternal blood volume is observed in the eighth or ninth month. A pregnant woman reaches her maximum cardiac output at a lower rate of work. Minute ventilation during exercise also increases, especially in the third trimester. Because of the increase of total body mass, additional oxygen is required to perform any given activity. Other usual physiologic alterations include a reduction of hematocrit and a slight decrease of hemoglobin concentration. Lordosis of the lumbar spine and relaxation of the cartilages of the symphysis pubis are other major changes. These are endocrine-based changes of carbohydrate and steroid hormone metabolism as well.

In general, exercise brings about similar physiologic alterations. Changes are most pronounced for the cardiovascular and respiratory systems and less marked for the musculoskeletal and endocrine systems. If pregnancy and exercise are combined, there is a doubled physiologic impact. This fact suggests that if a prospective mother has not been involved in an exercise program prior to pregnancy, she should not be encouraged to begin one during her pregnancy.

The assumption is made that the condition of the mother is not complicated by hypertension, diabetes mellitus, anemia, or other metabolic diseases, which in themselves affect management of the pregnancy. The few reported studies of exercise during pregnancy are limited to small numbers of subjects and all deal with healthy volunteers.

In summary, the physiologic changes brought about in pregnancy are similar to those produced through strenuous exercise. Thus, a pregnant woman should not begin an exercise program after she has become pregnant. If, on the other hand, she becomes pregnant while involved in an exercise program such as running, it would not be harmful to continue the program. Exercise may become self-limiting, as a result of the increasing size of the pregnant uterus. Additionally, musculoskeletal changes may limit exercise that requires rapid movement and coordination, for example, competitive tennis, soccer, or equestrian dressage. As these activities also predispose the pregnant woman to an accidental fall, with the risk of trauma to both mother and fetus, such activities should be discouraged during pregnancy.

TRIMESTER RECOMMENDATIONS

The effects of exercise on the developing fetus are not so easily evaluated in humans as in animals. A number of recent studies have looked at the impact of exercise on the developing maternal-fetal complex.

First Trimester

In the first trimester, strenuous exercise has no great effect on the mother, as she is essentially unchanged from her prepregnant condition insofar as either body mass or cardiorespiratory and musculoskeletal systems are concerned. For the developing fetus, the major concerns to the mother are (1) to avoid medications, drugs, tobacco, and alcohol use, and (2) to avoid hyperthermia (here defined as a body temperature over 40 to 41°C). G. Parker reported a trend toward increased meningomyelocele in newborns delivered of women who had exercised vigorously during the first trimester of pregnancy and had suffered heat stress. The risk of developmental anomalies is greatest during the first trimester. A mother who sustains an injury while exercising may, unless she knows she is pregnant, be exposed to a medication that might produce a teratogenic effect.

General recommendations given for the first trimester are to continue the usual exercise program, to avoid training during hot periods (ambient dry-bulb temperature greater than 27°C), and to be certain to replace fluids lost as a consequence of any workout. Summer exercise should be conducted in the cool morning hours, when there is light for outdoor activities but the temperature has not peaked. Running late in the evening (after sunset) may avoid the heat, but there is then an increased risk of injury because of darkness.

Second Trimester

During the second trimester of pregnancy, the regular exercise program may be continued, but it should be supplemented by exercises that strengthen the muscles to be used in labor. The mother also should augment her diet; she requires iron and calcium supplementation as the developing fetus begins to demand these elements in increasing amounts. The mother has probably had a physical examination by this time, and the degree of competency of the cervix has been ascertained. If an incompetent cervix has been diagnosed and a cerclage procedure has been employed, exercise should certainly be limited. An incompetent cervix is the main contraindication to strenuous exercise during the second trimester. As in the first trimester, the mother may continue jogging, walking, swimming, golf, and other exercises which do not require rapid directional change or increase the opportunity for an accident or a fall. Blood volume is increased at this stage, and anemia is a common occurrence, so that supplemental iron is recommended.

Third Trimester

The largest number of investigations have been conducted in the third trimester. J. Pomerance and associates monitored fetal heart rates before and after exercising in 54 normal pregnancies. Four of five subjects who showed a suspicious test (change in fetal heart rate of more than 16 beats/min) also had signs of fetal distress during labor. Other clinicians evaluated moderate exercise in 7 pregnant women who routinely ran 7.2 km per week before and during their pregnancies. In the third trimester, nonstress tests were performed immediately after a 2.4 km run. All nonstress tests remained reactive, although fetal tachycardia was present. All of the women concerned delivered healthy infants at term.

R. H. Dressendorfer studied the acute responses of fetal heart rate in five trained swimmers who performed graded exercise cycling in a semi-Fowler's position at 32 to 39 weeks gestation. The fetal heart rate averaged 142 beats/min before exercise and gradually increased during exercise to a peak of 149 beats/min. Maternal heart rate reached 146 beats/min during the same time period. They suggested that their findings portrayed a normal fetal heart rate response to dynamic submaximal effort. The aerobic exercise that raised maternal heart rate was approximately 80 percent of the maximum and did not produce fetal bradycardia or trachycardia.

Sibley et al studied a 10-week swim conditioning program. Experimental subjects were able to maintain their initial fitness levels, while a sedentary control group could not. Additionally, maternal blood pressure, pulse, and fetal heart tones remained, for all subjects, within clinically acceptable limits during both the conditioning program and treadmill testing.

In a retrospective questionnaire study of 67 healthy, experienced runners who continued jogging during pregnancy, Jarrett and Spellacy collated data on pre-pregnancy health status, pregnancy, and delivery, and running experience during pregnancy. No correlation was found between the distance run and infant "weight" or gestational age. The incidence of fetal and maternal complications was low. There was a prematurity rate of 4.4 percent and one reported spontaneous abortion (1.5%). The information gathered suggests that jogging during pregnancy by conditioned runners is not harmful to the infant.

Effects on the Mother

Research conducted at Emory University has examined the clinical course of pregnancy and fetal and neonatal outcome in young women who continued to run or jog during their pregnancy. The majority of runners decreased their mileage as their pregnancy progressed. Acute illnesses such as nausea, vomiting, fatigue, joint pain, ligament pain, uterine contractions, fear of harm to the fetus, and awkwardness were listed as reasons for a decrease of running distance. Also, training speeds decreased from 10.7 km/hr (5.6 min per km) to 8.0 kms/hr (7.5 min per km). The mean increase of maternal body mass was 11.2 kg for runners and 12.9 kg for nonrunner controls. Length of labor in the runners ranged from 8 hours 20 minutes to greater than 20 hours, as contrasted to controls whose labor ranged from 4 hours to 27 hours. Use of analgesics and anesthesia during labor and delivery was similar in both groups. All runners had episiotomies, except for those who had cesarean sections. Similar information was recorded for the controls. Infant birth "weights" averaged 3.39 kg for runners and 3.45 kg for controls.

Fetal Monitoring

Studies of simultaneous maternal and fetal heart rates during treadmill exercise demonstrated a transient fetal bradycardia in three technically acceptable tracings. This decline continued for 2 to 3 minutes, at an intensity of effort likely in submaximal training. Recovery of the fetal heart rate to a normal range of 120 to 160 beats/min occurred after the 3 or 3½ minute mark of exercise, before attainment of the target heart rate for the mother. These results suggest that moderate maternal exercise has no harmful effects on fetal heart activity.

PRACTICAL RECOMMENDATIONS

From the above studies, the following recommendations may be made for the third trimester. Activities should be avoided which might initiate uterine contractions or lead to a potential imbalance and fall by the mother. Other features to avoid include rapid change of direction, prolonged lying on the back, prolonged standing, and heavy lifting. There is no evidence from any of the studies cited that exercise has a detrimental influence on fetal development.

Each of the three trimesters of pregnancy carries specific recommendations. For the first trimester, hot baths, whirlpools, and saunas are to be avoided. The mother should not begin a strenuous exercise program after she knows she is pregnant. However, it is not necessary to make any radical changes in her ongoing exercise program. Finally, she should not take any medications unless necessary for treatment of medical illness and prescribed by a physician.

In the second trimester, unless directed by a physician, she should not resort to special diets; exceptions are made in the cases of maternal hypertension and/or diabetes mellitus. However, foods high in energy content and low in nutritive value should be avoided. A well-balanced diet is usually prescribed and, when followed, will be of advantage to both the mother and the developing fetus. The mother should remember that exercise during pregnancy is not intended to control body mass, but rather to preserve muscle tone. Strong muscles should shorten the period of labor, making delivery easier on both mother and baby and hastening the return to optimal physical fitness following delivery.

In the third trimester, the mother should avoid exercises that may compromise blood flow, particularly venous return. For this reason, she should avoid long periods of standing and/or lifting heavy objects.

Ideal exercises that may be conducted throughout pregnancy include certain yoga asanas, swimming (until near term, but certainly not after rupture of the membranes), and, most ideally, walking with good posture.

POSTPARTUM EXERCISES

Depending on the type of delivery and the normality of delivery events, an exercise program should be resumed as shortly after delivery as is felt comfortable by both mother and attending physician or nurse-midwife. Even before leaving the hospital, the mother can begin to restore muscular tone to her abdomen and pelvis. This will reduce the likelihood of urinary incontinence and prolapse of the uterus, while possibly enhancing a return to satisfactory sexual activity. Exercise also promotes blood flow, avoiding such complications as varicose veins, leg cramps, edema, and thrombus formation. Improved circulation promotes healing of traumatized pelvic tissues and strengthens uterine and pelvic ligaments and tendons. An added factor, not scientifically documented, may be a reduction of postpartum depression. Exercise has always been known to improve self-image, and this could be very helpful to the mother during the postpartum period.

In the postpartum period, Kegel exercises in which the muscles of the pelvic floor are exercised are recommended, as they are before delivery. Exercises that strengthen the pelvic floor, particularly the pubococcygeal muscles are of greatest benefit.

The major exercises to be avoided in the postpartum period are those that employ a knee-chest position. This position has been implicated in several maternal deaths and may be associated with air embolism or neurologic changes.

FETAL WELL-BEING

A major question, asked throughout the years, is the effect of maternal exercise upon fetal well-being. To date, there is no evidence to suggest that a healthy mother guarantees a healthy fetus. Nevertheless, a mother who has a strong health orientation in terms of exercise and diet, is a nonsmoker, and does not consume large quantities of alcohol will certainly deliver a baby that is healthier than a baby born of a mother who continues to smoke cigarettes and consume large amounts of alcohol and/or other drugs and medications during her pregancy. There is no suggestion that exercise during pregnancy is detrimental to fetal growth and development, nor is there evidence of reduced fetal mass, increased perinatal or neonatal mortality, or physical or mental retardation as sequelae to strenuous exercise performed during pregnancy. Because of the newness of this field, we must await future studies to determine the impact upon childhood development, although it appears safe to speculate that the parents' health orientation will most likely carry over to their children.

Guides

A number of popular books emphasize Kegel type exercises and yoga as being helpful to the mother. It is important that the attending physician and/or nurse midwife be familiar with these exercises so that he/she can discuss them with the patient, stressing why certain exercises will be helpful and why others should not be done. Whether the mother exercises strenuously or merely engages in daily recreational activity, the program does not have to be altered drastically during pregnancy. The pregnancy itself often serves to make the necessary adjustments in the exercise program. Exercise can be carried out alone, in a group, or with friends. It can be undertaken with the confidence that a healthy mother is the woman most likely to deliver and nurture a healthy baby.

EXERCISE IN CHILDHOOD

ODED BAR-OR, M.D., F.A.C.S.M.

PHYSIOLOGIC DIFFERENCES IN RESPONSE TO EXERCISE BETWEEN CHILDREN AND ADULTS

Although children and adults respond to exercise in essentially the same way, there are *quantitative* differences which depend on growth and maturation (see Bar-Or, O. Pediatric Sports Medicine for The Practitioner. New York: Springer-Verlag, 1983). The following is a brief overview focusing on characteristics of the exercising child which are relevant to exercise prescription (Table 1).

A question often asked is whether prolonged activities that require cardiorespiratory endurance ("aerobic" tasks) are more suitable for children than short-term, highly intense activities which require local muscular endurance ("anaerobic" tasks). Children, as a group, have a similar maximal aerobic power (expressed as maximal O_2 intake per kg body mass) to that of young adults. Prepubescent girls have an even higher maximal aerobic power than do older females. In contrast, the ability of girls or boys to perform intense anaerobic tasks that last 10 to 60 seconds is distinctly lower than in adults.

The foregoing characteristics have prompted the encouragement of children to participate in long-distance road races, including the gruelling marathon run. Indeed, increasing numbers of children are taking part in such races. Yet, when left to exert *spontaneously*, children

TABLE 1   Physiologic Characteristics of the Exercising Child, Which Have Relevance to Exercise Prescription

Function	Compared with Adults	Implication for Exercise Prescription
Metabolic		
Maximal oxygen intake per kg body mass	Similar	Can perform endurance tasks reasonably well
Submaximal oxygen demand in running or walking	Higher	Greater fatigability in prolonged high-intensity tasks; greater heat production
Rate of anaerobic glycolysis	Lower	Lower capability in intense "anaerobic" tasks of 10 to 60 seconds' duration
On-transients of oxygen intake and post-exertional recovery	Shorter	Well-suited to intermittent activities
Cardiovascular		
Cardiac output at a given oxygen intake	Lower	Potential deficiency of peripheral blood supply during maximal exertion and in hot climates
Respiratory		
Submaximal ventilation, ventilatory equivalent, and respiratory frequency	Higher	Early fatigability in tasks that require large respiratory minute volume
Thermoregulatory		
Sweating rate	Lower	
Acclimatization to heat	Slower	Greater risk of heat-related illness
Tolerance time in extreme heat	Shorter	on hot/humid days
Body cooling in water	Faster	Potential hypothermia
Body core heating during dehydration	Greater	Fluid intake to be enforced repeatedly in prolonged activities
Perceptual		
Rating of perceived exertion	Lower	Child willing to continue exercise when physiologically strained

prefer short-term intermittent activities with a high recreational component and variety to monotonous, prolonged activities. A child at the swimming pool, for example, would rather splash, dive, and play than swim lengths. This activity pattern can be attributed to children's temperament and relatively short attention span, but it may also reflect physiologic characteristics. Some are related to the on-transients at the beginning of exercise or upon an increase in exercise intensity: children reach metabolic steady state faster, and contract a lower O_2 deficit, than do adults. This enables them to recover faster after exercise, a pattern that is useful in intermittent activities. In contrast, children require a higher oxygen intake than do adults during identical submaximal running or walking, and they therefore operate at a relatively high percentage of their maximal aerobic power. This causes greater fatigue during prolonged activities. Furthermore, their high metabolic level causes excessive body heating. This, coupled with a poor sweating capacity and large surface-to-mass ratio, is the reason for children's short tolerance time when exercising in hot climates.

In conclusion, children can perform exercise over a wide range of intensities and durations, but they are best suited to repeated activities which last a few seconds each and are interspersed by short rest periods. The least suitable activities for children are those that are highly intense and last 10 to 60 seconds, such as a 300-meter run. Prolonged exercise (10 or more minutes) can be prescribed, but the child may not be able to sustain it at high intensities.

EXERCISE PRESCRIPTION IN PEDIATRIC MANAGEMENT

Healthy children are habitually more active than adults and, given opportunity and support, will not need a specific exercise prescription. In contrast, children with an illness or disability are often hypoactive and require a specific exercise prescription as part of their clinical management. The number of conditions in which exercise can be used in therapy is greater for children than it is for adults. Table 2 summarizes the rationale for such prescription and the activities most recommended for each illness.

Exercise is used in pediatric populations for the following purposes: (1) to increase maximal aerobic power, (2) for control of body mass and fat reduction, (3) to increase muscle strength and muscle endurance, (4) to increase range of movement, (5) to improve self-esteem and self-confidence, and (6) to combat specific pathophysiologic processes.

Increase of Maximal Aerobic Power. Due to their hypoactivity, patients are often detrained. Low maximal aerobic power is typical of such conditions as obesity, cerebral palsy, mental retardation, neurocirculatory asthenia, and spina bifida. For such patients, training that improves general stamina should be a major component of exercise prescription.

Control of Body Mass and Fat Reduction. Obesity, as an isolated illness or in combination with another illness, is highly prevalent among children and adolescents, especially in developed countries. More often than not, it is accompanied by hypoactivity and detraining.

TABLE 2 Exercise Prescription in the Management of Specific Pediatric Diseases

Disease	Purposes of Program	Recommended Activities
Anorexia nervosa	Means for behavioral modification; educate regarding lean mass versus fat.	Various; emphasize those with low energy demand.
Bronchial asthma	Conditioning; possibly reduction of exercise-induced bronchospasm; instill confidence	Aquatic, intermittent, long warm-up
Cerebral palsy	Increase maximal aerobic power, range of motion, and ambulation; control of body mass	Depend on residual ability
Cystic fibrosis	Improve mucus clearance, training of respiratory muscles	Jogging, swimming
Diabetes mellitus	Help in metabolic control; control of body mass	Various; attempt equal daily energy output
Hemophilia	Prevent muscle atrophy, contractures, and possibly bleeding into joints	Swimming, cycling; avoid contact sports
Mental retardation	Socialization; increase self-esteem; prevent detraining	Recreational, intermittent, large variety
Muscular dystrophies	Increase muscle strength and endurance; prevent contractures; prolong ambulatory phase	Swimming, calisthenics, wheelchair sports
Neurocirculatory disease	Increase effort tolerance; improve orthostatic response	Various; emphasize endurance-type activities
Obesity	Reduction of body mass and fat; conditioning; socialization and improved self-esteem	High in calorie uptake but feasible to child; emphasize swimming
Rheumatoid arthritis	Prevent contractures and muscle atrophy; increase daily function	Swimming, calisthenics, cycling, sailing
Spina bifida	Strengthen upper body; control of body mass and fat; increase maximal aerobic power	Arm shoulder resistance training, wheelchair sports (including endurance)

The increase of energy expenditure through exercise is therefore a logical means of inducing a negative energy balance. Loss of body mass through exercise alone is a prolonged, and often a frustrating, experience. A low-energy diet as the sole therapy, especially if extreme, may induce a negative nitrogen balance, which is contraindicated in the growing child or adolescent. Exercise reverses the negative nitrogen balance through its anabolic effect. A combined exercise-diet regimen is therefore the method of choice in control of body mass. Recommended activities are those that require moving of the whole body mass, such as walking, running, cycling, cross-country skiing, or swimming. The last-mentioned is particularly well tolerated, and enjoyed, by obese children due to their high buoyancy. One added advantage of swimming is that the child is submerged and an "ugly" body is not exposed to others.

Control of body mass is strongly recommended for adolescents with a compromised gait, as in cerebral palsy, muscular dystrophy, or paraparesis. While still young and lightweight, such individuals can walk, with or without the support of braces or crutches. However, once they reach adolescence and become heavy, many can no longer support their own body mass and they soon resign themselves to wheelchair status. In such individuals, a preventive exercise regimen should combine "weight control" with muscle strengthening.

Increase in Muscle Strength and Muscle Endurance. Some diseases are accompanied by a reduction in muscle strength or in the child's ability to sustain muscle contractions of high intensity. Examples include muscular dystrophy, myopathy, arthritis, and hemophiliac muscle atrophy. Such a reduction in physiologic performance is also detrimental to the child's walking ability and to other daily functions. Strengthening of specific muscle groups (resistive exercises) is indicated, in combination with walking and other "purposeful" movements.

Increase in Range of Movement. This is especially relevant to children who are liable to lose their joint flexibility and develop contractures. Typical examples include patients with rheumatoid arthritis, cerebral palsy, hemophilia, and muscular dystrophy.

Improved Self-Esteem and Self-Confidence. Exercise and play are important means of expression, more so in children than in adults. Children and adolescents who are deprived of this mode of expression may lose confidence in themselves. Often, a vicious circle may evolve in which the hypoactive child loses confidence in physical (and social) prowess, becoming even less active. To help in breaking this circle, an exercise should be prescribed which gives the child *attainable* goals, capitalizing on abilities rather than exaggerating current disabilities. The intensity and complexity of the prescribed tasks can be increased gradually as the child regains confidence.

Combat Specific Pathophysiologic Processes. Some data suggest that exercise reduces the impact of specific pathologic processes. While more research is needed both to validate such claims and to understand the underlying mechanisms, the following empirical findings are worth mentioning. It has been shown, for example, that bronchial mucus clearance in the child with cystic fibrosis is enhanced during and after running. Conditioning can also increase the endurance of the respiratory muscles in such patients (see chapter on *Exercise and Cystic Fibrosis*). The extent and prevalence of exercise-induced bronchoconstriction in the asthmatic child can be somewhat reduced with conditioning. Both symptoms and signs of neurocirculatory asthenia are alleviated following an endurance program. Children with insulin-dependent diabetes mellitus show an improved metabolic control (as manifested by the degree of glycosuria or by the concentration of hemoglobin A_1C) during periods when they are physically active. Furthermore, such patients then require less insulin and can markedly increase their dietary intake. Hemophilia patients have reported a decrease in the rate or intensity of intra-arterial and intramuscular bleeds while they are habitually active.

MENSTRUAL IRREGULARITIES

GUY R. BRISSON, Ph.D.

The increasing incidence of menstrual dysfunctions occasioned by the massive enrolment of girls and women in recreational or competitive sports has forced sports medicine to focus its attention heavily upon the female reproductive system. Sports participation now involves many adult women as well as peripubertal girls. Clinical symptoms thus include a varying degree of delayed menarche in adolescents and mild to severe secondary menstrual dysfunction in postpubertal women.

DELAYED MENARCHE

Menarche is a milestone upon a long continuum whereby complex and poorly understood metabolic processes ensure a gradual but progressive sexual maturation. Several factors affect the chronologic age at which menarche is attained. Of special interest is the increasing frequency with which participation in sports has been identified as a factor capable of delaying the onset of menarche.

Body Fat Hypothesis

At puberty, the energy demands occasioned by intensive physical training have been considered in the etiology of late menarche. For R. Frisch and her collaborators, nutritional factors could represent the most important extrinsic elements regulating pubertal development. Numerous studies reporting delays of menarche in anorexic or in malnourished patients point in that direction. Frisch proposed a "critical weight hypothesis", whereby a specific body mass had to be reached in order for pubertal growth to progress. Based on longitudinal studies, she and her associates calculated that menarche was bound to occur when a body mass of approximately 48 kg had been attained. The variability of that value was significantly reduced when they later expressed body mass in terms of total body water or lean body mass. Some 11.5 kg of body fat should be deposited for the first meses to occur. Thus, it could be argued that the energy expenditure associated with intensive practice of sports during the peripubertal period retards accumulation of sufficient body fat for maturation of the ovarian axis. The enormous energy requirements imposed by the practice of specific sports (ballet dancing, gymnastics, figure skating) are often coupled with a low energy intake (for subcultural, esthetic reasons). It is thus not surprising to find the largest incidence of late maturers among these young athletes.

Other Explanations

A. J. Ryan found no evidence that sports by themselves provoked any significant changes in the menstrual cycle. Malina suggested that the high incidence of late menarche in young athletes could reflect a tendency for physical training to be undertaken by an unusual population of delayed maturers, perhaps a cohort with a more linear physique, a body build that has been associated with late maturation. Abraham and coworkers noticed menstrual disturbances in 79 percent of female entrants to a professional ballet school. However, this may not be due simply to selection of a specific body type, since their sample of Australian dancers already had at entry (mean age ± s.d. 16.8 ± 0.8 yr) 3 to 13 years of ballet dancing experience. It appeared that deterioration of the menstrual pattern was related to strenuous physical exercise, rather than to any change of body mass. Studies by M. P. Warren have tended to confirm the intrinsic effect of exercise. She also emphasized that the critical body fat hypothesis may not be adequate to explain reproductive dysfunction, at least in ballet dancers. In her study of ballerinas, an acceptable body mass and composition were attained 4 to 8 months prior to menarche. She thus suggested that the decrease of weight-for-height observed in the dancers prior to menarche in the dancers could be considered as a relative weight deficiency, and that this was sufficient to delay the onset of the first menses. Sizonenke also argued against the weight-for-height concept, on the grounds that obesity was not associated with precocious menarche, even though obese adolescents were taller and heavier than control girls of the same age. In contrast, Montemagno and associates reported that menarchial age was consistently lower in patients with early-onset obesity compared with controls.

An Adaptive Strategy?

It has been postulated that the absence of menstruation is an adaptive strategy intended to avoid body iron depletion through an iron-rich menstrual flow. Several studies have pointed out iron deficiencies in athletic populations (Dewijn et al, 1971; Haymes, 1973). Dietary studies in our laboratory suggest that inadequate food intake rather than heavy exercise is responsible for deficiencies of serum iron transferrin and ferritin in young elite female athletes (Jolicoeur et al, 1983). Transferrin, a blood iron carrier protein, has also been associated with gonadal dysfunction in males. Eumenorrheic iron-deficient anemic patients do not seem to support such a concept, although it has been suggested that transferrin is involved in growth regulation, apparently through a feedback action upon growth hormone secretion.

PRIMARY AMENORRHEA

By the age of 15 or 16 years, a diagnosis of primary amenorrhea becomes more appropriate than one of delayed puberty. It is then of crucial importance to investigate the hypophyseal-gonadal-uterine axis thoroughly, to rule out causes of dysfunction other than intensive exertion, particularly if the training regimen is to be maintained. One should seriously consider hormonal supportive treatment.

SECONDARY MENSTRUAL DYSFUNCTION

Incidence

A high incidence of menstrual dysfunction is common among adult athletes actively involved in sports requiring physical effort and endurance. Menstrual abnormalities have been reported in connection with ballet dancing, middle and long distance running, swimming, bowling, weight lifting, fencing, and various field events.

Possible Causes

During regular training, many factors change simultaneously (stress, dietary habits, sleep patterns, body mass), and it is correspondingly difficult to isolate the causative variables. Competitive events probably involve sufficient stress to induce significant endocrine changes. Changes of body mass and composition have also attracted much attention.

Body Fat and Thermoregulation

After the age of 16, Frisch and McArthur (1974) suggested that the body mass should comprise at least 22 percent fat in order to sustain the menstrual cycles. Body mass and body height could thus be used to predict the onset of amenorrhea or the return of eumenorrhea.

A survey of 900 female participants in the Portland marathon pointed to body mass and to loss of mass as determinants of menstrual dysfunction. Young women weighing less than 52.3 kg and losing more than 4.5 kg were likely to develop menstrual problems. A low body mass, and/or a significant decrease of body mass apparently induced hypometabolic states from hypothalamus-mediated endocrine changes. Such hypometabolism could reflect altered function of hypothalamic thermoregulatory mechanisms. In support of this view, amenorrheic women who are exposed to hot environments experience a rise of core temperature, while normal women maintain body temperature, dissipating additional heat through sweating. In a cold environment, contrary to the behavior of normal women, amenorrheic women may not shiver; they thus experience a drop of core temperature. During exercise, anorexia patients show higher rectal temperature values than controls. A critical amount of body fat seems needed for adequate thermoregulation.

Thyroid Function

Several authors have investigated thyroid function during exercise and training, but no one has yet established that amenorrheic athletes convert thyroxine (T_4) into nonthermogenic reverse triiodothyronine (RT_3), a conversion that is well recognized in emaciated anorexia patients. After gain of body mass, the circulating RT_3 levels of anorexia nervosa patients are restored to normal. Lean athletes, in our experience, do not complain of feeling cold. When they experience hypometabolism, it seems that it is mainly from hypogonadism. Numerous studies of the endocrine system have sought an explanation for menstrual irregularities in athletes, but too often athletes have been investigated according to their availability or the hosting of a major sports event.

Limitations of Hormonal Assay

The evaluation of circulating hormone levels during exertion remains difficult. For any given analysis, marked differences of results exist from one laboratory to another. Findings must thus be interpreted with close regard for the normal values declared by a particular laboratory. Normal interlaboratory differences are greatly magnified when radioimmunological techniques are used to assay circulating hormones. Increasing specificity of steroid antisera provides more and more accuracy for androgen, estrogen, and progestogen determinations. A quantitative evaluation of circulating levels of gonadotropins (peptidic hormones) is only possible through radioimmunology. There is, of course, a need to calibrate techniques against an international reference standard. Recent reports in which biological titrations of gonadotropins have been conducted parallel with radioimmunologic assays strongly suggest a dissociation between immunologic (quantitative assay) and biologic (qualitative assay) determinants of LH and FSH molecules. These considerations, plus the probable existence of several forms of circulating gonadotropins could afford an explanation of the difficulties encountered in interpreting the involvement of the pituitary trophic hormone in exercising women. Finally, variations of hormonal concentration measured in the peripheral circulation could reflect a change of the metabolic clearance rate of the hormone and/or hemoconcentration, rather than a change in production of the hormone. Without underestimating fundamental information that can be obtained by examining the endocrine status of exercising athletes, the resting hormonal profile is probably of greater clinical significance. The resting profile is helpful in eliminating other potential causes of amenorrhea (e.g., hyperprolactinemia, thyroid dysfunction, hyperandrogenism, gonadal failure, and pituitary tumor) among athletes consulting for hypogonadism.

Hypoestrogenism

The usual finding in amenorrheic runners is hypoestrogenism. Estrogen deficiency after oophorectomy has been linked to a high incidence of clinical bone fractures in young women. Lack of estrogen has also been implicated in the skeletal calcium loss that affects postmenopausal women. Secondary amenorrhea associated with hyperprolactinemia causes a loss of bone density at a rate equivalent to that observed in postmenopausal women. To date, this has not been considered a problem for young amenorrheic athletes, although transient elevation of blood prolactin has been observed in exercising young women. We are still awaiting studies on the incidence of bone fractures in amenorrheic subjects with and without exogenous estrogen therapy, and with and without exercise. The view that exercise strengthens bones, thus compensating for a possible hypoestrogenic demineralization, is not supported by a recent animal study where treadmill running failed to prevent bone calcium depletion in ovariectomized rats. Osteoporosis (hardly a reversible process) thus remains a possible concern in hypoestrogenic athletes; steroid replacement therapy seems indicated, together with appropriate dietary calcium supplementation.

Therapy of Secondary Amenorrhea

Menstrual disturbances may, theoretically, be minimized by the use of oral contraceptive drugs; this tactic appeals to some athletes whose efficiency is disturbed by hormonal swings. However, one should not attribute menstrual dysfunction to exercise until a thorough gynecologic investigation has excluded other possible causes. Should secondary amenorrhea prevail for a year or more, an estrogen-progesterone regimen should be recommended, not only to prevent osteoporosis and stress fractures, but also to minimize the predisposition to vascular disease and to protect the endometrium.

PHYSIOLOGICAL CHARACTERISTICS OF FEMALE ATHLETES

BARBARA L. DRINKWATER, Ph.D.

The change in society's attitudes toward the athletic aspirations of women during the early 1970s coincided with the growth of the masters' programs, which provide opportunities for adults of both sexes to continue athletic competition throughout their lives. The result has been an interesting blend of age, ability, experience, and expectations among today's female athletes. Women born after 1960 have come through an educational system which offers similar athletic opportunities for boys and girls. Their level of skill and knowledge is quite different from that of many older women entering the sports world as novices. These enthusiastic converts to exercise often lack even rudimentary knowledge of conditioning techniques, how to select appropriate equipment and clothing, and how to protect themselves from overuse syndromes and other injuries. Both groups are of interest to the exercise physiologist; one group supplies information about gender differences in the physiological response to exercise when both sexes have had an opportunity to reach their biological potential, and the other group is a source of information regarding the role of physical activity in moderating the physiological changes usually associated with the aging female. Results from both groups have forced a reevaluation of what is a "normal" exercise response for women.

AEROBIC POWER

One of the most frequent observations is that habitual level of activity, not gender or age, is the primary determinant of an individual's cardiovascular fitness. For example, male and female athletes participating in the same sport are more similar in aerobic power ($\dot{V}O_2$ max) than are athletes of the same sex in different sports. The average $\dot{V}O_2$ max of male basketball players, 45.8 ml/kg/min, is almost the same as that reported for female players, 49.6 ml/kg/min. Both values are considerably less than that of men (78.3 ml O_2kg/min) and women (68.2 ml)$_2$/kg/min) on one national Nordic ski team. This does not mean that there are no sex differences in the potential for developing high levels of aerobic power. In all sports where endurance capacity is a factor for successful performance, the elite male athlete has a higher $\dot{V}O_2$ max than the elite female athlete. In those sports where the main workload is displacement of the athlete's body mass, relative $\dot{V}O_2$ max expressed as ml/kg/min is the appropriate basis of comparison, and reported differences between sexes generally range from 5 to 25 percent. It is possible to remove body fat from consideration mathematically by expressing $\dot{V}O_2$ max relative to lean body mass (LBM). This purely theoretical comparison minimizes the differences of $\dot{V}O_2$ max between the sexes, but still leaves approximately a 5 to 10 percent difference unaccounted for. The lower oxygen carrying capacity of the woman's blood, a reflection of her lower hemoglobin levels, is presumed to be a major factor in this difference.

Absolute levels of $\dot{V}O_2$ max are frequently higher for men because males are usually larger than females, and $\dot{V}O_2$ max is directly related to body size. This is a problem for women only in those sports or activities where both sexes must perform at the same absolute work rate. Since men and women seldom compete against each other in sport, the relationship between body size and work capacity is more relevant in the workplace. Even here, the woman can often compensate for her smaller size by training to increase both her $\dot{V}O_2$ max and her muscular strength.

The most important outcome of descriptive studies of female athletes has been the recognition that women can attain high levels of cardiovascular fitness, that they are physiologically capable of withstanding the physical stress of endurance sports, and that they do not, as many texts tell us, reach their peak fitness levels at age 15. While data on older female athletes are still sketchy, those which are available clearly show that the declining $\dot{V}O_2$ max values for average women beyond the age of 20 years are not mirrored by female athletes. The average aerobic power of 58 women runners in their 30s, 56.6 ml O_2/kg/min, was slightly higher than that of 50 younger distance runners in their 20s and almost double that of sedentary women in the 30 to 40 year age bracket. Eventually, aging does result in a diminished aerobic power, but the decrease across the years is less striking than the immediate effect of a sedentary lifestyle. Sedentary women in their 20s have the dubious distinction of having an average $\dot{V}O_2$ max equal to that of masters' swimmers in their 70s (37.6 ml/kg/min). In general, older female athletes can count on having levels of cardiovascular fitness equivalent to those of sedentary women a decade younger, while older women who train specifically for endurance events gain two decades or more.

Aging curves based on both cross-sectional and longitudinal data show a similar decrease in $\dot{V}_{O_2}$ max per decade for both active and sedentary women, but the practical consequences of starting the decline from a higher level of fitness are significant for the masters' athlete. Even more heartening are the results from women who were inactive during their early adult years and are now actively engaged in physical fitness programs. The training effect shifts them from the sedentary curve to the athlete's slope, or from their perspective, reverses the biological clock!

Numerous studies of aerobic training have reported a basic similarity in the response of men and women, an increase in $\dot{V}_{O_2}$ max ranging from 10 to 20 percent, an increase in maximal ventilatory volume, a decrease in resting and submaximal pulse rate, and a faster recovery following exercise. While all training programs should be individualized for each athlete, gender per se is not a factor which must be considered in prescribing exercise for women. The woman's initial level of fitness, her previous experience, and her level of knowledge and skill are far more important factors. The older female with no previous experience in sports will require much more guidance than the younger woman who has had competitive experience under the tutelage of an experienced coach. The basic principles of exercise prescription outlined in Part I, Chapter 4 apply equally to men and women, but there will be greater variability in the background of women seeking exercise advice.

STRENGTH

When weight training became part of the overall conditioning program for many sports, it was soon evident that the potential of women for developing strength had been greatly underestimated. Women benefit from strength training, not only through improved athletic performance, but also because strong muscles are a protection against injury. Although some women are competing in weight-lifting and body-building competitions, many others are concerned with society's aversion to well defined muscles on the feminine form. It is reassuring for these women to learn that they can obtain approximately the same percent increase in strength as men with only a fraction of the male increase in bulk. Unfortunately, this same gender difference in muscle mass provides men with a strength advantage that women are unlikely to overcome. While other factors, perhaps in the neural pathways, may contribute to increases in strength with training (Section I, Chapter 1), the cross-sectional area of the muscle is considered to be the main factor determining maximum strength. The anabolic properties of testosterone (the level is about ten times higher in males than in females) is presumed to account for the difference in muscle size between the sexes.

Numerous studies have reached the same conclusion; the overall strength of women is approximately two-thirds that of men. When body size is eliminated as a factor, the difference is less, with women showing approximately 80 percent of the male values. More important to the athlete is the variability in strength between specific muscle groups. Upper body strength of the female averages approximately 55 percent of the male's, while leg strength is almost identical when expressed relative to body mass. Training does not close the gap appreciably. It is unlikely that men and women can ever compete equally in events where success is determined primarily by strength or power.

Histochemical and biochemical analyses of muscle fibers from athletes and nonathletes have shown that gender differences lie in fiber size, not in fiber composition or enzyme activity. Among endurance athletes, the percentage of slow-twitch (ST) fibers is high for both men (63% ST) and women (60% ST), while in sprint events, where fast-twitch (FT) fibers predominate, men and women have 76 percent FT and 73 percent FT respectively. In contrast, untrained men and women have approximately 51 percent ST and approximately 49 percent FT fibers. The oxidative potential of the muscle, as indicated by succinate dehydrogenase (SDH) activity, also reflects training rather than gender; nor are there consistent differences between male and female athletes in the activity of the glycolytic enzymes, lactate dehydrogenase (LDH) and phosphorylase (PH).

The gender difference lies in the size of the muscle fiber. In untrained groups, women have 68 percent and 71 percent of male FT and ST fiber area respectively. Among athletes, the percentage varies according to the sport, but in each case the fiber area of the male exceeds that of the female. While fiber area can be increased with training, men still retain a biological advantage in fiber size as a result of the hormonal differences between the sexes.

Comparisons between male and female athletes are interesting, but should never be allowed to discourage women from developing their muscular strength to meet the demands of their sport. A woman can develop the strength to handle her own body mass, whether she be a mountaineer climbing up a fixed rope or a gymnast mounting to a handstand on the balance beam. Contrary to popular opinion, she can also do pull-ups and "men's" push-ups. In fact, developing upper body strength should be a priority for most female athletes, since study after study has found that a woman's arm and shoulder strength fall well below that of other muscle groups. It would also be wise to strengthen the quadriceps muscles. While not all reports of injury rates agree, there have been some that suggest women are more likely to suffer knee injuries than are men. An explanation for the difference usually revolves around the effect of the broader female pelvis on the θ angle. Whether or not women are anatomically more susceptible to knee injuries is debatable. However, they can minimize the possibility of such an injury by strengthening the muscles that stabilize the knee joint.

BODY COMPOSITION

In some sports, such as running, performance is

enhanced if the athlete can minimize the amount of nonessential fat she carries with her during a race. As a result, the percent body fat (% BF) of distance runners is at the lower range of the values recorded for female athletes. At the upper end of the curve are the athletes who believe that extra body mass, even if it be adipose tissue, is helpful in their event. The range between these two extremes can be as much as 25% BF. In general, endurance athletes such as runners or cross-country skiers average 12 to 18% BF, with some individual marathon runners down in the 6 to 8% BF range. Athletes in team and individual sports, such as basketball, lacrosse, volleyball, tennis and swimming, average 18 to 24% BF. None of these figures should be considered optimal for a specific athlete; they are averages representing wide variations among individual women. Part of this variation is due to individual differences, but part is also due to different techniques in estimating % BF. Hydrostatic weighing to determine body density and conversion of density to % BF by the Siri or Brozek equation is usually considered the most accurate technique for assessing % BF. However, even this method may not be valid for athletes or for all ages. When anthropometric methods are used to predict % BF, the error can be even larger unless the prediction equation has been validated and cross-validated on similar athletic groups. Since some women are likely to interpret a high % BF as a rationale for severe dietary restriction, it is important to emphasize that these figures are merely estimates and only one aspect of the athlete's physiological profile.

The older female athlete is likely to be delighted with her % BF, which may be as much as 10 to 15 percent below that of sedentary women in her age group. Female distance runners in their 30s average approximately 15% BF, while sedentary 30 year olds average 27% BF. Tennis players (20.3% BF) and mountaineers (18.7% BF) in the same age range also have values that are closer to those of active 20 year old women (20% BF) than women of their own age. An increase in % BF is not an inevitable consequence of aging for the active woman.

HEAT TOLERANCE

One of the reasons women were discouraged from participating in endurance sports for so long was the pervasive belief that they were unable to tolerate heat stress as well as men. That myth still flourishes, even though it is now apparent that older studies of gender difference in thermoregulation had confounded heat tolerance with work tolerance. In retrospect, it is evident that indices of heat strain, core temperature and heart rate, were higher for women in thermoregulatory studies because they were exercising at a higher percentage of their maximal workload. Both variables are a function of relative (% $\dot{V}_{O_2}$ max), not absolute, workload. When men and women are matched on $\dot{V}_{O_2}$ max and exercise at the same % $\dot{V}_{O_2}$ max there is no difference in their ability to tolerate work in the heat.

Both $\dot{V}_{O_2}$ max and % $\dot{V}_{O_2}$ max must be considered, because most endurance-trained athletes are partially heat acclimated. Female marathon runners, for example, have a lower resting core temperature (Tc), an earlier onset of sweating, a larger plasma volume, and a lower heart rate, Tc, and mean skin temperature ($\bar{T}$sk) than age-matched controls when exercising in a hot-dry environment. Women who train at an intensity greater than 50% $\dot{V}_{O_2}$ max for only 8 to 12 weeks will not only improve their tolerance to heat but will find that they can acclimate to heat in a shorter time than untrained women. These advantages appear to be limited to those athletes whose training results in a sustained elevation of core temperature with its attendant stimulation of the sweating response. Athletes should be warned that physical training is not a substitute for heat acclimation; they are not immune to heat illness. High-intensity exercise in combination with a high external heat load is a dangerous combination, no matter how well trained one is. The best protection for an athlete is to acclimate gradually to the specific environmental conditions in which she will be competing.

As recently as 1979, women were told they could not acclimate to heat as well as men. Research has shown the opposite to be true; men and women who are matched on cardiovascular fitness, body surface area, and surface area to mass ratio acclimate successfully to heat in both hot-dry and hot-wet conditions. Tolerance times increase, heart rate and core temperature decrease, and both sexes increase sweat-sensitivity and capacity. The latter point is particularly important, since the observation that women usually sweat less than men was formerly used to bolster the belief that women had more difficulty coping with heat stress. Three points must be considered in assessing differences in the sweating response between individuals or groups. First, the need for heat loss through evaporation of sweat is related to absolute, not relative, workload. An 80 kg male running with a 55 kg woman should produce more sweat, because he is producing more heat even though both may be running at the same % $\dot{V}_{O_2}$ max. Second, regardless of gender, the person who is acclimated to heat or who is a well conditioned endurance athlete will sweat sooner and in greater amounts than the person who is not. Third, calculating the ratio of sweating required to dissipate heat to the amount of sweat produced may be a better way of assessing the adequacy of the sweating response. Using this technique, a recent study found sweating efficiency higher for women in humid heat and no gender differences in dry heat. In both conditions, the men and women finished exercising with the same core temperature and heart rate.

At one time it was believed that estrogen exerted an inhibitory effect on the sweating mechanism, and that this effect plus a higher core temperature during the luteal phase of the menstrual cycle would put women more at risk for heat illness during that phase of her cycle. Numerous studies have failed to find any evidence that changes in cyclic hormones or basal temperature markedly affect the core temperature, cardiovascular stability, or sweat rate of women working in the heat. There may be some subtle changes in fluid shifts, but there is no evidence that these affect heat tolerance. Apparently the combined stress of heat and exercise mask the cyclic changes observed at rest in normal environments.

While gender per se is no longer credited with determining thermoregulatory response, some women are at risk in the heat. Overfat women and those begin-ning exercise after years of sedentary living should be warned of the potential hazards of exercising strenuously in hot weather. Older women in particular often elect to wear warmup suits or full leotards while they participate, because they are self-conscious. They should be alerted to the effect that clothing has on heat dissipation. As a matter of course, all exercise prescriptions should be accompanied by tips on how to exercise safely in both heat and cold.

HEAD AND FACE INJURIES

HEAD INJURIES IN ATHLETICS

LEONARD A. BRUNO, M.D.,
THOMAS A. GENNARELLI, M.D.,
JOSEPH S. TORG, M.D.

The athlete who receives a blow to his head or a sudden jolt to his body that results in a sudden acceleration-deceleration force to the head should be carefully evaluated. If the injured individual is ambulatory and conscious, the entire spectrum of intracranial damage, ranging from a grade I concussion to a more severe intracranial condition, must be considered. Initial on-field examination should include evaluation for the following: (1) facial expression; (2) orientation to time, place, and person; (3) presence of post-traumatic amnesia; (4) presence of retrograde amnesia; and (5) abnormal gait.

Traumatic injuries to the brain can be classified into focal brain injuries and diffuse brain injuries.

The immediate and definitive management of athletically induced trauma to the brain depends on the nature and severity of the injury. Those responsible for managing such injuries must understand these problems from the standpoint of the basic pathomechanics.

DIFFUSE BRAIN INJURIES

Diffuse brain injuries are associated with widespread or global disruption of neurologic function and are not usually associated with macroscopically visible brain lesions. Diffuse brain injuries result from the shaking of the brain within the skull and are thus lesions that are caused by the inertial or acceleration effects of a mechanical input to the head. Both theoretic and experimental evidence point to rotational acceleration as the primary injury mechanism for diffuse brain injuries.

Since diffuse brain injuries, for the most part, are not associated with visible macroscopic lesions, they have historically been lumped together to include all injuries not associated with focal lesions. Recently, however, diagnostic information has been gained from CT scanning, as well as from neurophysiologic studies, which enables us to more clearly define several categories within this broad group of diffuse brain injuries. These injuries are discussed in detail.

Three categories of diffuse brain injury are now recognized:

1. *Mild Concussion*. Several specific concussion syndromes exist that involve temporary disturbances of neurologic function without loss of consciousness.
2. *Classic Cerebral Concussion*. Classic cerebral concussion is a temporary, reversible neurologic deficiency caused by trauma that results in temporary loss of consciousness.
3. *Diffuse Axonal Injury*. Diffuse axonal injury is prolonged traumatic brain coma with loss of consciousness lasting more than 6 hours. Residual neurologic, psychologic, or personality deficits often result because of structural disruption of numerous axons in the white matter of the cerebral hemispheres and brain stem.

Mild Cerebral Concussion Syndromes

The syndromes of mild cerebral concussion are included in the continuum of diffuse brain injuries. They represent the mildest form of injury in this spectrum. Mild concussion syndromes are those in which consciousness is preserved, but with some degree of noticeable temporary neurologic dysfunction. These injuries are exceedingly common and, because of their mild degree, often are not brought to medical attention; however, they are the most common brain injuries encountered in sports medicine.

A grade I mild concussion, the mildest form of head injury, results in confusion and disorientation unaccompanied by amnesia. This temporary confusion, without loss of consciousness, lasts only momentarily after the injury. This concussion syndrome is completely reversible and is associated with no sequelae. An individual with a grade I mild concussion is confused and has a dazed look on his face. There may also be mild unsteadiness of gait. However, post-traumatic and retrograde amnesia are not prominent features. This clinical picture is best described by the athletes themselves who say, "I had my bell rung." Usually the state of confusion is short-lived, and the athlete is completely lucid in 5 to 15 minutes. When his mind is clear, he may return to the activity under the watchful supervision of the team physician or trainer. However, associated symptoms such as vertigo, headaches, photophobia, and labile emotions should preclude returning to the game.

A grade II mild concussion is characterized by confusion associated with retrograde amnesia that develops after 5 to 10 minutes. Again, this is an extremely frequent event, particularly in sports medicine. Athletes may experience such a "ding" and, although confused, continue coordinated sensorimotor activities after the accident. If examined immediately, these players have total recall of the events immediately prior to impact. However, retrograde amnesia develops 5 to 10 minutes later, and thereafter the player does not remember the impact or events immediately before impact. The amnesia usually covers only several minutes before the injury, and although it may diminish somewhat, the player always has some degree of permanent, though short, retrograde amnesia despite resumption of a completely normal consciousness. The confusion and disorientation completely resolve in a matter of moments.

Individuals manifesting amnesia should not be permitted to return to play that day. These athletes require postinjury evaluation. They may develop the "postconcussion syndrome", which is characterized by persistent headaches, inability to concentrate, and irritability. In some instances, these symptoms may last for several weeks postinjury, and participation in the sport is precluded as long as symptoms are present.

As the mechanical stresses to the brain increase in the grade III mild concussion, confusion and amnesia are present from the time of impact. Athletes can usually continue to play while having no recollection of prior events. By this stage, some degree of post-traumatic amnesia (forgotten events after the injury) also occurs in addition to retrograde amnesia (forgetting events before the injury). The patient's length of confusion may last many minutes, but then his level of consciousness returns to normal, usually with some permanent degree of retrograde and post-traumatic amnesia.

These three syndromes of mild cerebral concussion have been witnessed frequently and described in detail. Although consciousness is preserved, it is clear that some degree of cerebral dysfunction has occurred. The fact that memory mechanisms seem to be the most sensitive to trauma suggests that the cerebral hemispheres, rather than the brain stem, are the location of the mild injury forces. The degree of cerebral cortical dysfunction, however, is not sufficient to disconnect the influence of the cerebral hemispheres from the brain stem activating system, and therefore consciousness is preserved. No other cortical functions except memory seem at jeopardy, and the only residual deficit that patients with mild concussion syndromes have is the brief retrograde or post-traumatic amnesia. However, since definite alteration of brain function has occurred, athletes who sustain a mild cerebral concussion should not be permitted to participate in the remainder of the contest.

Classic Cerebral Concussion

The classic cerebral concussion involves the "knocked out" player. This individual is in a paralytic coma, usually recovers after a few seconds or minutes, and then passes through states of stupor, confusion with or without delirium, and finally an almost lucid state with automatism before becoming fully alert. This individual will most certainly have retrograde and post-traumatic amnesia. If the loss of consciousness lasts for more than several minutes or if there are other signs of a deteriorating neurologic state, the patient should be immediately transported to a hospital.

Initial evaluation of the athlete who has been rendered unconscious should involve the determination of whether he is breathing, whether he has a pulse, and the level of consciousness. If unobstructed respirations and an adequate pulse are present, there is no immediate need to do anything other than to keep in mind that head and neck injuries are frequently associated. Therefore, the player should be protected from injudicious manipulation or movement.

Such patients frequently remain semistuporous for more than several minutes. It should be emphasized that these individuals should be carried off the field on a spineboard or stretcher rather than be permitted to stagger off. An athlete who has been rendered unconscious for any period of time should not be allowed to return to contact activity, even if he is mentally clear. Overnight observation in a hospital should be seriously considered for these athletes.

Insufficient attention has been placed on the precise events of recovery from classic cerebral concussion. Although, by definition, the loss of consciousness is transient and reversible, sequelae of concussion are commonplace. Certainly, some sequelae such as headache or tinnitus may reflect injuries to the head, inner ear, or other noncerebral structures. However, subtle changes in personality and in psychologic or memory functioning have been documented and must be of cerebral cortical origin. Thus, although the majority of patients with classic cerebral concussion have no sequelae other than amnesia for the events of impact, some patients may in fact have other long-lasting, though subtle, neurologic deficiencies, which must be investigated further.

Brain Swelling

Brain swelling is a poorly understood phenomenon that can accompany any type of head injury. Swelling is not synonymous with cerebral edema, which refers to a specific increase in brain water. Such an increase in water content may not occur in brain swelling, and current evidence favors the concept that brain swelling is due in part to increased intravascular blood within the brain. This is caused by a vascular reaction to head injury, which leads to vasodilation and increased cerebral blood volume. If this increased cerebral blood volume continues for a long enough time, vascular permeability may increase and true edema may result.

TABLE 1   Brain Swelling

Acute swelling
  Associated with focal lesions
    Acute subdural hematoma — hemispheric
    Contusions — focal
  Associated with diffuse brain lesions

Delayed swelling
  Associated with lethargy
  Associated with light coma
  Associated with deep coma

Although brain swelling may occur in any type of head injury, the magnitude of the swelling does not correlate well with the severity of the injury. Thus, both severe and minor head injuries may be complicated by the presence of brain swelling. The effects of brain swelling are thus additive to those of primary brain injury and may, in certain instances, be more severe than the primary injury itself.

Despite the lack of knowledge of the precise mechanism that causes brain swelling, it can be conceptualized in two general forms (Table 1). It should be remembered that many different types of brain swelling exist, and that acute and delayed brain swelling represent phenomenologic rather than mechanistic entities.

Acute brain swelling occurs in several circumstances. Swelling that accompanies focal brain lesions tends to be localized, whereas diffuse brain injuries are associated with generalized swelling. Focal swelling is usually present beneath contusions, but does not often contribute additional deleterious effects. On the other hand, the swelling that occurs with acute subdural hematomas, though principally hemispheric in distribution, may cause more mass effect than the hematoma itself. In such circumstances, the small amount of blood in the subdural space may not be the entire reason for the patient's neurologic state. If the hematoma is removed, the acute brain swelling may progress so rapidly that the brain protrudes through the craniotomy opening. Every neurosurgeon is all too familiar with external herniation of the brain, which, when it occurs, is difficult to treat.

The more serious types of diffuse brain injuries are associated with generalized rather than focal, acute brain swelling. Although not all patients with diffuse axonal injury have brain swelling, the incidence of swelling is higher than in patients with either classic cerebral concussions or one of the mild concussion syndromes. Because of the serious nature of the underlying injury, it is difficult to determine the extent of swelling in these patients. The swelling, though widespread throughout the brain, may not cause a rise in intracranial pressure for several days. This late rise in pressure probably reflects the formation of true cerebral edema, and it may be that diffuse swelling associated with severe diffuse brain injuries is deleterious because it produces edema. In any event, this type of swelling is different from the type of swelling associated with acute subdural hematomas.

Delayed brain swelling may occur minutes to hours after head injury. It is usually diffuse and is often asso-ciated with the milder forms of diffuse brain injuries. Whether delayed swelling is the same or a different phenomenon than the acute swelling of the more serious diffuse injuries is unknown. However, in less severe diffuse injuries there is a distinct time interval before delayed swelling becomes manifest, thus confirming that the primary insult to the brain was not serious. Considering the high frequency of the mild concussion syndromes and of classic cerebral concussion, the incidence of delayed swelling must be low. However, when it occurs, delayed swelling can cause profound neurologic changes or even death.

In its most severe form, severe delayed swelling can cause deep coma. The usual history is that of an injury associated with a mild concussion or a classic cerebral concussion from which the patient recovers. Minutes to hours later the patient becomes lethargic, then stuporous, then finally lapses into a coma. The coma may either be a light coma with appropriate motor responses to painful stimuli, or a deep coma associated with decorticate or decerebrate posturing.

The key difference between these patients and those with diffuse axonal injury is that in the latter the coma and abnormal motor signs are present from the moment of injury, whereas with delayed cerebral swelling there is a time interval without these signs. This distinction is significant, however, since with diffuse axonal injury a certain amount of primary structural damage has occurred at the moment of impact, but is not present in cases of pure delayed swelling. Therefore, the deleterious effects of delayed swelling should be potentially reversible, and if these effects are controlled, the outcome should be good. However, control of the effects of brain swelling may be difficult. Vigorous monitoring of, and attention to, intracranial pressure is necessary, and prompt and vigorous treatment of raised intracranial pressure is required in order to control brain swelling. If this is successfully accomplished, the mortality rate from increased intracranial pressure associated with diffuse brain swelling should be low.

FOCAL BRAIN SYNDROMES

In discussing the occurrence of intracranial hematoma as a result of athletic injury, two major points must be emphasized. First, owing to recent developments in clinical evaluation of patients and animal research correlation, we have a satisfactory understanding of the mechanism of occurrence of focal intracranial hematoma, which is somewhat different from older concepts of head-injured patients. Second, management of head-injured patients has advanced rapidly and changed dramatically over the last decade from what was accepted medical practice in the past.

The entire spectrum of traumatic intracranial hematomas occurs in sports injuries. These include cerebral contusions, intracerebral hematomas, epidural hematomas, and acute subdural hematomas. The presentation of athletic head-injured patients who have had serious trauma is similar in most instances. Management depends on definitive diagnosis and varies depending on the underlying pathologic process.

Intracerebral Hematoma and Contusion

Athletic injuries of this type occur in patients with impressive intracerebral injury who have never suffered loss of consciousness or focal neurologic deficit, but who do have persistent headache or periods of post-head-injury confusion and post-traumatic amnesia. As with any head-injured patients, athletic head-injured patients with such symptoms should have a CT scan to permit early differentiation between solid intracerebral hematoma and hemorrhagic contusion with surrounding edema.

Epidural Hematoma

With epidural hematoma the middle meningeal or other meningeal arteries are often embedded in bony grooves in the skull, and skull fractures, crossing this bony groove, frequently tear the blood vessel at that site. Because bleeding in these instances is arterial, accumulation of clot continues under high pressure; thus bleeding does not stop early enough to prevent serious brain injury.

The classic picture of an epidural hematoma is that of loss of consciousness at the time of injury, followed by recovery of consciousness in a variable period, after which the patient is lucid. This is followed by the onset of increasingly severe headache, decreased level of consciousness, dilation of one pupil (usually on the same side as the clot), and decerebrate posturing and weakness (usually on the side opposite the hematoma). In our experience, however, only one-third of the patients with epidural hematoma present with this classic history. Another one-third of patients do not become unconscious until late in their course, and the other third are unconscious from the time of injury and remain unconscious throughout their course.

The absence of a classic clinical picture of an epidural hematoma cannot be relied upon to rule out this diagnosis, and the best diagnostic test for evaluating these patients is a CT scan.

Acute Subdural Hematoma

Athletic head injuries result from lower inertial loading than that involved in serious head injuries caused by vehicular accidents or falling from heights. Thus, an acute subdural hematoma also occurs much more frequently than an epidural hematoma in athletes. In head-injured patients in general, the incidence of acute subdural hematomas is approximately three times that of epidural hematomas.

Acute subdural hematomas have been clearly identified as two main types: (1) those with a collection of blood in the subdural space, which apparently are not associated with underlying cerebral contusion or edema, and (2) those with collections of blood in the subdural space, but associated with an obvious contusion on the surface of the brain and hemispheric brain injury with swelling. The mortality rate for simple subdural hematomas is approximately 20 percent, but this increases to more than 50 percent for subdural hematomas with an underlying brain injury.

Patients with an acute subdural hematoma are typically unconscious, they may or may not have a history of deterioration, and they frequently display focal neurologic findings. Patients with simple subdural hematomas are more likely to have a lucid interval following their injury and are less likely to be unconscious at admission than those patients with hemispheric injury and brain swelling. It is necessary to obtain a CT scan or angiogram to diagnose an acute subdural hematoma. The size of the subdural clot relative to the size of the midline shift of the brain structures can be evaluated best by CT scan. Of patients with acute subdural hematoma, 84 percent also have an associated hemorrhagic contusion or intracerebral hematoma with associated brain swelling.

The term "acute subdural hematoma" raises the image in most physicians' minds of a large collection of clotted blood in the intracranial cavity, compressing the brain substance and causing compromise due to the space-occupying hematoma. Although not an infrequent consequence of closed head trauma, this type of subdural hematoma is more common in adults who have a degree of cortical atrophy.

Young athletes, and especially children, frequently develop only minimal subdural hematomas with underlying cerebral hemispheric swelling. This type of brain injury is not the result of a space-occupying mass from clotted blood causing brain compression, but rather swollen brain tissue causing consequent rises in intracranial pressure. The advent of CT scanning permits accurate differential diagnosis between these two conditions, which frequently cause similar clinical pictures. The modalities of treatment of these two distinct types of acute subdural hematomas are quite different.

PRINCIPLES OF MANAGEMENT

As our knowledge of physiology and pathophysiology has increased, so has our ability to successfully resuscitate seriously ill or severely injured people. We began in the 1950s to successfully treat acute respiratory and postoperative problems, followed by satisfactory cardiac resuscitation and emergency cardiac care in the 1960s. We extended innovations in critical-care medicine in the form of brain resuscitation in the 1970s. Such care is based on the concept that the degree of permanent neurologic, intellectual, and psychologic deficits after brain trauma with coma is only partly the result of the initial injury, and is certainly due in part to secondary postinsult changes, which can be worsened or improved by the quality of the supportive care. Head injuries, by their very nature, require resuscitation, i.e.,

TABLE 2   Treatment Protocol for Head Injury

First Aid: Hyperventilation
Diagnosis: CT Scan

Surgery: For epidural hematoma, large subdural hematoma, or
large intracerebral hematoma

No Surgery: For small subdural hematoma, confusion, diffuse
injury, most intracerebral hematomas

ICP Monitoring and Treatment
Goal: Keep ICP less than 15 mm Hg
Modalities: Hyperventilation (PCO_2 22 to 30 mm Hg)
Corticosteroids (1 mg/kg)
Mannitol (1 g/kg, serum osmolality 330 to
320 mOsm/L)
Barbiturates (30 mg/kg loading and 0.5 to
3 mg/kg/h maintenance)

therapy initiated after the insult. The proper care of
head-injured patients, athletic or otherwise, depends on
the full appreciation and use of brain resuscitation measures in an intensive care setting.

Treatment for focal intracranial hematoma consists of removal of the hematoma and recognition and
treatment of any underlying brain injury. Included in
this concept of treatment for the underlying brain injury
is that of resuscitation of the brain, which is designed to
have specific neuron-saving potential once general
resuscitation methods and supportive care have begun.
Our current management and treatment protocol is
outlined in Table 2.

First aid should consist of getting the patient safely
into a supine position and determining vital signs and
the significance of any associated injuries. Initial treatment should consist of establishing an adequate and
useful airway and beginning hyperventilation maneuvers. This can be accomplished by using a manual resuscitation bag with supplemental oxygen, if it is available.
The patient should then be transferred as quickly as
possible to a medical facility where diagnosis and treatment of brain injury can begin. Although these measures are important for all patients who have suffered
concussion, they are of extreme importance for the
patient who remains comatose following trauma. The
use of an initial dose of corticosteroids given parenter-
ally is specifically indicated, and 100 mg dexamethasone
or 1 g methylprednisolone sodium succinate can be
administered to the average adult. Once the patient
arrives in the emergency room and it is determined that
he or she is stable from a cardiorespiratory point of
view, endotracheal intubation is immediately performed
on comatose patients and a CT scan is obtained as soon
as possible. The CT scan provides an immediate diagnosis of the intracranial situation, and as can be seen from
the management schema, patients are then divided into
either a surgical or nonsurgical category, depending on
the size of the intracranial hematoma present.

Initial evaluation of all head trauma patients
includes determination of their coma state by numerical
ranking on the Glasgow Coma Scale (Table 3). This
coma scale is based on the patient's response to stimulation by eye-opening, best motor response, and best
verbal response. Scores of 15 to 3, from normal neurologic status to deeply comatose, are possible.

Patients with a Glasgow Coma Scale of 7 or lower
should have immediate intracranial pressure (ICP)
monitoring as part of their treatment. Intracranial
hypertension, defined as a pressure over 15 mmHg, is
seen in 50 percent or more of severely head-injured
patients. The poor correlation between alterations in
ICP and the patient's neurologic status has been well
described in the past. Therapy to treat intracranial
hypertension can only be given correctly when the pressure is known. We are firmly convinced of the usefulness
of continuous ICP monitoring in the intensive care of
the severely head-injured patient. Because intermittent
waves of increased pressure, which commonly occur
without other signs or symptoms, can be diagnosed and
treated before significant neurologic deterioration
occurs, ICP monitoring facilitates titration of therapy.

TABLE 3   Glasgow Coma Scale

Eyes	Open	Spontaneously	4
		To verbal command	3
		To pain	2
		No response	1
	To verbal Command	Obeys	6
	To painful stimulus*	Localizes pain	5
Best motor response		Flexion-withdrawal	4
		Flexion-abnormal (decorticate rigidity)	3
		Extension (decerebrate rigidity)	2
		No response	1
Best verbal response†		Oriented and converses	5
		Disoriented and converses	4
		Inappropriate words	3
		Incomprehensible sounds	2
		No response	1
		Total	3–15

* Apply knuckles to sternum; observe arms.
† Arouse patient with painful stimulus if necessary.

The Glasgow Coma Scale, based upon eye opening and verbal and motor responses, is a practical means of monitoring changes in the level of
consciousness. If response on the scale is assigned a numerical value, the responsiveness of the patient can be expressed by totaling the figures.
Lowest score is 3; highest is 15.

When muscle paralysis or barbiturates are used to control elevated ICP, it is impossible to follow the patient's neurologic state. Other than brain-stem evoked potentials, ICP is the only parameter that can be followed. It would be inappropriate to use muscle paralysis or barbiturates without continuously recording ICP. Ideally, the ICP should be monitored from the earliest possible time after the patient's arrival in the hospital. In our unit, it is usually possible to obtain a CT scan within one hour of admission in all severe head injuries. The ICP monitor is usually inserted after the CT scan and within 2 hours of admission.

However, if any delay in diagnosis is foreseen or if the patient is rapidly deteriorating, an ICP bolt is inserted immediately following emergency resuscitation. This early insertion is especially important in patients with signs of shock from other injuries who require rapid fluid replacement. In other cases, we begin to monitor pressure in the emergency room with a portable recording system.

The ICP monitoring system must be simple, easily inserted, and reliable. The subarachnoid bolt, which can be easily inserted and maintained and does not require an operating room procedure, can be inserted at bedside with local anesthesia.

We monitor ICP in comatose head-injured patients whether they are operated on initially for decompression or not. We rarely intervene surgically to remove contused brain, believing that if ICP can be controlled, the removal of potentially functional brain tissue is unacceptable as it may limit the patient's recovery. After surgical intervention in patients with hematoma, we routinely insert subarachnoid bolts and monitor ICP for possible further therapy.

The following principles of management of head-injured patients apply both to those who do not have indications for surgical intervention and to those who have undergone surgery. This management is guided by the monitored variables, and its goals are to prevent three major complications which cause most deaths if the patient is alive on arrival at the hospital: (1) intracranial hypertension, (2) inadequate cerebral oxygenation, and (3) systemic medical complications. These must be attacked vigorously for optimum results. Treatment for intracranial hypertension is also designed to maximize cerebral oxygenation, and the modalities are those previously listed.

Of all therapies for high ICP, hyperventilation is the first one that we use, and it is extremely effective. With the patient intubated, we keep the Pco_2 at 22 to 30 mmHg and note that the fall in ICP is rapid after hyperventilation and, in some instances, is all that is necessary for control.

Corticosteroids in large doses (1 mg/kg dexamethasone *q6h*) are given routinely. Hyperosmotic agents decrease ICP by removing brain water due to an induced osmotic gradient from the brain to the intravascular component. Although slightly less rapid in its action, 20 to 25 percent mannitol has largely replaced 30 percent urea in this country because of less rebound after administration. Two forms of hyperosmotic ther-

apy are available; intermittent bolus use and continuous infusion therapy. High-dose bolus therapy, 1 to 2 g/kg mannitol, is reserved for initial emergency control of ICP, usually in patients who have a rapid decrease in level of consciousness, dilating pupils, or decerebration. Maintenance therapy can then be carried out with smaller boluses of 0.15 to 0.3 g/kg mannitol every 1 to 2 hours or whenever the ICP exceeds 15 mmHg. Close attention must be given to the serum osmolality so that it does not rise above 320 mOsm/L. Significant cardiopulmonary and renal complications are frequent and often irreversible with serum osmolality above these levels. Clinicians utilizing this therapy should have a thorough understanding of the hyperosmolar state.

The most recent contribution to ICP control is the use of the barbiturates. When initially used to protect the brain by lowering metabolism, it became apparent that reductions of ICP occurred regularly. Although the mechanism of barbiturate action on elevated ICP is not known, its successful use when other forms of therapy have failed to lower ICP is encouraging. The doses of barbiturates required have varied. Pentobarbital has been the most widely used agent, usually with loading doses of 10 to 30 mg/kg. Thereafter, infusions of 0.5 to 3 mg/kg/hr are maintained. We have been impressed with the wide variation of serum levels obtained by similar doses in different patients and no longer rely solely on serum levels as criteria. We prefer to titrate the dose until a burst-suppression pattern is present on the EEG monitor. Therapy is then closely regulated to keep the burst-suppressions of equal length. At this physiologic end point, the serum pentobarbital level may vary from 2.5 to 5.0 mg/dl. Care must be taken to prevent barbiturate cardiac toxicity and subsequent hypotension. This has not been a problem except in older patients, and the cerebral perfusion pressure can be adequately maintained without the use of pressor agents.

For the duration of barbiturate therapy, monitoring must be intensive because neurologic signs are abolished. Spontaneous respiratory activity is not present, and all other neurologic signs are generally absent. Although we have continued barbiturate therapy for as long as 21 days, the usual course is less than 5 days. By this time the ICP rarely rises when an attempt is made to discontinue the barbiturate infusion. Once a patient's ICP is less than 15 mmHg for longer than 48 hours, we discontinue therapy in a sequential manner, stopping barbiturates first, then decreasing hyperosmolar therapy, and finally, ceasing hyperventilation.

The accepted treatment of a patient with acute subdural hematoma remains controversial. Some neurosurgeons believe that the majority of patients with acute subdural hematoma are not helped by an operation, and that the major problems are the control of brain swelling and elevated intracranial pressure. Others believe that because of obvious deterioration of the patient, evacuation of the hematoma, no matter how large or small, improves intracranial compliance and the neurologic state.

In patients whose CT scans show a large localized

subdural clot with an equal or large shift of the midline structures, we surgically evaluate the hematoma. In patients with a "smear subdural", a few millimeters thick over the entire lateral aspect of one hemisphere, with the midline shift greater than the thickness of the subdural, we probably would not operate, but would aggressively control ICP. Disagreements arise when a state between these two is seen. The argument against surgical intervention is that the major cerebral problem is brain injury, which cannot be helped by an operation. If there is a disruption of the blood-brain barrier with vasogenic edema, craniotomy decreases tissue pressure, increases hydrostatic pressure gradients between capillaries and tissue, and may therefore cause a marked increase in edema in the decompressed hemisphere. Thus, even if the clot is removed, the increased edema may cause swelling of the hemisphere, which rapidly returns the intracranial volume-pressure relationships to where they were prior to the operation.

If an operation is performed, we recommend a large temporofrontoparietal craniotomy flap, with evacuation of the clot and control of the hemorrhage from bridging veins and cortical laceration. The patient with a sizable subdural hematoma should have an operation for evacuation of the clot followed by management of ICP. A patient with a small subdural hematoma along the outside of the left hemisphere is best managed by aggressive treatment of brain swelling and therapy for increased ICP.

The mortality rates for the surgical treatment of acute subdural hematoma reported in the last 10 years vary from 42 to 63 percent. One important variable seems to be the level of consciousness of the patient at the time of the operation. We do not believe that an operation is necessary in all patients with acute subdural hematoma, but we do feel it is vital that all patients, including those who have had surgical intervention, have postoperative ICP monitoring and control. Of patients who died after surgical intervention, 25 percent died from uncontrollable elevated ICP. Thus, postoperative ICP monitoring plays a major role in the care of patients with acute subdural hematoma. We firmly believe that this will improve mortality rates and the quality of life.

HEAD INJURIES IN BOXERS

ALAN R. HUDSON, M.D., B.S., F.R.C.S.(Ed), F.R.C.S.(C)

STRUCTURE AND FUNCTION

A great deal of information has accrued over the years concerning the relationship of the function and structure of the brain. While much remains to be discovered, certain general statements can be made with confidence. The brain is the seat of consciousness, which is to say, if a person's brain is functioning normally, that person is alert and is able to relate to his environment in a rational manner. Progressive impairment of the function of the brain results in drowsiness, and subsequently unconsciousness, and finally death. The abilities to reason, process abstract concepts, display judgment, and create new ideas are undoubtedly related to the presence of a normally functioning brain. Indeed, the very qualities that determine an individual's personality, his ability to relate to other people, and his ability to earn his living are directly related to the structure and function of the brain.

A concept of fundamental importance is that of lack of regeneration of brain substance. Brain heals by scarring and not by replacing damaged brain with new, normal brain. Thus, repeated injuries result in a cumulative effect. The brain loses substance in the normal process of aging, and it is not unusual for the appearance of obvious clinical abnormalities to be delayed until many years following the receipt of numerous head injuries, such as those sustained in the boxing ring. Presumably, this is related to the additive effect of the aging process and the preexisting injury.

For many years it was thought that it was possible to damage the function of the brain temporarily, e.g., with a knockout blow, without significantly damaging the structure of the brain. The vast majority of experts in head injury disagree with that point of view. The modern view is that if a person is knocked out, his brain has received structural damage.

Bearing in mind these rather sobering facts, it is reasonable to examine some of the factors surrounding head injuries suffered by boxers in greater detail.

MEASUREMENT OF BRAIN FUNCTION

The most widely used scale of measurement of consciousness is the Glasgow Coma Scale (see chapter on *Head Injuries in Athletics*). This scale is derived from measuring the alertness of the contestant. It is obtained by adding numbers derived from three different tests. Values ascribed to the response are indicated in parenthesis. The first test measures the person's speech in response to an appropriate question such as "Where are you?" "What is the date?" The response may indicate that the patient is oriented (5); the conversation may indicate confusion (4); the person may use inappropriate words (3); all that may be obtained are incomprehensible sounds (2); or no response (1).

The next test is to observe motor response to a command such as "Raise your right arm". The boxer may obey (6). If the fighter is unconscious, but reaches up to try to remove the hand applying a painful stimulus, he is said to localize (5). The unconscious fighter may not respond in this way, but may withdraw a limb if a painful stimulus is applied (4). A deeply unconscious fighter may respond with abnormal flexion (3), or abnormal extension (2), of a limb in response to pain. If there is absolutely no response, the score is (1).

The final test relates to eye opening. Eye opening may be spontaneous (4); in response to speech (3); in response to pain (2); or nil (1).

The numbers from the three categories are added together and thus a normal person will score 15 and a deeply unconscious person will score 3. While it is immediately obvious that an internationally accepted method of measuring consciousness is a great advantage in that this type of scoring should be applied to a fighter who has been knocked out and who does not immediately regain his senses, it is also immediately apparent that this international system does not test any of the finer elements of cerebral function which have already been referred to and which distinguish us as human beings. Unfortunately, testing of these functions requires a battery of detailed psychometric evaluations which take many hours to complete. In other words, such tests are impossible to apply to a fighter between rounds of a contest. It should also be noted that such tests cannot possibly be administered with any degree of accuracy in the time usually allotted to a pre-fight examination of a contestant.

WHAT IS BRAIN INJURY?

The reader should appreciate that a continuum exists, ranging from very minor injury at one extreme to lethal brain injury at the other. Every time a fighter receives a significant head injury, the exact brain injury he receives will fall somewhere within this continuum. It is emphasized that such injuries are additive over a period of time because of the lack of regeneration of the brain following injury. The brain may be injured directly by bruising or tearing or by pressure from hemorrhage, which may complicate either. The brain may be further injured as a result of swelling of the brain, which may complicate head injury. Blood vessels on the surface of the brain may be broken, giving rise to surface hemorrhages, which are called subdural hematomas or extradural hematomas.

These matters have been studied in a variety of areas. The brains of world champions have been examined carefully following death. The brains of fighters who have died following head injury in the ring are routinely examined by the coroner. A great deal of experimental evidence has accrued following animal experimentation and, to a lesser extent, biomedical engineering experimentation.

If one could produce a significant head injury and not damage the brain, this would be a most surprising result. Virtually all the evidence derived from the aforementioned studies indicates that what common sense tells one is true, i.e., that a significant head injury damages the brain. That the most extreme form of brain damage results in death is merely a matter of record, and it is the occasional ring death which causes significant publicity. Far greater attention needs to be focused, however, by fighters, trainers, and promoters, on the effect of sublethal, repetitive head injury sustained by a boxer in the ring. Very little scientific evidence is available with relationship to these injuries. This is not surprising as no university ethics committee could possibly consent to the performance of an experiment in which human volunteers were hit on the head so that the effects could be measured. The likely consequence is so predictable as to render the experiment quite unethical. The scientific evidence related to animal experiments points to a frightening conclusion. When the degrees of severity of brain injury are compared with the acceleration of the head following a known injury, it is seen that of the time/acceleration curves required to produce lethal brain injury, those required to produce recognizable but sublethal brain injury are alarmingly closely drawn. Thus, any fighter who is capable of knocking out his opponent is capable of killing him. Any fighter who is capable of being knocked out is capable of being the recipient of lesser blows which may yet cause brain damage. The effects of that immediate brain damage may not be visible in the clinical sense until many years have passed following the injury.

In that most fighters are trained to cause head injury in their opponent and in that one of the surest ways of winning a contest is to knock their opponent out, all those involved with boxing should clearly understand that neither the aggressor nor the defender, in the excitement of a contest, is capable of determining what the result of a head shot will be, with reference to the degree of brain damage it will cause.

MINIMIZING THE DANGER OF HEAD INJURY

The express purpose of most boxing matches is that of causing a head injury to one's opponent. Is there any way in which the effect of such a head injury can be minimized?

It is apparent that the most significant method of injury is that of sudden rotation of the skull. The brain is suspended in a fluid cushion and does not rotate until a fractional second later, and similarly, when the skull reaches the end of its rotation, the brain rotates fractionally longer. It is this mechanism (akin to shaking a soft kilogram of butter within a shoe box) which results in the most damage. Thus, the only way that such an injury can be completely avoided is to ban punches to the head in a boxing contest. The wearing of safety headgear, of course, can in no way prevent the sudden rotation of the head which follows a blow to the jaw or temple. While the wearing of headgear may lessen the number and severity of soft tissue cuts, such minimal, although sometimes spectacular, injuries are really of very small account in comparison to the danger of brain damage which cannot be prevented by any external device unless it firmly fixes the head upon the shoulders. Such a device would, of course, prevent a boxer from either adequately defending himself or attacking his opponent.

The effect of lessening the impact by increasing the weight of the gloves has a more rational basis, but the safety factor derived from such a maneuver has probably been grossly exaggerated.

Clearly, every precaution should be taken to lessen the effect of a secondary head injury which a fighter might sustain in falling down following the receipt of a punch. Unfortunately, the provision of adequate ring structure, designed to lessen the effect of a secondary head injury, can in no way prevent the effect of the primary head injury which follows sudden acceleration and rotation of the skull on receipt of a significant blow.

All fighters should be aware of the fact that, with one possible exception, there is virtually no physical exercise which can be performed which will prevent brain damage. In a society which gives so much attention to physical fitness, there is a spurious suggestion that if a fighter is physically fit, he is less likely to suffer from brain damage. A fighter who is physically fit is, of course, far more capable of sustaining a prolonged and repetitive attack and of sustaining the power of his punches round after round. The argument is far more compelling that a physically fit fighter is more capable of causing brain damage than he is of preventing its occurrence in himself. The one possible exception to this argument is that of building up the power of the neck muscles. It is a reasonable conclusion that a head which is freely mobile on a supple neck will sustain a greater degree of brain damage as a result of a blow which will do far less damage to a head which is firmly fixed by muscular action. It is a common sight to see a fighter taking punishment start to lose control of his neck muscles, so that each successive blow causes greater and greater damage prior to the final knockout.

THE DOCTOR AT THE RINGSIDE

The doctor at the ringside lends a totally false sense of safety to the proceedings. The fact that a head injury is witnessed by a doctor in no way can lessen the severity of the head injury. Beyond securing the airway of an unconscious fighter (a task which can be performed by a well-trained paramedic), there is really nothing that a doctor can do immediately to reverse the effect of the brain damage which he has just witnessed. The question of future liability of a doctor who has just pronounced a fighter fit to receive brain damage is a matter which undoubtedly will be one of medical/legal interest. The question of liability of a doctor who has pronounced a fighter fit to receive repetitive, sublethal head injuries, whose effect may not be apparent for many years, is one

of considerable interest. While it may be extremely difficult to prove that an ex-fighter who suffers personality change, marital disharmony, and loss of his job has undergone these changes as a result of the numerous head injuries he has sustained in his youth, the medical evidence is steadily mounting, so that one day it may be possible to provide irrefutable medical evidence to sustain such an action. Although calls for the banning of boxing by various national bodies may be based as much on moral and ethical grounds as on the presence of scientific evidence, doctors at the ringside should be aware of the fact that the vast majority of brain surgeons feel that the evidence currently available is sufficiently compelling. Even if the final proof is lacking, a doctor should ask himself whether he really is capable of stopping a fight before a brain-damaging blow is struck. The answer to this question is quite clearly in the negative.

SUGGESTIONS FOR THE MANAGEMENT OF THE HEAD-INJURED BOXER

1. *Informed Consent*: All those involved in boxing, whether they be fighters, trainers, promoters, or rulemakers, should be aware of the current state of knowledge with reference to head injuries sustained in the ring. Thus, those who wish to take the risk of receiving or causing brain damage should be fully conversant with the fact that the risk is a significant risk. They should be aware of the fact that this risk cannot be removed by having a fighter in excellent physical condition, by having up-to-date first-class equipment in the ring, or by having a doctor at the ringside.

2. *Training*: Fighters should be thoroughly schooled in the defensive arts. A man who repeatedly takes excessive punishment en route to securing a victory may be regarded as courageous in some quarters and excessively stupid in others.

3. *Training Sessions*: Training sessions should be devised to minimize the occurrence of head shots. A fighter who has been the recipient of numerous stiff left jabs to the face is just as surely at risk in the gym as he is in a public contest. In promoting a contest, promoters must do everything in their power to ensure that fighters are as evenly matched as possible. Referees and corner men should stop a contest at the very first sign that a fighter is in trouble. These signs are well known to the boxing community and include a fighter who is failing to respond to repeated attacks, a fighter who is slightly confused, a fighter whose reflexes have obviously been dulled, a fighter whose mobility around the ring seems to have been impaired, and a fighter whose head appears to be snapping backwards on receipt of each successive blow. To allow the fight to continue in the hope that the injured fighter can clear his head and continue the contest assumes the risk of additive damage, which is really not conscionable in the light of present-day knowledge. The concept of the standing 8-count, initially regarded as a breakthrough in the concern for the safety of fighters, should be examined with care. It is probable that if a

fighter requires a standing 8-count, the fight should be terminated then and there.

4. On no account should ringside handlers attempt to revive a confused contestant or one whose mobility of legs or hands has been impaired as the result of the punishment he has taken in the previous round. Handlers should be aware that they might well be sending their man to his death or to the receipt of serious brain injury if their fighter is pushed out into the ring in such circumstances at the beginning of the following round. Any fighter who has been knocked out must be examined by a doctor who is conversant with the subtleties of a neurologic examination. Fighters who have been even briefly unconscious should receive a detailed neurologic examination by a neurologist or neurosurgeon on the day following the contest and should receive an electroencephalographic (EEG) examination and a computerized tomographic (CT) examination at the same time.

5. The question of the duration of lay-off following a knockout blow is frequently raised. In reality, the answer is that any fighter who is knocked out should never fight again if he values normal brain function for the rest of his life. In reality, few fighters will accept this, and present suggestions are that, provided a fighter has a completely normal neurologic examination, a normal EEG, and a normal CT scan, he should not receive further head injuries for at least another 60 days.

6. It is difficult to comprehend how any doctor can state that a fighter is fit to receive further head injury if he has been knocked out more than twice.

OCULAR INJURIES IN SPORT

ROBERT C. PASHBY, M.D., F.R.C.S.(C),
THOMAS J. PASHBY, C.M., M.D., C.R.C.S.(C)

Eye injuries account for 1 percent of the total related to sports. They can end the career of a professional athlete and change the life style and earning power of others. Their prevention is possible, as proved first in hockey and now in racquet sports. When they do occur, they must be recognized, their severity assessed, and treatment instituted. The team physician, trainer, or first aid attendant should have a basic knowledge of eye anatomy and physiology (Fig. 1) and the necessary equipment to carry out on the spot examination. He must decide whether the injury can be treated and the patient released or whether ophthalmologic consultation is necessary.

EXAMINATION

A minimum list of equipment required for ophthalmologic examination includes:

1. Vision card
2. Pen light
3. Sterile fluorescein strips
4. Sterile eye pads
5. Eye shield
6. Tape
7. Sterile Q-Tips
8. Sterile irrigating solution

To determine the severity of an eye injury, a routine eye examination is carried out. By oblique illumination of the eye with a pen light, damage to the conjunctiva, cornea, anterior chamber, iris, pupil, and lens can be determined. Intraocular examination behind the lens requires the use of an ophthalmoscope and the ability to interpret findings.

The steps in the examination are as follows:

1. Inspection of the soft tissues for laceration, bruising, or hematoma.

2. Inspection of the conjunctival sac for hemorrhage, laceration, and foreign bodies. In many cases eversion of the upper eyelid reveals a foreign body, which is easily brushed away. Displaced contact lenses often are found.

3. Examination of the cornea by oblique illumination for foreign body, abrasions, and lacerations. Abrasions are readily outlined by a fluorescein strip dipped into the tears exposed as the lower lid is pulled downward.

4. The clarity and depth of the anterior chamber is compared with the fellow eye.

5. Pupillary size, shape, and reaction to light are compared with those of the other eye.

6. The iris colors of each eye are compared.

7. Intraocular examination with an ophthalmoscope (if available) may reveal lens, vitreous, and retinal damage.

8. Visual acuity is tested in each eye separately, using a reading card or book; corrected vision less than 20/40 is referred.

9. Peripheral vision is tested by having the patient fix on the examiner's nose and, after occluding the fellow eye, by asking for identification of the number of fingers held up in all fields of gaze. A normal visual field extends to 90° temporally, 65° downward, 60° nasally, and 45° upward. Any loss of field demands referral.

10. Ocular movements are tested by having the patient follow a light to his right, then upward, then downward, then similarly to his left. Both eyes should move together. Any diplopia must be referred.

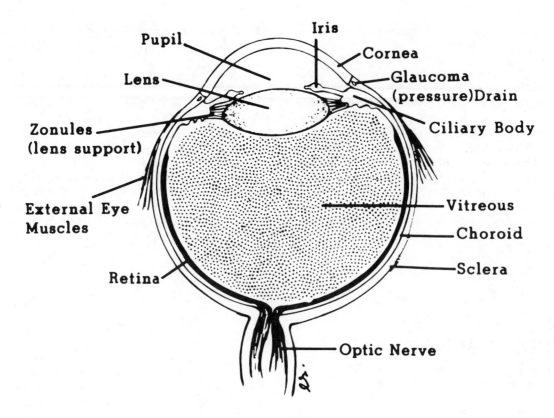

Figure 1 Cross section of the eye

11. Facing the patient, determine whether one eye is sunken (narrowing the palpebral aperture) or proptosed (enlarging it). The former suggests an orbital floor fracture while the latter suggests an orbital hemorrhage.

Should there be any doubt about the function of the eye or seriousness of the injury, referral is indicated.

In our series of almost 2400 eye injuries caused by sports, gathered over the past 10 years, all of which required ophthalmologic care, 12 percent resulted in a legally blind eye (20/200 or less), and most suffered severe intraocular damage.

The sport causing most eye injuries varies from country to country (Table 1). In Canada, hockey has been responsible for most eye injuries, although since the hockey mask was introduced, racquet sports are rapidly catching up (Table 2).

Examining the hockey injuries in more detail proves the benefit of wearing certified protective equipment.

Before hockey face masks were introduced, an average 272 hockey eye injuries, including 32 blinding injuries, were reported annually. Since masks have been required in minor hockey, the annual average number of eye injuries has dropped to 79 and the number of blinding injuries to 14. No eye injury has been reported to a player wearing a Canadian Standards Association certified mask.

An analysis of 2089 sports-related eye injuries reveals that over 50 percent are intraocular in type (Table 3).

TREATMENT AND MANAGEMENT

Orbital Hemorrhage

This type of injury usually results from blunt trauma. Bleeding into the orbit causes swelling and proptosis. It is wise to check for intraocular damage before the swelling becomes extensive. Central and peripheral

TABLE 1 Causes of Sports-Related Eye Injuries in United States and Canada

Canada (COS Study)*	Sport	United States (CPSC)†
39%	Hockey (post, mask)	4%
30%	Racquet sports	20%
11%	Baseball	27%
8%	Ball hockey	1%
4%	Football and soccer	7%
1%	Basketball	20%

* Canadian Ophthalmological Society
† Consumer Product Safety Commission

TABLE 2 Number of Eye Injuries According to Sport

Sport		Injuries	Blind Eyes
Hockey	(10 years)	1,140	172
Racquet sports	(8 years)	466	17
Baseball	(8 years)	175	10
Ball hockey	(8 years)	124	16
Football	(8 years)	65	2
Golf	(8 years)	20	7
Skiing	(8 years)	9	6
Other sports	(8 years)	90	11

TABLE 3   Types of Sports-Related Eye Injuries

Soft tissue	34%
Orbital fractures	4%
Corneal injuries	9%
Hyphemas	27%
Other intraocular injuries	23%
Ruptured globes	3%

vision, pupils, iris color, and the presence of diplopia must be recorded. Most injuries resorb without treatment, but severe hemorrhage may embarrass the blood supply to the optic nerve and cause visual loss. Such injuries must be referred. Application of an ice pack is suggested.

Corneal lacerations present, again, with similar symptoms. If the eye can gently be opened without undue squeezing and without pressure on the globe, the pupil will appear irregular, the anterior chamber shallow, and the iris probably attached to or prolapsed outside the corneal wound. A sterile eye pad is gently applied, and the patient is referred to the hospital for immediate ophthalmologic repair.

Injuries to the Lens

The lens can be injured by blunt trauma interfering with lens metabolism or causing a split in the lens capsule, allowing aqueous to enter the lens, rendering it opaque. The lens may also be involved in penetrating injuries. Cataract changes may occur immediately or develop over weeks or months. The lens is suspended within the eye by radiating zonular fibers attached to the ciliary body. Zonular rupture is not unusual following injury, and this allows vitreous to herniate into the anterior chamber. If the zonular rupture is extensive, the lens may subluxate. The iris will jiggle (iridodonesis).

Removal of the cataractous or dislocated lens and replacement with an implant or the fitting of a contact lens usually restores vision to normal. Lens injuries, of course, demand specialized care.

Traumatic Glaucoma

Intraocular tension often fluctuates above and below normal for days after ocular trauma. Should there be no structural damage inside the eye, intraocular tension then settles back to normal. More severe trauma may produce a split in the anterior chamber angle. The ciliary body is damaged, the anterior chamber deepened, and the aqueous outflow channels are embarrassed. Should the remaining undamaged aqueous outflow channels be unable to adequately handle aqueous production, ocular hypertension ensues. Glaucoma will develop in 10 percent of split angles early or even after many years. Once anterior chamber angle damage has been identified, the intraocular pressure should be followed at regular intervals.

Secondary glaucoma commonly complicates lens dislocation and occurs with hyphemas, especially after secondary hemorrhages. Normalization of pressure is necessary to prevent optic nerve damage and peripheral field loss. Secondary glaucoma complicating hyphema requires early attention to prevent blood staining of the cornea. Evacuation of the blood and blood clots from the anterior chamber is indicated.

Hyphema

Hyphema is a collection of free blood in the anterior chamber. It is a very common ocular sports injury. Over 550 hyphemas are listed in our series. It is important that the person rendering first aid recognize this type of injury because immediate referral and hospitalization is required. Aspirin should be avoided.

Lid Lacerations

With any lid laceration, damage to the globe, ocular muscles, and orbit must be ruled out. Bleeding can be controlled by direct pressure. Close inspection is necessary to reveal lacerations of the lid margin, of the puncta, or into the lacrimal apparatus. Such lacerations demand meticulous closure to prevent epiphora. Primary repair using the microscope is indicated. Examination of the globe and a record of visual function is necessary.

Conjunctival Injuries

Minor lacerations of the conjunctiva do not require suturing. Foreign bodies may be removed with a moist, sterile Q-Tip. A sterile eye pad is applied for 24 hours when follow-up examination is made.

Foreign bodies commonly lodge under the upper lid margin. Eversion of the upper eyelid will expose them. They too can be wiped away with a moist Q-Tip.

Conjunctival Hemorrhage

Although the bright red blood covering the white sclera is an alarming sight, such uncomplicated injuries are not serious. Eye function is recorded, and if it is normal, no treatment is needed. The redness gradually disappears over 10 days.

Orbital Fractures

These injuries usually result from blunt trauma. The most common fracture occurs to the orbital floor where the bone is thinnest. Blunt trauma forces the eye back into the orbit increasing the orbital pressure and causing a "blow out fracture" of the orbital floor. The inferior ocular muscles may be caught in the fracture, causing limitation of upward and downward gaze with resulting diplopia. Enophthalmos is usual. Eye function is recorded, and x-ray studies including tomograms are arranged. Some recover spontaneously; others require freeing of the inferior ocular muscles and insertion of a Teflon plate along the orbital floor to cover the fracture. Fractures into the sinuses cause leakage of air into the orbit producing crepitus, a crackling sound, with finger pressure over the swelling. X-ray examination reveals air in the tissue. Spontaneous resolution is usual. Roof fractures require immediate neurosurgical care because they involve the anterior cranial fossa.

Corneal Injuries

Corneal injuries cause sudden severe pain accompanied by tearing, photophobia, and blepharospasm. Superficial corneal foreign bodies can be irrigated off with sterile solution or brushed off with a moist Q-Tip. Eye function is recorded, a sterile eye pad applied, and the eye re-examined in 24 hours. Embedded foreign bodies will not irrigate or brush off the cornea and require removal by an ophthalmologist using a sterile needle or eye spud under slit lamp magnification. Eye function is recorded, a sterile eye pad applied, and recheck in 24 hours arranged.

Corneal abrasions produce similar symptoms. Fluorescein outlines the denuded area. Should no foreign body be present, visual function is recorded, a sterile eye pad applied, and follow-up examination in 24 hours carried out.

When the injured eye is first examined, the blood appears as a haze in the anterior chamber. The pupil is usually irregular in shape and sluggish in reaction to light. The anterior chamber may be deepened. These diagnostic points are readily appreciated by comparing the injured to the fellow eye. Vision is blurred. On bed rest the blood settles down by gravity and appears the next day as a level in the anterior chamber. Continued bleeding may occur, however, and if severe, the anterior chamber appears black, the so-called "8-ball eye". Most hyphemas clear in 5 days, but 15 percent suffer secondary bleeds, usually within 2 to 5 days. Prompt recognition and referral is necessary. Conservative treatment includes hospitalization, sedation, and binocular bandages, especially for children. Secondary glaucoma occurs in 50 percent of secondary hemorrhages. Irrigation of the anterior chamber is indicated to relieve the increased intraocular pressure and prevent blood staining of the cornea.

Injuries to the Posterior Pole

These injuries commonly result from a blunt blow to the front of the eye, producing a pressure wave which travels to the posterior pole and crushes the choroid and retina against the tough sclera. This contra-coup force commonly causes a choroidal split or tear. Should the split occur across the macular area, visual acuity is markedly reduced. Less severe contra-coup forces may cause macular edema with reduced visual acuity.

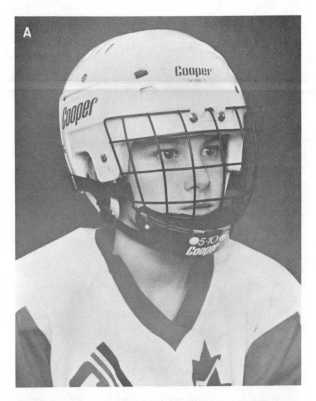

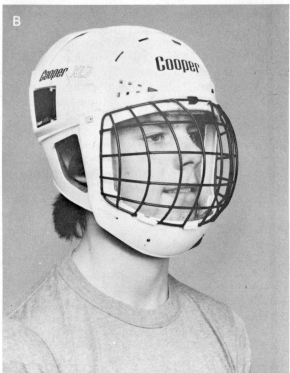

Figure 2 A, Mask-helmet for 5- to 10-year-old hockey players. B, Mask-helmet for older players.

Depending on the severity of the blow, resolution may occur, but usually the edema creates a macular cyst, which then may rupture and leave a macular hole. Central vision is then markedly reduced.

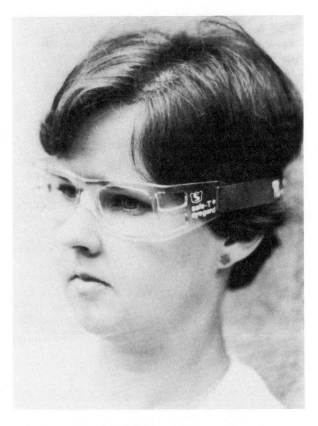

Figure 3 Eye protector for racquet sports participants.

Retinal injuries may result in hemorrhages or detachments. One-third of traumatic retinal detachments are sports related. Recovery of visual function depends on early recognition and treatment. Once the detachment involves the macula, normal vision will not be restored, although the retina is successfully reattached.

No outward sign of retinal detachment is evident. Some blurring of vision, when tested, with some loss of peripheral field is diagnostic. For this reason, eye injuries of even moderate degree deserve ophthalmoscopic examination at the time of injury, certainly on recheck the following day. The patient is warned to report any loss of visual function, especially to the sides, up, or down.

Ruptured Globe

These injuries destroy vision and usually result in removal of the eye. Over 70 such injuries have been recorded in our series. The offending weapon is usually a hockey stick or puck, a golf ball or club, a ski tip, a squash ball or racquet, or a tennis ball or baseball. At the time of injury, pain causes orbicularis spasm. If the lids can be gently opened, the eye will appear soft and sunken in the orbit. Vision will usually be reduced to perception of hand movement or light. Treatment requires gentle application of a sterile eye pad and transport to a hospital for immediate ophthalmologic care.

PREVENTION

Prevention is the key. Modifying rules and the wearing of certified protective equipment have done much to reduce the number of eye injuries in Canadian hockey. Racquet sports eye protectors with polycarbonate lenses are saving eyes in squash and racquetball as well (Figs. 2A,B; Fig. 3).

EAR, NOSE, AND THROAT INJURIES

J. SIMON McGRAIL, M.D., M.S., F.R.C.S.(C)

The head and neck areas of the body are vulnerable to injury in sports that involve bodily contact. This contact can be with an opponent's head, fist, or other parts of his anatomy, or with a foreign object held by the opponent, such as a hockey stick.

As with injuries from any cause, they can be classified into soft tissue injuries with or without involvement of the underlying bone or cartilage. Soft tissue injuries include skin, subcutaneous tissue, muscles, nerves, and blood vessels. Each of these must be thought about when an injury is being evaluated.

THE NECK

Injuries to the neck are usually blunt injuries and do not involve laceration of the skin and underlying soft tissues. By far the most important structure in the neck to consider is the airway. The larynx can be injured by blunt trauma; for example, a crosscheck from a hockey stock or a karate chop.

In this type of injury the head is usually extended, bringing the larynx closer to the surface where it is much more vulnerable to the assault. Immediately the player complains of discomfort in the neck, but more importantly, he can have different degrees of airway obstruction. If he has immediate hemoptysis, a mucosal tear is present, and with this combination of events the player must be immediately removed from the scene of his activity and carefully and thoroughly assessed.

The first consideration is the adequacy of his airway. If his breathing is noisy but he can inflate his chest well, there is time to get this player to a hospital where he can be properly examined. If his breathing is such that he has gross airway obstruction, indicating a badly smashed larynx, an airway has to be secured. Fortunately the majority of laryngeal fractures involve the thyroid cartilage, and placing an airway into the cricothyroid membrane alleviates most of the obstruction. A hypodermic needle placed in the cricothyroid membrane can act as a very adequate first aid measure until the player can be moved to a hospital. Alternatively, in the past I have employed a stab incision over the cricothyroid membrane and inserted the outer casing of a ballpoint pen, which gives a very adequate airway. Any time a cricothyrotomy is carried out, a tracheostomy must be done later in an orderly manner, but there is no urgency in this provided the revision is done within 24 hours. However, in the case of a badly smashed larynx, a tracheostomy almost certainly would be necessary anyway to assist in the rebuilding process.

An alternative cricothyrotomy instrument is the Fisher tube, which is part of a standard intravenous set.

The majority of sports injuries to the neck fall short of this dire emergency, but certainly can be worrisome to the attending physician and/or trainer. Any player who has received a neck injury and has any degree of airway problem should be sent as soon as possible to the nearest hospital where indirect laryngoscopy can be carried out. The usual finding in such a case is some degree of laryngeal edema, with or without submucosal hemorrhage, the degree of edema being reflected in the amount of airway obstruction present. As the edema is likely to progress for a period of up to 12 to 24 hours, these players should be kept under close observation in a hospital setting until the airway has returned to normal.

The majority of such injuries do not require surgical intervention. They subside with rest, steam, and reassurance. I do not advocate sedatives in these cases because of their respiratory depressant action, and I find that most players respond well to a full explanation of this, together with the reassurance already mentioned. The majority of cases need a 3- to 4-day stay in the hospital. As soon as the larynx has returned to normal, the player can resume his full normal activities.

If a mucosal tear is suspected because of hemoptysis, nothing further need be done unless the tear can be seen. If it can be visualized on indirect laryngoscopy, the larynx should be carefully assessed under general anesthesia, as a compound fracture of this nature may require an open reduction.

Finally, I would not recommend intubation of a suspected laryngeal fracture until the extent of the injuries can be assessed fully. It is better to establish an airway below the area of fracture, and then assess the degree of damage. Intubation may be difficult because of edema and also may cause further damage and displacement of laryngeal fragments. If available, Heliox is always useful in the treatment of airway obstruction, but the vast majority of such injuries subside without heroic measures, particularly if a calm reassuring attitude can be maintained.

Sharp injuries (e.g., from a skate blade) can cause significant lacerations to the neck and, if deep enough,

can cut the sternocleidomastoid muscle and the underlying jugular vein. Fortunately this type of injury is relatively uncommon, but it is a very dramatic one when it does occur. In recent years a jugular vein was cut during a hockey game, and the player's life was saved by the quick action of the trainer, who was able to exert pressure on both sides of the laceration and occlude the jugular vein until this could be surgically repaired.

A more common injury is the superficial laceration, which can usually be primarily sutured. As with all lacerations, care should be taken to clean the wound to ensure that no foreign particles have been left behind.

Lacerations around the upper neck, the ear, and the face may damage the facial nerve. In the immediate evaluation of the injury, it is sufficient to document whether facial nerve function has been affected. If the player is asked to close the eyes tight, wrinkle his forehead, screw up his nose, smile, and whistle, any facial asymmetry should be recognized during these maneuvers. If there is injury to the facial nerve, this should be mentioned so that appropriate exploration and nerve repair can be carried out within a few hours of the injury.

THE MOUTH

Injuries to the mouth include those of the lips, the teeth, and the tongue.

Injuries to the lip follow the principles that Dr. Douglas has outlined in his chapter on *Facial Injuries*, and it is worth noting that most mucosal injuries heal spontaneously, often with minimal morbidity. If a laceration includes skin and mucosa, this laceration must be carefully sutured, preferably in a hospital setting.

Trainers of sports teams are usually taught good first-aid procedures, and for a lip laceration the most important measure is to squeeze it tightly on either side of the laceration to cut down on what is often very free bleeding. Sucking an ice cube and placing this next to the laceration also helps. Similar principles apply to lacerations of the tongue, which are not uncommon hockey injuries. They usually occur in a player who, while skating hard with his mouth open and his tongue out, receives a blow under the jaw to cause a self-inflicted bite injury to the tongue.

These bleed freely, but firm pressure on either side of the cut controls the bleeding until hemostasis can be secured and the tongue sutured. Because of the possible edema that can result from this type of injury, it should be treated in a hospital setting and the player kept under observation for 24 hours to be sure that there is no airway problem.

THE EAR

Injuries to the ear are relatively uncommon, occurring most often in wrestlers. We are all familiar with the classic cauliflower ear of the wrestler and boxer, and this should be an entirely preventable result of injury. It follows from a subperichondrial hematoma that is not treated and finally absorbs the underlying cartilage, resulting in a grotesque abnormality. If a hematoma is recognized in the auricle, the correct treatment is immediate incision. The hematoma is drained, and to prevent its reformation, careful localized packing is placed in the different nooks and crannies of the auricle and a firm pressure bandage applied over the ear and head. This should be inspected daily until it is clear that the hematoma is not reforming. If this treatment is carried out expeditiously, the ear will suffer no anatomic damage. The patient should be given antibiotics because the danger of perichondritis is high, and this in itself can cause severe deformities.

THE NOSE

Lacerations to the nose will be discussed by Dr. Douglas in his chapter on *Facial Injuries*. I mention them here only to reinforce the view that a laceration to the nose that involves a through-and-through injury with underlying mucosal damage must be treated in a hospital setting. Treatment consists of careful intranasal mucosal approximation by suturing, followed by suturing of the skin laceration. If this type of injury is neglected, adhesions within the nose can cause significant nasal obstruction in the future.

Perhaps the most important injury of the nose is that affecting the nasal septum. Careful evaluation is necessary to see whether a septal hematoma is forming. If a bulge in the septum is noticed, particularly bilaterally, this must be drained immediately. This is done by a sharp incision through the nasal septal mucosa and suctioning out the blood that is present. Through this incision a small wick is inserted, and the nose is packed fairly firmly to hold the septal mucosa together and prevent reformation of the hematoma. If a hematoma is over-looked or neglected, a septal abscess is likely to develop, causing loss of bone and cartilage in the nose and leaving a nose that is difficult to correct from both a cosmetic and a functional point of view. Antibiotics should be given when a septal hematoma is diagnosed in an effort to prevent infection.

Although nasal fractures will be discussed, I will describe here the first-aid treament of the nosebleeds that so frequently accompany nasal fractures.

After any injury to the nose with epistaxis, the player is instructed to sit forward with his head down and to gently blow one nostril at a time. This measure is expected to remove clots, allow the vessels to contract and retract, and stop the nosebleed. If the nose is then gently pinched, if this is possible (that is, if there is no associated fracture), the nosebleed stops quickly, in which case the player can probably resume his activity. If there is an associated fracture that prevents pressure from being applied, ice is applied to the back of the neck in the hope of causing a reflex vasoconstriction, and a small amount of packing into both sides of the nose usually helps. When there is an associated fracture, the player is sent to hospital where a reduction of the fracture can be performed, either within 24 hours or within the next 7 to 10 days, depending on the degree of edema and bruising.

Although the majority of nosebleeds are caused from septal blood vessels, a significant nosebleed can be caused by injury to the anterior ethmoidal artery. This is seen with a blunt injury to the root of the nose and the medial canthal area of the eye, as from a fist or hockey puck. This can result in a brisk hemorrhage which needs careful and thorough packing in the roof of the nose to control it. This type of bleeding tends to persist even after adequate packing, and it is not unusual to explore the ethmoid sinuses through an external incision and clip the anterior ethmoidal vessel.

FACIAL INJURIES

LEITH G. DOUGLAS, M.D., F.R.C.S.(C), F.A.C.S.

Injuries to the face are common in many sports, particularly those involving body contact. In my experience as team plastic surgeon with the Toronto Maple Leafs of the National Hockey League for some 15 years, I have seen approximately 100 per season. The main instrument of injury has been the hockey stick, accounting for about 80 percent of cases. The puck, the ice, skates, goalposts, the glass surrounding the rink, and fists accounted for the remainder. The incidence has remained approximately the same, but the seriousness of the injuries has decreased now that almost everyone in the National League wears a helmet.

PREVENTION

Body contact sports will always be responsible for some facial trauma. This can probably still be reduced to some degree. The use of properly fitting helmets in hockey and football is mandatory, and their value is self-evident. Face guards may become popular in hockey in the future if they can be made lighter and easier to wear. Penalties for improper use of hockey sticks, and deliberate attempts to injure in any way, should be increased and will act as a deterrent to violence-minded players. Football goalposts have been made much safer, so consideration might be given to altering the construction of goalposts in hockey. The removal of the deep central tongue of the net and the introduction of the new magnetically seated net are steps in the right direction.

Facial injuries can be broadly classified into those involving soft tissue only and those involving the facial bones.

SOFT TISSUE INJURIES

The types of soft tissue injury are (1) contusions, (2) abrasions, (3) puncture wounds, and (4) lacerations (simple and complicated).

Contusions

The majority of contusions are simple and require no treatment other than the application of an ice bag. However, some of them may result in hematoma formation. A small hematoma is completely absorbed in a few weeks, but larger ones that become encapsulated require incision and drainage. Incisions for these should be placed so that the resulting scar is minimized and no vital structures are damaged. Sometimes it is necessary to insert a small Penrose drain in the incision for 24 to 48 hours. It is best to evacuate hematomas at the "currant jelly" stage rather than go on for many weeks waiting for full liquefaction. I have not found proteolytic enzymes given systemically to be of any help in liquefying hematomas.

Hematomas of the external ear must be promptly and properly drained and prevented from reaccumulating or developing a seroma. Failure to do so results in the formation of a cauliflower ear.

Abrasions

These vary from simple brush burns of the epidermis to those that go through the epidermis and into the dermis. The former require nothing other than cleansing with a good detergent and the application of an antibiotic cream for a few days. With deeper abrasions the area should be fully cleansed and any foreign material removed. The time to do this is at the initial treatment. Foreign material left in a wound not only contributes to the incidence of infection, but may result in traumatic tattooing. It becomes fixed to tissues in about 12 hours and becomes extremely difficult to remove without a formal surgical abrasion procedure. The use of local, and even general, anesthesia may be necessary to permit proper cleansing. A soft brush may be required to remove deeply embedded material. The area should then be covered with an antibiotic ointment and suitably dressed. Most abrasions heal in about a week unless they become infected.

Puncture Wounds

The principles of treatment are the same as for puncture wounds anywhere on the body. The track of the puncture should be followed, and the possibility of deep injury to nerves, vessels, or other vital structures ruled out. It is particularly important to determine whether foreign bodies are retained in the wound. X-ray examination should be done as indicated. Narrow puncture wounds are best not sutured, particularly if they are deep and there is a possibility of the development of infection. The track should be irrigated with saline or hydrogen peroxide and covered with a dry dressing.

Bite wounds are a special type of puncture wound. They may occur when a player strikes his face on an opponent's teeth or, fortunately infrequently, as a result of malicious intent. These are very serious wounds and have a very high potential for infection. They should be copiously irrigated with hydrogen peroxide and saline, getting to the depths of the wound with the liquid. They should be left open in all except the rare case in which a vital function is compromised as, for example, in a complete tear of a lower lip. In these cases, loose closure is done, with definitive repair carried out secondarily or as a delayed primary procedure.

Penicillin and cloxacillin are started immediately in moderately high dosage; cephalosporins are used in patients with penicillin allergy. The wound is re-examined in 24 hours, and may be secondarily closed in a few days if it remains clean. Evidence of developing infection warrants admission to hospital, where high-dose intravenous antibiotic therapy is administered.

Lacerations

Simple Lacerations

These may be linear lacerations due to hockey sticks and other sharp objects, but are frequently of the bursting type caused by a bony prominence of the face coming in contact with a blunt object. With these there is also an element of contusion.

They should be cleansed with a good antiseptic solution, such as aqueous Hibitane, then irrigated with saline. Needless to say, no material should be used on the face which is poisonous, stains the skin, or is dangerous to the eyes.

Examination of the wound for foreign material and for damage to blood vessels and nerves is then carried out. A judicious debridement may be necessary if there are small tags of nonviable tissue or ragged edges in bursting wounds, but this should be very judicious.

The vast majority of simple facial lacerations may be repaired under local anesthesia. I usually use 1 percent lidocaine without epinephrine. Infiltration with a No. 25 or 27 needle through the wound is adequate. Many athletes prefer not to have the area anesthetized, arguing that it swells more and is more prone to infection afterward. I have no evidence to support this claim, but I respect their wishes and have repaired more lacerations in hockey players without anesthetic than with it. The area is usually much less sensitive initially owing to the contusion, and thus it is not really so barbaric as it sounds.

If an adequate clinic room is available at the arena or stadium, most simple facial lacerations can be repaired there without compromising good medical practice. There should be adequate space with a good light and a quiet environment. One must have an assistant to help with the supplying of materials and possibly to cut sutures and sponge as indicated. Antiseptic solutions, saline, gauze dressings, drapes, and sterile instruments are required. I have been using disposable paper drapes with a small window cut out for some time, and they are excellent for this purpose. Instruments needed are a suitable needle holder, Adson forceps, about 6 hemostats, curved and straight iris scissors, the necessary syringes and needles, and suture material.

My choice of suture material for facial lacerations is 5-0 or 6-0 nylon on the surface, sometimes supplemented by deep sutures of 4-0 or 5-0 polyglycolic acid material.

Any small bleeders should be caught and ligated as necessary. Wound closure should be done somewhat more loosely than in a clean surgical wound, as the element of contusion leads to more swelling, causing the sutures to tighten and cut in. Interrupted suture technique is usually employed, although subcuticular closure with a continuous suture may be possible in some clean, incised linear wounds.

Simple lacerations are usually dressed with a small adhesive dressing strip. Sometimes an antibiotic ointment may be applied over the suture line. When there is contusion, the application of ice over the dressing is indicated.

I recommend removal of dressings in 24 hours and gentle daily washing after that. My infection rate in such wounds has been practically zero.

Complicated Lacerations

These include more extensive lacerations requiring more than 10 or 12 sutures as well as those involving specialized structures.

Lacerations of the eyelids and of the alar margin and complex lacerations of the ears are probably best dealt with in the Emergency Department of a hospital rather than in a clinic room. The technique remains the same, i.e., cleansing, anesthetizing properly, very judicious debridement, and accurate closure. Closure of lacerations crossing anatomic boundaries, such as the vermilion border of the lip and the eyebrow, should be done very carefully, in order to restore the anatomy as perfectly as possible. This is not always as easy as it sounds and frequently requires considerable effort. Incidentally, one *never* shaves an eyebrow!

Also included in this group are lacerations with actual soft tissue loss. If this is minimal the wound may be closed by simply advancing the edges. Other more complicated situations with avulsion of flaps should be treated in hospital and, in rare instances, may require skin grafting to restore the deficit.

The trap door flap or U-shaped laceration is always a problem. The dimensions of the flap may be such that the length-to-width ratio leads to compromising of its circulation. It may therefore be necessary to excise the questionable part and close it by advancing the edges. In curved lacerations, direct closure frequently leads to a pincushion effect with the central part becoming heaped up in relation to the surrounding tissues. This is due to contracture along the line of the scar and sometimes to a

degree of edema, which makes it stand out even more prominently. This is particularly true if the flap is in a true U-shape based superiorly rather than an inverted U-shape, as this tends to act as a barrier to normal lymphatic drainage. Despite this problem, there is no place for Z-plasties and excisions of tissue at the initial procedure. The best plan is to simply close the wound as carefully as possible, revising it later only if necessary. Since it is not possible to predict just how good or how bad a given flap is going to be, it is always wisest to wait.

With simple lacerations, the player is usually able to return to the game, but with the more complicated ones, it is prudent to give them a chance to heal without danger of further trauma. A simple laceration heals in a few days, with sutures being removed at 4 or 5 days. In more complicated ones, a few sutures may be left in place for 2 or 3 days more. Lacerations that have transgressed the facial nerve or parotid duct and other such serious injuries are beyond the scope of this discussion. They should be dealt with in the same manner as they would be in non-sports practice.

Antibiotics are employed only when dictated by common sense. In simple lacerations they are not indicated unless there is gross contamination. They should be employed in the more complicated ones, those involving eyelids and ears, and those in which there has been considerable contamination or in which there is a question whether the wound has been cleansed adequately.

The patient's tetanus immunization status should be determined and supplemented as indicated.

It is necessary to carry out a proper examination of vital structures, such as the eyes if the eyelids are injured, the internal structure of the nose if the nose is injured, or the teeth and underlying bone if the mouth area is involved. Facial nerve injuries do not occur frequently, but function should be tested if there is any possibility of damage.

The cardinal principles are (1) a full assessment of the injury, (2) thorough cleansing, (3) hemostasis, (4) judicious debridement, and (5) anatomic closure with fine sutures.

FRACTURES OF THE FACIAL BONES

These may be classified as closed (simple) fractures and open (compound) fractures. By far the greater majority are compound. This compounding is from within rather than from without in most cases. For example, nasal bone fractures and fractures of the zygoma and maxilla almost invariably involve tears of the mucoperiosteum of the nasal cavity or the maxillary antrum. Most fractures of the mandible, being through tooth-bearing areas, are also compound. Fractures may be further classified as linear or comminuted, displaced or undisplaced, and stable or unstable.

The Nose

The nose is the most commonly injured bony structure on the face. Fractures may be due to blows from the side or directly end-on. The former type of injury usually produces simple fracturing with deviation to one side, whereas end-on blows may result in comminution of both bone and cartilage.

Diagnosis usually is not difficult. The patient may have heard or felt a crack in his nose at the time of the injury. There is usually epistaxis, which may be profuse, and a clinical deformity of the nose may be obvious to both the patient and the attending physician. Roentgenograms are helpful, but the decision to treat and the assessment of the results of treatment are a matter of clinical judgment.

It may be possible to manipulate a fractured nose quickly back into position in a relatively painless manner if the physician sees the patient immediately after the injury. This has the effect of reducing the bleeding, reducing bruising and edema, and affording considerable comfort to the patient.

A good clinical examination of the internal as well as the external nose is mandatory. If the nasal septum is fractured, it is possible to develop a septal hematoma. The characteristic bluish bulge on the septum should alert the physician, and appropriate drainage with packing should be carried out without delay. The mucoperichondrium may be dissected off the underlying cartilaginous septum by the hematoma. This can lead to resorption of the cartilage and loss of tip support. In some cases, cartilage is laid down as it is in a cauliflower ear, producing a mass that obstructs the airway. Septal abscess formation is also possible. Septal hematomas are of vital importance in children, as loss of cartilaginous tip support in a growing nose may lead to a severe "snub nose" deformity.

Reduction of the fracture, if necessary, may be done under local or general anesthesia after the swelling has subsided—usually within 4 or 5 days. Intranasal packing and plaster splinting are usually necessary in complex injuries involving comminution or septal hematomas, but the simpler fractures may be treated without them.

It is usually inadvisable for a player to resume playing for at least a week after a nasal fracture of any consequence. Before he returns it is necessary to be sure that there is no significant swelling and no possibility that bleeding will recur, and that the fracture is stable and does not require external support.

An external protective device is usually required for at least 4 weeks after such an injury. The wearing of helmets in hockey facilitates the attachment of a face guard, and in football it is, of course, already worn.

Antibiotics usually are not necessary in the treatment of nasal fractures unless there has been gross comminution or operative intervention such as the drainage of a septal hematoma.

The Zygoma and Orbit

Blows to the prominence of the cheek may result in zygomatic fractures. These may involve only the arch laterally or, more commonly, cause the classic fracture through the frontozygomatic, zygomaticomaxillary, and zygomaticotemporal suture lines, with the zygoma being displaced medially and inferiorly.

Diagnosis may be made by inspection alone when there is obvious flattening of the cheek on the affected side. The patient complains of pain and, frequently, of trismus due to the impingement of the displaced zygomatic arch on the coronoid process of the mandible. He may also complain of diplopia due to displacement of the lateral canthal ligament of the eye, which is attached to the zygoma. There may be loss of sensation on the tip of the nose and the upper lip on the affected side due to impingement of the fracture site on the infraorbital nerve. Unilateral epistaxis is also seen due to the fracture crossing the antrum and thus tearing its mucoperiosteum and causing bleeding, which spills over through the ostium into the nose. In addition to these symptoms and signs, palpation over the fracture sites will reveal the characteristic steps in the bone.

X-ray examination shows the fractures at these three sites, opacification of the antrum due to blood, and an alteration of the contour of the lateral wall of the maxilla.

The majority of these are sufficiently displaced to warrant surgical intervention. Most can be managed by simple elevation, with an elevator being passed down behind the zygomatic arch in the temporal area and the bone levered up into normal position. Although this measure is usually sufficient, some of these fractures may be unstable, and interosseous wiring may be required.

Blow-out fractures of the orbital floor also occur. The surrounding bony framework of the orbit itself need not be fractured, and the damage may be confined to the orbital floor. This occurs when a blow to the eyeball forces it backward, compressing the orbital fat so that it finally bursts out through the inferomedial part of the floor, which is its weakest part. Herniation of the orbital contents into the antrum may occur, producing enophthalmos. This constitutes a significant cosmetic deformity and may also produce diplopia. It is also possible for the extraocular muscles to become caught up on the bony margin of the blown-out segment, thereby becoming tethered and limiting upward gaze. Presence of these signs and symptoms should be sought in any player after a blow to the eye. Facial roentgenograms show antral opacity and air in the orbit suggesting the injury, but tomograms are necessary to fully delineate the damage. Surgical exploration is usually required. The defect in the floor may be repaired by replacing the fracture fragments with bone from the anterior wall of the antrum or with a sheet of silicone rubber. Obviously, a full ophthalmologic examination is mandatory in such cases. Sometimes the blow may only cause a small crack between the ethmoid sinus and the orbit. When the patient blows his nose, air is forced back up through this into the orbit, and the eyelids rapidly inflate with surgical emphysema, causing the patient considerable alarm. There is no specific treatment other than to refrain from blowing the nose for 2 weeks or so while the opening closes spontaneously. Antibiotic cover is prescribed.

This phenomenon may sometimes be seen in fractures of the zygoma, particularly if the patient has engaged in vigorous nose-blowing.

Players with a fractured zygoma or orbit should not engage in contact sports for at least 3 weeks, and then should wear a protective face mask to avoid further injury for at least another 3 weeks.

The Maxilla

Fractures of the maxilla are classically divided into three types:

1. *LeFort Type I*: extends horizontally across the maxilla at the level of the floor of the nose, thereby shearing off the hard palate and upper dental alveolus.
2. *LeFort Type II*: also called a pyramidal fracture, extends obliquely upward and medially through the body of the maxilla toward the apex of the nose on both sides, thereby fracturing out a pyramid-shaped section of bone.
3. *LeFort Type III*: also called a craniofacial separation. This describes the injury in that the fracture extends from one frontozygomatic suture line across the craniofacial junction to the other side. This shears the facial bones completely away from the cranium. It is usually due to a blow from straight ahead, and the wedge-shaped face is driven posteriorly and downward along the inclined plane of the base of the skull, producing a dish-face deformity or an "equine facies". Combinations of these types may occur, e.g., LeFort II on one side and III on the other or bilateral II and III.

The deformities may be evident on inspection, and palpation of the bones reveals the fracture sites. In most cases mobility may be demonstrated in the fractured segment. X-ray examination confirms the clinical findings.

These are very serious injuries, particularly the craniofacial separation, and require reduction and appropriate interosseous wiring and suspension of the fracture fragments. A tracheotomy is frequently necessary at the time of surgery. The wiring is usually maintained for at least 6 weeks. It may be a matter of many months before any consideration can be given to a return to sports following such an injury. Residual deformity is frequent despite adequate surgery. Loss of sense of smell is also frequent due to tearing of the olfactory bulbs.

It is obviously possible for one to suffer an associated craniocerebral injury with fractures of the maxilla or, indeed, with any facial injury. One extremely important finding, which should be sought at the time of the original examination, is the presence of CSF rhinorrhea, indicating a fracture in the area of the cribriform plate of the ethmoid and tearing of the dura mater. Neurosurgical consultation should be sought in all patients with significant facial trauma whether or not they show signs of head injury.

The Mandible

Fractures of the mandible may be simple or compound. The latter is the rule, as most of them occur through the tooth-bearing area, thus opening a free passage from the mouth down to the root level. They may be unilateral, bilateral, or have multiple sites. They may also be classified anatomically, i.e., condylar neck, ascending ramus, angle, body, coronoid process, or parasymphyseal.

The diagnosis is usually straightforward. The patient may have actually heard or felt the bone fracturing at the time of the injury. There is usually significant pain. In the case of a compound fracture, bleeding may be noted in the mouth. The patient may complain of malocclusion, and crepitus and mobility may be noted at the fracture site. X-ray examination usually confirms the diagnosis. It is sometimes necessary to employ special x-ray techniques, such as the Panorex view, but this is not common.

Single undisplaced fractures of the condylar neck and the ascending ramus, or of the body in an edentulous patient, may warrant a trial period of conservative management employing only soft diet and avoidance of trauma without wiring of the teeth. This is sufficient if the patient is comfortable. The majority, and certainly all compound fractures, should be immobilized in some way. The simplest form of immobilization for single undisplaced fractures is the application of islet loops with cross wiring to hold the teeth in occlusion. With instability or displacement, some form of arch is necessary to hold the fragments in place prior to wiring the teeth into occlusion. A cable arch made up of twisted 24-gauge wire (Risdon's method) or patent arches of the Erich or Winter type may be used. These latter have an added advantage in that elastic band traction may be employed with them and the cross elastics or wires may be more readily removed for access to the mouth in an emergency. In fractures that are unstable or unfavorable in their angulation, an open reduction with interosseous wiring as well as interdental wiring is done. Patients with partial or full dentures should have them in place to maintain spacing and for stability during the period of immobilization.

The presence of fractures of the roots of teeth is significant, and a dental consultation may be sought to determine whether certain teeth are salvageable and to extract fractured roots. Fragments of teeth, fillings, and dentures should always be sought in the patient's mouth at the time of injury to prevent his swallowing or aspirating them. It is necessary to obtain a chest roentgenogram of a patient with a missing tooth, denture, or tooth fragment to rule out the possibility of its having been aspirated, particularly if he has been unconscious.

Fractures of the mandible may constitute a life-threatening injury under some circumstances, particularly in patients with bilateral, displaced, unstable fractures of the body. The patient, in effect, loses control of his tongue and may be unable to swallow properly. This, plus the presence of blood and saliva, and possibly vomitus in the mouth, may constitute a threat to his airway. Such patients should be cared for initially in the sitting position or, failing this, while prone with their face turned to one side to allow free drainage from the mouth. A tensor bandage around the face under the chin may temporarily hold the mandible immobilized in occlusion, thus affording considerable comfort to the patient and helping him to retain some control over his airway.

Compound fractures of the mandible rarely become infected nowadays, but this is indeed possible. All patients require appropriate antibiotic coverage.

Immobilization of most fractures is required for approximately 6 weeks. In simpler fractures in which an arch bar has been applied to the lower dentition, it may be possible to open the interdental fixation earlier and rely on the arch alone for stability.

Contact sports are out of the question during this 6-week period, and the patient should wear an appropriate face protector for at least a further 6 weeks to prevent another injury.

Maintenance of proper nutrition may be a problem with patients who have their teeth wired into occlusion, particularly those who do not have any gaps due to missing teeth through which solid food can be passed. Food reduced to the fine consistency of baby food by a food processor is required.

Dislocations of the Mandible

These may occur if the patient is struck while his mouth is open wide. They may also result from simply opening the mouth very widely in a shout or a yawn as in non-sports practice.

To reduce a dislocated mandible, first be seated behind the patient, cradling his head against the chest. Place both *well-padded* thumbs just posterior to the last lower molars. Then exert downward and posterior traction with the thumbs, at the same time rolling the mandible upward and anteriorly so that the condyles slip back into position.

Some persons have very lax temporomandibular joints and suffer periodic dislocations. Reduction is usually easy in them.

It may be necessary to employ sedation for sufficient relaxation to carry out the reduction in some patients, particularly if they are having a considerable amount of pain or are very apprehensive.

After-care should include resting the mandible and avoidance of maneuvers that might lead to another dislocation.

This has been a brief summary of facial injuries in sports. There are many aspects which could not be covered due to space limitations. The interested reader is referred to the standard texts for further information.

SPINAL INJURIES

ATHLETIC INJURIES TO THE CERVICAL SPINE

JOSEPH S. TORG, M.D.,
JOSEPH J. VEGSO, M.S., A.T., C.

Of the variety of injuries that can occur to the athlete, those involving the head and neck are the most difficult to evaluate and manage on the field. Because of the actual or potential involvement of the nervous system, risks can be high, and consequently the margin for error is low. The initial clinical picture frequently may be misleading. Patients with significant intracranial hemorrhage may at first present with minimal symptoms only to follow a precipitous downhill course. On the other hand, short-lived problems such as neurapraxia of the brachial plexus may at first present with paresthesia and paralysis, raising the question of a significant spinal injury, only to resolve within minutes with the individual returning to his activity. Fortunately, the more severe injuries that can occur to the neck are infrequent. Consequently, most team physicians and trainers have little, if any, experience in dealing with them.

Managing the unconscious athlete or one suspected of having significant injury to the cervical spine is a process that should not be done hastily or haphazardly. Being prepared to handle this situation is the best way to prevent actions that could convert a reparable injury into a catastrophe.

Thus, the single most important point to remember is: *prevent further injury*. Adequate preparation will alleviate indecisiveness and second-guessing. Immediately immobilize the head and neck, check first for breathing, and then for level of consciousness.

If the victim is breathing, simply remove the mouth guard, if present, and maintain the airway. Once it is established that the athlete is breathing and has a pulse, simply maintain the situation until transportation is available, or until the athlete regains consciousness. If the athlete is face down when the ambulance arrives, change his position to face up by logrolling him onto a spine board. Make no attempt to move him except to transport him or to perform cardiopulmonary resuscitation (CPR) if it becomes necessary.

The transportation team should be familiar with handling a victim with a cervical spine injury. It is important not to lose control of the care of the athlete. Therefore, prior arrangements with an ambulance service should be made.

Lifting and carrying the injured athlete require five individuals: four to lift and the leader to maintain immobilization of the head.

The same guidelines apply to the choice of a medical facility as to the choice of an ambulance: be sure it is equipped and staffed to handle an emergency neck injury. There should be a neurosurgeon and an orthopaedic surgeon to meet the athlete upon arrival.

NERVE ROOT AND BRACHIAL PLEXUS NEURAPRAXIA

The most common cervical injuries are the pinch-stretch neurapraxias of the nerve roots and brachial plexus. The key to the nature of this lesion is its short duration and the presence of a full, pain-free range of neck motion. Although the majority of these injuries are short-lived, they are worrisome because of the occasional plexus axonotmesis that occurs. However, the youngster whose paresthesia completely abates, who demonstrates full muscle strength in the intrinsic muscles of the shoulder and upper extremities, and who, most importantly, has a full pain-free range of cervical motion, may return to his activity.

The occasional athlete who experiences recurrent episodes of root or plexus neurapraxia should have cervical spine roentgenograms and electromyographic studies. If these, as well as the physical findings, are negative, an intensive isotonic neck muscle strengthening program should be initiated. It will take several months for the benefits of such a program to be realized. The susceptible individual should continue the program on a year-round basis. Also, a cervical neck roll should be worn.

If the electromyogram demonstrates involvement of the deltoid, infraspinatus, supraspinatus, and biceps, the lesion should be considered an axonotmesis.

Persistence of paresthesia, weakness, or limitation of cervical motion requires that the individual be protected from further exposure and that he undergo neurologic, electromyographic, and roentgenographic evaluation. These athletes with evidence of associated

155

axonotmesis should be withheld from contact sports until they have achieved full muscle strength and have a repeat electromyogram that shows evidence of axonal regeneration. This usually takes a minimum of 4 to 6 weeks. In addition to protection from further injury, treatment consists of a neck and upper extremity muscle strengthening program with emphasis placed on the involved muscles. Also, these individuals should wear a neck roll.

ACUTE CERVICAL SPRAIN SYNDROME

Acute cervical sprains are frequently seen in contact sports. The patient presents with limitation of cervical spine motion and without radiation of pain or paresthesia. Neurologic examination is negative and roentgenograms are normal.

Stable cervical sprains and strains eventually resolve with or without treatment. Initially, the presence of a serious injury should be ruled out by a thorough neurologic examination and determination of the range of cervical motion.

The athlete with less than a full, pain-free range of cervical motion, persistent paresthesia, or weakness should be protected and excluded from further activity. Subsequent evaluation should include appropriate roentgenographic studies, including flexion and extension views, to demonstrate fractures or instability.

In general, treatment of athletes with "cervical sprains" should be tailored to the degree of severity. Immobilization of the neck in a soft collar, application of heat, and use of analgesics and anti-inflammatory agents until there is a full, spasm-free range of neck motion is appropriate. It should be emphasized that individuals with a history of collision injury, pain, and limited cervical motion should have routine cervical spine roentgenograms. Also, lateral flexion and extension roentgenograms are indicated after the acute symptoms subside. If the patient has pain and muscle spasm of the cervical spine, hospitalization and head-halter traction may be indicated.

CERVICAL VERTEBRA SUBLUXATION WITHOUT FRACTURE

Axial compression-flexion injuries incurred by striking an object with the top of the head can result in disruption of the posterior soft-tissue supporting elements with angulation and anterior translation of the superior cervical vertebrae. Fractures of the bony elements are not demonstrated on roentgenograms, and the patient will have no neurologic deficit. Flexion-extension roentgenograms demonstrate instability of the cervical spine at the involved level manifested by motion, anterior intervertebral disc-space narrowing, anterior angulation and displacement of the vertebral body, and fanning of the spinous processes. Demonstrable instability on lateral flexion-extension rotentgenograms in a young, vigorous individual requires

vigorous treatment. When soft-tissue disruption occurs without an associated fracture, it is likely that instability will develop despite conservative treatment. When anterior subluxation greater that 20 percent of the vertebral body is due to disruption of the posterior supporting structures, a posterior cervical fusion is recommended.

CERVICAL FRACTURES AND DISLOCATIONS: GENERAL PRINCIPLES

Fractures or dislocations of the cervical spine may be stable or unstable and may or may not be associated with neurologic deficit. When fracture or disruption of the soft-tissue supporting structure immediately violates or threatens to violate the integrity of the spinal cord, implementation of certain management and treatment principles is imperative.

The first goal is to protect the spinal cord and nerve roots from injury through mismanagement. Second, the malaligned cervical spine should be reduced as quickly and gently as possible to effectively decompress the spinal cord. When dislocation or anterior angulation and translation are demonstrated roentgenographically, immediate reduction is attempted with skull traction utilizing Gardner-Wells tongs. These tongs can be easily and rapidly applied under local anesthesia, without shaving the head, in the emergency room or with the patient in his hospital bed. Since these tongs are spring-loaded, it is not necessary to drill the outer table of the skull for their application. The tongs are attached to a cervical-traction pulley, and weight is added at a rate of 5 pounds per disc space or 25 to 40 pounds for lower cervical injury. Reduction is attempted by adding 5 pounds every 15 to 20 minutes and is monitored by lateral roentgenograms.

Unilateral and bilateral facet dislocations, particularly at the C3-C4 level, are not always reducible by means of skeletal traction. In such instances, closed skeletal or manipulative reduction under nasotracheal anesthesia may be necessary. The expediency of early reduction of cervical dislocations must be emphasized.

It has been proposed that the presence of a bulbocavernous reflex indicates that spinal shock has worn off and that, except for recovery of an occasional root at the injury, neither motor nor sensory paralysis will resolve regardless of treatment. The bulbocavernous reflex is produced by pulling on the urethral catheter. This stimulates the trigone of the bladder, producing a reflex contraction of the anal sphincter around the examiner's gloved finger. Although the presence of a bulbocavernous reflex is generally a sign that there will be no further neurologic recovery below the level of the injury, this is not always true. The presence of this reflex does not give the clinician license to handle the situation in an elective fashion. The cervical spine malalignments and dislocations associated with quadriparesis should be reduced as quickly as possible, by whatever means necessary, if maximum recovery is to be expected.

In most instances in which a vertebral body burst fracture is associated with anterior compression of the cord, decompression is logically effected through an anterior approach with an interbody fusion. Likewise, traumatic intervertebral disc herniation with cord involvement is best managed through an anterior discectomy and interbody fusion. In cervical fractures and dislocations, posterior cervical laminectomy is indicated only rarely when excision of foreign bodies or bony fragments in the spinal canal is necessary. Realignment of the spine is the most effective method for decompression of the cervical cord.

Indications for surgical decompression of the spinal cord have been delineated. A documented increase in neurologic signs is the clearest mandate for surgical decompression. Further observation, expectancy, and procrastination in this situation are contraindicated. Persistent partial cord or root signs, with objective evidence of mechanical compression, are also an indication for surgical intervention.

Management of cervical spine fractures and dislocations requires the generous use of parenteral corticosteroids (dexamethasone) to decrease the inflammatory reactions of the injured cord and surrounding soft-tissue structures. Initially, 100 mg of dexamethasone should be given intravenously in a single bolus followed by 1 mg/kg/day intravenously in divided doses for 10 days. Drugs that inhibit norepinephrine synthesis or deplete catecholamines have been advocated to prevent autodigestion of the cord, but there is no evidence as yet that this is of value in improving the prognosis for cord recovery. Procedures such as durotomy, myelotomy, and rhizotomy require extensive laminectomy, adding further instability, and are contraindicated.

The third goal in managing fractures and dislocations of the cervical spine is to effect rapid and secure stability, thus preventing residual deformity and instability with associated pain and the possibility of further trauma to the neural elements. The method of immobilization depends on the postreduction status of the injury. Indications for nonsurgical and surgical methods for achieving stability may be summarized as follows:

1. Patients with stable compression fractures of the vertebral body, undisplaced fractures of the lamina or lateral masses, or soft-tissue injuries without detectable neurologic deficit can be adequately treated with traction and subsequent protection with a cervical brace until healing occurs.

2. Stable, reduced facet dislocation without neurologic deficit can also be treated conservatively in a halo jacket until healing has been demonstrated by negative lateral flexion-extension roentgenograms.

3. Unstable cervical spine fractures or fracture-dislocations without neurologic deficit may require either surgical or nonsurgical methods to ensure stability.

4. Absolute indications for surgical stabilization are an unstable injury without neurologic deficit and late instability following closed treatment.

5. Relative indications for surgical stabilization in unstable injuries without neurologic deficit are anterior subluxation greater than 20 percent, certain atlantoaxial fractures or dislocations, and unreduced comminuted vertical compression injuries.

6. Cervical spine fractures with complete cord lesions require reduction followed by closed or open stabilization as indicated.

7. Cervical spine fractures with incomplete cord lesions require reduction followed by careful evaluation for surgical intervention.

The fourth and final goal of treatment is rapid and effective rehabilitation started early in the treatment process.

TRANSIENT QUADRIPLEGIA

An infrequently occurring and not well-documented phenomenon is that of transient quadriplegia. This characteristically occurs to an athlete, most often a football player, who sustains either forced hyperextension or hyperflexion to his neck and cervical spine. A painless paralysis ensues which may manifest itself as weakness or complete absence of motor function in all four extremities. The episode is brief, lasting 5 to 10 minutes. The involvement of sensory function has not been established. Roentgenograms do not demonstrate findings indicating acute trauma to the cervical spine. However, examination of the lateral films reveals either a congenital fusion or a developmental decrease in the sagittal diameter of the spinal cord, which is increased on lateral flexion and extension roentgenograms.

There is no evidence that those who experience one or more episodes of transient quadriplegia are prone to more severe injury, namely, permanent quadriplegia. However, they are susceptible to recurrence of the transient episodes, and therefore it is recommended that they avoid certain contact activities.

CERVICAL SPINE INSTABILITY

The spectrum of late cervical spine instability following an injury is a necessary consideration when an athlete is injured. If possible, it is well to avoid subsequent permanent or transient narrowing of the spinal canal with compression of the neural elements. For each particular injury it is not possible to accurately predict whether late instability will result in structural malalignment, with or without neurologic deficit. However, the recent work of White, Southwick, and Punjabi in establishing guidelines regarding this problem is noteworthy.

They performed a series of cadaver studies in which the various supporting structures were systematically cut and resulting instabilities in the spine were noted. The supporting structures of the lower cervical spine can be divided into two groups, anterior and posterior. The anterior group includes soft-tissue supporting structures anterior to and including the posterior longitudinal ligament. These are the anterior and posterior longitudinal ligaments, the intervertebral disc, and the annulus fibrosus. The posterior group consists of the facet capsular ligaments, ligamentum flavum, and the interspinous and supraspinous ligaments. White et al have devised a check list for the diagnosis of clinical instability of the lower cervical spine. If point values are assigned to the elements in Table 1 and the points total 5 or more, then the spine should be considered clinically unstable. It should be noted that evaluation of the first two entities, the status of the anterior and posterior elements, is based on clinical history, evaluation of radiographs, and interpretation of flexion-extension films.

TABLE 1   Check List for Diagnosis of Clinical Instability in Lower Cervical Spine

Element	Point Value
Anterior elements destroyed or unable to function	2
Posterior elements destroyed or unable to function	2
Relative sagittal plane translation > 3.5 mm*	2
Relative sagittal plane rotation > 11°†	2
Positive stretch test	2
Spinal cord damage	2
Nerve root damage	1
Abnormal disc narrowing	1
Dangerous loading anticipated	1
Total of 5 or more = unstable	

* As measured on lateral flexion-extension films
† As measured on lateral films
From Spine 1:15, 1976.

ACTIVITY RESTRICTIONS

Physicians involved in the management of athletes who have sustained significant cervical spine injuries are ultimately faced with the question whether the patient can return to his or her activity. Since few, if any, attempts have been made to formally address this question, the following guidelines are offered which are based on clinical experience.

Youngsters who have been diagnosed and successfully treated for cervical sprains, intervertebral disc injuries without neurologic involvement, and stable wedge compression fractures may return to all activities when they are symptom-free, have a full range of cervical motion, full muscle strength, and stability of the cervical spine as demonstrated by flexion and extension films.

Those with lesions of the cervical spine resulting in subluxation without fracture should be excluded from further participation in contact sports despite lack of motion on lateral flexion-extension films. Flexion and extension films are a static demonstration of stability and not an adequate measure of the stability of the spine when it is subjected to the forces involved in contact sports.

Individuals who have undergone a successful one-level anterior interbody decompression and fusion for herniated nucleus pulposus or anterior instability may return to all activities provided they have a full range of motion and strength. However, they should be fully apprised of the possibility of intervertebral disc herniation at an adjacent level.

Individuals who undergo more than one-level anterior fusion or posterior fusion for cervical spine injury should be evaluated on an individual basis with regard to return to noncontact sports. However, these individuals should not be permitted to return to contact activity regardless of how "solid" the fusion appears on roentgenograms. Altered biomechanics of the cervical spine with more than a two-level fusion presents several problems. The decrease in motion will, in itself, deprive the spine of its capability of dissipating force through motion. Also, it would appear that there is a higher risk of injury because of the increased torque on the lever arm on the level above and below the fusion mass. The effect of cervical fusion as a precipitating cause of degenerative disease at other levels is also a question that is unanswered but should be considered.

SPINAL DEFORMITIES AND THE ATHLETE

LYLE J. MICHELI, M.D.

The physician dealing with sports-related injuries must have a working knowledge of the normal contour of the spine as well as structural deformities that may enhance the potential for spinal injury or compromise spinal function in the course of athletic activities. The importance of the spine in normal function cannot be overemphasized. It is the structural centrum from which extremity motion initiates, and it contains important elements of the central nervous system and the origin of the peripheral nerves.

The four major issues pertaining to spinal deformities are:

1. The detection of spinal abnormalities that may render sports participation ineffective or even dangerous to the child.

2. The early detection of spinal deformity in the child athlete, with the initiation of ongoing assessment or bracing.

3. The effective management of relatively mild spinal deformities with bracing or electrical stimulation techniques while a child continues to participate in sports.

4. Determining the level of athletic participation that is safe and effective for a child who has required a spinal fusion.

There is a range of "normal" contour of the human spine. The spine, consisting of a series of 7 cervical vertebrae, 12 dorsal vertebrae, and 5 lumbar vertebrae perched upon the sacrum, is designed for both stability and movement. In the sagittal plane, this semirigid column has a normal dorsal kyphosis or posterior angulation and lumbar lordosis or anterior angulation. The cervical spine is capable of a wide range of motion, but normally is postured in a position of slight lordosis. The "range of normal" of the dorsal kyphosis or lumbar lordosis is a matter of some debate. In general, when a person is standing, a dorsal kyphosis of 20 to 50 degrees is considered to be the normal range. Deviations outside this limit are either hypokyphosis ($<$ 20 degrees but $>$ 0 degrees) or hyperkyphosis or simply kyphosis (greater than 50 degrees). Similarly, the range of "normal" lumbar lordosis is described as 20 to 50 degrees (Fig. 1).

These "normal" curves of the spine are in the sagittal plane. Any curvature of the spine in the coronal plane is defined as scoliosis. Although 10 percent of the population may have a mild scoliosis (up to 10 degrees) in some portion of the spine the condition is not present normally and is in fact a deformity. At present, all measurements of degree of deviation or angulation of the spine are done with the Cobb technique (Fig. 2). With this technique, the angle subtended by the top of the most tilted vertebra above and the bottom of the most

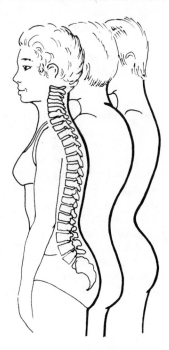

Figure 1 "Normal" lumbar lordosis and dorsal kyphosis in the sagittal plane is 40 degrees.

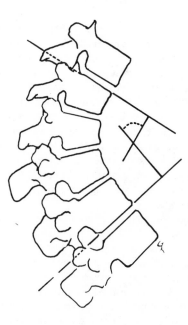

Figure 2 The Cobb technique for determining spinal curve measures the angle between the top of the most tilted vertebral body at the superior limit of the curve and the bottom of the most inferior vertebral body.

tilted vertebra below is defined as the angle of curvature, with the intervening spine seen as a portion of a complete circle.

Scoliosis, while always "abnormal", may be functional in origin—the result of muscle spasms, or postural angulation of the spine, or such extraspinal factors as leg-length discrepancy or pelvic obliquity. In functional scoliosis, there is no true deformity of the spine, and if the paraspinal or extrinsic factor is corrected, the spine will once again be straight.

Structural scoliosis is a fixed deformity of the spine, but even so may lend itself to partial correction with mechanical techniques such as a pulsion pressure or traction. Structural scoliosis may have multiple etiologies, including (1) paralytic disorders such as poliomyelitis or myodysplasia, (2) congenital abnormalities of the spine in which there is true deformity or abnormality of the structure of the spine, or (3) idiopathic scoliosis. The last-mentioned is by far the most common type of scoliosis encountered in North America.

Idiopathic scoliosis often is familial, risk being increased five-fold in family members. Idiopathic scoliosis is noteworthy in that it becomes apparent at a specific time in the growth and development of the child. We subdivide this deformity into (1) infantile onset scoliosis, which is evident in the first year of life, (2) juvenile onset scoliosis, which has its onset during the prepubescent period, and (3) adolescent-onset scoliosis, which can develop rapidly and progressively with the onset of adolescence.

Since most conditions that cause scoliosis occur during childhood or adolescence, scoliosis may be a consideration in the child's participation in sports for two reasons: (1) the spinal deformity may influence the child's ability to engage in sports safely and effectively, and (2) the sports environment, particularly organized team sports, provides an excellent opportunity for the detection and early recognition of a developing spinal deformity. An important part of the pre-participation physical examination, which really should be done on an annual basis for any child involved in organized sports, is the assessment and careful measurement of the posture and contour of the body, with special attention to the contour of the spine, torso, and pelvis. The child who shows evidence of symmetric posture on one examination may, a year later, show evidence of the development of progressive spinal scoliosis or dorsal roundbacking and early kyphosis.

In school screening, which is now mandated in more than half the states in the United States as well as in Canada, abnormalities of posture and contour are carefully assessed. These screening programs are at least 85 percent effective in the early detection of spinal abnormalities and, when combined with an effective bracing or electrical spinal stimulation program, can prevent the progression of spinal curvature and the acute need for surgery.

DIFFERENTIAL DIAGNOSIS

Spinal deformities or structural abnormalities (congenital and acquired) may significantly increase the risk of injury from sports participation. Certain congenital conditions, such as Down syndrome or Morquio's disease, are associated with an increased incidence of instability of the upper cervical spine.

This instability is of particular concern in Special Olympics competition. In these children a lateral flexion/extension radiograph is recommended to rule out measurable mechanical instability of the cervical spine. An excursion greater than 5 mm of C1 on C2 is a reflection of ligamentous instability or laxity of the atlas on the axis. Opinions vary whether prophylactic fusion is indicated, but in cases of detected laxity, there is general agreement that contact sports and such activities as heading the ball in soccer must be contraindicated. Klippel-Feil syndrome, characterized by shortness of the neck or webbing, may be associated with congenital abnormalities of the cervical spine. In these cases also, plain radiographs and, if indicated, lateral flexion/ extension views of the cervical spine may be necessary to confirm the mechanical stability of the spine.

In the lumbar spine, spondylolysis or spondylolisthesis may result in relative postural deformity or even scoliosis. Increased tightness of the hamstrings, relative flattening of the lumbar spine with posture, and pain on hyperextension of the spine may also be findings in this condition. Radiographs of the lumbar spine, including obliques, generally are diagnostic (Fig. 3). If a frank lack of continuity of the neural arch is detected at the level of pars intraarticularis, a standing lateral radiography of the lumbar spine is recommended to determine the

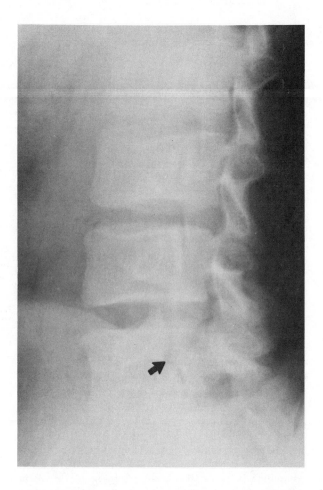

Figure 3 Spondylolysis, a defect in the pars intraarticularis of the vertebra, is best seen on the oblique view.

amount of stability at this site and the coexistence of spondylolisthesis. In our experience, symptomatic spondylolysis or grade I spondylolisthesis in young athletes may actually be a stress fracture of the lumbar spine and rarely progresses to frank instability of the lumbar spine. This condition can be treated effectively with exercises or with bracing, which flattens the lumbar spine, relieves pain, and promotes healing of the defect (Fig. 4). Once the child becomes asymptomatic and free of pain, with concomitant increase in the flexibility of the hamstrings, he or she can safely and effectively participate in sports even while wearing the antilordotic brace.

Certain other conditions in the young athlete present as a spinal deformity, but this may actually be a reflection of more significant disease, such as localized spinal infection, discitis, or spinal tumor. Tumors or infections of the lumbar spine or disc space may present initially as scoliosis. The incidence of bony tumors or infections is much higher in the young athlete than in the adult. Any spinal deformity or spinal scoliosis that persists beyond 3 weeks and is associated with muscle spasm and pain must be investigated thoroughly and not simply ascribed to a minor back strain or sports injury.

EARLY DETECTION OF SPINAL DEFORMITY

As noted, the pre-participation evaluation provides an excellent opportunity for scoliosis screening. Symmetry of shoulder and pelvic heights, balance in the sagittal or coronal plane, and the symmetry of contour between the two sides of the back or lumbar spine are noted. On forward bending, asymmetries of the height of the torso may be a reflection of idiopathic scoliosis reflecting with the axial rotation of the spine and torso that usually is seen in addition to the curvature.

Once we have eliminated leg length discrepancies or functional causes for possible spinal asymmetry, we usually obtain a standing PA and lateral x-ray film of the dorsal lumbar spine in cases of coronal or sagittal

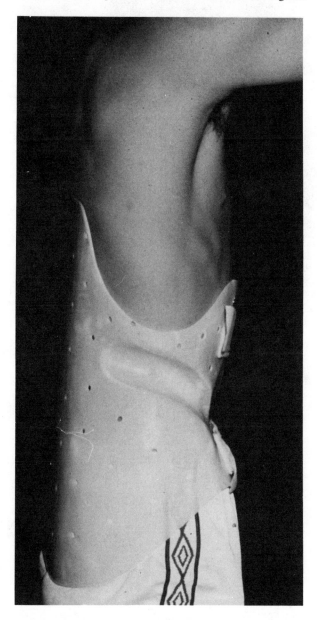

Figure 4 Thermoplastic "low profile" brace used to treat spinal deformities or certain cases of low back pain in young atheletes.

decompensation. If these radiographs show a scoliosis curvature that is less than 15 degrees or a dorsal kyphosis less than 50 degrees (Fig. 5), we recommend a program of directed exercises aimed at increasing the strength and flexibility of the spine and pelvis. In addition, we usually institute dorsal extension or asymmetric lateral bend exercises in the case of kyphosis or scoliosis, respectively.

It is essential to continue regular follow-up of even a small curvature. We initially re-evaluate the child in 3 to 4 months. This re-evaluation usually consists of clinical assessment only. If Moire topographic photography is available in the office or clinic, an initial Moire photograph and a subsequent follow-up Moire photograph can be useful in determining further asymmetry of the torso in association with scoliosis progression. If this is not available, the clinical examination can reliably determine the need for additional radiographs at follow-up—if the spinal asymmetry appears to have progressed. For scoliosis, a posteroanterior radiograph of the spine is all that is necessary. If the primary problem is the dorsal kyphosis, a lateral radiograph will suffice. This must always be a standing radiograph comparable to the initial set of radiographs. If the curvature of scoliosis has progressed beyond 15 degrees, and at least 3 degrees since the last radiograph, bracing or electrical muscle stimulation should be instituted.

In most cases, spinal bracing is the most effective and the most readily available technique for preventing progression of the curvature. The Milwaukee brace has been the standard of treatment in North America for the management of progressive spinal disorders. However, in the past 10 years a number of different low-profile orthoses have been developed, and these appear to effectively manage spinal deformities while allowing a significant increase in function. In our experience, these orthoses can adequately prevent progression of a spinal curvature if the apex of curvature is below D/9.

Electrical muscle stimulation for scoliosis must be considered experimental. The two different techniques being used at present hold obvious advantages for the sports-active child. The treatment, which is applied at night, consists of intermittent pulses used to stimulate the muscles in the convexity of the curve. The sports-active child obviously continues in full sports participation without problems throughout the day.

In most cases, full-time brace treatment has been required to prevent progression of the curvature. In our own clinic, this involves 23 hours a day of treatment, including use at night, with an hour out of the brace to permit exercising and bathing. Exceptions to this full-time use pertain to the sports-active child, whom we allow to remove the brace during times of active sports participation or practice for a maximum of 2 additional hours a day. There have been no ill effects such as increased rate of progression or brace failure. Most children can participate in sports while wearing the low-profile brace, including physical education in school and most recreational sports activities such as climbing, riding bicycles, and running.

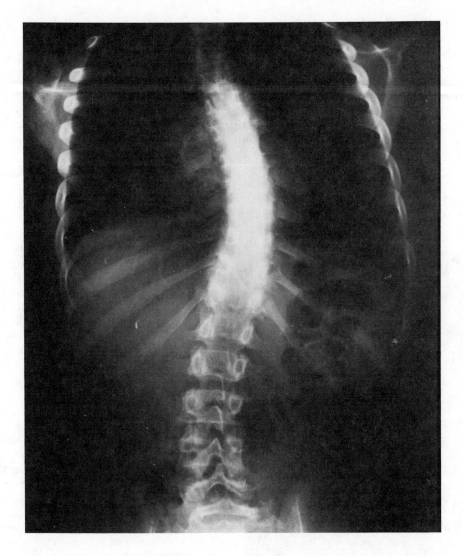

Figure 5 Mild scoliosis in the skeletally mature adolescent is no contraindication to full sports participation.

Most physicians treating scoliosis of the juvenile onset idiopathic type report a dramatic mechanical response to bracing treatment over a period of 3 to 6 months, after which a part-time bracing regimen (usually 12 hours a day) is adopted. Ongoing follow-up is the rule to determine whether there is loss of correction with this regimen. We prescribe this part-time brace for younger patients with juvenile onset scoliosis who must wear it until skeletal maturity has been attained, sometimes for 5 to 6 years. The part-time bracing regimen has been extremely successful in allowing an essentially normal life style while preventing progression of the curvature.

The incidence of dorsal kyphosis appears to have increased among athletically active adolescents, particularly males. There is some controversy about the naming of this condition, the traditional designation being Scheuermann's kyphosis. Scheuermann's kyphosis is defined as a dorsal kyphosis of more than 50 degrees in which there is at least 15% wedging of at least three vertebral bodies and narrowing of disc space with struc-

tural changes in the vertebral bodies. While there may be a congenital predisposition, this condition may also be acquired, the result of repetitive microtrauma on the anterior aspects of the vertebral bodies in the dorsal spine with resultant wedging. In many instances, the precondition appears to be a tight lumbar lordosis which does not allow adequate forward flexion of the lumbar spine. As a result, particularly with forward bending, the injuries occur in the anterior aspect of the vertebral bodies, with secondary structural deformation and dorsal roundbacking.

Early detection is imperative because of the dramatic reversal afforded by prompt and early bracing techniques if growth still remains. Although scoliosis generally requires bracing until growth ceases, Scheuermann's kyphosis or dorsal roundbacking can be treated effectively in as short a period as 9 to 12 months, with reconstitution of anterior vertebral height and restoration of a relatively normal contour of the spine. In addition to treating the dorsal roundbacking with mechanical bracing, specific attention must be paid to restoring the strength and flexibility of the lumbar spine and hamstrings. The one particular disadvantage of this bracing regimen for dorsal roundbacking or Scheuermann's kyphosis is that it usually requires a full brace with neck ring to adequately treat this condition, particularly in the young male adult.

In the fully mature athlete with pre-existent scoliosis, a scoliosis curve even as great as 40 to 50 degrees is no contraindication to full active sports or dance participation. We mention dance because the incidence of mild scoliosis curves in dancers is really quite high. As many as 25 to 30 percent of serious young amateur dancers or professional dancers in modern dance or ballet have scoliosis curvatures. Despite this, there appears to be no increased incidence of backache or subsequent long-term disability in these individuals.

If a young candidate for dance participation is noted to have a scoliosis curvature and is fully mature, it is our practice to obtain a standing PA roentgenogram of the DL spine to document the degree of curvature before encouraging full dance or sports participation in conjunction with a full back exercise regimen.

Another spinal deformity noted in young athletes is hyperlordosis or swayback. If the child has hyperlordotic posturing of the low back but is fully flexible on forward bending and not only flattens but reverses the lumbar spine on forward bending, without evidence of excessive tightness of lumbodorsal fascia or hamstrings, an antilordotic exercise program is instituted, and the child reassessed at regular intervals. For fixed lumbar lordosis, however, we initially institute a directed exercise program of antilordotic strengthening, lumbodorsal fascia and hamstring flexibility exercises. If exercises alone are not effective, we add an antilordotic bracing program. Certain sports appear to increase the tendency to develop lumbar lordosis, e.g., figure skating, gymnastics, and ice hockey. Participants in these activities need a prophylactic program of abdominal strengthening and lumbar flattening exercises, with particular emphasis on the pelvic tilt.

The presence of lordosis increases the risk of spondylolysis, and there is some evidence that hyperlordotic posturing, either continuous or intermittent, increases the chance of disc herniation. Therefore, young athletes who are performing hyperlordotic maneuvers should be on the prophylactic antilordotic exercise program.

In the case of a young athlete who has hyperlordosis and back pain, a complete work-up is necessary to rule out spondylolysis and disc or other etiologies before making the diagnosis of mechanical back pain. If exercises alone are insufficient to relieve the back pain, antilordotic bracing should definitely be considered. The response to antilordotic bracing is often dramatic, with progressive reposturing of the lumbar spine and loss of pain, while allowing full participation in sports activities. We ask the young athlete to participate while wearing the antilordotic low-profile brace, but once pain relief has been obtained and the patient remains asymptomatic

during sports participation, the brace can safely be removed for active sports participation or practice, but it must be worn the rest of the day. At least 6 months of treatment are required to attain a satisfactory realignment of the spine. Bracing treatment for spondylolysis, however, is done full-time.

SPINAL FUSION

Fusion of the spine may be required in certain cases of severe or progressive spinal deformity such as dorsal roundbacking and scoliosis. Furthermore, localized fusion may be required for a previous spinal injury or deformity with resultant instability. In such cases, concern is naturally expressed about the possibility of returning to sports participation following spinal fusion. Spinal instrumentation, which is now commonly used in conjunction with the spinal fusion, has enhanced our ability to straighten the spine and has appeared to increase the rate of fusion from such procedures (Fig. 6). In some instances, external casting or brace support may no longer be required following this spinal fusion. Despite the increased sophistication of this internal instrumentation, however, it is generally agreed that attainment of a stable spinal fusion requires approximately 12 months and that vigorous sports participation should not be resumed earlier. By vigorous sports participation, we mean participation that involves twisting, turning, or potential impact to the back or spine. We do allow swimming early in the postoperative period—in some cases, as early as 6 to 8 weeks following spinal fusion while plastic orthotic braces are worn postoperatively.

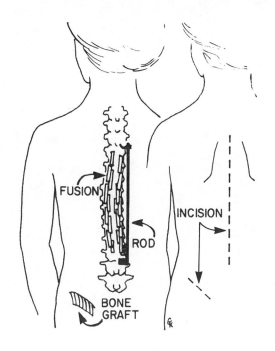

Figure 6 Extensive spinal fusion with instrumentation is a contraindication to contact sports, but many other sports and fitness activities are allowed.

A child or adolescent who has had spinal instrumentation and fusion of more than 2 segments of the spine should be strongly counseled against participation in high impact sports such as gridiron football or rugby, even after solid fusion has been attained. On the other hand, moderate contact sports such as basketball, soccer, or field lacrosse are generally allowed.

In the case of more localized fusions such as single level fusion of the cervical spine for antecedent trauma, or fusion across the lumbosacral junction for spondylolysis, return to sports participation must be individualized. When the site of fusion is the spine, there is an increased risk of long-term problems due to deterioration of the spinal elements immediately above or below the area of fusion. Such deterioration may be hastened by vigorous sports participation, particularly if sports participation involves active impacting or use of the head and neck. The presence of associated neurologic symptoms or compromise at the time of the initial injury must also be a factor in the decision to continue sports participation.

Following lumbosacral fusion, return to full sports participation, including contact sports participation, is generally allowed at the end of one year if it is certain that a stable fusion has been attained and there are no sequelae or neurologic compromise in the lower extremities. In some instances, if newer techniques of localized instrumentation of the fractured pars interarticularis are used, return to sports participation as early as 3 months following fusion has been allowed, but decided on an individual basis.

BACKACHE

IAN MACNAB, M.B., Ch.B., F.R.C.S.,
F.R.C.S.(C)

REFERRED PAIN

A major factor that has clouded and confused the diagnosis of soft tissue lesions of the back is the phenomenon of referred pain. When a deep structure is irritated, whether by trauma, by disease, or by the experimental injection of an irritating solution, the pain resulting may be experienced locally, referred distally, or experienced both locally and radiating to a distance. It is important to recognize that tenderness may also be referred to a distance as has been shown by the injection of hypertonic saline into the lumbosacral supraspinous ligament. Under such circumstances, pain may not only radiate down the leg but also may be associated with tender points, which are commonly situated over the sacroiliac joint and the upper outer quadrant of the buttock (Fig. 1).

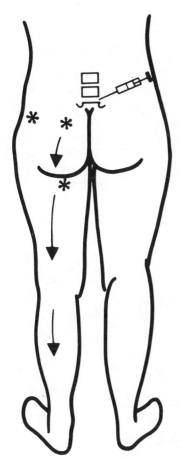

Figure 1. The injection of hypertonic saline into the supraspinous ligament between L5 and Sl gives rise to local pain and pain referred down the back of the leg in sciatic distribution. Usually, this does not extend below the knee, and there are points of tenderness in the lower limbs, most commonly noted at the sites marked by the asterisks.

The complaint of pain and the demonstration of local tenderness may obscure the fact that the offending lesion is centrally placed and may lead the clinician to believe erroneously that the disease process underlies the site of the patient's complaints. This erroneous belief may apparently be confirmed by the temporary relief of pain on injection of a local anesthetic when in reality there is no local problem at all. These points must be borne in mind when considering the site and nature of soft tissue injuries giving rise to low back pain, for a failure to do so will only lead to diagnostic and therapeutic errors.

MYOFASCIAL SPRAINS OR STRAINS

Partial tears of the attachment of muscles may occur, giving rise to local tenderness and pain, generally of short duration. There is always a history of specific injury, either a blunt blow or a forceful movement, usually rotation. The pain and tenderness are always away from the midline. This is a young man's injury with strong muscles guarding a healthy spine. A similar injury sustained by an older man with weaker muscles and with degenerate discs is much more likely to result in a posterior joint strain.

These lesions heal with the passage of time despite, rather than because of, treatment.

Injections of local anesthetic (with or without the addition of local steroids) in and around the area of maximum tenderness certainly afford temporary relief of varying duration, but it is doubtful whether they speed the resolution of the underlying pathology. The symptoms may persist for about 3 weeks in varying degree, during which time the patient is well advised to avoid provocative activity. If symptoms persist beyond this period, the problem should be carefully reassessed lest some more significant underlying lesion be overlooked.

TENDINITIS

Tendinitis has come by custom to be associated with athletic activities. However, it must be remembered that tendinitis is just a clinical syndrome, the pathologic basis of which is inadequately defined. Clinically, it is recognized that well-localized areas of tenderness may develop at the attachment of tendons, fascia, or ligaments to bone, anywhere in the body.

In the spine, breakdown changes of this nature may occur at the attachment of muscles to the sacrum or iliac crest, or the supraspinous ligaments may give rise to pain after having been subjected to moderate to mild trauma. On examination, the areas of breakdown present a small but well-localized area of tenderness. Pressure over the area not only elicits tenderness, but when maintained, reproduces the patient's symptoms.

The pathologic basis of this syndrome is probably a local area of tendon breakdown or degeneration, which invokes an inflammatory or autoimmune response. It is possibly the vascular reaction associated with localized edema that accounts for the pain and tenderness. Empirically, it has been found that gratifyingly rapid relief of pain can be obtained by the injection of steroids.

KISSING SPINES: SPRUNG BACK

Approximation of the spinous processes (kissing spines) and the development of a bursa between them has been indicted as a cause of low back pain after hyperextension injuries. "Sprung back" is a term coined by Newman to describe rupture of the supraspinous ligament following a sudden flexion strain applied to the spine with the pelvis fixed, as in falling on the buttocks with the legs outstretched. It is doubtful whether either of these entities is, of itself, a cause of low back pain (Fig. 2) in the absence of disc degeneration allowing excessive movement at the segment.

With a normal disc, extension of a segment is limited by the anterior fibers of the annulus, and at the limit of normal extension the spinous processes do not come into contact. Contact between the spinous processes is only seen with abnormal mobility associated with disc degeneration. Although apposition of the spinous processes and the development of a painful bursa may aggravate and intensify the symptoms derived from segmental instability associated with degenerative disc disease, it is never the sole source of symptoms. Tearing of the supraspinous ligament, thought to be the basis of "sprung back", can only occur in the presence of disc degeneration allowing an abnormal degree of flexion, or with an injury severe enough to disrupt the posterior fibers of the annulus and the capsule of the posterior joints.

Separation and apposition of the spinous processes when symptomatic are indicative of segmental instability associated with disc degeneration, and the treatment of such lesions is, therefore, the treatment of the associated disc degeneration.

DISC DEGENERATION

It is necessary to discuss briefly the changes associated with disc degeneration and the manner in which they predispose to symptoms following minor to moderate injury.

The intervertebral discs are composed of a combination of the annulus, the nucleus pulposus, and the hyaline cartilage plate, which makes for a very efficient coupling unit, provided all the structures remain intact. Normally, the vertebral bodies roll over the incompressible gel of the nucleus pulposus whose structural integrity is maintained by the annulus, with the posterior joints guiding and steadying the movement. Once degenerative changes involve any one of the components of the disc, such as inspissation of the nucleus pulposus, a tear in the annulus, or a rupture of the hyaline cartilage plate, the smooth roller action is lost and the movement between adjacent vertebral segments becomes uneven, excessive, and irregular. Although these changes occur most commonly at about the age of 40, they may affect the younger age groups, especially those with a family history of low back pain.

Normally on flexion of the spine, the discal borders of the vertebral bodies become parallel above the level of L5. This is the maximal movement permitted. In the stage of segmental instability, excessive degrees of extension and flexion are permitted and a certain amount of backward and forward gliding movement occurs as well (Fig. 3). This abnormal type of movement can be shown

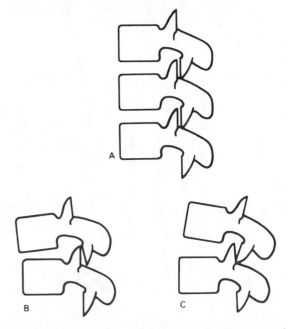

Figure 3. In the early stages of degenerative disc disease, excessive degrees of flexion and extension are permitted at the involved segment. This abnormal mobility is associated with rocking of the posterior joints (*B* and *C*).

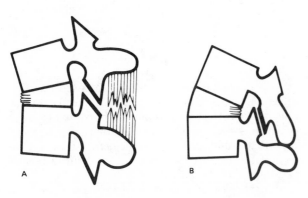

Figure 2. *A*, An acute flexion injury of the spine may produce a tear of the supraspinous ligament. This lesion has been referred to as a "sprung back". It is unlikely, however, that this lesion can occur in the absence of gross disc degeneration which, by itself, is probably the source of the patient's complaint. *B*, the radiologic demonstration of apposition of the spinous processes has been referred to as "kissing spines". This anatomic disposition of the spinous processes cannot occur in the absence of an unstable disc segment. In the balance of probabilities, it is the associated disc degeneration rather than the bony apposition of the spinous processes that is the cause of the patient's symptoms.

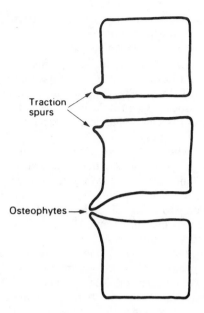

Figure 4. The traction spur projects horizontally from the vertebral body about 1 mm away from the discal border.

clinically by roentgenograms taken with the patients holding their spines in full extension and in full flexion. One problem posed by motion studies is the fact that when a patient is in pain, the associated muscle guarding does not permit adequate flexion and extension films to be taken. However, there are two radiologic changes that are indicative of instability, the Knuttson phenomenon of gas in the disc and the "traction spur".

The traction spur differs anatomically and radiologically from other spondylophytes in that it projects horizontally and develops about 2 mm above the vertebral body edge (Fig. 4). It owes its development to the manner of attachment of the annulus fibers. With abnormal movements, an excessive strain is applied to the outermost annulus fibers and it is here that the traction spur develops. It is a small traction spur that is clinically significant in that it is probably indicative of present instability.

Segmental instability by itself is probably not painful, but the spine is vulnerable to trauma. A forced and

unguarded movement may be concentrated on the wobbly segment and produce a posterior joint strain or a posterior joint subluxation. Repeated injuries may, indeed, produce osteochondral fractures and loose bodies in the posterior joints.

In the next stage of disc degeneration, segmental hyperextension occurs. Extension of the lumbar spine is limited by the anterior fibers of the annulus. When degenerative changes cause these fibers to lose their elasticity, the involved segment or segments may hyperextend (Fig. 5). A similar change may be seen in the next stage of disc degeneration, disc narrowing. As the intervertebral discs lose height, the posterior joints must override and subluxate (Fig. 6). In both segmental hyperextension and disc narrowing, the related posterior joints in normal posture are held in hyperextension, and this postural defect is exaggerated if the patient has weak abdominal muscles and/or tight tensors.

When the posterior joints are held at the extreme of their limit of extension, there is no safety factor of movement, and the extension strains of everyday living may push the joints past their physiologically permitted limits and thereby produce pain.

On the premise that the majority of backaches occur before the age of 40, the roentgenograms of 300 40-year-old laborers, who had been engaged in heavy work all their lives, were reviewed. Of these, 150 denied any history of low back pain and 150 were under treat-

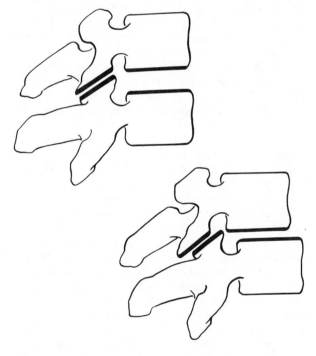

Figure 6. As the intervertebral discs lose height and the vertebral bodies approach one another, the posterior joints must override and assume the position normally held in hyperextension. It is to be noted that owing to the inclination of the posterior joints, as the upper vertebral body approaches the vertebral body beneath it, it is displaced backward, producing a retrospondylolisthesis. This posterior displacement of the vertebral body, indicative of posterior joint subluxation, is readily recognizable on routine x-ray examination of the lumbar spine.

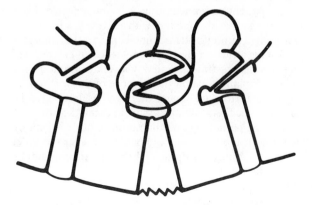

Figure 5. When the anterior fibers of the annulus lose their elasticity, the involved segment falls into hyperextension, permitting subluxation of the related posterior joint.

ment for backache at the time of the review. A careful statistical analysis of the films showed no difference in the incidence of anatomic variants and the incidence of degenerative changes in the two groups studied. This is important because the mere demonstration of an anatomic anomaly or a minor pathologic change is no reason to prevent the athlete from continuing with his sports activities.

With our present stage of knowledge regarding disc degeneration, only the following may be stated: (1) disc degeneration may occur and may remain asymptomatic; (2) disc degeneration may be associated with changes within the disc itself, which may be productive of pain; and (3) disc degeneration may give rise to mechanical instability which renders the spine vulnerable to trauma, as a result of which pain may arise from ligamentous or posterior joint damage.

The pain experienced may remain localized to the back, or there may be both local pain and referred pain, or referred pain only.

DISC RUPTURES

An intervertebral disc separating two vertebral segments may be likened to the old-fashioned motorcar tire, with a hard, outer fibrous casing and an inner tube—in this case filled with jelly. A ruptured disc may occur in one of two forms—either similar to a blister in the motorcar tire with a weakening of the outer casing or, on occasion, as a complete blowout (sequestration) of the inner tube through the hole in the outer fibers of the annulus.

In 1934, Mixter and Barr suggested that sciatic pain could result from irritation of a lumbar nerve root by a prolapsed intervertebral disc. Although skeptically received at first, this concept soon become universally accepted and founded the "dynasty of the disc", during which time the complaint of sciatic pain tended to become uncritically equated with a diagnosis of disc herniation. Surgical exploration of patients with evidence of lumbar nerve root irritation revealed the fact that there are, indeed, several sources of nerve root compromise of which a ruptured intervertebral disc is but one example.

A ruptured intervertebral disc produces nerve root pressure and this presents as radicular pain, that is to say, pain radiating from the buttock to the ankle, associated with paresthesia, associated with signs of root tension and, on occasion, with evidence of impairment of root conduction. This lesion does not commonly result from a sport-related injury.

If the person has a mechanically insufficient spine and sustains a vigorous strain, the symptoms resulting, as stated previously, may be backache with pain *referred* down the leg in sciatic distribution. This referred pain rarely goes below the knee; it is not associated with paresthesia; it is not associated with signs of nerve root tension, such as limitation of straight leg-raising; and it is never associated with any evidence of impairment of root

conduction, as reflected by changes in reflex activity, sensory appreciation, or motor power.

If a patient is just about to suffer from a prolapsed disc, he may well sustain the prolapse as he is going down a ski slope, but the sport of skiing is not of itself commonly associated with the production of a ruptured disc. The back injuries associated with athletics are the injuries of joint sprains and associated muscle and fascial damage. The pain resulting from this varies in severity. Characteristically, while the patient is carrying out his normal activities in sports, he is suddenly seized with back pain and cannot move. ("I was paralyzed with pain.") The lumbar spine is splinted rigidly, and the patient can move only with painful caution, clutching his back and walking with his trunk leaning forward, keeping his hips and knees slightly bent.

Examination reveals that all movements of the spine are limited by pain and muscle spasm, but there is no evidence of nerve root tension. The clinical picture is explosively dramatic and threatening to the patient. The physician must not overreact. The physician must constantly remind himself that even if he elected to treat the patient by rolling peanut butter on each buttock, in the balance of probabilities, the patient would get well fairly quickly.

In the majority of such cases, the patient is suffering from a "sprain" of one of the zygoapophyseal joints. When trying to rationalize treatment, one should compare the lesion with a severely sprained ankle in a patient who has only one leg and who is unable to wear a prosthesis. There is only one way to treat a sprained ankle in such a patient: the patient has to be put to bed. Theoretically, the patient with an acute low back strain should also be treated by strict bed rest. However, theoretical treatment must be tempered by reason, and you must allow your reasoning to be tempered by the patient's reaction to your therapeutic suggestions.

Let me repeat: you are treating a patient and not a spine, and the experience of the lay world is that many (in fact, the majority) will get better by just creeping around with their pain mollified by analgesics. Some patients, however, cannot cope; their pain is too severe. In such instances, if they cannot do their normal daily work, they should be sent to bed.

A patient with pneumonia is ill and defeated. He is happy to go to bed. A patient with a severe low back pain feels well in himself and does not want to go to bed. He is mad at his affliction, and your insistence on bed rest will increase his frustration unless you take care and take time to explain in detail the purpose of this apparently neglectful form of management. It is advisable to give the patient some literature explaining in detail the probable underlying pathology and the rationale of treatment by bed rest. You must advise the patient in regard to toilet facilities. Using a bedpan at home is an impractical acrobatic feat. The use of crutches makes it easier for the patient to get to the bathroom, and the purchase of a high toilet seat is essential.

To relieve the pain, local ice application has definite merit for the first 48 hours. Local application of ice over a muscle probably acts on the muscle's spindle system. A muscle that retains its extensibility through its normal resting length is usually pain-free. When it does not retain its extensibility, it is considered to be in "spasm" and a source of pain. Ice applied to the overlying skin probably sends impulses to the cord that "compete" with the pain, producing impulses that are conveyed by much slower fibers. The ice-produced impulses temporarily cause a refractory period in the other impulses, and the muscle spasm is momentarily relieved. Stretch of the muscle is now possible, which decreases the spasm. If ice is applied for too long a period, the muscle may become literally chilled, and this increases muscle spasm and adds to the pain.

There are very few orally administered muscle "relaxants" that have any effect on skeletal muscles. If they were truly effective, the eye muscles would also be grossly relaxed, and the patient would develop nystagmus. Their major action is as a tranquilizer. Analgesics in sufficient doses can be given, but they must be given on a time-dependent basis and not on demand. These patients must not be allowed to pop pills for pain; otherwise the physician is just inducing a habituation. In the vast majority of patients, after 2 or 3 days, the "smoke clears away" and the patient can get around each day with increasing comfort.

If, on neurologic examination, there is no evidence of nerve root compression or irritation and no evidence of impairment of root conduction, the resolution of symptoms may be speeded by a flexion manipulation (Fig. 7). The patient lies on his back, and the physician raises the patient's legs, maintaining the knees in flexion. By applying pressure on the heels, the physician then pushes the patient's knees toward the shoulders. This movement is done very slowly. The degree of flexion obtained is determined by the discomfort the patient experiences. The movement is then repeated slowly and rhythmically over a period of 5 minutes. In the majority of instances, the range of movement that can be achieved by this passive manipulation gradually increases, and at the conclusion of the manipulation, the patient is instructed to flex his knees fully and allow his feet to come down to the bed, soles first.

The patient then carries out a series of passive flexion manipulations of his spine once an hour. He does this by lying on his back and pulling his knees slowly up to his

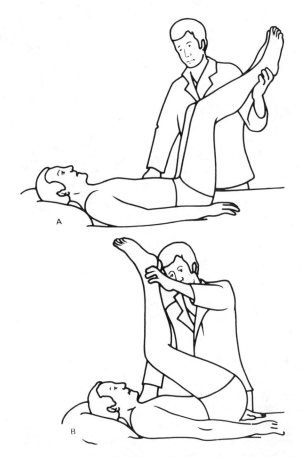

Figure 7. *A,* Flexion manipulation by the physician. The physician raises the patient's legs maintaining the knees in flexion. *B,* By applying pressure to the heels the physician then pushes the patient's knees towards the shoulders.

chest (Fig. 8). He should maintain this position for 5 minutes. In very acute attacks with severe pain, the patient may find it easier to assume the same position lying on his side. By the second day, the patient should be able to carry out the flexion manipulations of his back himself (Fig. 9).

Once the attack is over, the patient and his physician are now faced with the difficulty of trying to prevent recurrent episodes. Adequate trunk muscles are the major guardians against repeated attacks. It must be remembered that the spinal column is not a self-

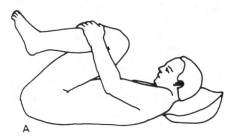
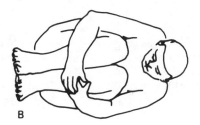

Figure 8. A patient may abort an acute episode of low back pain by lying on his back and pulling his knees slowly up to his chest, *A.* He should maintain this position for 5 minutes. If pain is severe the patient may find it easier to assume the same position lying on his side, *B.*

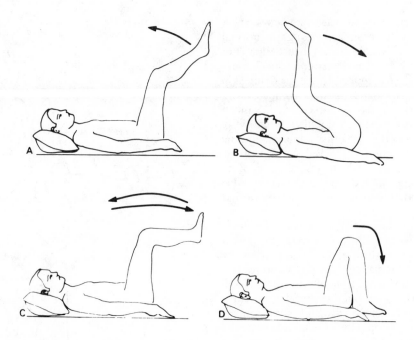

Figure 9. Flexion exercise-manipulation of the lumbar spine. The patient lies on the bed with the head supported by a pillow. *A*, The hips are flexed to 90° and the knees slightly flexed. *B*, The patient now attempts to kick the feet over the head, raising the buttocks approximately 6 inches off the bed. *C*, After each "kick-up" the patient returns to the starting position. *D*, After five kick-ups, the patient rests by lowering his legs with the knees fully flexed, thereby putting his feet on the bed, soles first. It is very important that he should not lower the legs with the knees fully extended because this places a painful hyperextension strain on the spine.

supporting structure. If the trunk and abdominal muscles are paralyzed, as in infantile paralysis, the spine collapses. The spine is supported by muscle action in much the same way the mast of a ship is supported by stays (Fig. 10). In addition to this, the abdominal cavity acts as a hydraulic sac, dissipating loads by pressing upwards on the diaphragm and downwards on the pelvic floor, thereby unweighting the spine (Fig. 11). Because of this, the tone and strength of the abdominal muscles are of vital importance in protecting the spine against weight-bearing and extension strains.

The exercise program is started by pelvic tilting. This is best carried out with the patient lying supine on a firm surface. The patient lies in a comfortable position with his hips and knees flexed, keeping the soles of both feet flat on the bed or floor. The patient now presses his lower back down flat against the floor so that he obliterates the lumbar lordosis. This movement is achieved by a combined contraction of the abdominal muscles and the glutei. In order to help the patient get into this habit, it is often easier to ask him to put his hands behind his back and press his spine back onto his hands.

Once the lumbar spine is pressing against the floor, the pelvis is rotated by raising the buttocks from the floor. As the buttocks are being raised, the lower back must not be permitted to leave the floor. Raising the buttocks away from the floor reverses the lumbar lordosis. Patients may find it easier if they put one hand on the symphysis pubis and the other on the zyphoid process and then try to bring their hands together whilst they are doing the exercises. As the patient becomes more adept at this exercise, he should practice the movement rhythmically, initially with the hips and knees flexed before trying the same exercise with the hips and knees flat.

Pelvic tilting can also be practiced with the patient standing with his back flat against the wall and his feet about 2 feet away from the wall. Holding his lumbar spine flat against the wall (checking this with a hand placed between his spine and the wall), he then gradually brings his heels toward the wall and tries to straighten his knees. To begin with, this is difficult, but when he can achieve this easily, he has managed to learn the art of pelvic tilting in a manner that will overcome a tendency to hyperlordosis.

When flexion exercises are started, the patient should lie on his back with his hips and knees bent and his feet *supported*. He should put his hands forward to touch his thighs and then gradually crawl up his thighs until his hands are on the top of his knees. He should then take his hands away from his knees and let his back fall gently into the supine position. Flexion exercises should never be performed with the patient holding his knees fully extended. The only way it is possible to get up with the knees extended is to whip the back up because the weight of the trunk is greater than the weight of the legs. A person has to put an extension strain on the lower back to begin the movement and then the rest of his spine is flung forward, as with a whiplash.

At this stage, it is necessary, in the prevention of recurrence of back pain, to test for the flexibility of the hamstrings and the heel cords. The supine position is again used. One leg is fully flexed at the hip with the knee and thigh against the chest. The leg, undergoing the

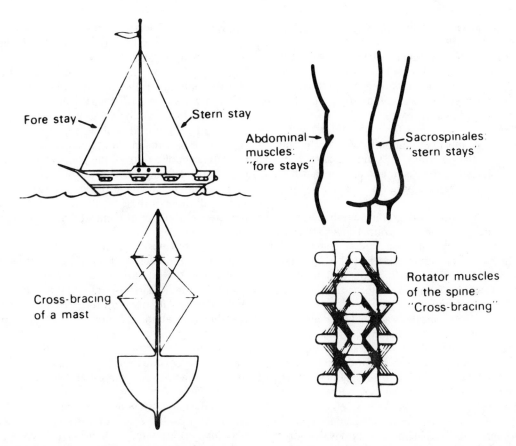

Figure 10. It is interesting to note the similarity between the bracing used to support the mast of a ship and the muscular bracing of the human spine.

stretching of the hamstrings, is maintained in full extension. The patient now tries to sit up slowly and reach toward the toes of the extended leg. The fixed, flexed leg prevents the occurrence of hyperlordosis during the act of sitting up. If the heel cords are found to be tight, the extended leg should be placed in such a manner that the sole of the foot is flat against the wall. The heel cords can also be stretched by leaning foward against the wall, keeping the feet flat on the floor, and the force applied to

the heel cords can be increased by getting the patient to squat down.

On occasion, a tight tensor fascia femoris causes anterior pelvic rotation, and this increases the lumbar lordosis. This needs passive stretching by a physiotherapist.

As in all therapeutic exercises, initially a few specific exercises are directed toward the lesion being treated, but once the discomfort starts to subside, it is of vital importance that the patient engage in a general controlled physical exercise program.

Figure 11. The abdominal cavity acts in a manner similar to a hydraulic sac. By increasing intra-abdominal pressure, the diaphragm is pushed up and the pelvic floor is pushed down. This tends to "elongate" the lumbar spine, thereby taking some of the weight off the discs and the posterior joints.

FURTHER INVESTIGATION

The question is often asked, "When should you take an x-ray?" Probably the following criteria are adequate:

1. Severe back pain following significant trauma.
2. Incapacitating back pain.
3. The excessively anxious patient. In such people, an x-ray examination is an essential part of treatment. They cannot be reassured by clinical examination alone.
4. Patients in whom the history and examination are suggestive of an early ankylosing spondylitis. A specific request should be made for oblique views of the sacroiliac joint.

5. Patients with a clinically apparent spinal deformity.

6. Patients with significant root tension and patients presenting with evidence of impairment of root conduction. It must be remembered that being very athletically inclined does not prevent these young people from having a tumor of the cauda equina.

7. If severe pain persists for longer than 2 weeks despite treatment, an x-ray examination is indicated, not only to exclude the possibility of some obscure spinal abnormality, but also to reassure the patient that he is not suffering from a serious progressive disease.

On occasion, the radiograph reveals a spinal anomaly. Of the spinal anomalies once believed to cause back pain, such as sacralization of L5, spina bifida occulta, the ossicle of Oppenheimer, and a unilateral iliotransverse joint, all are now recognized as being incidental findings and having no influence on the development of low back pain.

There remains just one bony anomaly that gives rise to concern. If the patient's radiograph reveals a spondylolysis of L5 with or without a listhesis, the question always arises whether this defect in the pars interarticularis developed as a result of repeated trauma on the football field or whether this boy had this defect before he started playing football.

It has been reported, and convincingly demonstrated radiographically, that linebackers may develop in the course of the season, as a result of the vigorous hyperextension strains they place on each other, a stress fracture through the pars interarticularis, giving rise to a spondylolysis. Without specific therapy and certainly without surgery, over the course of the next 6 months, these stress fractures heal by themselves and will not be the source of further disability.

In patients in whom a routine x-ray examination reveals a spondylolisthesis of grade I or more, the question is always raised whether it is safe to let the young athlete continue with contact sports. There is no evidence that vigorous physical contact will cause an increasing slip. These patients may have pain derived either from the subjacent disc or from the syndesmosis at the site of the isthmic defect or, most probably, from degenerative disc changes occurring at the level above the slip. Any one or all three of these factors may be responsible for repeated episodes of discomfort while playing and may markedly interfere with the patient's competence.

In these cases, there are two choices. Either they must give up contact sports or, if this is going to be their profession, the question is raised whether the patient should be admitted to hospital for more detailed analysis of the source of his discomfort to see whether it would be possible stop abnormal movement at the level of the defect and stabilize the degenerative disc above the slip by a localized intertransverse fusion. It must always be remembered, of course, that it will take at least 9 months to one year before this young man returns to competitive sports.

In the diagnosis and management of a patient presenting with low back pain, the orthopaedic surgeon must play many roles: family practitioner, internist, radiologist, physiatrist, orthotist, psychiatrist, social worker, and friend. He should rarely find it necessary to play the role of his chosen avocation–an orthopaedic surgeon.

DISCOLYSIS FOR HERNIATED NUCLEUS PULPOSUS

JOHN A. McCULLOCH, M.D., F.R.C.S.(C)

Discolysis with chymopapain requires, as does all surgery, the careful selection of patients and proper performance of the procedure.

Chymopapain's only effect is on the proteoglycans of nucleus pulposus tissue. Chymopapain breaks down the proteoglycan structure so that its ability to imbibe water is impaired. This hydrolysis of the nucleus pulposus, in effect, reduces the pressure within a disc herniation. This pressure reduction is associated with relief of nerve root compression and thus relief of any symptoms, such as sciatica, associated with nerve root compression. Chymopapain has little effect on annulus fibrosis, nor will it dissolve osteophytes or scar tissue or relieve emotional strains!

INDICATIONS

The classic indication for chemonucleolysis is a herniated nucleus pulposus that is causing sciatica. The classic location for a herniated nucleus pulposus is posterolateral, with pressure being applied to one nerve root. At the L4–L5 level, the fifth lumbar nerve root is compressed, and at the L5–S1 level, the first sacral nerve root is compressed. The clinical features include leg pain greater than back pain, specific paresthetic discomfort, significant straight leg-raising changes, two of four neurologic signs, and a positive myelogram (Table 1). A patient who has four or five of the criteria listed in Table 1 is most likely to have sciatic discomfort in the leg on the basis of a soft disc herniation. It is this patient who will respond to the injection of chymopapain. The less than classic indications include:

1. A lateral disc herniation of L5–S1 involves the fifth lumbar nerve root, and of L4–L5 which involves the fourth lumbar nerve root. It is a lesion often missed on myelography, especially in the days of oil-based myelography. The straight leg-raising changes are not so dramatic as with a posterolateral herniated nucleus pulposus. Otherwise, the presentation is similar. Some believe that a lateral or foraminal disc herniation automatically implies an extruded or sequestered disc and thus precludes a successful chymopapain injection. Such is not always the case.

**TABLE 1   Criteria for Diagnosis of
Herniated Intervertebral Disc**

Leg pain is a more dominant symptom than back pain. It affects one leg only, and follows a typical sciatic (or femoral) nerve distribution.

Paresthesiae are localized to a dermatomal distribution.

Straight-leg raising is reduced by 50% of normal, and/or pain crosses over to the symptomatic leg when the unaffected leg is elevated, and/or pain radiates proximally or distally with digital pressure on the tibial nerve in the popliteal fossa.

Two of four neurologic signs are present (wasting, motor weakness, diminished sensory appreciation, or diminution of reflex activity).

A contrast study or CT scan is positive and corresponds to the clinical level.

2. A midline disc herniation. This entity exists and can be supported by a CT scan. Diagnosis is difficult because of the inclusion, based on clinical criteria, of patients with degenerative disc disease, facet joint syndrome, and degenerative spondylolisthesis in its very early stages. The diagnosis should be made only on the basis of (a) absence of degenerative changes on x-ray examination, but intermittent episodes of severe back pain with sciatica scoliosis in a young patient; (b) bilateral leg pain— sometimes simultaneous, sometimes alternating; (c) bilateral straight leg-raising changes (reduction, bowstring, crossover); (d) minimal neurologic changes (occasionally neurologic symptoms); and (e) a positive CT scan. The best support for the diagnosis comes when one leg tends to dominate and the CT scan defect is eccentric to that side.

RELATIVE CONTRAINDICATIONS

Spinal Canal Stenosis.   Although there are very few indications for the use of chymopapain in canal stenosis, the patient with a symptomatic canal stenosis may sometimes suffer a herniated nucleus pulposus that will respond to chymopapain injection. More often, a herniated nucleus pulposus in spinal stenosis is merely part of the downhill chain of events that will eventually require surgical intervention, and as such will not respond to chymopapain injection.

Lateral Recess Stenosis.   There are even fewer indications for the use of chymopapain in lateral recess stenosis. The compromise of a narrowed lateral recess by a herniated nucleus pulposus should respond, theoretically, to the injection of chymopapain, but this is rarely the case.

Post-Surgery Recurrence.   Chymopapain will not dissolve away your surgical failures, unless, of course, you operated at the wrong level!

Most post-surgery recurrences of herniated nucleus pulposus occur at the same level on the same side. In such cases, chymopapain is effective if (1) previous surgery was done for sciatica, (2) the patient was better after surgery for at least 4 to 6 months before symptoms recurred, and (3) major symptoms and signs are sciatic in nature.

If a post-surgery patient has a disc herniation at a different level, or on the opposite side, it should be treated as a virgin disc.

There is a slightly increased risk of subarachnoid injection in patients with a history of previous surgery. A recurrent herniated nucleus pulposus may penetrate a scarred, immobile dural sheath.

Age.   The older the patient, the more likely it is that the back ailment is due to degenerative conditions rather than a herniated nucleus pulposus. However, older patients may have "young" discs and present with a syndrome of herniated nucleus pulposus.

Chymopapain is safe to use in adolescent patients.

The stenotic patient, the post-surgery patient, and the older patient are less likely to be encountered in the athletic community, but it is important to understand the condition in these patients to properly appreciate the indications for chymopapain injection.

ABSOLUTE CONTRAINDICATIONS

Listed below are the absolute contraindications to chymopapain discolysis:

1. Signficant emotional involvement
   Symptoms: multifocal, nonmechanical spinal pain; weak, numb legs; legs that give way; unusual treatment responses; and multiple intervention (hospital, doctor, surgery)
   Signs: superficial nonanatomic tenderness; simulated movement; distraction tests; nonanatomic neurologic changes; and academy award performance
2. Signficant neurologic deficit
   Usually accompanied by a significant myelographic or CT scan defect
3. A sequestered disc
   The only reliable diagnostic test is a myelographic or CT scan defect that is largely behind the vertebral body
4. Known allergy to chymopapain
5. Previous injection of chymopapain (role of skin test?)
6. Neurologic lesion of cord (e.g., multiple sclerosis)
7. Bladder or bowel involvement of cauda equina syndrome
8. Pregnancy
9. Disc lesions at spinal cord levels

Most of the foregoing contraindications do not pertain to the athletic population. Exceptions are (1) a significant neurologic deficit resulting from a disc herniation, and (2) a sequestered disc. Athletes so affected should be excluded from chymopapain treatment, and undergo standard surgical treatment. Only patients who have failed to respond to adequate conservative treatment for HNP should be selected for discolysis.

PREOPERATIVE INVESTIGATION

Although I generally rely on the CT scan alone as the preoperative investigation, in the following circumstances a myelogram, alone or in combination with a CT scan, is essential: (1) doubt regarding the diagnosis, (2) older patients (over age 50 to 55 years), (3) bilateral symptoms suggesting a midline defect, (4) previous surgery (with or without metal), and (5) poor scan in an obese patient. CT scanning alone as a preoperative test is sufficient only in the classic patient with a herniated nucleus pulposus who is young, who has had no previous surgery, and has the classic story of unilateral, dominant leg pain with marked reduction in straight leg-raising and with neurologic symptoms and signs.

Finally, investigation can be impeded by poor technique. In this age of outstanding CT scan technology, I still see scans that are done poorly and/or done on machines that are technically outdated.

TECHNIQUE

Some caveats regarding technique are:
1. Never cross the midline (subarachnoid space) with a needle that will be used to inject chymopapain.
2. Do not inject chymopapain until you are sure the needle tip is in the middle of the nuclear area.
3. Obey instructions in the product brochure.
4. When inserting the needle leave the stylet of the needle out after the skin is pierced. If you inadvertently cross the subarachnoid space while advancing the needle, or enter the subarachnoid space in the axilla of the nerve root, you will know immediately because of the backflow of cerebrospinal fluid. If this backflow occurs, abort the procedure and wait at least one week before rescheduling it.

Anesthesia

Local (augmented with neuroleptic agents) anesthesia is preferred because (1) it is safer; (2) it is efficient, shortening operating room time and shortening hospital stay; (3) it spares the patient the complications of general anesthesia and intubation, (4) it allows for earlier intervention in the event of complications such as anaphylaxis; and (5) it preserves discometry or discography as a test.

In the face of a negative skin test, it is highly unlikely that a patient will experience an immediate hypersensitivity reaction. Thus, the main reason for suggesting general anesthesia is eliminated.

Prophylactic Premedication with Antihistamines and/or Steroids and Test Dose

I do not use premedication or a test dose. Rather than assume that all patients are at risk and premedicate, I try to identify potential reactors by (a) an allergic history and (b) skin testing. Other tests, such as the RAST test (Pharmacia Laboratories) or the ChymoFAST test (Allergenetics Reference Laboratory) are available.

My reasons for not premedicating are:

1. The incidence of anaphylaxis, which is generally low (0.5%), is even lower when skin-test positive patients are eliminated from chymopapain treatment (O anaphylaxis in over 600 patients–personal experience).
2. There is no scientific evidence that premedication lowers the incidence of anaphylaxis below our experience (0.35%).

3. Many patients are being given unnecessary medicine.
4. Prophylactic programs, in general, should contain the most effective agent; the most effective agent in anaphylaxis is epinephrine, and obviously it cannot be included in a prophylactic program.
5. Patients who have been premedicated according to Smith Labs' recommendation have experienced severe anaphylactic reactions.
6. Patients who have received a test dose of chymopapain according to Smith Labs' recommendation have experienced severe anaphylactic reactions.
7. Anaphylaxis requires aggressive treatment with larger doses of medication than the recommended regime and the addition of epinephrine.
8. The best defense against anaphylaxis is (a) identification and exclusion of the hypersensitive patient (skin test), and (b) an alert, well-prepared team of assistants who are not lulled into a false sense of security by premedications.

Operating Room or X-Ray Department

The operating room (OR) has the greatest collection of skilled associates for managing the complications of discolysis. Although complications are rare, the occurrence of one in the radiology department does not allow for the smoothest, most effective management of the complication with the least upset in a department routine. Just the opposite is true in the OR, where there is an adequate staff with a depth of experience in managing emergencies. Obviously, if the operating room does not have good image intensifier capabilities, the radiology department will have to be considered.

Prone or Lateral Position

The lateral position is the choice of most surgeons. The prone position is acceptable, provided the needle insertion site is not too far lateral. Theoretically, the bowel has not fallen away from the lateral abdominal gutter in the prone position. In the lateral position, the bowel falls away from the lateral gutter, and a needle insertion site 10-12 cm from the midline is very safe. The needle can be used without the stylet as a precaution against entering the subarachnoid space.

Guidelines for the Lateral Approach

1. Maintain proper position of the patient.
2. Select the correct disc.
3. Select the correct insertion site (10-12 cm from the midline).
4. Approach the disc at the proper angle (60°).
5. Position the needle tip in the middle of the disc.
6. Inject the proper amount (2 cc or 4000 units) of active chymopapain into a clean disc space.

POSTOPERATIVE MANAGEMENT

The patient should be observed in the Recovery Room for at least one hour for any untoward effects. If the postinjection course has been uneventful for one hour, it is highly unlikely that any further complication will occur. The patient is then returned to the floor for early ambulation.

Early ambulation within a few hours of the procedure serves to reduce the back spasm that is so common after chymopapain injection (20% of cases) and allows for early discharge from the hospital. Early ambulation in corset support permits most patients to be discharged from the hospital on the day of or the day after the procedure. Most patients, especially the active young athlete, are pleased with the support that a canvas corset gives them during the first month. At the end of the first month, in most cases, the corset is discarded, analgesic medication is discontinued, and the patient becomes interested in a higher level of physical activity. It is at this time that the patients start a flexion exercise program designed to return them to their previously active life style. Most patients can start a swimming or bike-riding program 4 to 6 weeks after injection and are permitted heavier athletic activities (such as jogging) 3 months after injection.

High levels of physical activity, such as those pursued by the athlete, place significant demands on the low back. For a number of months after chymopapain injection, there is a sensation of weakness or instability in the low back that does not allow the achievement of high levels of physical activity such as professional contact sports. As a general rule, a professional athlete involved in contact sports requires 6 months to one year of rehabilitation before returning to that level of athletic activity after a chymopapain injection.

RESULTS

Results range from "no good" to 90 to 95 percent satisfactory. In my practice, the "good" result rate is approximately 70 percent, slightly higher for younger patients and at the L5–S1 level.

The most common cause of failure is an extruded, sequestered disc that responds nicely to microdiscectomy. You will be guaranteed a failure if you relax the criteria for the selection of patients.

MICROSURGICAL LUMBAR DISCOTOMY

WILLIAM J. HORSEY, M.D., F.R.C.S.(C), F.A.C.S.

Injuries to the low back are common in athletes. Most of these do not obviously involve the intervertebral discs. A few do result in herniation of the nucleus pulposus with sciatic nerve root interference. When sciatica occurs in persons active in sports, the onset is not often in the context of a recognizable precipitating solitary event of an accidental nature.

Most patients with sciatica improve with nonoperative management. Discotomy is reserved for the relief of intractable nerve root compression by a protruding intervertebral disc. This is its sole role, and it has no place in the treatment of other spinal conditions such as segmental instability and spinal stenosis.

Since Mixter and Barr's demonstration that the pain of sciatica could be relieved by the surgical removal of protruding intervertebral discs of the spinal canal, numerous technical modifications of the procedure have been developed. These have been prompted by advances in diagnostic methods which now render exploratory surgery almost obsolete, and by refinement of surgical technique engendered by better understanding of the purposes and limitations of the procedure. One of these refinements is the introduction of microsurgical technique.

Most disc protrusions consist of posterolateral herniation of the nucleus pulposus through a defect between fragmented interlacing fibers of the annulus fibrosus. Fragments that extrude through the full thickness of the annulus may remain confined by the posterior longitudinal ligament, which in turn may be lifted away from the annulus and from the posterior surface of the vertebra above or below. Pieces of disc tissue that break through the posterior longitudinal ligament lie sequestrated in the spinal canal. The protruding disc stretches, compresses, and irritates the adjacent nerve root, provoking pain, paresthesias, and neurologic deficit referable to that root. It is uncommon to have more than one nerve root involved by a herniation, and it is rare for more than one disc to herniate and cause symptoms simultaneously.

It is difficult to define the role of trauma in herniation. In young persons, it seems that the disc prolapse is associated with significant injury more frequently than in older individuals. Many of the latter refer to minor trauma, such as twisting the back at the onset of complaints, which may come on very rapidly. Conversely, in patients with significant trauma, disablement may be delayed for weeks or months, during which time only mild low back pain or buttock pain may be noticed. Young individuals with large herniations often complain of much pain but, despite the evidence of nerve root irritation, have remarkably little neurologic deficit. Consequently, they frequently are not treated adequately, especially in the early phases of the condition, because objective evidence of nerve root dysfunction is disproportionately small in comparison to the complaint. In adolescence, dislocation of a vertebral epiphysis is an uncommon result of injury, but it is important to recognize it, for it almost invariably demands surgical excision of the displaced fragments.

In about 60 percent of cases, the pain of sciatica caused by lumbar nerve root irritation due to a prolapsed disc subsides with nonoperative management, the mainstay of which is bedrest. The time required for remission varies considerably and is related to the severity of the pain, the severity of neurologic deficit, and the size of the prolapse, as shown on myelography or computerized tomography. In an initial attack, many authorities advise a period of 6 weeks of nonoperative management before considering investigation with a view to a surgical procedure, but in practice this is modified by the severity of the discomfort and the patient's ability to withstand it. The appearance of worsening motor deficit often demands early intervention. Pain that has subsided may return repeatedly, and if it recurs with intolerable frequency, surgical treatment may be required. In patients who have large central herniations, with disc fragments compressing the cauda equina and interfering with sphincter function, surgical treatment is carried out as soon as possible on an emergency basis.

The effectiveness of any therapy depends on the accuracy of diagnosis. The recognition of nerve root pain in a typical case is not difficult, especially if physical examination reveals appropriate motor, sensory, and reflex abnormalities in conjunction with signs of nerve root tension on straight leg raising and the bowstring test. The identification at the bedside of the particular root(s) involved and the disc responsible is not quite so certain. Characteristically, a low lumbar disc ruptures posterolaterally, and the root that it involves is the one that will emerge through the intervertebral foramen immediately below the level of the disc that is ruptured (e.g., the first sacral nerve root is involved in herniation of the lumbosacral disc). However, a laterally placed extrusion, especially if it extends cephalad, may involve the root emerging at the level of the disc. Furthermore, there are anatomic variations in segmentation and root distribution.

Radiographic studies are therefore needed to establish the level of the prolapse. Plain radiographs of the lumbar spine are a necessity if one is to have an appreciation of the anatomic features that must be known prior to any operative procedure. Not infrequently, they are normal, or nearly so, especially in younger individuals with herniations. Even when evidence of disc collapse and degenerative change is present, plain films in themselves do not provide sufficient information to allow one to proceed to operative therapy.

Myelography remains the principal investigative method in patients with disc disease. Computerized tomography is extremely useful and growing in its application. In many centers it has become the initial investigative technique, and it has largely displaced discography and epidural venography in the study of patients with problems affecting their nerve roots. When metrizamide myelography is inconclusive, much infor-

mation can be obtained by computerized tomography with the contrast medium in place.

It is undeniable that the traditional operation for the removal of prolapsed intervertebral discs is effective. It is equally incontestable that results are by no means uniformly good even when the diagnosis is accurate. There is a risk of damage to the roots and to the apophyseal joints, and there is a significant morbidity in the postoperative period. Even in cases judged to be successfully treated in the early phases, there may be continuing or recurrent disability due to reherniation or involvement of the nerve root in scar. Although many of these problems can be attributed to mechanical derangements, some are undoubtedly related to tethering or compression of the root by scar formation. Subarticular entrapment and pedicular kinking of the root may be significant sequelae of degenerative change.

Proponents of microsurgery believe that this modification minimizes problems inherent in traditional discotomy. It is claimed that there is less damage to the paraspinal muscles with the smaller exposure. By lessening the extent of removal of the ligamentum flavum, there is reduction in the area of scar dorsal to the dura covering the cauda equina. With less vigorous retraction on the root and the preservation of epidural fat, there is less opportunity for injury to the root and for scar formation with binding of the spinal muscles to the root and the dura. Following the removal of the extruded sequestrated fragment, there is no incision into the annulus fibrosus as the nucleus is removed through the defect in the annulus through which the herniation has occurred, allowing a small amount of fibrous tissue to reconstitute the integrity of the annulus.

Methods of carrying out microdiscotomy have been described by a number of authors, many of whom opine that different details of techniques are of great significance. Williams uses high magnification, avoids removal of bone, does not coagulate epidural veins, and does not incise the annulus fibrosus or curette the disc space. Under lower magnification, Wilson carries out a minimal removal of bone, coagulates the epidural veins if they obstruct access to the herniation, and carries out curettage of the disc space. Their published results are comparable. Seeger is unique in advocating a transverse incision. All recognize that special retractors and discotomy forceps facilitate the procedure.

AUTHOR'S TECHNIQUE

The patient is anesthetized, intubated, and placed prone on the operating table on bolsters or in the knee-chest position on a frame with the spine flexed. The hips and knees are not acutely bent. A stout hypodermic needle is inserted vertically into the skin at the level of the interspinous ligament judged to correspond to the level of the herniation. A lateral radiograph is used to confirm the position of the needle. The line of the incision is then marked on the skin. It is usually about 4 cm in length, although in obese persons it may be longer. At the lumbosacral level, the incision is centered over the interspinous space. At L4–L5, the incision is made from the upper margin of the spine of L4 to the upper margin of the spine of L5. At L3–L4, the incision is similarly marked. The back is then prepared and draped. The initial cut through the skin and subcutaneous tissues exposes the lumbodorsal fascia, which is then separated from its attachment to the spinous process and inter-spinous ligaments. (Alternatively, the fascia may be raised as a flap based on the spinous processes and reflected medially to expose the attachment of muscle to the bone and interspinous ligament.) The muscle is then separated from the bone and interspinous ligament on the side of the herniation by means of elevator or a cutting diathermy. Hemostasis is secured as muscle is dissected. The laminae and ligamentum flavum are exposed. A Williams microdiscotomy self-retaining retractor is then inserted. With a small elevator the lower margins of the lamina above, where it overhangs the ligamentum flavum, is cleared and a small amount of bone removed with an angled Kerrison-style rongeur. If necessary, the bone is waxed for hemostasis.

The microscope, with a 300-mm objective lens, is then brought into position and the ligamentum flavum incised longitudinally no more than 1 cm from its lateral limit. By means of a Kerrison-style rongeur, that portion of the ligament lateral to the incision is removed piece-meal. The epidural fat is exposed. Care is taken not to damage the apophyseal joints. A small amount of bone may be removed in the process of clearing the exposure laterally. With a small elevator, such as a Penfield No. 4 dissector, the floor of the spinal canal is palpated and the herniation and the nerve root identified by touch. In this way, the epidural fat is teased away from the disc, although every effort is made to preserve it where it covers the dura mater and root. The lateral edge of the nerve root is identified and eased medially to expose the herniation. Occasionally, sharp dissection is needed if these structures are firmly adherent. (More centrally placed herniations may be approached in the angle between the nerve root and the dural sac.) The summit of the bulging disc is visualized, and if necessary, a very superficial vertical incision, no more than 1 mm in depth, is made in the posterior longitudinal ligament. Only occasionally is it necessary to make a cruciate incision. The herniated portion of nucleus pulposus is then seen. It is grasped with a toothed Williams discotomy rongeur, and with the root well protected, the herniated nucleus pulposus is extracted. Usually, it comes in one or two substantial pieces, removal of which is followed by dramatically reduced tension on the nerve root. Irksome venous bleeding usually subsides, although it may be necessary to control it with a bipolar coagulator. The defect in the annulus through which the nucleus has come is often readily identified at this stage. It is not often necessary to make an incision in the annulus, as the Williams discotomy rongeurs can usually be introduced into the disc space easily in order that more nucleus may be removed. It is frequently necessary to loosen portions of the nucleus close to the defect in the annulus with a

3-mm ring curette. Typically, there is very little nucleus remaining in the disc space. No attempt is made to accomplish total removal of this material through the small opening in the annulus, which will probably heal soundly. A careful search is made with a blunt hook for sequestrated fragments or pieces of disc material which have extruded, lifting the posterior longitudinal ligament and migrating upward or downward posterior to the vertebral body. The root must appear slack and rounded before the quest for extruded tissue is abandoned.

If, as usually happens, some of the epidural fat has been lost from around the root, it is replaced with a free graft of subcutaneous fatty tissue. Hemostasis is secured and the wound closed with absorbable sutures in the fascia and subcutaneous tissues followed by a fine sub-cuticular, absorbable suture for the skin. A small dressing is applied.

Postoperatively, the patient is encouraged to be active. He is usually out of bed on the first postoperative day. The minimal dissection of muscle reduces postoper-ative pain, allowing for active cooperation in physio-therapy, including rapid mobilization and strengthening exercises. Injected analgesics are seldom needed after the first postoperative day. Postural retraining is often necessary, especially in those with lengthy disability. It is particularly important to prevent tethering of roots by scar, and to this end, active straight leg raising is begun as soon as it is tolerated. With the increasing level of activ-ity, good back hygiene is emphasized.

With the foregoing regimen of patient selection and treatment, over 90 percent of the patients have an excel-lent or good result and are able to resume within 3 months all the activities in which they engaged prior to the onset of sciatica. However, in the athlete it must be recognized that herniation of a lumbar intervertebral disc is a significant event. It indicates that there is an abnormal spinal segment with degenerative disease. These may remain symptomatic or vulnerable to further stresses. Loss of nucleus pulposus reduces the volume of contents of the annulus fibrosus so that the latter must bear more vertical compression force between the verte-brae. In comparison with traditional discotomy, the microtechnique allows for the addition of less damage to the annulus during the operation and therefore better preservation of that structure.

Although many athletes are able to resume sports, it is unusual for a person to return to body-contact games and competition in which exceptional muscular strength is required, e.g., rugby, football, wrestling, and weight-lifting. In these activities, there is a possibility of injuring the abnormal spinal segment in which degeneration has begun and has already caused significant problems. Although many persons with degenerative disc disease escape further difficulties on returning to strenuous activity, there are those who suffer a relapse in which the predominant symptom is low back and buttock pain rather than sciatica. Still others, who take exceptional care to protect themselves, have a return of symptoms. With the aforementioned notable exceptions, it is not justifiable to proscribe all or even most forms of athletic endeavor, provided the patient can tolerate them. In comparison to traditional discotomy, microsurgery seems to offer an improved likelihood of continuing with a life of relatively little restriction of activity.

Notwithstanding the relief of sciatica due to nerve root irritation, some patients have continuing back pain for several weeks following the procedure. It is almost invariably associated with paravertebral muscle spasm and sciatic scoliosis. There is no evidence on investigation of the majority of these that there is any infection. With judicious rest, postural retraining, and graded exercise, most of these patients fare very well. The complaints are probably related to a mechanical derangement at the segment. Resumption of vigorous activity by these individuals is regulated cautiously.

SHOULDER INJURIES

SHOULDER ARTHROSCOPY AND ATHLETIC INJURIES

A.M. WILEY, M.Ch., F.R.C.S., F.R.C.S.(C)

The accurate diagnosis of soft tissue lesions of the shoulder is primarily dependent on thoughtful and regulated clinical examination. Such examination is often necessarily repeated at intervals and supplemented by routine and special x-ray examinations: arthrotomography for the labrum, contrast and double-contrast arthrography, and even "bursography" of the subacromial bursa. There are a number of conditions which remain less than well defined; depending upon the etiology, these have been called "supraspinatus tendinitis", "rotator tendinitis", or, in the swimmer, "swimmer's shoulder". The term "instability", when applied to the shoulder, may quite accurately refer to dislocations, to subluxations, to the much more obscure condition of hypermobility, and to giving way due to intra-articular "seizure". Whereas the first two varieties obviously imply a gross disarticulation, it is surprising how they are defined in the literature in varied terms. This matter is given some consideration merely to emphasize the imprecision with which certain soft tissue lesions of the shoulder are described, especially in cases involving athletes.

Hypermobility implies overlaxity, which may be either congenital (in fibroelastosis) or acquired from injury or repeated stress, such as in swimmers and certain throwers. A shoulder may be hypermobile if there has been muscular paralysis, in which case it may sublux inferiorly to the confusion of an unwary radiologist; this may even occur temporarily after exploring the joint.

In an effort to define this subject with more clarity, Figure 1 presents these conditions in the form of a diagram, the use of which may enable the clinician, when testing the shoulder, to categorize the abnormality and direct treatment. Especially in athletic injuries, the development of arthroscopy has proved of value in defining shoulder conditions, in detecting their severity and planning management, and as means of endoscopic treatment.

TECHNIQUE OF ARTHROSCOPY

Initial experiments with the arthroscope suggested the use of a small-size sheath (3.8 mm), but subsequently it was found quite simple to use a standard 5-mm sheath. Posterior instrumentation is recommended; the patient should be given a general anesthetic to enable the arm to be distracted and maneuvered by an assistant. This may be especially important if the joint has to be enlarged to permit instrumental surgery. A pulley may be attached to the arm for this purpose, but brachial plexus lesions

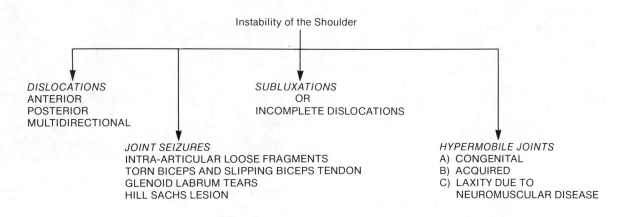

Figure 1   Instability of the shoulder

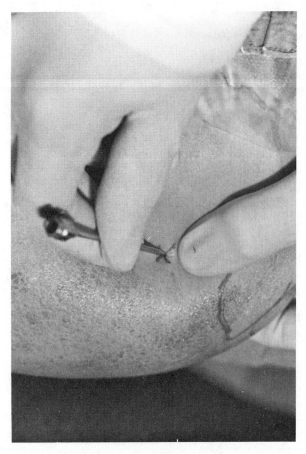

Figure 2   Insertion of the arthroscope

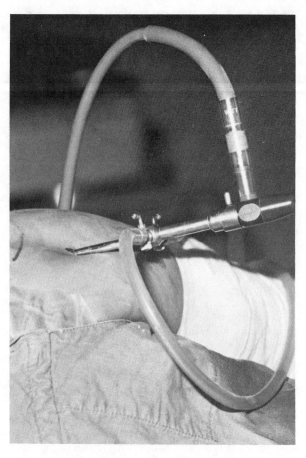

Figure 3   The arthroscope in position

have been recorded. An assistant seems to be a better solution; he can also support the articulated arm of a television camera. The instrument is inserted 2 centimeters below the angle of the acromion, with the patient in the lateral sit-up position on the operating table. Local anesthesia, using Marcaine, may be used in unusual circumstances but usually obviates the important manipulative maneuvers. The shoulder may be examined in three segments, supraglenoid, glenoid, and infraglenoid (Figs. 2, 3).

In the supraglenoid view, the long head of the biceps and the undersurface of the rotator cuff are seen. The head of the humerus and its posterosuperior aspect should be carefully searched for the depression which may deepen into an ulcer, known as Hill-Sachs lesion. In the glenoid view, the labrum is seen. Slow withdrawal of the telescope reveals the posterior labrum. Anterior advancement reveals the glenohumeral ligaments which are often torn (Figure 4). In the infraglenoid recess are often found loose bodies, but seldom is the space obliterated.

The examiner should take the opportunity to measure the capacity of the joint when first distending it prior to inserting the arthroscope. Normally, the joint accepts 35 ml; amounts greater than this suggest a rotator cuff leak or a voluminous capsule associated with "hyper-mobility". A capacity of less then 35 ml is noted both in frozen shoulders and postsurgical contractures.

At the conclusion of the examination and not

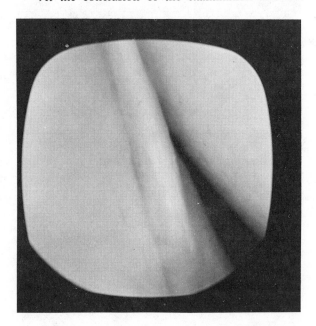

Figure 4   The glenoid labrum seen in glenoid view

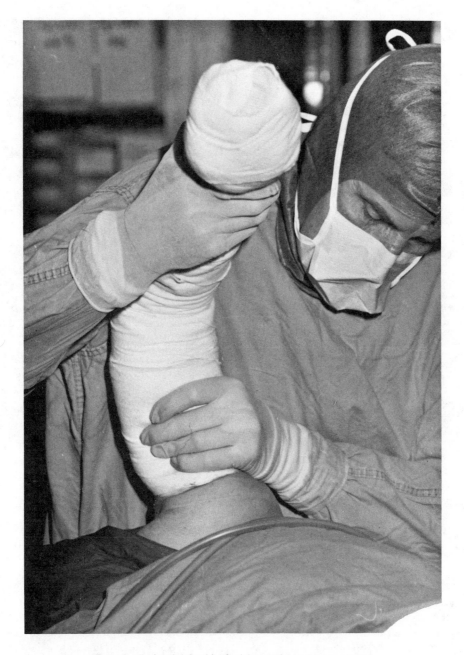

Figure 5 Testing the shoulder for labrum click and for instability

before, so as to avoid intra-articular bleeding, the examiner should test the joint for anterior, posterior, and inferior dislocation. This maneuver requires practice. I have been struck with indecision in cases where the shoulder slips from posterior dislocation into the glenoid cavity, thus mimicking an *anterior* dislocation, or vice versa, an anterior dislocation relocates backward suggesting *posterior* displacement. Even more perplexing may be the appearance of multidirectional dislocations which require complex management. These maneuvers may be assisted by viewing under the image intensifier. With the patient in the arthroscopy position, the C-arm

may be quite easily applied, though testing in this position requires that he be firmly immobilized by chest rests or supports to avoid displacement from the field of vision of the x-ray.

Finally, the surgeon may compress the humeral head against the glenoid while rotating the arm and thereby elicit a "labrum click". He may be able to demonstrate joint contracture and restriction indicative of "frozen shoulder" or postoperative contracture (Figure 5). A proportion of patients suffering from definitive intra-articular abnormality actually experience symptomatic relief (usually transitory) after these maneuvers.

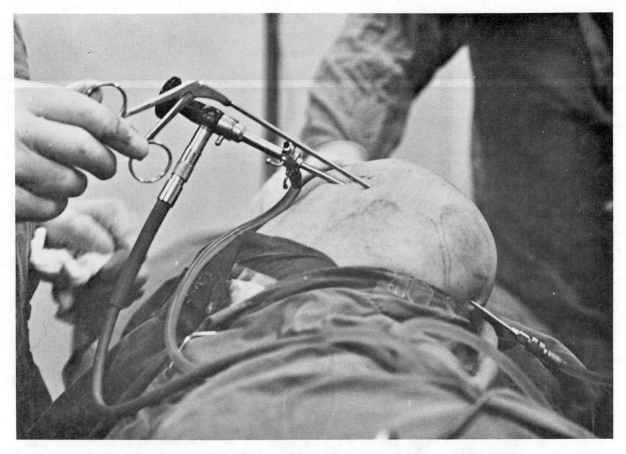

Figure 6   Posterior instrumentation using curved or straight scissors

ADVANTAGES AND DISADVANTAGES

There are five advantages to arthroscopy.

(1)   The procedure provides extended diagnostic facility.
(2)   There is negligible morbidity (two complications in 500 procedures; no infection).
(3)   The procedure affords a high degree of accuracy. (Fifteen cases of rotator cuff injury explored; arthroscopy found accurate in 14.)
(4)   There is less discomfort for the patient than results from arthrography.
(5)   Arthroscopy provides recognizable therapeutic benefit to patients with stiffening of the shoulder.

There are two disadvantages to arthroscopy.

(1)   General anesthesia is required.
(2)   This is an invasive procedure, although no infections have been reported so far.

ARTHROSCOPIC SURGERY OF THE SHOULDER

The facility with which the shoulder may be arthroscoped with standard equipment has prompted the handling and manipulation of intra-articular lesions.

Technique

Two portals are commonly used for bimanual instrumentation. As in the knee joint, operating arthroscopes have proved to be less versatile than instruments inserted through separate portals. Also, 7-mm operative arthroscopes are too large for the shoulder.

Portal 1.   Curved instruments (2–5 mm) can be inserted posteriorly 3 to 4 cm lateral and superior to the sheath of the examining instrument. This enables a rotator cuff to be debrided or a glenoid labrum to be resected (Figure 6).

Portal 2, the anterior portal.   The telescope of the examining instrument is thrust across the joint to shine through the capsule. A small incision enables a trocar to be inserted for a probe, a curette, or a basket or powered chondrotome. Use has been made of this route to insert pegs or staples into the labrum and glenoid margin in the repair of recurrent shoulder dislocation (Figure 7).

SHOULDER ARTHROSCOPY IN THE ATHLETE

The foregoing account of the technique of arthroscopic shoulder surgery emphasizes the role that such instrumentation will undoubtedly play in the future in both diagnosis and treatment of shoulder conditions in both young and old patients. The instruments are now

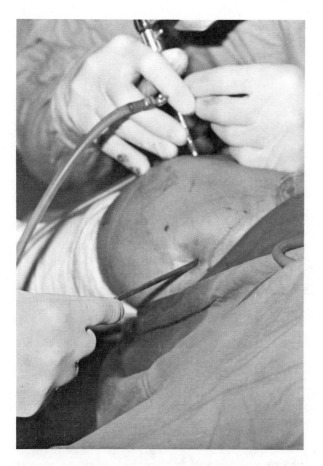

Figure 7 Using an anterior portal to introduce a straight instrument

usually available in orthopaedic departments; expertise can result only from practice. Although the special x-ray techniques are no doubt useful, many are painful. Some become complicated and few are as accurate as direct visualization.

I have used the arthroscope extensively in the diagnosis and management of rotator cuff tears, the vast majority of which occur in middle-aged and elderly patients. I have, of course, encountered both incomplete and complete cuff tears in the young athlete and recommend open surgery for the latter. Arthroscopic debridement of incomplete cuff tears is currently under review.

SHOULDER INSTABILITY

Direct visualization and manipulation under the image intensifier may reveal dislocation, subluxation, hypermobility, or intra-articular loose bodies. I have reviewed 51 patients with dislocation or subluxation who have had either a Bankart operation, a Putti-Platt procedure, or a Bristow procedure. The decision as to which procedure would be used was based on the arthroscopic findings. Thus, when a Bankart lesion was discovered, a Bankart procedure was carried out. A lax capsule prompted a Putti-Platt procedure. Hypermobility was treated by a Bristow procedure, particularly when limitation of rotation was to be avoided, for example, in the

throwing athlete. Multidirectional dislocation was treated by simultaneous anterior and posterior repair.

In a review of results, only one patient had a recurrence. He had a Putti-Platt procedure for a Bankart lesion (an error). One patient became subject to repeated subluxation after having been a habitual "dislocator": he had a Bristow procedure. A large Hill-Sachs lesion was missed at arthroscopy.

THE TORN GLENOID LABRUM AND BICEPS TENDON LESIONS

This is a lesion that occurs in throwing athletes. The examiner must be careful to search for dislocation. In the absence of dislocation, the clicking phenomenon with or without joint "seizure" may derive from a torn labrum. The patient may benefit from removal of the torn labrum. Of 15 cases so treated, 13 were improved and required no further surgery. A long-term follow-up of such cases is in progress.

Encountered also in some athletes were incomplete tears of the long head of the biceps; local debridement may be beneficial. In some instances, particularly when there had been previous subacromial surgery, the long head of the biceps was found adherent to the undersurface of the rotator cuff. The clinical implications of this lesion are undetermined at present. It seems quite possible that some residual symptoms after acromioplasty, especially a dragging sensation after excessive elbow flexion, may be the result of this lesion. This condition appears not to have been described in the literature; it is readily treatable with an intra-articular scissors.

LOOSE BODIES

Loose bodies may or may not be radiopaque. Searching joints in the athlete with the arthroscope has often revealed a surprising number of loose fragments; these are quite common where instability is neglected or, alas, untreated! Loose bodies are removable by grasping (again using curved instruments introduced posteriorly) or by suction, either through a separate portal or applied to the arthroscopic sheath without the telescope.

ARTHROSCOPIC SURGERY FOR RECURRENT DISLOCATION

Eight patients have had a more complicated endoscopic repair following persistent instability after a previous repair performed elsewhere. Three maneuvers were used: (1) arthroscopic intra-articular curettage of the anterior glenoid labrum; (2) the same, with resection of the labrum (in both instances I placed the arm postoperatively by the side with internal rotation for 3 weeks); and (3) stud wiring of a loose glenoid labrum. To date, a review of these patients shows that all those treated by "pinning" the labrum to the glenoid margin have remained satisfactory, whereas those treated by curettage, with or without labrum excision, followed by

immobilization of the arm, have presented continuing symptoms.

DISLOCATIONS OF THE SHOULDER: ACROMIOCLAVICULAR AND STERNOCLAVICULAR JOINTS

R.PETER WELSH, M.B., Ch.B., F.R.C.S.(C), F.A.C.S.

Dislocations of the glenohumeral and acromioclavicular (AC) joints are relatively common in contact sports, whereas dislocation of the sternoclavicular joint is a relatively uncommon injury.

Dislocation of the shoulder usually results from a fall on the outstretched arm. Longitudinal loading along the axis of the limb drives the humeral head out of the glenoid, tearing the anterior or anteroinferior capsule and detaching the glenoid labrum from the glenoid rim to create a Bankart lesion.

Separation of the shoulder is indeed an apt eponym for dislocation of the acromioclavicular joint, for the injury is usually incurred in a fall on the point of the shoulder. Here the shoulder is driven downward, the force of the impact separating, as it were, the upper extremity from the rest of the torso. With complete dislocation there is disruption not only at the acromioclavicular joint, with tearing of its capsule and meniscus, but a disruption of the conoid and trapezoid ligaments of the coracoclavicular complex as well as tearing of the adjacent deltoid and trapezius musculature.

Sternoclavicular disruption, though uncommon, can be life-threatening in that the posterior displacement of the clavicle can compromise the airway by tracheal impingement. Direct trauma, as in a blow to the chest, is the most common cause of injury, but with a fall on the shoulder the transmission of loads through the clavicle may induce disruption of the sternoclavicular joint with medial and posterior displacement of the clavicle relative to the sternum.

GLENOHUMERAL DISLOCATION

A traumatic dislocation of the shoulder should be reduced as soon as possible whether it occurs in the gymnasium, on the basketball court, or on a ski hill. Early reduction, done before muscle spasm makes things too tight, can usually be effected by the Hippocratic technique, with gentle traction on the extremity and a counter force from a stockinged foot placed in the axilla.

A careful neurovascular evaluation should be made before and after the maneuver, for occasionally there may be associated damage to the brachial plexus or axillary nerve.

Should there be a delay in reduction, laying the patient prone with the weight suspended from the dependent limb may encourage muscle relaxation sufficient to allow spontaneous reduction. Should this fail, it may be necessary to resort to closed reduction under sedation or anesthesia. Open reduction is rarely necessary, but if there is an associated fracture, manipulation alone may not be effective. However, even under these circumstances, manipulative reduction should be attempted as a first-line treatment.

Protection in a shoulder immobilizer for 5 to 6 weeks should be practiced with all primary dislocations in young athletes. A period of intense rehabilitation follows, concentrating on gentle mobilizing exercises with pendulum and pulley drills and pushup and punching bag activity for strength. External rotation and overhead stretch and abduction are restricted for 3 months from the time of injury; contact sports can be resumed thereafter as strength and mobility return to normal levels. In a study of over 300 athletes suffering primary dislocation who were treated in this manner, only 17 percent had recurrence of their dislocation. This is a vast improvement on figures generally quoted for this injury and amply demonstrates the efficacy of conservative treatment in primary traumatic dislocation.

Recurrent Dislocation

In those athletes who suffer subsequent episodes of dislocation, immobilization is ineffective, and if strengthening exercises and modification of activity fail to control the situation, surgical stabilization may be necessary. There are several types of surgical repair in common use, each technique having its proponents and detractors. The objectives, however, are similar, that is, to stabilize the shoulder with minimal restriction of motion afterwards. In all cases, the pathology must be fully addressed, first with closure of the Bankart lesion, then reefing of the redundant capsule, and, finally, tightening of the envelope musculature. Occasionally, in longstanding cases with bony involvement of the humeral head or rarely of the glenoid rim, more elaborate techniques with bone grafting need to be employed.

Immobilization after surgery should be limited in most instances to no more than 3 weeks, followed by a conservative program of exercise, progressing to resisted strengthening and overhead work by 6 weeks. Contact sports should be restricted for 12 weeks.

In reviewing a large number of surgically stabilized shoulders, the major impediment to a return to optimal athletic performance was the restriction of overhead reach and external rotation. In throwers, a persistent sense of loss of power in overhead throwing was also a common complaint. In undertaking surgical repair in the throwing athlete, this possible limitation on subsequent performance may be encountered even though the shoulder has been stabilized and adequate range and recovery achieved.

ACROMIOCLAVICULAR DISRUPTION

In a partial shoulder separation, the AC joint capsule is severely strained, and, with partial rupture of the coracoclavicular ligament, the joint becomes unstable in a horizontal plane. The clavicle subluxates posteriorly, particularly when the arm is abducted across the chest or when the patient lies on the affected side. This movement is extremely painful, and control can be obtained with a figure 8 type shoulder harness for 3 to 4 weeks. Following immobilization, overhead movement is restricted until the sixth week, and contact sports should not be resumed until the eighth week.

With complete separation of the AC joint, the coracoclavicular ligaments and AC joint capsule are totally disrupted; and the clavicle becomes unstable in the vertical plane, with the outer end of the clavicle presenting prominently. This injury can be treated conservatively in all but extreme cases with a figure 8 harness for 4 to 6 weeks. A complete reduction is seldom maintained; but a reduction in the size of a lump at the AC joint is achieved, and functional return is excellent although return to contact sport should be restricted for 2 months.

In those extreme cases where the clavicle is grossly prominent, surgical reduction can be undertaken. Additionally, internal fixation will be required either across the AC joint with pins or screws or by stabilization of the clavicle to the coracoid with a screw, fascia, or, as has been advocated by some, a loop of prosthetic ligament.

It has been shown, however, that operative treatment is associated with a far greater morbidity than when this third-degree lesion is treated conservatively. A return to work or sports has been found to be delayed twice as long in those treated surgically, so that it is recommended that only those with the grossest instability should be treated per primum in this manner.

Late Acromioclavicular Instability and Degenerative Change

A few adolescents who have sustained injury to the AC joint may show autolysis of the outer end of the clavicle and supervening degenerative change. Older patients may have mild residual instability and go on to develop degenerative changes also. Clinically, they show localized pain at the AC joint, pain on overhead reach, and pain on resisted abduction of the shoulder or adduction of the arm across the chest. This group, along with those with continuing symptomatic instability of a more major degree, are all very well handled by late stabilization of the AC joint by means of modified excisional arthroplasty as recommended by Carter Rowe.

Technique

The 10-cm surgical incision centered at the AC joint is made along the line of the clavicle, continuing laterally over the acromion. The soft tissues are incised in a similar line to expose the outer end of the clavicle. Here, adequate resection of the clavicle tip ($\sim$ 1 cm) is carried out and the prominence bevelled to remove the bump. The clavicle is then reduced and the carefully preserved soft tissue envelope closed in layers. Protection in a sling is maintained for 3 weeks with light sports activity at 6 weeks and contact sports by 3 months.

STERNOCLAVICULAR DISLOCATION

Acute posterior dislocation of the clavicle requires emergency reduction. Until this is achieved, the patient should be maintained supine with shoulders braced backward, a bolster or sandbag between the shoulder blades, and with careful attention paid to maintaining the patient's respiratory status.

General anesthetic with endotracheal intubation should be practiced and reduction undertaken, closed if possible, using towel clips to grasp the clavicle and manipulate the reduction. Open reduction may be necessary in refractory cases, in which instance stabilization is further enhanced with screw fixation and, perhaps, fascial reinforcement. Excision of this joint should never be undertaken since it leads to a gross and disabling instability pattern.

Occasionally, a partial subluxation of the sternoclavicular joint may be encountered; if the subluxation proves stable, it can be left in an unreduced state since it will often stabilize in location. A CT scan will be required, however, in order to clearly evaluate the exact status of this joint which is very difficult to visualize with standard x-ray techniques.

Occasionally, persistent late instability of the sternoclavicular joint can arise, in which case stabilization is necessary, utilizing fascia or subclavius tendon in order to rebuild the ligamentous support.

SHOULDER SUBLUXATION IN THE ATHLETE

CARTER R. ROWE, M.D.

One of the most disconcerting shoulder problems to the athlete is transient subluxation. I recall in the 1950s and 60s athletes who were seen because of sudden, unexplained pain and weakness of their shoulder following a forceful hyperextension of their arm or direct blow to the shoulder. They complained of a "dead arm" due to pain and loss of the functional capacity of the arm in overhead activities. X-ray studies would be normal and physical examination unrevealing. Some of the athletes were, unfortunately, considered "no longer productive", "uncertain and undependable", and a few were even marked as having lost their spirit as a player. The athletes, to say the least, were frustrated, as were their referring physicians.

My first introduction to this syndrome was with an athlete in the early 1960s who, after seeing a number of consultants and was no better, requested that we "look into" his shoulder. To our surprise, we found a well-developed Bankart lesion, which, after repair, returned this young man to full athletic performance. Interestingly, he gave no history of instability or looseness of his shoulder joint following his injury.

In 1969, Blazina and Satzman reported on a number of patients with recurrent anterior subluxation of the shoulder and brought this problem to the attention of doctors treating athletes. However, this report covered only those patients who were *aware* of their shoulders slipping in and out during the use of their arms. There remained the athletes with the same shoulder problem, but who were *unaware* that their shoulders were unstable. Their only complaint was a sudden "severe pain" when attempting to throw, serve in tennis, or swim forcefully overhand due to a temporary "dead arm".

In 1981, my associate, Dr. Bertram Zarins, and I reported our experience with the "dead arm" syndrome, reviewing 60 shoulders in 58 patients who had recurrent transient anterior subluxation of the shoulder. Of specific interest was the identification of two separate groups with this problem: group I, consisting of 26 patients who were aware of their shoulder subluxation, and group II, consisting of 32 patients who were not aware that subluxation was occurring, but only of a painful paralyzing pain. Identification of the cause in group II was much more difficult than in group I. It is interesting that both groups had similar mechanisms of injury, similar symptoms and physical findings, comparable pathologic lesions at operation, and similar results after the same surgical treatment. Other authors have reported their experience with recurrent transient subluxation.

DIAGNOSIS

Pain and dysfunction of the athlete's arm may be due to a number of conditions. It is most important to consider carefully the mechanics of injury. Was the injury due to a direct or indirect injury? In what position was the arm when injured? Was it due to repetitive or forceful use of the arm? Also, on examination, how did the patient reproduce the pain? What positions of his arm does he avoid? In the differential diagnosis, a number of conditions should be considered, such as:

1. Impingement syndromes (subacromial tendinitis and bursitis)
2. Bicipital tendinitis

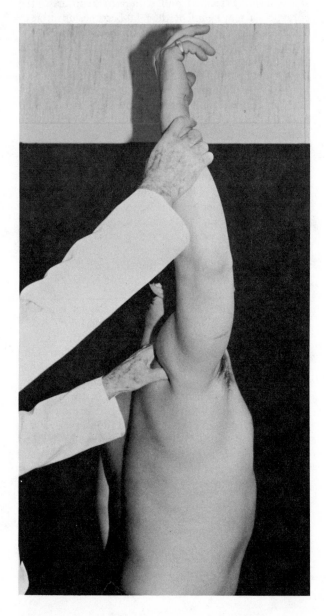

Figure 1 The "apprehension" test with the patient standing, the arm in elevation and external rotation, and pressure applied posteriorly to the humeral head.

3. Rotator cuff tears
4. Thoracic outlet syndrome
5. Suprascapular nerve pressure
6. Cervical disc and other causes of referred pain
7. Circulatory deficits
8. Acromioclavicular instability or traumatic changes.

The characteristic features of recurrent transient anterior subluxation of the shoulder are:

1. The *history* of a forceful hyperextension or over-extension of the elevated arm, such as a quarterback being "sacked" in football, or a direct blow to the posterior aspect of the shoulder, a fall on the outstretched arm, and, in some instances, excessive pitching or serving in tennis, or excessive swimming using the butterfly or breast stroke.

2. On *physical examination*, reproduction of pain with the patient standing by putting stretch on the anterior capsule with the arm in elevation and external rotation and pressure applied posteriorly to the humeral head. This is referred to as the "apprehension test" (Fig. 1). This, in fact, is the position in which the athlete delivers power in throwing or serving in tennis or in forcefully swimming.

3. Reproduction of instability and pain with the patient lying supine with the arm abducted and elevated and posterior pressure applied to the humeral head (Fig. 2).

4. Absence of pain when the arm is used anterior to the coronal plane, or below shoulder level.

5. Absence of pain on palpation of the rotator cuff, bicipital groove, or the acromioclavicular joint.

6. Absence of neurologic findings.

It is of interest that in group II, 55 percent of the patients had been previously diagnosed as having some condition other than subluxation when first seen by us, such as "pinched" nerve, bursitis or tendinitis, or impingement or subluxation of the bicipital tendon. Fourteen percent had had incorrect surgical procedures performed on their shoulders. When the diagnosis is in

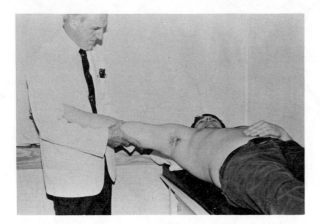

Figure 2   Pressure applied to the anterior or posterior capsule with the patient supine.

doubt, arthroscopy or arthrotomography should give additional information. We did not, however, find it necessary to depend on the demonstration of instability of the shoulder, either clinically or by fluoroscopy, to make the diagnosis.

PATHOLOGIC FINDINGS

Bankart lesions were found in 64 percent of our operated shoulders, mild in 17, moderately severe in 10, and severe in 5. Excessive laxity of the anterior capsule was present in 13 shoulders or 26 percent of the 50 surgical repairs. Increase of the interval between the subscapularis and supraspinatus tendon was found in 20 of the 37 shoulders in which the superior aspect of the shoulder was explored at the time of surgery. Hill-Sachs lesions of the humeral head were present in 40 percent of the 60 shoulders, and traumatic changes of the anterior glenoid rim were present in 45 percent in which the true axillary view was taken.

TREATMENT

Conservative Treatment

We have found that in roughly 13 percent, a program of specific resistive exercises in abduction, external rotation, and internal rotation restored functional stability and eliminated the need of surgical repair.

Operative Treatment

When a Bankart lesion was present at surgery, a standard Bankart procedure was performed (Fig. 3). When a Bankart lesion was absent and the pathology was due to excessive laxity or redundancy of the capsule, a modified capsulorrhaphy was performed (Fig. 4). We did not find it necessary to use other surgical procedures, although the capsulorrhaphies of Neer and Protzman have been reported successful. If a Bankart procedure is to be used, specially designed instruments are necessary and helpful. The head retractor must be a correct one, in order to give adequate exposure. The rim of the glenoid must be freshened and the holes in the rim carefully completed with proper instruments which are now available. We have avoided using any type of metal such as staples, screws, or pins. We emphasize the value of careful layer-by-layer exposure of the shoulder joint as only by careful dissection can the surgical lesion be identified. Without careful separation of the subscapularis tendon and muscle from the capsule, one would not be able to determine the degree of laxity of the capsule and whether it was a factor in the shoulder's instability. In throwing sports, the only pathologic lesion may be abnormal redundancy or laxity of the capsule, in which case a modified capsulorrhaphy is indicated. Thus, the routine of careful anatomic exposure, identification of the lesions, correction of the lesions, and returning the muscle layers to their original insertions with as little trauma to the tissues as possible will go far to ensure preservation of strong, stable, rhythmic, and coordinated shoulder motion. The surgical procedure should be designed to restore complete range of motion to the shoulder, rather than to depend on restriction of motion for stability.

Postoperative Care

The postoperative management is similar to that used after surgical repair for recurrent anterior dislocation of the shoulder. A sling is used for only 2 or 3 days, after which the arm is free. We have found that early motion of the shoulder has eliminated the need for physical therapy. The patient is instructed in gentle pendulum exercises, and the use of the arm and shoulder as tolerated. At 6 weeks, the patient is instructed in gradual resistive exercises in abduction to 50 degrees, inward and outward rotation of the arm, and water therapy if available. At 3 months, with increasing range of motion, swimming, rowing, and taking part in light sports is advised. At 6 months, complete range of motion is expected and contact sports and heavy labor are permitted if, at that time, the patient is not apprehensive and has strong muscles and functional range of motion.

Results

The results of surgery for transient subluxation of the shoulder over a 4-year follow-up period (ranging from 2 to 16 years post operation) were: 70 percent, excellent results; 24 percent, good results; and 6 percent, fair results. All results were graded on a 100-unit rating system.

With an *excellent* result (90 to 100 units) there was no limitation of function in sports or work, and the patient was able to throw a baseball or football hard, to serve hard in tennis, and to swim forcefully, with no pain, no instability, and 95 to 100 percent of motion. A *good* result must register 70 to 89 units, and a *fair* result must register 40 to 69 units. *Poor* results were those with 39 units or less. We had no poor results in our series. Of the 33 dominant shoulders, 64 percent were able to return to throwing hard in baseball or football. One of this group returned to pitching for a large state university, relieved of his so-called "dead arm", which had disabled him for 2 years. Seven patients were unable to pitch in baseball, but could play football, use their shoulders forcefully overhead, and play tennis. Two patients returned as professional tennis instructors, and two patients continued playing in the national hockey league without recurrence. Of the 15 nondominant shoulders, 87 percent had no limitation in sports or work and returned to all activities in which they had participated before injury. It is interesting that of eight patients operated on, whose injury was produced by hard throwing, four were graded excellent and could throw hard and four had good results but were unable to pitch. They could throw a football a long distance and play tennis.

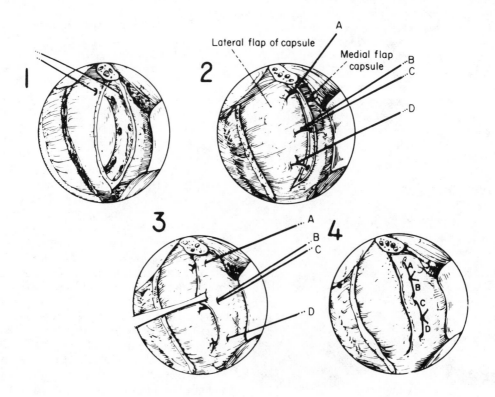

Figure 3   The standard Bankart procedure (when a Bankart lesion is present): 1, Three holes in the freshened anterior glenoid rim. 2, Suturing the lateral flap of capsule to the rim. 3, Passing the sutures through the medial capsule. 4, Tying sutures A to B, and C to D, thus double-breasting the capsule securely along the rim of glenoid.

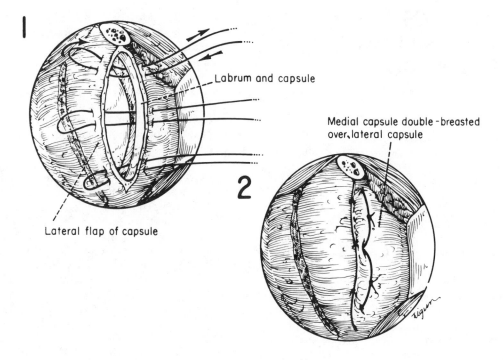

Figure 4   Modified capsulorrhaphy (when a Bankart lesion is not present): 1. The suture is passed under the attached labrum out through the lateral capsule and back under the labrum at three or four levels, thus double-breasting the lateral capsule under the medial capsule. 2. When there is multidirectional instability, the repair can be carried further inferiorly and posteriorly.

Complications

There were no infections or serious complications in the 50 shoulders that had undergone operation. One patient experienced a postoperative hematoma which after evacuation healed per primum. One patient developed a postoperative thrombophlebitis of his cephalic vein which resolved. No patient experienced recurrence of subluxation or dislocation after surgical repair.

Late Radiographic Changes

Our experience in surgery for transient anterior subluxation was similar to that for shoulders with recurrent anterior dislocations in 1978, in which no significant degenerative changes of the joint were present at follow-up examination. One patient had mild degenerative changes preoperatively from an initial severe blow to the shoulder; 5 years following our repair, these changes had not increased.

DISCUSSION

In an athlete who has experienced a sudden over-extension of his shoulder, or a fall on the outstretched arm, or who subsequently is unable to throw overhead, serve hard in tennis, play basketball, or swim forcefully overhead because of a sudden sharp piercing pain in his shoulder, anterior transient subluxation of the shoulder should be considered. The athlete with this condition frequently refers to his arm as being "dead". As a rule, no conservative treatment has benefited him. He is usually frustrated and discouraged. A positive apprehension test, in which the patient's symptoms are reproduced with the arm in elevation and external rotation, should strongly suggest transient subluxation and a deficit of the anterior capsular mechanism.

Differential diagnosis must be carefully considered, especially subacromial impingement of the rotator cuff or a thoracic outlet syndrome. We have not encountered instability or subluxation of the long head of the biceps in the young active athlete. Increase in the interval between the subscapularis and supraspinatus tendon should be noted, as this may be a factor in above-shoulder functions of the arm.

A question frequently asked is whether it is necessary to demonstrte subluxation of the shoulder before diagnosis can be made. We have not found this to be necessary. Much more significant is the history and examination of the patient.

During the past few years, in questionable cases of whether the disease is located under the acromion or in the glenohumeral joint, arthroscopy has proved to be a great help, as the glenoid rim can be adequately examined, the course of the biceps tendon identified, the articular surface of the rotator cuff clearly inspected, and disease to the anterior capsule identified. Although double-contrast arthrography or arthrotomography has proved helpful, we obtain more information from arthroscopy.

RECURRENT POSTERIOR LUXATION AND DISLOCATION OF THE SHOULDER

VIRGIL R. MAY, Jr., M.D., F.A.C.S., A.A.O.S., C.O.A.

The shoulder is the most mobile joint of the musculoskeletal system and thus lacks stability under certain stresses. It allows all functions of the forearm and hand and all reflex protective motions of the arms. All parts of this complex system of at least seven joints must be in harmony with each other to meet the demands of work and recreation, especially in athletic endeavors. Strenuous athletic competition is now the world-wide way of life.

Posterior traumatic dislocations are much less common than anterior traumatic dislocations. Wilson and McKeever, in their review of 260 dislocations of the shoulder, found four instances of posterior dislocations —an incidence of 1.5 percent. McLaughlin reported an incidence of 3.8 percent in a review of 581 shoulder dislocations, 22 of which had posterior dislocations. Wood reported three posterior dislocations from a series of 115 dislocations of the shoulder joint from the Massachusetts General Hospital—an incidence of 2.6 percent. The incidence of the recurrent disabling type is even lower. In the initial luxation or dislocation, fracture of the lesser tuberosity or an inferior avulsion fracture from the glenoid may occur, causing either capsular tears with fragmentation of the posterior glenoid rim or stripping of the periosteum and capsule from the scapular neck posterior. These pathologic occurrences all lead to recurrent posterior luxations or dislocations. Associated arterial and nerve compromise is rare.

In the treatment of this entity the objective is to restore the anatomy of the shoulder joint and improve its function as completely as possible. To accomplish this, one must understand the mechanism of injury. Careful systematic examination of the structures and their functions must be fully comprehended as the examiner reviews the functional anatomy. Documentation of the extent of injury to the soft tissues and bone by history, physical examination, roentgenograms, computer tomography, and arthroscopy is necessary for decision-making with regard to the appropriate treatment, be it surgical repair or a conservative regimen of muscle building and improvement of range of motion. Counseling the patient as to participation in athletic endeavors or job change is also appropriate.

ETIOLOGY

Trauma by direct and indirect forces may produce lesions to the soft supporting tissues and bone. Acute disruptive lesions may cause painful malfunction of the shoulder joint. At the time of impact, the severity of posterior traumatic dislocation is influenced by the position of the hand, forearm, and humerus at the glenohumeral joint. Abnormal positioning of the arm at the glenohumeral joint produces stress on the posterior shoulder capsule and on the glenohumeral ligaments. A fall on the internally rotated hand or forearm with the elbow flexed and the humerus adducted at the shoulder joint results in posterior dislocation of the shoulder. A direct posterior blow to the shoulder may also create a posterior dislocation (Fig. 1). If the shearing force is great enough as the humeral head is swept over the posterior rim of the glenoid, a fracture occurs through the anatomical neck, or through the lesser tuberosity or at the posterior glenoid rim (Fig. 2). The natural architecture of the shoulder joint makes it less vulnerable to posterior recurrent luxations and dislocations than to anterior recurrent dislocations. The acromion process and the normal angle of anterior glenoid tilt act as a buffer against the posterior force. The angle of the scapula as it glides over the posterior rib cage in a 45-degree angulation tends to protect the glenohumeral joint from posterior disruption. The severity of the initial trauma determines whether recurrences will ensue through capsule avulsion or tears. Inadequate immobilization (a period of 6 weeks is the rule) and excessive mobilization exercise prevent proper tissue healing and thus recurrent luxations and dislocations. If the arm at the glenohumeral articulation is forcefully internally rotated and adducted in repetitive throwing, posterior recurrent luxation may occur. Soreness, in varying degrees, which may last for 7 to 14 days, along with a weakness secondary to the acute pain in the posterior shoulder muscles are precursors of recurrent luxations. Once an initial dislocation has occurred, a recurrent lesion can be expected at some time.

In rare instances, spontaneous atraumatic posterior luxation and dislocation are seen; in these cases posterior instability develops spontaneously as a result of appar-

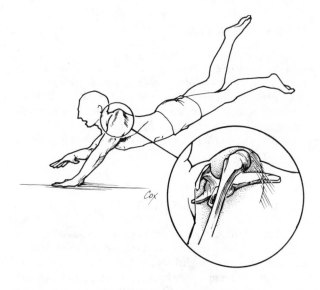

Figure 1 A fall on an internally rotated arm in adduction at the glenohumeral joint causes posterior dislocation.

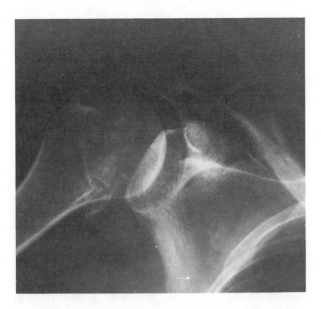

Figure 2   An anteroposterior roentgenogram shows a reduced posterior dislocation of the humeral head with a reduced fracture through the anatomical neck.

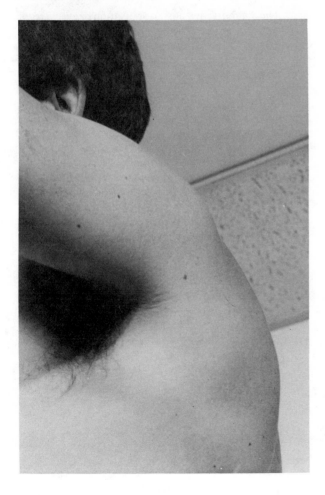

Figure 3   A painless recurrent posterior luxation of the shoulder may occur spontaneously. The humeral head can be felt to slide over the posterior rim of the glenoid.

ently insignificant trauma. This disorder develops at an early age and may be present in one or both shoulders, usually producing no pain or functional disorder until traumatic arthritic changes occur. Spontaneous reduction usually occurs at the will of the patient. Possible causes include congenital glenoid or humeral head malformation, connective tissue dysplasia, neuromuscular imbalance, and even a familial trait (Fig. 3). The surgeon who contemplates a repair in these "double-jointed" patients must carefully evaluate the patient for any psychologic disorders. Despite an excellent repair, frequent follow-up, and an intensive exercise program, symptoms in the operated shoulder may persist.

An entity that is sometimes overlooked is the uncontrollable and involuntary inferior luxation or multidirectional instability of the glenohumeral joint due to the redundancy of the ligaments, particularly the inferior part of the capsule. Subluxation becomes pronounced on traction downward with the patient's arm at his or her side or with the humeral head at right angles to the glenoid fossa and downward pressure on the upper third of the humerus. Symptoms exhibited by these patients are pain, fatigue, and weakness of the shoulder muscles. These symptoms are particularly inhibiting when the patient attempts to carry heavy loads or to throw, swim or engage in overhead movements of any type. Conservative therapy has been recommended, including change in the work load on the shoulder coupled with muscle-strengthening exercises. A surgical procedure described by Neer and Foster for this entity consists of obliterating the inferior pouch and capsular redundancy on the side of the surgical approach. Laxity of the capsular tissues on the opposite side may also be accomplished. The inferior capsular shift is done on either the anterior or posterior side, depending on the direction in which the shoulder demonstrates loosening in repetitive motions. (Fig. 4).

PATHOLOGY

The posterior capsular and muscular mechanism is composed of the synovial membrane, the periosteum, the labrum, and the posterior capsule. Overlying these structures are the posterior superior rotator cuff muscles and tendons, which include the supraspinatus, infraspinatus, and teres minor. In recurrent posterior luxation and dislocations, the labrum may be eroded, split, detached, or fragmented. The posterior capsule is elongated and forms an enlarged pouch with attachment to the periosteum of the posterior scapula. An arthrogram of the shoulder demonstrates this phenomenon. Enlargement in the synovial capsular pouch is generally less pronounced than that seen in recurrent anterior dislocations (Fig. 5). This is due to less excursion of the humeral head in posterior dislocations and less elongation of the posterior capsule mechanism. Occasionally, loose bone fragments from the posterior glenoid rim are found within the synovial cavity.

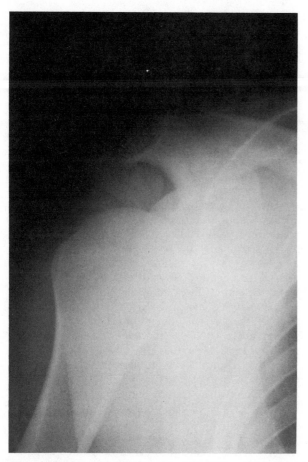

Figure 4 Involuntary inferior luxation of the glenohumeral joint due to gravity pull.

Dorgan has attempted to classify the lesion into groups according to dependence on anatomic displacement rather than abnormalities of function. The following are included in his anatomic criteria:

1. When the humeral head impinges on the posterior glenoid rim, there is humeral rotational subluxation with the head pointing posteriorly and the greater tuberosity anteriorly.

2. Subacromial retrograde dislocation may be present with internal rotation of the arm.

3. Complete posterior dislocation may occur with the humeral head in the subacromion spine position.

In traumatic recurrent posterior luxations and dislocations there has been an episode of disruption of the glenohumeral joint posteriorly. This action predisposes the humeral head to recurrent posterior luxations and dislocations. Often an osteochondral fracture of the humeral head occurs at the initial traumatic experience (Fig. 6). With each succeeding dislocation, a notching of the superior medial aspect of the humeral head increased in depth. The greater the defect observed in the humeral head, the more likely a posterior recurrence because with each impingement the defect deepens. Continued pain and limitation of motion have been misinterpreted as adhesive capsulitis.

DIAGNOSIS

The diagnosis of a posterior luxation or even a frank dislocation is often missed as one may not suspect that this uncommon condition is present. The physician is distracted because the classic physical signs may be masked by swelling, obesity, hematoma, heavy musculature, and inability of the patient to allow a detailed examination because of acute pain. Since these cases are usually seen in emergency facilities, the examining physician is provided with no more than a single anterior posterior plain roentgenogram, which fails to show salient features. A frequent finding on examination is lack of external rotation. More internal rotation is allowable if the humeral head is not locked by impingement on the rim of the glenoid fossa. Spasm of the surrounding intrinsic muscles, such as the trapezius, the

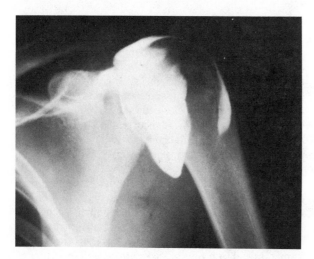

Figure 5 An arthrogram of the shoulder shows some increase in the capsular pouch in posterior luxation or dislocation. This increase is generally less than that seen in recurrent anterior luxations or dislocations.

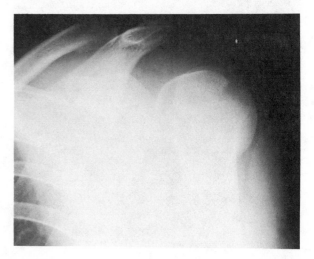

Figure 6 A roentgenogram of a posterior luxation shows impingement of the humeral head on the posterior rim of the glenoid with internal rotation of the humerus. A trough line of humeral head indentation is observed. (Orthop Clin N Amer 1980; Vol 11, No 2.)

deltoid, and the pectoral group, may or may not be present. The arm is held in neutral or fixed internal rotation and there is lack of abduction. The coracoid process is prominent. The head of the humerus is palpated below the spine of the scapula, and there is an abnormal space below the acromion and humeral head. The head shows a decreased anterior palpable prominence. When spasm accompanies the recurrence, winging of the scapula is present in many cases (Fig. 7).

Many patients with recurrent posterior luxations or dislocations experience minimal pain. Relocation of the glenohumeral joint is voluntarily accomplished when the arm is brought upward and forward, and then externally rotated. There is usually a snapping sensation of the humeral head as it reduces in the glenoid fossa. The arm is then brought back to its normal position. The luxation cannot be produced when the arm is held in external rotation. Patients with voluntary luxation or dislocation following an episode of trauma are not considered to be habitual dislocators.

Roentgenography

The routine x-ray examination of the shoulder, which consists of anteroposterior views, usually is satis- factory for the diagnosis of traumatic disorders, but not of posterior luxations or dislocations, confirmation of which requires additional views. Axillary and scapular "Y" projections demonstrate the abnormal posterior position of the humeral head. In many cases the axillary view is not feasible because of severe pain and spasm, which make positioning of the arm impossible. Unless the humerus is abducted to 90 degrees, the coracoid process is difficult to visualize, and the humerus appears foreshortened on the film, obscuring details of the pathology.

Another view, the upright anterior oblique view, is technically easy and the patient does not have to be recumbent. In this projection the scapula and coracoid are seen tangentially, so that posterior dislocation of the shoulder is easily identified. This view is obtained with the patient standing at a 45-degree angle to the film (Fig. 8).

Transthoracic lateral views of the shoulder are more difficult to interpret because the rays traversing the dense tissues of the chest cause confusing shadows. In this view one must recognize the normally smooth arch formed by the axillary border of the scapula and the inferior medial wall of the humeral head and the neck. This arch may be distorted if a true right-angle transthoracic view is not

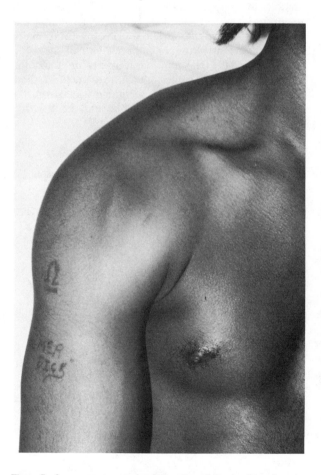

Figure 7 In recurrent posterior dislocation of the shoulder, there is frequent spasm and winging of the scapula. Anteriorly the shoulder joint is flattened and the coracoid is prominent. (Orthop Clin N Amer 1980; Vol 11, No 2.)

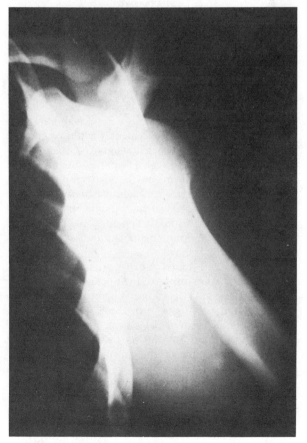

Figure 8 A tangential roentgenogram shows the humeral head posterior to the glenoid with the humeral head internally rotated in recurrent posterior shoulder dislocation.

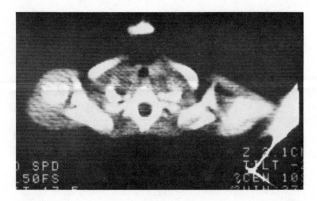

Figure 9   A CT scan in a posterior dislocation of the shoulders shows excellent detail of the pathology. (Orthop Clin N Amer 1980; Vol 11, No 2.)

obtained. This view is more valuable in the slender patient.

Although not readily available in the initial dislocation, computerized tomography is helpful in the recurrent posterior luxated and dislocated shoulder. This study readily establishes the diagnosis, especially with the updated machines (Fig. 9).

TREATMENT

Taylor and Wright reported six acute posterior dislocations treated by manipulation and immobilization without any known recurrences.

Conservatism is recommended for patients who have experienced painless recurrent posterior luxations and dislocations, particularly if these episodes do not interfere with the patient's daily activities and are relatively infrequent. The displacement is seldom complete, and the findings are not so definite as in complete posterior subspinous dislocations. The patient feels the head "slip out of joint" as it engages the posterior glenoid rim, and he is able to reduce the shoulder himself. A daily program of vigorous calisthenics should be maintained to keep the complex muscle system of the shoulder in condition for smooth, painless, and synchronous movement.

Athletically inspired patients, whether luxators or dislocators, require operative treatment, for which there are many designed operations. Such procedures can be classified into soft tissue procedures, glenoid arthroplasty, internal fixation devices of crossed Kirschner wires, Steinman pins through the humeral head into the glenoid, and stapling of the capsule to the posterior glenoid neck.

Combination soft tissue and bone block procedures are more logical because they correct two areas of weakness—capsule and musculotendinous laxity—and include correction at the glenoid rim and humeral head. Hohman, in 1933, used a posterior graft from the iliac crest. Several other authors report one to several cases of posterior recurrent luxation or dislocation in which they used a posterior graft from the iliac crest.

Feore and Mialaret have obtained grafts from the eighth rib. Even tibial grafts have been used to form a strong bone buttress.

Operative Procedure

The procedure recommended is one that tightens the posterior capsular structures at the infraspinatus and the inferior portion of the supraspinatus at their musculotendinous junctions. It also provides a more stable posterior bone buttress in preventing posterior luxation and dislocation. This procedure carries some of the advantages of double reinforcement as has been described for anterior recurrent dislocations using the modified Bristow operation.

With the patient in a lateral prone position, the posterior scapular incision is made to adequately expose the pathology of the posterior shoulder joint and the donor site of the bone block graft. This incision has been made popular by Rowe and Yee (Fig. 10). It begins at the junction of the medial one-third and middle one-third of the scapular spine, extends laterally over the spine and posterior aspect of the acromion, and curves laterally and downward over the shoulder joint 2 to 3 inches. The deltoid, by sharp dissection, is separated subperiosteally from the spine and lateral aspect of the acromion. The muscle is retracted inferiorly, exposing the infraspinatus muscle, the short musculotendinous cuff of the infraspinatus, and the teres minor as it inserts into the posterior humeral head. An inferior portion of the supraspinatus and the infraspinatus is sectioned 2 cm from the insertion, preserving a flap to tighten and reef the infra-

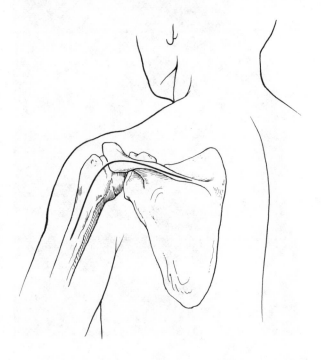

Figure 10   Diagram of the incision is shown for the repair of recurrent posterior luxation and dislocation of the shoulder.

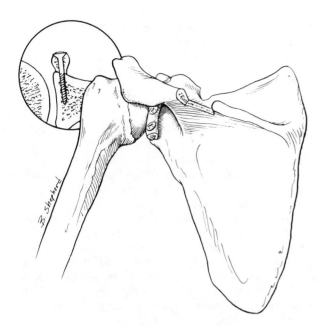

Figure 11 The scapular spine graft source site, with positioning of the graft just behind the shoulder capsule, is secured with two screws.

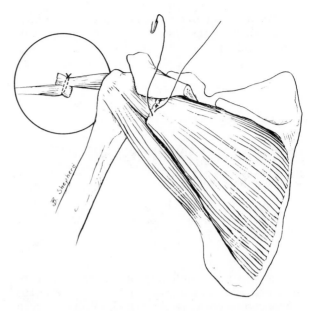

Figure 12 The infraspinatus is sectioned at its musculatendinous junction and reefed to eliminate the capsule and muscle laxity. The teres minor is not sectioned.

spinatus. In preserving the teres minor, we protect the posterior branch of the axillary nerve as it passes through the quadrilateral space. The infraspinatus and the teres minor are exposed and separated along the direction of its fibers. Care is taken, when raising the flap of the infraspinatus, to carefully retract it medially to preserve the supraspinatus artery and nerve as they sweep around the inferior portion of the acromion and scapula spine to primarily supply this muscle. The infraspinatus fossa is exposed. The capsule is then opened transversely to expose the joint, which is then explored for loose bone chips or labrum fragments. Should the labrum be frayed, torn, or detached it is smoothed, or it may be removed. The anterior portion of the joint can also be inspected.

A 3-cm long full-thickness bone block is removed from the midportion of the scapular spine. A bed for its insertion is made just posterior to the attachment of the posterior glenoid capsule by decorticating the glenoid neck on the posterior aspect of the glenoid. Two cancellous screws are used to secure it to the glenoid neck (Fig. 11).

With the arm now held in some extension and external rotation of at least 30 degrees, the capsule is reefed and overlapped with the supraspinatus and infraspinatus musculotendinous cuff. The deltoid is carefully reattached to the acromion. No difficulty in reattachment of the deltoid has been encountered over the graft source site (Fig. 12).

Following closure, the arm is held in a shoulder spica with the arm in 30-degree external rotation and 20-degree extension and abduction (Fig. 13).

Immobilization is continued for 6 weeks and isometric exercises are instituted. After all external immobilization is discontinued, active range-of-motion, pendulum, pulley, and wheel exercises are begun to increase motion and strengthen muscles. Progressive resistive

exercises are discouraged until 10 weeks postoperatively. Overstretching of the tightened elements of lifting weights, contact sports, and forceful throwing are discouraged for 6 months.

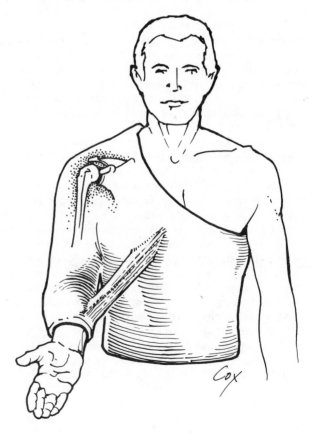

Figure 13 A shoulder spica of 20 degrees forward flexion and 30 degrees external rotation is maintained for 6 weeks.

The advantage of this operation lies in its effectiveness in stabilizing the posterior laxity of the soft tissue elements and in providing an additional support through a posterior bone buttress to prevent recurrent posterior luxation and dislocations.

SHOULDER IMPINGEMENT SYNDROME

GARY W. MISAMORE, M.D.
RICHARD J. HAWKINS, M.D., F.R.C.S.(C), F.A.C.S.

Impingement syndromes are among the most commonly encountered disorders of the shoulder. The rotator cuff tendons pass through the relatively limited space underneath the coracoacromial arch (coracoacromial ligament and anterior acromion) in their course to their distal insertion on the proximal humerus. Many athletic activities require repetitive use of the shoulder in the elevated position, and this can result in hypertrophy or swelling of the rotator cuff tendons, with resultant impingement due to the increased volume of the soft tissues passing under the unyielding coracoacromial arch.

The human shoulder is not particularly well designed to withstand many of the repetitive abuses to which it is commonly subjected in many sporting activities, as well as in many vocations. Activities requiring repetitive use of the arm above the horizontal level of the shoulder joint may produce an impingement syndrome. The functional arc of elevation of the shoulder is forward, not lateral. With forward elevation, impingement occurs predominantly against the anterior edge of the acromion and the coracoacromial ligament. The throwing motion involved in baseball pitching, quarterbacking, and serving and overhead strokes in tennis, can lead to repetitive minor trauma to the subacromial structures. Likewise, many of the arm motions in swimming, weightlifting, gymnastics, and volleyball result in impingement.

Cadaver studies of the microcirculation of the rotator cuff have demonstrated a relatively avascular zone ("critical zone") near the supraspinatus tendon insertion. The biceps tendon, which passes through the intertubercular groove deep to the supraspinatus insertion, also has a relatively avascular zone in the segment of the tendon adjacent to the "critical zone" of the supraspinatus. It is this "critical zone" of the rotator cuff, and the biceps tendon, which are subjected to impingement. Therefore, chronic microtrauma to this "critical zone" from impingement, combined with the relatively poor nutrition and healing ability of that portion of the tendon due to the impaired circulation, set the stage for the "impingement syndrome".

Chronic irritation of this relatively avascular region can lead to an inflammatory reaction with resultant tendinitis of the rotator cuff. This inflammatory state can also often involve the biceps tendon, subacromial bursa, and acromioclavicular joint. The natural history of prolonged impingement and tendinitis is often one of gradual attrition of the tendon. With time, this process can result in rupture of the rotator cuff. Since gradual attrition of the rotator cuff is generally a primary factor leading to complete rupture of the cuff tendons, this affliction is relatively uncommon in young athletic patients, occurring more commonly in patients over 50 years of age who have had longstanding problems with impingement tendinitis. Rarely, younger patients can suffer ruptures of the rotator cuff tendons, but a violent injury or repetitive significant trauma is necessary to cause cuff rupture in those patients.

CLINICAL STAGES OF IMPINGEMENT

The course of impingement syndrome is variable. Progression or remission depends on the patient's anatomy, the functional demands placed on the shoulder, and the treatment modalities employed. There are three commonly recognized stages of the disorder.

Stage I. Stage I involves relatively mild tendinitis which is usually reversible. This usually is found in younger athletes (less than 25 years old), but can occur in all age groups. Pain occurs predominantly during or after exercise or strenuous activity in which the arm has been used in the overhead position. The pain is generally a vague, dull diffuse aching about the shoulder. The problem can progress to the point where significant pain occurs during activity, and may even be severe enough to affect the patient's athletic performance. A typical patient is a young adult involved in throwing or racquet sports or, in many cases, swimming. The duration of symptoms prior to seeking medical consultation is usually fairly short, as these patients are often aggressive athletes. However, stage I impingement is not uncommon among 40-year-old weekend tennis players.

Stage II. Stage II involves more severe tendinitis, usually with some residual scarring so that the disorder is more refractory to conservative treatment. In many cases, the changes that occur in the cuff and subacromial bursa may not be totally reversible. Generally, the pain is more significant than in stage I, and may occur after as well as during activity. Pain often occurs during the night, particularly when the patient lies or rolls onto the involved shoulder. Patients with stage II impingement usually are within the 25- to 40-year old range, although all ages can be affected. The typical patient with this stage of impingement syndrome is a young or middle-aged adult involved in recreational athletes (playing tennis several times each week).

Stage III. Stage III represents the end stage of the impingement process—rupture of the rotator cuff. These patients are usually over 40 years of age and have had shoulder symptoms for many years. They usually complain of activity-related pain, as well as night pain. Frequently they complain also of stiffness and weakness (features not typically seen in stage I, and only occasionally seen in stage II). In our experience, rupture of the rotator cuff is infrequent in athletes. They either seek treatment before this stage is reached, or they are forced to curtail their athletic activity because of the pain long before reaching this stage.

PHYSICAL EXAMINATION

Each of the stages of impingement has relatively specific findings associated with it. However, since the disorder represents a continuum from mild, reversible tendinitis to rupture of the rotator cuff, the patient may show findings consistent with more than one stage as he progresses between stages. Despite such variations, most patients can be classified into one of the typical stages based on the history and physical examination. Often the inflammatory process spreads to involve the biceps tendon, subacromial bursa, and acromioclavicular joint, producing some variation in the signs and symptoms.

Stage I. The important clinical signs of stage I impingement are (1) point tenderness over the greater tuberosity at the supraspinatus insertion, (2) tenderness over the anterior acromion, (3) a painful arc of abduction, and (4) positive impingement signs. The impingement signs are maneuvers designed to reproduce the impingement by forcing the greater tuberosity against the anterior acromion and coracoacromial ligament. The most reliable impingement maneuver is performed by forcibly forward-flexing the arm at the extreme of elevation (forcing the "critical zone" of the rotator cuff against the anterior acromion). An alternative method involves forceful internal rotation while the arm is forward-flexed to 90° (forcing the "critical zone" against the coracoacromial ligament). A positive test results in reproduction of the patient's shoulder pain, as well as a fairly typical facial grimace. Often the biceps tendon is involved, in which case there is also (1) tenderness over the biceps tendon, (2) a positive straight arm-raising test (resisted forward flexion with the elbow extended—Speed's test), and (3) a positive resisted supination test (resisted supination with the elbow flexed 90°—Yergason's test).

Stage II. As the shoulder progresses into stage II, the same physical findings are present. In addition, there is usually soft tissue crepitus from the scarring of the subacromial bursa. Significant findings of biceps involvement are noted more frequently at this stage. In addition, there is slight limitation of motion of the shoulder owing to significant pain at the extremes of motion. If motion is significantly limited, the impingement signs may be difficult to demonstrate.

Stage III. When rupture of the rotator cuff occurs, the end stage of the impingement syndrome has been reached. Patients with stage III impingement generally have some limitation of motion, with passive motion being greater than active motion. Most have subjective and objective weakness. If the rupture of the cuff tendons has been present for more than a few weeks, wasting of the infraspinatus and supraspinatus muscles is apparent. There is usually more soft tissue crepitus than is found in stage II. Impingement signs usually are present, but occasionally cannot be demonstrated because of limitation of motion and pain occurring throughout a large portion of the arcs of motion. Biceps tendon involvement is common at this stage. Biceps attrition is so advanced in approximately one-third of these patients that tendon rupture occurs in association with rupture of the rotator cuff.

Probably the greatest diagnostic problem regarding impingement syndrome comes in trying to distinguish stage II from stage III. This distinction often is critical, since many patients with rupture of the rotator cuff may best be treated with early surgical intervention. A subacromial injection of local anesthetic can be useful in making the diagnosis of impingement, and often even more useful in distinguishing stage II from stage III disease. Elimination of the pain and the impingement signs following injection of a local anesthetic confirms the diagnosis. Patients with rupture of the rotator cuff obtain good pain relief with the injection, as do stage II patients, but stage III patients have continued weakness and limitation of motion.

RADIOGRAPHS

Radiographs of the shoulder are generally normal during stage I and stage II impingement. Abnormalities often are present on plain radiographs during stage III (and occasionally in stage II), consisting of (1) sclerosis and osteophytes along the anterior-inferior acromion, (2) cystic changes in the greater tuberosity, and narrowing, sclerosis, and osteophytes at the acromioclavicular joint. If a large and longstanding rotator cuff tear is present, the humeral head may migrate proximally, reducing the normal distance between the humeral head and the acromion. An acromiohumeral gap of less than 5 mm is highly suggestive of a massive rotator cuff tear.

Arthrograms are generally diagnostic of rotator cuff tears. However, the clinical signs and symptoms must be correlated with the arthrographic findings since both false-positive and false-negative arthrograms do occasionally occur.

DIFFERENTIAL DIAGNOSIS

The diagnosis of impingement syndrome is relatively straightforward in patients with typical symptoms and signs, especially when the impingement tests are obviously positive. However, in somewhat atypical cases, several other disorders should be considered in the differential diagnosis. Acute traumatic bursitis or tendinitis can have features much like those of impingement tendinitis. Following a direct blow to the anterior aspect of the shoulder, the athlete may develop traumatic bursitis or tendinitis. This disorder usually resolves with rest. If not treated promptly, swelling and inflammation can occur with resultant development of a classic impingement syndrome.

Instability of the shoulder often occurs without actual dislocation. Instability problems can cause vague, aching shoulder discomfort, much like that of impingement tendinitis. In addition, some patients with significant instability develop secondary rotator cuff tendinitis because of the chronic irritation occurring each time the shoulder subluxes. If the instability and secondary tendinitis are not treated, these patients can also develop a typical impingement syndrome along with their instability. Most patients with shoulder instability are aware that their shoulders "come out of joint".

Primary acromioclavicular disorder can cause similar symptoms; however, physical examination should reveal tenderness, and often crepitus and osteophytes, at the acromioclavicular joint. The other typical findings of impingement syndrome will not be present. There usually is a history of previous acromioclavicular injury.

Presenting symptoms of glenohumeral arthritis in older patients can be much the same as those of impingement syndrome. This disorder is rarely seen in athletic populations. However, young patients can develop one of the inflammatory arthritides or post-traumatic arthritis following a severe injury. In general, patients with arthritis are elderly, have bony rather than soft tissue crepitus, have limitation of passive motion (particularly in rotation), and do not have tenderness localized to the area of the greater tuberosity. Radiographic evaluation reveals typical changes of arthritis in the glenohumeral joint.

Cervical disease can cause radicular pain to the shoulder area which is not totally unlike the vague ache of impingement tendinitis. Patients with cervical disorders generally have painful and limited motion of the neck, often with tenderness along the posterior aspect of the cervical column. Motor, sensory, and reflex examination may reveal findings consistent with a neurologic problem, but the typical physical findings of impingement are lacking. Occasionally both disorders occur concomitantly, presenting a diagnostic and therapeutic challenge.

Disorders of the suprascapular nerve can cause vague shoulder discomfort as well as weakness of abduction and external rotation, combined with atrophy of the spinati muscles. Suprascapular nerve palsy can result from trauma or from chronic entrapment as the nerve passes over the scapula. These patients do not have positive impingement signs. Electromyography is needed to confirm this diagnosis, which is rare in our experience.

In some patients, there may be findings consistent with more than one of these disorders. When doubt remains following a thorough history and physical examination, subacromial injection with local anesthetic may be necessary for clarification. Only patients with impingement syndrome or acute traumatic bursitis/tendinitis are afforded relief by the injection, whereas with the other disorders in the list of differential diagnoses, the pain remains unchanged.

TREATMENT

The majority of patients with impingement tendinitis of the shoulder obtain good relief with conservative management, especially those in stage I of the disorder.

Stage I

Rest. The inflamed rotator cuff tendons must be protected from continued overuse and abuse. This occasionally requires complete cessation of the aggravating activity. However, usually the patient can continue with sports with some modifications. Athletes need thorough evaluation by their coaches to search for flaws in technique. Often a small change in the throwing technique, swimming stroke, or tennis serve provides relief of the impingement problem.

Medications. Anti-inflammatory medications help to reduce the inflammatory response about the rotator cuff tendons. As swelling of the cuff tendons subsides, impingement is reduced. Analgesics may be necessary for some patients.

Ice/Heat. Athletes should utilize heat modalities (hot packs, linaments, or ultrasound) prior to workouts to increase the local blood supply. To minimize the inflammatory reaction that results after strenuous use of the arm, athletes should perform ice massage of the shoulder following workouts.

Stretching and Strengthening. A well-structured exercise program is often beneficial. Stretching of the muscle-tendon units which comprise the rotator cuff should be routine prior to sporting activities. Strengthening exercises working specifically on the rotator cuff musculature should be performed. Strengthening exercises must be done in such a fashion that the positions in which impingement occurs are avoided. Physical therapists and athletic trainers should be able to direct such an exercise program.

Stage II. Conservative treatment for stage II impingement includes all of the same modalities utilized for stage I patients. In addition, stretching by means of range-of-motion exercises should be performed to maintain full motion of the shoulder.

Stage III. The same treatment program is utilized for patients with stage III impingement syndrome. For these patients, however, emphasis is placed on range-of-motion and strengthening exercises.

Surgical Treatment

Surgical intervention for impingement syndrome is considered only for refractory cases that are not responsive to prolonged conservative management. Surgical intervention in stage I is unusual since the process is still reversible and should respond to aggressive nonsurgical management. Patients with stage II impingement who are not relieved by conservative modalities are candidates for decompressive surgical procedures. Decompressive surgery implies surgical alteration of the coracoacromial arch to reduce the impingement, with no surgery directed at the rotator cuff tendons themselves. The most common procedure done to achieve that includes anterior acromioplasty and resection of the coracoacromial ligament. Some surgeons advocate resection of only the coracoacromial ligament in younger athletic patients. Surgical decompression provides good results in approximately 90 percent of patients with stage II impingement syndrome. In athletes, however, such as swimmers and throwers, only a small percentage are likely to return to their previous level of performance following surgical decompression. The primary indication for surgical intervention following rupture of the rotator cuff (stage III) is pain. An additional consideration when considering surgical intervention for rotator cuff rupture should be prevention of progression of the process. Many patients with torn rotator cuffs have progressive deterioration of shoulder function. Although the initial cuff tear may be small, the size of the tear can gradually increase as the edges are retracted by the continued pull of the affected muscles. On this basis, some surgeons advocate repair of all rotator cuff tears in active patients as soon as the diagnosis is made. However, many patients with rupture of the rotator cuff seem to function quite adequately with minimal symptoms. In young and active patients, such as are found in an athletic population, a more aggressive approach toward surgical repair of ruptured rotator cuff tendons should be followed. Surgery undertaken to improve strength or motion, or to return an athlete to sporting activities, often results in a dissatisfied patient. Pain relief should be the primary goal of surgery.

Regardless of the stage of the impingement process and the specific treatment modalities employed, cooperation on the part of the patient is critical to the successful treatment of this problem. Whether surgical or nonsurgical methods are utilized, the patient must understand the rehabilitation program if optimal results are to be achieved.

BICEPS TENDON RUPTURE IN THE ATHLETE

LOUIS U. BIGLIANI, M.D.
IRA N. WOLFE, B.A.

Rupture of the biceps tendon is an infrequent problem in the athlete. However, depending on the type of rupture, the location, and the activity in which an athlete may participate, it can be disabling. It can occur in a wide range of sporting activities, from violent contact sports (football, rugby) to noncontact sports which either place excessive amounts of stress across tendons (weight lifting, gymnastics) or require multiple less stressful repetitive movements (tennis, squash). The etiology of biceps rupture is either a direct blow on a contracted muscle or an indirect force through the tendon while performing a stressful activity. In contact sports, a direct blow is usually the mechanism of injury. The mechanism producing an indirect force may be violent from a very strenuous activity or subtle from repetitive less stressful activities. In the latter instance, the tendon is usually weakened from abnormal wear, and this degeneration can allow rupture with only subtle actions. Lifting a heavy weight and catching a heavy object are examples of a violent mechanism, while swinging a racquet as in tennis is an example of a subtle mechanism.

CLASSIFICATION

A simple classification of biceps tendon ruptures is presented in Table 1 in an attempt to clarify the treatment of different ruptures. The two main types are proximal rupture and distal rupture. Anatomically, the proximal biceps has two heads, the short and the long head. Rupture of the short head is extremely rare. The most common biceps tendon rupture is that of the long head of the biceps. This type of rupture can be further divided into two distinct types, the rare low type and the more common high type. The low type of rupture occurs at the musculotendinous junction in younger athletes, usually secondary to a violent direct or indirect trauma as seen in football, basketball, or weight-lifting. The more com-

TABLE 1   Biceps Tendon Ruptures

Classification	Patient Age
Proximal	
Short (Rare)	
Long	
1. High type (Most common)	>40
2. Low type	<40
Distal (Less common)	
1. Partial	
2. Complete	

mon high type, usually seen in middle-aged and older athletes, occurs in the impingement area between the undersurface of the anterior acromion and the greater tuberosity of the humerus. The impingement area extends to the bicipital groove, and the degenerated biceps tendon ruptures within either the glenohumeral joint or the proximal bicipital groove.

Rupture of the distal biceps tendon is much less common than proximal rupture. It usually occurs in younger athletes participating in sports such as body building, gymnastics, and weight lifting. The rupture can be either partial (more common) or complete.

Biceps tendon ruptures can also be classified according to the length of time from the injury to diagnosis and treatment. An acute rupture is seen within 6 weeks of injury; a chronic rupture is one seen more than 6 weeks after an injury.

TREATMENT

Rupture of the Proximal Biceps

Rupture of the short head of the biceps is rare, but if encountered acutely, it should be repaired. The short head is responsible for a significant amount of the biceps power necessary for elbow supination and flexion while performing strenuous activity. We have recently seen a young man with a chronic short head rupture who was having biceps muscle fatigue with spasm and pain after strenuous activity. Approximately one year following injury, the contracted short head was mobilized and reattached to the tendon of the long head. He is now stronger and his symptoms have disappeared.

Treatment of long head rupture is more complex since there may be an underlying shoulder disorder. This is usually the case in the high type and not in the low type. The low type is usually free of shoulder symptoms, therefore we will discuss this treatment first.

The treatment of the low type of long head rupture is direct, end-to-end suture. Ideally, this should be performed within 10 days of injury, while the tendon is mobile and minimally retracted. The torn proximal tendon and distal tendon or distal muscle belly are in close approximation of one another. The portion of the proximal tendon within the bicipital groove is undamaged and functional. Therefore, reattachment of the distal muscle belly should achieve an excellent result.

A short, slightly oblique, 5-cm incision is made starting at the distal aspect of the bicipital groove and extending distally. A Bunnell-type of cross stitch with nonabsorbable nylon suture, such as Tevdek, is preferable. The rotator cuff need not be explored unless there are significant shoulder symptoms. Usually, patients in this category are young and free of shoulder pain. The arm should be protected in a cylinder cast with elbow flexed to 90° for 6 weeks. The distal part of the cast should be well molded so as not to allow supination or pronation. After the cast is removed, passive assisted and gentle active motion of the elbow are allowed for 3 weeks. This is followed by progressive resistive exercises (to be described).

The high type of rupture of the long head of the biceps is usually associated with a subacromial impingement lesion. It is seen in older, active athletes who frequently have a history of shoulder pain and disability. There is wear on the tendon of the long head as well as the supraspinatus tendon in the critical area of impingement. This can lead to tendon degeneration and make the long head of biceps and supraspinatus more susceptible to injury. It is important to be aware of this combined lesion so that the treatment rationale will include both the underlying subacromial impingement lesion and the possible rotator cuff tear. Athletes with an acute high type should have surgical reattachment of the tendon to the bicipital groove since end-to-end repair is not feasible. Several drill holes are placed in the groove or anterior humerus, and the tendon is sutured with nonabsorbable sutures. If a tear of the rotator cuff is suspected, the patient should have a shoulder arthrogram prior to surgery. However, the rotator cuff can and should be inspected at the time of biceps tenodesis. If surgical repair of the biceps is deferred, an arthrogram is essential in order to assess the rotator cuff in all patients with a history of shoulder pain or who may develop shoulder pain. If the arthrogram is positive, immediate repair and decompression of the rotator cuff as well as the biceps tenodesis is advised, in order to minimize retraction and facilitate mobilization of the cuff and biceps.

Some older, active athletes with chronic long head biceps ruptures develop persistent shoulder pain and disability. These patients should also be evaluated by means of an arthrogram; if the arthrogram is positive, they should have a decompression and cuff repair. The biceps repair is optional since it is retracted distally and shortened, making it difficult to mobilize. The functional improvement from tenodesis of this attenuated tendon and muscle is minimal, and only cosmesis is improved. The only indication for tenodesis is spasm and pain in the biceps muscle belly.

The detailed technique of subacromial decompression and cuff repair will not be discussed since the subject matter of this chapter is biceps repair. However, if there is a combined lesion, the approach to the shoulder for anterior acromioplasty, as described by Neer, should be made first. In some acute long head ruptures, the distal tendon may be pushed into the wound by flexing the elbow and squeezing the distal biceps. If this maneuver is unsuccessful, a second 5-cm incision is made along the anterior edge of the deltoid starting at the distal aspect of the bicipital groove and extending distally. The biceps tendon is dissected free, pushed up into the proximal wound, and attached to the most proximal part of the groove to which it will extend. The danger of injuring the musculocutaneous nerve in this step must be recognized. A second incision would be needed to explore all chronic biceps ruptures and unravel the contracted muscle and tendon. We do not recommend this since the tissue is of poor quality, and the risk of nerve injury is high. All of the athletes we have encountered have had symptoms in their shoulder and not in the distal biceps. They have had excellent, pain-free results after their shoulder problems

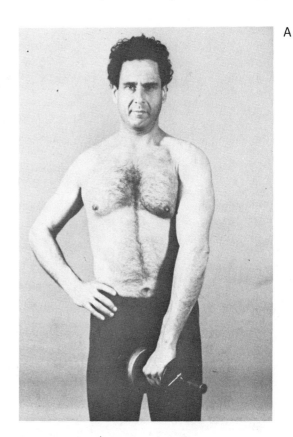

A

were corrected and have had no residual problems from the unrepaired chronic biceps rupture.

If the shoulder is asymptomatic, the distal approach for biceps tenodesis is performed first. This incision may be extended a little proximally and a small split made in the deltoid to explore the rotator cuff for a partial-thickness rotator cuff tear. Following repair of high type biceps ruptures, the same postoperative regimen that is used for low type biceps repairs is recommended.

We have seen several patients develop rotator cuff tears after transfer of the long head of the biceps to the coracoid. This procedure should be avoided in active athletes since it can accelerate impingement.

Rupture of the Distal Biceps

Treatment of the less common distal biceps rupture depends on whether the rupture is complete or partial. The specific athletic activity may also be a factor. An acute complete rupture should be repaired in active athletes of all ages. An unrepaired complete distal biceps rupture will result in weakness of elbow flexion and supination (Figure 1). Morrey, using a torque dynamometer, has demonstrated significant weakness of elbow flexion and supination in patients with unrepaired distal biceps ruptures. Most partial ruptures can be treated conservatively unless the athlete is involved in a highly stressful sport such as olympic weight lifting, power lifting, or throwing field events (shotput, discus, javelin, hammerthrow). These activities demand enormous strength, and if a large portion of the tendon is torn, repair should be considered. We have seen several body builders with a partial rupture due to their tendency to isolate joint activity to increase the amount of stress across the muscle. Rupture in these athletes is a unique problem in that they require perfect muscle shape and definition, but scars will detract from their appearance, especially in competition. Therefore, we carefully explain the option of an irregular biceps or a long scar. All have chosen conservative treatment, since there is minimal weakness and functional loss with a partial distal biceps rupture.

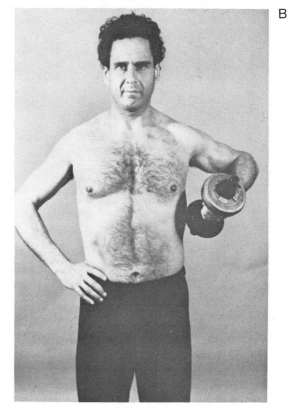

B

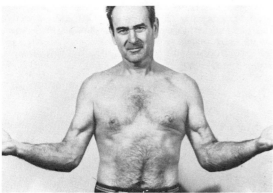

Figure 1 Bilateral, chronic, complete distal biceps ruptures in a 51-year-old former competitive gymnast and gymnastic coach. The injuries had occurred 5 and 7 years earlier while the patient was catching athletes during gymnastic maneuvers. Despite his strength, he complains of weakness of elbow flexion and supination.

C

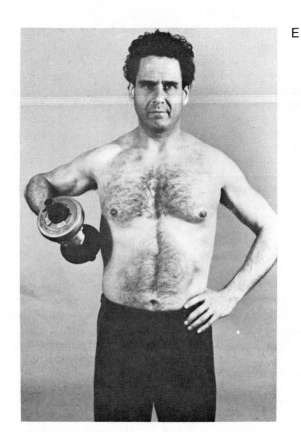

E

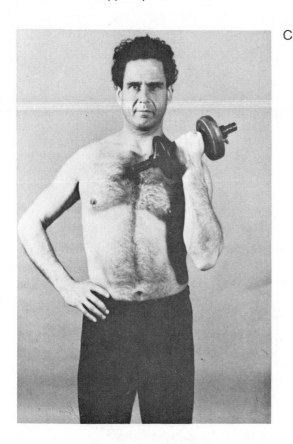

D

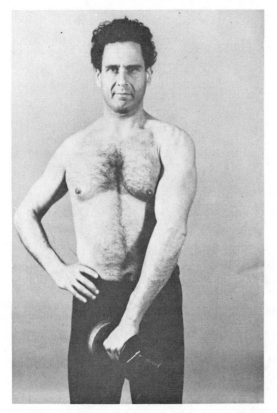

Figure 2 A, The starting position of the modified biceps curl (MBC). The elbow is extended and pronated with the arm slightly adducted across the body. B, Movement is initiated by simultaneous supination and flexion of the elbow. The shoulder is moved into extension as the elbow continues to supinate and flex. This is continued until maximum elbow flexion, forearm supination, and shoulder extension are achieved. C, The shoulder then moves to a neutral position, thereby placing the elbow under the hand. D, The second phase of the exercise is initiated by hyperextending the shoulder. This maneuver places the hand holding the resistance distal to the axilla again. E, The elbow is extended and pronated as the shoulder is returned to neutral, and the arm is slightly adducted across the body to the starting position. The exercise is repeated.

Several technical considerations are important in repairing a complete distal biceps rupture. First, the tendon should be resutured to the radial tuberosity so that both elbow flexion and supination are restored. The biceps is the chief elbow supinator. Also, the radial nerve must not be injured while dissecting out the proximal forearm about the radius. This injury is usually obviated by performing two incisions and by avoiding an extensive anterior approach. The approach recommended by Boyd and Anderson allows for adequate exposure without increasing the risk of injury to the radial nerve. We immobilize the arm in a cylinder cast in approximately 100° of flexion and full supination. A subcuticular 4–0 Dexon suture is used in the skin and the cast is removed at 6 weeks. Screws and hardware should be avoided in this repair. A pull-through stitch is preferred.

REHABILITATION

Rehabilitation of a repaired or torn biceps tendon must strengthen the remaining or repaired biceps muscle while minimizing stress across the tendons. The standard biceps curl is a single-joint exercise which tends to maximize the stress across the biceps muscle and tendons. A more ideal exercise is the modified biceps curl (MBC) described by Robert Narcessian. It is the primary exercise that we use for rehabilitation of this injury. The MBC shortens the lever arms at the elbow, approximates physiological motion, and minimizes unwanted strain across the muscle and musculotendinous junctions while strengthening the muscle.

To perform the MBC, the resistance is held in the affected arm. It may be rubber tubing fastened to the patient's contralateral foot, a dumbbell, or even a soup can or partially filled plastic jug. Start the exercise in a standing position with the elbow extended and pronated. The arm is slightly adducted across the body (Figure 2a). Movement is initiated by simultaneous supination and flexion of the elbow. The shoulder is moved into extension as the elbow continues to supinate and flex. The resistance should travel a path as close to the frontal midline of the body as possible. The elbow remains parallel to or higher than the hand until a position of maximum elbow flexion, forearm supination, and shoulder extension is achieved (Figure 2B). At this point, the hand will approach the axilla. The shoulder then moves to neutral position, thereby placing the elbow under the hand (Figure 2C).

The second phase of the exercises is initiated by hyperextending the shoulder (Figure 2D). This maneuver places the hand holding the resistance distal to the axilla again. The elbow is then extended and pronated as the shoulder is returned to neutral (Figure 2E). The arm is slightly adducted across the body to the starting position. The exercise is then repeated. The MBC should be performed with a moderate resistance for multiple repetitions at a controlled tempo (6 seconds/repetition).

ELBOW, FOREARM AND HAND INJURIES

OVERUSE INJURY TO THE ELBOW IN THE THROWING SPORTS

FRED L. ALLMAN, Jr., M.D.

In the throwing sports, as in other activities, the basic power unit of performance is the musculotendinous unit; therefore, most elbow problems that arise during or as a result of throwing are related to muscular activity. The main offender is a dynamic overload to the musculotendinous unit and may occur over an extended period of time as the result of late effect of microtrauma.

In order to properly treat elbow injuries that result from the act of throwing, it is necessary for the physician, trainer, or coach to have insight into the basic qualities of muscle function, and the intricate mechanism of throwing as it relates to the various sports, as well as a working knowledge of the clinical characteristics of each of the various types of injury which may occur.

An understanding of the basic qualities of muscle function is necessary if one is to correctly evaluate these injuries. Clinically, there are three basic qualities of muscle function:

1. Strength—the ability of a muscle to contract.
2. Elasticity—the ability of a muscle to give up contraction and to yield to passive stretch.
3. Coordination—the ability of a muscle to cooperate with other muscles in proper timing and with appropriate power and elasticity.

It is usually possible to explain a deficiency in muscle action as the consequence of one, two, or all three of these basic qualities of muscle function.

A muscle acts best from an elongated position because the elastic force of the muscle augments its contractile force. A muscle contracts best from its full length; therefore, overuse and overloading leads to fatigue. With fatigue, the muscle relaxes more slowly and more incompletely than normal and enters into a state of temporary myostatic contracture. It is during this period of myostatic contracture that injuries are likely to occur. The resulting injury might be a minor strain to the

muscle or tendon, or if repeated over and over again, actual tears may take place in the muscle. Attempts at repair result in fibrosis, and this fibrosis in turn results in a permanent loss of elbow extension.

A basic knowledge of the biomechanics of throwing is essential if these injuries are to be properly understood. The mechanism of throwing has been called intricate and fascinating.

The throwing act consists of four essential steps for proper execution. After the initial stance, we have the preparatory phase or windup, the initial forward action of the arm and, lastly, release and follow-through. Injury usually occurs during the forward motion and follow-through phases.

Stresses upon the elbow vary somewhat according to the various sports. Dr. James Bateman has noted that in baseball the most common injury is a tear or partial avulsion of one of the tendon insertions, often the result of medial overload produced by the valgus strain on the elbow.

In football, the windup is less than in baseball; the foward fling is shorter, and the follow-through is in a different arc and not as powerful.

Hammer throwing and shot-putting place tremendous traction stress on the heavy muscles of the elbow and shoulder because of the momentum of the follow-through and the heavier projectile which is being propelled.

The javelin is released with a powerful extension of the elbow and with forcible pronation of the forearm. The pronation is extreme and it is necessary to prevent the whip of the javelin. In the follow-through, the thrower may almost completely turn around.

Studies by the late Jay Bender at Southern Illinois University demonstrated that there may be at least three distinct patterns of throwing. Each pattern can be highly successful within itself; however, the methods of teaching throwing attempt to have a throw made in a more or less standard pattern, which means changing a subject's own basic pattern. This not only causes a confusion in technique but also leads to frustration, and often injury.

Shands, nearly 50 years ago, showed that trauma to hyaline cartilage produced a definite hyperplasia. The elbow of a pitcher often shows evidence of such hyperplasia. The margins, the tip of the olecranon, and the adjacent surfaces of the condyles of the humerus are constantly traumatized by the act of throwing. The result is a definite osteochondritis with exfoliation of the cartilage, which may produce loose bodies, synovial thickening, or semiattached cartilaginous masses which obstruct and limit the extension of the elbow.

A working classification of injuries involved in the throwing sports might be related to the structure involved, or the classification might be related to the mechanisms as described by the late Don Slocum: (1) tension overloads to the inner side of the elbow which is muscular, ligamentous, and capsular; (2) lateral compression injuries—the fractured capitellum, osteochondral fractures, and traumatic arthritis; and (3) injuries to the extensor mechanism—acute traction injuries, disorders resulting from repetitive extensor action, and doorstop action of the olecranon fossa. We would therefore have strains of the flexor muscles and pronator; sprains of the collateral ligament and joint capsule; fractures of the medial epicondyle and of the olecranon (the olecranon fractures representing avulsions), as well as those to the medial epicondyle; and fractures to the radial head and capitellum, being mainly the osteochondritis type of injury.

Tension overload is seen frequently in young players as well as in more experienced players early in the season. Tightness develops on the medial aspect of the involved elbow. The medial muscle mass becomes tense and sore, and temporarily there is a loss of extension. If this pitcher is allowed to continue under these conditions—namely, while in a state of myostatic contracture—a more serious injury usually follows as extensive fibrosis results from multiple tearing throughout the muscle with resultant permanent loss of elbow extension.

Although rest, application of ice, gentle massage, anti-inflammatory agents, and other physical modalities are helpful, the main effort in treatment should be directed to the cause of the condition rather than to the resultant effect; that is, the musculotendinous unit must be slowly and gradually stretched and strengthened to withstand the stress of pitching, without producing an undue overload. Stated in different terms, the treatment of such conditions is restoration or improvement of the impaired quality of muscle function. If the muscle is weak, it must be strengthened. If the muscle is inelastic, the elasticity must be improved. If the muscle has lost its proper timing and synchronous action, the goal should be to restore proper coordination. The problem may be related to all three qualities—strength, elasticity, and coordination.

It has been said that the great Dizzy Dean was forced to stop pitching because of injuries to his elbow that resulted not from an initial elbow injury, but rather were due to altered form while pitching with an injured big toe.

Many ailing pitchers can relate the exact moment of the beginning of their pitching demise, although the demise may be drawn out over a period of years. In many cases, the onset of the demise was initiated by pitching too hard, too soon in the season, or too soon after a previous exhausting game. "I felt something pop and the elbow became sore" is often the phrase that pitchers use to explain their first traumatic episode.

Tension overload on the medial aspect of the elbow may ultimately produce traction spurs. These spurs, which are initially asymptomatic, usually become symptomatic in time. They arise from the medial aspect of the ulnar notch and extend proximally. The site of the pain is usually about one inch below the medial epicondyle, but the pain may also be located anteriorly over the joint. If the spur is of sufficient length, ulnar nerve symptoms and findings may occur.

Treatment for early cases without ulnar nerve involvement is rest, ice, and rarely injection with steroids. If symptoms become prolonged, if performance is notably altered, or if nerve involvement is present, surgical excision is indicated.

Tension overload in the "Little League" age group most often results in alterations of the medial epicondylar epiphysis. These might be physiologic hypertrophy, minute avulsion, or complete avulsion of the epiphysis. Those avulsions with minimal displacement are best treated symptomatically and with rest. Often the position of the player should be changed from that of a pitcher to that of shortstop or first baseman for the remainder of that season. Cases of avulsions with displacement are best treated by open reduction, with anatomic restoration of the fracture fragments and fixation with suture or pin. Three weeks of immobilization are usually adequate.

Lateral compression injuries are the result of impaction of the head of the radius against the capitellum in the act of throwing. Roughening and degeneration of the cartilage often results from such repeated insults to the articular cartilage. There is perhaps less resistance to this articular damage in the "Little Leaguer" than in the older player, and certainly the earlier the changes occur, the more guarded is the prognosis.

Again, treatment is symptomatic—initially with rest, ice, anti-inflammatory agents, and rarely steroids. Loose bodies should be surgically removed if they interfere with normal joint dynamics and function.

Extension injuries also constitute a frequent problem in pitchers. Chronic intermittent overload by the extensor mechanism results in hypertrophy of the ulna, the humerus, and the triceps muscle. It also results in a decrease in the size of the olecranon fossa. The tip of the olecranon and the olecranon fossa are the most common sites of osteochondral bodies in professional baseball pitchers.

Treatment is usually conservative, but surgical intervention might be indicated if pain cannot be controlled by more conservative means and especially if the pitcher shows a decline in performance and effectiveness. Two points should be stressed if surgery appears to be indicated. First, do not expect to gain full extension following surgery if there is a limitation of motion prior to surgery, even if large amounts of debris are removed from the olecranon fossa; second, do not hesitate to remove a generous portion of the olecranon process at the time of surgery. Probably the most gratifying surgery about the elbow is removal of loose bodies from the olecranon fossa.

It should also be noted that the repeated throwing motion in pitchers can result in tears in the ligaments about the elbow. Bleeding, swelling, and eventual calcification and ossification may develop. Continued stress to these areas can result in rupture, either incomplete or complete, in the involved ligament.

Rehabilitation of overuse injuries involving muscles and tendons should always include static stretching after a good warm-up. Next, a progressive resistive exercise program should follow. Progressive overload is essential if strength is to be increased. The progressive resistive exercise (PRE) program should include both concentric contractions and eccentric contractions, with greater emphasis on the latter. As strength increases and symptoms lessen, the speed of contractions can be increased.

In conclusion, it is important to remember the great individual variations in the human species. To my knowledge, there is no way that we can distinguish at an early age those youngsters who are most susceptible to elbow damage as a result of the stress of throwing. Certainly Satchel Paige, even with the best medical advice available, could not have improved his pitching longevity. Phil Neikro, Hoyt Wilhelm, Early Wynn, Gaylord Perry, and Warren Spahn are other classic examples of durability on the mound. However, we are all familiar with other pitchers who have not been nearly so durable and who showed rather pronounced symptomatology at a very early age as a result of their stressful occupations.

The danger signals include tightness, soreness, tenderness, swelling, pain, loss of control, and loss of motion. Contraction, fatigue, and weakness are other danger signals.

It is at this stage that the player must be given a careful evaluation by a competent physician who can best make a judgment as to what restrictions and/or treatment might be indicated.

The vast majority of elbow problems which are related to throwing could be prevented by a proper conditioning program, in conjunction with more judicious care of the arm before, during, and after competition.

Treatment of the various pathologic conditions about the elbow will never enable the athlete to achieve a performance level as high as he might achieve if the condition could have been prevented by proper action instituted at the proper time. Careful analysis of any problem is therefore essential.

OVERUSE SYMPTOMS ABOUT THE ELBOW

R. PETER WELSH, M.B., Ch.B., F.R.C.S.(C), F.A.C.S.
CHRIS R. CONSTANT, M.B., B.Ch., B.A.O., F.R.C.S.(I)

The overload syndrome affecting the forearm extensor origin at the bone tendon junction about the elbow is classically known as "tennis elbow", whereas a similar state on the medial side bears the eponym "golfer's elbow". Other overuse syndromes also occur in relation to the triceps and biceps insertions where a localized tendinitis may prevail. Another troublesome entity is that of the olecranon impaction syndrome with discomfort centered in the olecranon fossa at full extension of the elbow.

These periarticular elbow syndromes may cause major disability to the throwing athletes.

CLINICAL FEATURES

Pain located at the site of the tendon attachment is the hallmark of the condition in all instances, particularly on impact loading, when there is a sharp exacerbation of pain over and above the background nagging ache present in the chronic state.

In medial and lateral epicondylitis or flexor and extensor tendinitis, direct local trauma may be an initiating factor, but in many instances it is just repetitive impact loading of the extremity that provokes the condition. The use of a racquet or a club is really an extension of the arm, and force is transmitted up the shaft of the implement to the forearm musculature to be concentrated at the site of stress concentration, which is at the tendon origin. Here repeated microtrauma leads to a mild degenerative reaction with an associated low-grade inflammatory response. It is this persistent inflammatory process that is characteristic of these conditions and so often difficult to settle, for the body never really seems able to mount an effective repair effort to quell the reaction and cure the condition.

In examining the patient, the site of specific tenderness should be identified and maneuvers of resisted loading undertaken to confirm the specific clinical entity. Shoulder and elbow and forearm function should be assessed as well as the neurovascular status of the extremity. In most instances, the range of motion of the elbow is completely normal and the examination other than for the local tenderness completely clear. Occasionally, however, a radial nerve entrapment syndrome may masquerade as tennis elbow, or an ulnar nerve neuritis or subluxation of the ulnar nerve may be misdiagnosed as a "golfer's" elbow. Care should be taken in assessing the function of these nerves.

The olecranon impaction syndrome is specifically reproduced, with marked tenderness in the fossa, at hyperextension impact of the elbow. In this condition, there may well be a limit to full extension with a 5-degree or so flexion contracture of the elbow.

X-ray studies are of value in ruling out any associated disease in the elbow joint or bone structure. Rarely is an abnormality seen with tendinitis alone and only occasionally are calcific deposits noted in relation to the epicondyle. The only condition in which some structural change may be identified is the olecranon impaction syndrome, in which a beak or spur on the olecranon tip may be seen in addition to an occasional loose body.

EMG and nerve conduction studies should be undertaken if any concern exists regarding the status of the nerve function around the elbow.

MANAGEMENT OF ELBOW OVERUSE SYNDROMES

Modification of Activity

Unfortunately, simply stopping the provocative activity does not necessarily result in resolution of the syndrome. It may be necessary for many athletes to continue with their particular sport, even though their activity may have to be modified in some way and undertaken at a reduced level of competitiveness. Particular attention has to be paid to aspects of technique which may be particularly provocative of the injury, as in the tennis backhand stroke.

Not only need the activity be modified, but occasionally modification to the equipment employed may be necessary. Attention should be paid in tennis players to the size of the grip, and the flexibility or rigidity of the shaft of the racquet. Likewise, the tension in the stringing of the racquet may be important. Subtle modifications in this area can be of significant benefit, considering that it is the repetitive overloading of the bone-tendon junction which in many instances causes the condition to persist.

Physical Treatments

Exercises. In the amateur sportsman there is often a marked imbalance between the strength of the forearm flexors and that of the extensor group. Strengthening exercises aimed at building all forearm muscle groups should be undertaken, endeavoring to strengthen any obvious points of weakness. Two simple exercises that may be employed are (1) isometric strengthening of the flexor group by squeezing a soft squash ball in the hand and holding the contraction, and (2) strengthening of the extensor group by stretching a firm elastic band, spreading the fingers against the resistance of the rubber.

Restoration of normal flexibility in the forearm musculature is essential to prevent reinjury and to minimize the impact loading at the bone-tendon junction. The muscles of the forearm are, after all, the shock absorbers of the system and must absorb loads and redistribute stress so that impact at the bone-tendon junction is minimized. Stretching exercises are therefore aimed at both the flexor and extensor groups and should be part of a normal warm-up routine.

Local Pain Control. Ice friction therapy with an ice cube wrapped in a piece of muslin can be most effective when rubbed with firm pressure steadily over the epicondylar area for about 5 minutes both before and after sports activity is undertaken. This simple modality of treatment offers benefits by controlling both the pain and the inflammatory response.

Physiotherapy. Other methods employed in controlling the inflammatory response are the use of ultrasound and microwave modalities. These techniques may reduce the inflammation and promote in some way the revascularization process and ultimately, it is hoped, the resolution of the process. However, a limit should be placed on the utilization of such treatments; if, after 6 or 8 treatments, little benefit is shown there is clearly no reason for continuing the program. Likewise, if improvement has been shown, the benefits are not cumulative, and there is no real rationale for continuing on an indefinite basis.

Forearm Splints and Braces. A variety of splints or braces designed to dissipate the impact load through the musculature of the forearm and thereby reduce the impact-stress concentration at the bone-tendon junction are being promoted. These various devices all have their devotees, and there is no doubt that forces on the affected area can be reduced by the use of these splints and their use has a real place in the management of this troublesome condition. However, they should not be applied too tightly, as this will only impede the muscle reaction, and the correct position for their application is around the bulk of the muscle and not over the area of tenderness. These devices are designed to share the load with the musculature and are not meant as braces or supports in the same sense as one would utilize a knee brace.

Medications

Nonsteroidal anti-inflammatory drugs are most effective when used in the acute stages, in which high-dose administration for a limited time (7 to 10 days) is indicated. For the chronically established situation, these agents may modify symptoms to some extent, but the overall course of the condition is not generally modified significantly by their use.

Local Injection with Steroid. This is possibly the only justified application of cortisone steroid into the site of a bone-tendon junction. There may be some tendon degeneration and breakdown as a consequence of the injection, but this is not as serious as it would be were the drug to be administered to a structure such as the Achilles tendon. Such agents definitely halt the inflammatory reaction and give the body a chance to mount its own repair effort. The effect of corticosteroid may be cumulative, and multiple injections should not be necessary. However, if a recurrence of the condition necessitates another injection, this may safely be carried out. An arbitrary limit of three injections over a 6-month period will handle all but the most refractory cases. If the condition continues beyond this time, recourse to a surgical solution should be considered.

Surgical Intervention

Surgery for tennis elbow has proved most gratifying in instances in which the condition remains refractory to other modalities of treatment. For those disabled from participation in both sport and work activity, one can almost invariably anticipate an improvement in capability following surgical intervention.

Surgery for Tennis Elbow

A lateral incision over the epicondyle and radial head exposes the extensor origin and proximal tendon. The tendon is released from the epicondyle for about 2 cm above, and the joint itself is opened and the tendon attachment to the annular ligament released from the anterior aspect of the neck of the radius. A portion of the annular ligament is excised. The tip of the epicondyle is then excised and the bed drilled (akin to the forage procedure to relieve venous hypertension in bone) before the fascia is closed.

A soft dressing is worn for one week, during which a light exercise program of stretching and strengthening exercises is introduced. Thereafter this program is continued for 3 weeks before work or sport is resumed. Although it may take 3 to 4 months for resolution of major symptomatology, a graduated return to work and sport can generally be anticipated. Complete success has been achieved in 30 of 34 patients so treated.

Surgery for "Golfer's" Elbow

Release on the medial side follows a similar format, easing the flexor origin from the epicondyle, excising and drilling the medial epicondylar bed, and reconstituting the fascia.

Surgery for Olecranon Impaction Syndrome

A triceps tendon split exposes the tip of the olecranon. This is excised, and the synovium in the depths of the fossa is cleared. Any loose body should be excised, and at full extension of the elbow, there should be no bony impingement in the depth of the fossa. Following this procedure, hyperextension loading of the elbow is restricted for 6 weeks.

ULNAR NEURITIS AND MEDIAL COLLATERAL LIGAMENT INSTABILITIES IN OVERARM THROWERS

FRANK W. JOBE, M.D.

Athletes who participate in overarm sports can sustain a host of injuries to the elbow. Ulnar neuritis and medial collateral ligament problems in particular are commonly caused by overuse. Many overarm activities (e.g., baseball pitch, tennis serve, javelin throw) require similar movements: rapid, forceful extension of the elbow, frequently accompanied by valgus stress and pronation of the forearm. The slight, normal valgus angle of the elbow in extension may predispose the medial aspect of the elbow to overuse injuries. The speed, power, and repetitiousness of these movements all contribute to the microtrauma that occurs.

ULNAR NEURITIS

Etiology

In the upper arm, the ulnar nerve courses subfascially, anterior to the medial intermuscular septum. At the arcade of Struthers, it moves posterior to the septum, passing behind the medial epicondyle in the cubital tunnel. The boundaries of the tunnel are formed by the posterior band of the medial collateral ligament, the medial edge of the trochlea, the medial epicondylar groove, and the arcuate ligament (which acts as the tendinous arch of the insertion of the two heads of the flexor carpi ulnaris). The nerve continues into the forearm, passing between the humeral and ulnar heads of the flexor carpi ulnaris muscle.

During elbow flexion the ulnar nerve elongates an average of 4.7 mm and can be pushed over 7 mm medially by the medial head of the triceps. Cubital tunnel volume is reduced by concomitant stretching of the arcuate ligament and bulging of the posterior portion of the medial collateral ligament. Tightening of the aponeurosis of the flexor carpi ulnaris during flexion may also compress the ulnar nerve. Thus, the proximity of several other mobile structures endangers the mobility of the ulnar nerve. Entrapment may be caused by pathologic (tensile and compressive forces on the medial aspect of the elbow) or physiologic (hypertrophy of bone, muscle, or ligament) factors. Entrapment and/or dislocation of the ulnar nerve are conditions seen most often in athletes whose arms repeatedly perform a throwing motion that results in valgus stress at the elbow. This group includes baseball pitchers, javelin throwers, gymnasts, and football quarterbacks. Biomechanical analysis of arm motion in these athletes reveals three kinds of basic pathologic stresses to the ulnar nerve: compression, friction, and traction. Of course, in any one lesion a combination of these stresses may be present.

Compression of the ulnar nerve may occur in association with several conditions. Hypertrophy of the medial head of the triceps or anconeous epitrochlearis muscle is occasionally encountered in the top level pitcher or weight lifter. Entrapment of the ulnar nerve beneath a thickened arcuate ligament—the so-called Osborne lesion—is particularly common. This condition can occur in conjunction with forearm flexor hypertrophy that causes increased pressure on the underlying nerve. Pechan and Julis demonstrated elevation of intraneural pressures by direct measurement in the ulnar nerve with the wrist extended and the elbow at 90 degrees. Increased pressures are caused by both the physiologic stretch of the nerve and external compression from the overlying aponeurosis of the flexor carpi ulnaris muscle. Further flexion of the elbow, extension of the wrist, and abduction of the shoulder, such as occurs in the early stages of the overhead pitch, can elevate intraneural pressures to six times that in the relaxed nerve.

Friction neuritis commonly results from recurrent dislocation of the ulnar nerve anterior to the medial epicondyle of the humerus. Childress noted that 16.2 percent of the population demonstrates recurrent dislocation of the ulnar nerve as the elbow moves from complete extension to full flexion. This hypermobility is often secondary to congenital or developmental laxity of the soft tissue constraints that normally hold the nerve in the epicondylar groove. Childress also found that those nerves that incompletely dislocate over the medial epicondyle are more susceptible to direct trauma, whereas those that completely dislocate are more prone to develop friction neuritis.

Traction neuritis may develop when an attenuated ulnar collateral ligament allows the medial side of the joint to "open up" excessively, thus placing abnormal stress on the ulnar nerve and creating a valgus deformity. The nerve may also become tethered by fixed flexion deformity, scar formation, traction spurs, calcific deposits, or an irregular ulnar groove secondary to degenerative changes or an old medial epicondyle separation.

Clinical Presentation

A thorough history—including standard parameters such as duration of symptoms, severity of pain, frequency of pain, and aggravating factors—is particularly important in recognizing this type of injury. The chief clinical symptom is pain in the elbow, radiating down the ulnar aspect of the arm and into the hand. Numbness and tingling in the fourth and fifth fingers are common. Weakness of the flexor carpi ulnaris and flexor digitorum is rarely seen because the motor fibers to these muscles lie deepest in the cubital tunnel and are usually uninvolved. There may be some clumsiness and heaviness of the hand, especially after throwing. These symptoms may disappear with rest and then recur with return to activity. Recurrent dislocation of the ulnar nerve may cause a painful snapping or popping sensation when the elbow is rapidly flexed and extended, with sharp pains radiating into the forearm and hand. Tenderness to palpation over the ulnar nerve at the elbow—not over the ulnar collateral ligament—is most common. A history that reveals instances of sudden pain generally indicates subluxation rather than entrapment of the ulnar nerve.

Neural abnormalities in regions innervated by the ulnar nerve, including hypoesthesia, interosseous muscle wasting, and dry skin, should be carefully considered. Tinel's sign, when present proximal to the elbow, usually is not significant, but when present distal to the elbow, is indicative of an ulnar lesion. Evidence of nerve compression lesions at other levels must also be investigated. Cervical rib, scalenus anticus syndrome, superior sulcus tumor, cervical disc protrusion with radiculopathy, compression at Guyon's canal, or compression of the deep branch of the ulnar nerve can all produce symptoms along the ulnar nerve distribution and should be specifically ruled out. A thorough neurologic examination should be performed to investigate the possibility of spinal root distribution problems or thoracic outlet syndrome. Neural conduction studies occasionally are negative in the milder cases, but an impulse slowing across the elbow is the usual finding.

Electromyography may be helpful, but findings are often inconclusive owing to the intermittent nature of the problem. A complete series of roentgenograms, including a cubital tunnel view, should be performed. Upon palpation, the ulnar nerve itself may feel thickened or "doughy", and can often be subluxed manually. Additional symptoms of associated pathologic conditions (e.g., ligament laxity, loose bodies, degenerative changes in the elbow) should also be investigated, and the condition of the whole joint complex must be considered in decisions regarding treatment and rehabilitation.

Treatment

Acute cases of ulnar neuritis, in which the symptoms are not yet severe, may respond well to conservative treatment. Rest and ice should be applied and the joint immobilized with a splint for 2 to 3 weeks. Anti-inflammatory medications may also be helpful. In most cases surgical intervention is not required. When surgery is indicated, anterior transposition of the ulnar nerve deep to the flexor muscle group provides ample protection from direct and indirect trauma occasioned by throwing. Simple decompression is not sufficient for the long term.

Ulnar Nerve Transfer

A medial incision is made over the elbow, extending approximately 2 inches in either direction from the medial epicondyle. The intermuscular septum is cut proximally, as far as and including the arcade of Struthers, to free the nerve for anterior relocation. Special care must be taken to preserve the branches of the medial antebrachial cutaneous nerve during dissection. A portion of the medial intermuscular septum is excised to prevent impingement of the transferred nerve; the nerve is then freed up and retracted with a Penrose drain. If there is a great deal of scar tissue or hourglass constriction of the nerve, it may be necessary to perform a neurolysis.

At this point the posterior aspect of the joint may be inspected for loose bodies and/or osteophytes and treated accordingly. An incision is then made in the superficial flexor-pronator muscle mass, perpendicular to the direction of its fibers and approximately one centimeter from its insertion; this incision is extended proximally to the medial collateral ligament. The top margin of the flexor group, in the interval just short of the brachioradialis, is elevated and retracted distally, leaving a carpet of muscle fiber on the ligament to provide a bed of muscle for the nerve. The nerve should be freed of its fascial covering for at least 2 inches distal to the medial epicondyle, then placed in the flexor muscle fringe and covered with the muscle belly. To ensure that no entrapment occurs, a small section is cut out of the muscle fascia around the new course of the ulnar nerve. There must be no tethering of the relocated nerve either distally, where it should lie in a bed of muscle, or proximally, where it should lie in a bed of fat. The flexor muscles are reattached to the epicondyle either by direct suture to a soft tissue cuff or through drill holes in the bone. Closure is accomplished with absorbable sutures for the deep structures and 4.0 clear nylon subcuticular sutures for the skin.

Key Points. To recapitulate the most important points in this procedure: (1) the nerve should be decompressed for 2 inches distal to the medial epicondyle to prevent tethering; (2) the intermuscular septum should be opened as far as the arcade of Struthers; (3) a portion of the intermuscular septum should be removed to prevent impingement; (4) a carpet of muscle fibers should be left on the medial collateral ligament for the nerve, to prevent tethering; and (5) the ulnar nerve should be relocated next to muscle.

Rehabilitation

After closure, the joint should be splinted at 90 degrees of flexion, leaving the wrist free, for 10 days. The patient should begin squeezing a sponge or soft ball as soon as comfort permits. Range-of-motion exercises should begin at 2 weeks after surgery, followed by gradually increasing strength exercises. At about 2 months postoperatively, the patient may begin to toss a ball easily, gradually increasing the speed and power over the next 3 to 4 months. Return to full activity may be permitted at about 6 months after surgery. The earlier in the progress of the disease that surgical intervention takes place, the better is the prognosis for a return to full preoperative ability.

MEDIAL COLLATERAL LIGAMENT INSTABILITY

Etiology

The anterior oblique portion of the medial collateral ligament is the major stabilizing agent at the elbow. Injury or laxity of this structure results in instability of the medial aspect of the elbow joint under valgus stress. Injuries to the medial collateral ligament in athletes are primarily caused by overuse. Inadequate conditioning, warm-up, and body mechanics can predispose to "microfailures" in the fibers of the ligament as the result of repeated small stresses. If the rate of failure is greater than the rate of repair and reproduction, there will be pain, inflammation, and eventually disruption of the bone-ligament junction. Reinjury to the weakened area can then occur with less stress.

Diagnosis

The primary symptom of injury to the medial collateral ligament is pain on the medial aspect of the elbow during throwing. Patients may also exhibit tenderness to palpation and swelling of the medial area. Often there is a sensation of the elbow "opening" while throwing, and many patients show decreased range of motion at the elbow. There is often a single episode of "giving way", which probably represents only the final insult. Valgus instability at the elbow can be diagnosed clinically by first flexing the patient's arm 20 to 30 degrees, to unlock the olecranon from its fossa, then applying a gentle valgus stress. Instability of the joint will allow the medial side of the joint to open. A radiographic gravity stress test of the elbow may confirm the diagnosis.

Four stages of the disorder have been identified: edema; scarring and dissociation of ligament fibers; calcification; and ossification. If detected in the early stages, conservative treatment is appropriate. Rest—for a longer time than may ordinarily be recommended—is crucial. Heat and ice should be applied alternately, and injections of Xylocaine and steroids may be helpful. Injection should not be *into* the ligament, but rather on *top* of the ligament, to bathe it. I prefer to give no more than three injections, and not more often than once a month.

Scarring, calcification, and ossification are all stress raisers that focus biomechanical stresses on already weakened areas, thus increasing the likelihood of further damage. If scarring and calcification are present, and if they are accompanied by pain that does not respond to rest, the calcifications should be removed and the ligament repaired. If only stability of the joint is required, surgery is not necessary; however, if the patient desires to continue participation in a sport requiring throwing or other overarm movements, surgery may be necessary. Surgical reconstruction of the medial collateral ligament with a tendon graft is indicated (1) in cases of acute rupture in throwers, (2) where it is desired to re-establish valgus stability in the presence of chronic laxity that is symptomatic, or (3) following debridement for calcific tendinitis, if there is not sufficient viable tissue remaining to effect a primary repair in an athlete.

Repair

Using a tourniquet for hemostasis, a standard medial incision is made and carried down through the subcutaneous tissue to the muscle, taking care not to damage the sensory nerves. An incision is made into the fascial covering of the origin of the flexor muscle mass, in line with the muscle fibers; the flexor muscle mass is retracted to both sides to expose the anterior oblique portion of the medial collateral ligament. An incision is made in the ligament, again in line with the fibers, and the ligament is debrided to remove all calcifications. At this juncture, the elbow should be flexed 20 to 30 degrees and a valgus stress applied; the medial aspect of the elbow joint should open easily. If there is sufficient ligamentous tissue remaining, a simple primary repair can be effected; otherwise, it will be necessary to reconstruct the ligament.

When the ligament has been debrided it should be reattached to the periosteum. Slack in the ligament can be tightened using a figure-of-eight suture on both sides of the longitudinal split, then testing for snugness. The two halves of the ligament are then approximated and sutured. If the ligament has been torn off its bony inser-

tion, the bone should be rongeured to provide a good base for reattachment. Holes are then drilled in the bone, sutures are passed through the holes, and the ligament is sutured securely to the bone.

If it is necessary to reconstruct the ligament, the flexor muscles should be cut approximately 1 cm distal to the medial epicondyle, leaving a fringe of ligament for reattachment. Holes are drilled in the medial epicondyle and ulna, adjacent to the insertion of the anterior oblique ligament. These holes connect at their base to form a U-shaped passage for the tendon graft. The tendon graft is harvested from either the palmaris longus or the plantaris tendon. The graft is sutured at each end to facilitate its placement in the osseous passage. When properly placed, the graft forms a figure-of-eight, functionally replicating the anterior oblique part of the medial collateral ligament. Finally, the graft is sutured to itself. Viable ligamentous tissue should be sutured over the graft to provide additional strength. As already described, the ulnar nerve should be transferred anteriorly to protect it from damage during and after surgery; the flexor muscle mass is placed over the nerve, to help keep it in place, and sutured to the medial epicondyle.

Rehabilitation

After closing, the arm should be placed in a posterior splint in 90 degrees of flexion, leaving the wrist free, for 7 to 10 days. The patient should begin squeezing a sponge or soft ball as soon as comfort permits. Range-of-motion exercises should be initiated immediately after the splint is removed. A brace is not necessary or advisable. At 3 to 4 months after surgery, the patient may begin to toss a ball, lightly. Speed and power can then be increased gradually until at one year after surgery a few innings may be pitched. The average time to return to preoperative ability is 18 months for a professional pitcher. Athletes who play other positions require a shorter period of rehabilitation.

FRACTURES AND DISLOCATIONS IN THE HAND AND WRIST

C. STEWART WRIGHT, M.D., F.R.C.S.(C)

Hand and wrist injuries occur commonly to the athlete and may be frustrating for both trainer and physician because of difficulties in making diagnoses and obtaining a successful outcome. Acute injuries are usually caused by impact or rotational forces such as a fall

on an outstretched hand, and these may result in strains, fractures, or dislocations.

THE WRIST

Fractures of the distal radius or wrist usually result from a considerable force, e.g., falling from a height or flying off a speeding vehicle such as a bicycle or motorcycle. Distal radius and ulna fractures may be extra-articular, the so-called Colles' fracture, or extend into the joint. In either instance, accurate reduction of the distal radius is important, and if closed reduction fails, operative reduction may be necessary. Fracture-dislocations of the wrist may take the form of volar lip (Barton's fracture) or dorsal lip (reverse Barton's) radius fractures and involve a subluxation or dislocation of the carpus. These can usually be easily reduced by closed means, but may need pin fixation to maintain the reduction. A third variation of the wrist fracture-dislocation involves a fracture of the radial styloid (chauffeur's fracture). This also may require pin fixation if closed reduction cannot be maintained with plaster.

The distal radioulnar joint is usually injured by a rotational force applied to the forearm through the hand although impact may also be important. This injury can result in dislocation of the distal ulna dorsally or volarly. This force results in an injury to the triangular fibrocartilage complex which may take the form of a tear in the articular disc, in the dorsal or volar radioulnar ligaments, or in the ulnar collateral ligament. The joint may appear to be stable on examination, and pain on rotation of the forearm may be the only clue to the injury. Acute injuries with any subluxation should be immobilized to maintain proper reduction. Dorsal displacement is stabilized in full supination, and volar subluxation is maintained in neutral position. In both instances, a long arm cast will be necessary to maintain the reduced position. A transverse Kirschner wire may occasionally be necessary in addition to the cast.

There is a spectrum of injuries to the carpus. At one end are sprains, strains, flake fractures, and undisplaced carpal bone fractures. A ligamentous strain can occur between any of the carpal bones, but most often involves the scapholunate ligaments. The most common flake fracture occurs dorsally from the triquetrum and really represents a ligamentous injury. Ligamentous injuries can result in carpal instability, which may be difficult to diagnose on plain roentgenograms. Multiple views, including flexion-extension and radial-ulnar deviation, are helpful, as are cineradiography and arthrography. Wrist arthroscopoy is still in its infancy, but may prove to be a useful diagnostic tool as more experience is gained.

The next level in severity consists of scaphoid fractures that are not displaced. These scaphoid injuries may not be seen on x-ray examination at the time of injury and should be treated on clinical grounds initially by cast immobilization. A repeat roentgenogram or bone scan 7 to 10 days later is appropriate if tenderness persists directly over the scaphoid in the anatomic snuff box. An often overlooked carpal bone fracture is that of the hook of the hamate. This may be caused by a direct blow or by repetitive trauma as with using a baseball bat or a golf club. Like fractures of the scaphoid, this fracture may be difficult to demonstrate radiographically. A carpal tunnel view may be helpful, but a CT scan of the wrist is usually necessary to make this diagnosis. Ulnar nerve function must be examined because nerve compression may occur following this injury.

More severe carpal injuries are displaced scaphoid fractures and scapholunate dissociation with rotatory subluxation of the scaphoid. These often require surgery to obtain and maintain reduction of the malalignment. The most severe carpal injuries are those having a perilunate component. This may be a pure lunate or perilunate dislocation or have other associated fractures. The three most common are transcaphoid, transcapitate, and transradioulnar perilunate fracture-dislocations or a combination of the three. These generally require open reduction and internal fixation of the injury. It is important to check median nerve function, as this nerve is commonly injured during these carpal disruptions. Acute compression of the median nerve should be released by division of the transverse carpal ligament even if the physician decides to treat the fracture at a later date after the swelling has subsided.

Finally, one should be alert to an injury that occurs in the adolescent, Salter type I epiphyseal injury of the distal radius and ulna. Although these appear normal radiographically, there is tenderness just proximal to the radial and ulnar styloids. These injuries can be very painful and may require cast immobilization for 10 to 14 days.

THE HAND

The jammed finger is a common athletic injury and is usually caused by an impact force. This entity may involve any of the digits or the thumb at the carpometacarpal (CMC), metacarpophalangeal (MCP), or interphalangeal (IP) levels.

Carpometacarpal (CMC) Joint

The CMC joint may sustain a sprain, fracture, dislocation, or fracture-dislocation. These usually require casting until healed; some require open reduction and internal fixation. Bennett's fracture is an intra-articular injury to the CMC joint of the thumb. A fragment of the volar metacarpal base is held by the volar ligament while the remainder of the thumb is displaced owing primarily to the pull of the abductor pollicis longus and secondarily to that of the adductor pollicis longus.

Accurate anatomic reduction is essential to avoid the sequelae of post-traumatic osteoarthritis. A similar entity occurs at the base of the fifth metacarpal, the so-called "Baby Bennett's" fracture. Again, a volar fragment remains intact while the remainder is displaced by the pull of the extensor carpi ulnaris. This injury also should be accurately reduced and stabilized as necessary. Dislocations of the other three CMC joints may be unstable after reduction and may need pin fixation.

Metacarpophalangeal (MCP) Joint

MCP joint injuries of the thumb most commonly involve the ulnar collateral ligament, the so-called "gamekeeper's" or "ski-pole" thumb. This is usually caused by a fall on an outstretched hand with hyperabduction of the thumb. Strap bindings on ski poles are probably the most common cause of this injury. Most hand surgeons believe that a complete tear of the ligament should be surgically repaired. Surgery is warranted if there is a large intra-articular fragment attached to the ligament and the piece is significantly displaced. It may also be indicated for late cases of pain and instability of the joint. Strains of this ligament need to be taped during athletics and immobilized with a C splint during the day. This regimen usually suffices when a player cannot take the time away from sports for cast immobilization. A similar injury may occur to the radial collateral ligament, and the principles of treatment are the same as for the ulnar collateral ligament.

Dislocations of the MCP joint are most commonly dorsal and caused by hyperextension forces, although they may occur in any direction. The so-called "complex" or "locked" dislocations may be difficult to reduce by closed means or may remain subluxed after attempted reduction. Careful attention must be paid to postreduction roentgenograms for this residual subluxation, the presence of which usually necessitates an open reduction of the joint and freeing of the interposed soft tissues.

Collateral ligament or volar plate injuries of the digital MCP joints may be very slow to heal and require long-term use of buddy splinting (adjacent finger-strapping). The volar plate injuries often require extension block splinting in addition to the buddy taping. This involves the use of a dorsal splint, which blocks extension at a preset angle, but still allows for full flexion of the digits. Intra-articular steroids may also be needed to resolve these injuries if they become chronic. In spite of these measures it may take several months for symptoms to subside. The MCP collateral ligaments most often injured are on the radial side of the index and the ulnar side of the little fingers. Joint instability or a large bony fragment attached to the ligament usually requires surgical repair.

Proximal Interphalangeal (PIP) Joint

Beware of the "swollen" PIP joint. Serious injuries are often missed, and therefore not properly treated. One must carefully assess all four sides of the joint and determine the integrity of (1) the volar plate, (2) the radial collateral ligament, (3) the ulnar collateral ligament, and (4) the extensor mechanism. Any or all of these may be disrupted and require specific treatment. Digital block is helpful if pain limits proper examination.

Collateral ligament injuries occasionally occur alone, but are usually associated with an injury to the volar plate secondary to a hyperextension force. The collateral ligament injury can be treated by buddy taping to the adjacent finger. Injuries to the volar plate may require the use of extension block splinting for the first 7 to 10 days. Large bony fragments with associated joint instability require surgical repair.

With sufficient force the PIP joint may dislocate, most commonly in a dorsal dislocation. Three variations

of this injury include (1) volar plate avulsion from the middle phalanx and a major longitudinal split of the collateral ligaments, (2) fracture-dislocation with a volar fragment from the base of the middle phalanx less than 40 percent of the articular surface, and (3) a volar fragment of the middle phalanx greater than 40 percent of the articular surface. The first two can usually be managed by closed reduction followed by the use of extension block splinting. The third variation is usually unstable. Accurate closed reduction is difficult as the volar plate and collateral ligaments are no longer attached to the middle phalanx. This injury usually requires open reduction and reattachment of the fragment with a pull-out wire. If there is considerable comminution of the base of the middle phalanx, a volar plate arthroplasty, as described by Eaton, may be necessary.

Volar dislocations are much less common, but may have an associated dorsal lip fracture from the base of the middle phalanx. If this fragment is large and cannot be accurately reduced, open reduction of the piece is necessary. In either instance, this injury must be treated with the PIP joint in extension to allow for healing of the extensor apparatus.

Boutonniere deformities are often the result of catching a basketball or softball on the fingertip. They occur at the PIP joint following disruption of the extensor tendon central slip mechanism. This allows volar subluxation of the lateral bands and a flexed posture of the PIP joint. The subluxated lateral bands and oblique retinacular ligament can then produce hyperextension of the DIP joint through their pull. When seen immediately following injury, most boutonniere deformities are passively correctable and can be managed by splinting the PIP joint in extension. The DIP joint is left free, and flexion of this joint is encouraged. It may be necessary to splint the PIP joint for 6 to 8 weeks full time.

An uncommon variation of the boutonniere deformity occurs when a collateral ligament is also torn and becomes trapped inside the PIP joint. The joint then becomes irreducible passively and requires an open reduction and repair of the collateral ligament.

Distal Interphalangeal (DIP) Joint

At this level the most common injury is the mallet finger deformity that can be caused by catching a hard ball on the tip of a finger. Most of these injuries can be managed by splinting (see chapter on Tendon Injuries in the Hand). Many athletes are able to continue participation in their sport while wearing their splint.

Dislocations of the DIP are usually in a dorsal direction and easily reducible for the most part. The exception to this occurs when the volar plate becomes trapped in the joint, and these may require open reduction. Volar subluxation or dislocation is usually part of an intra-articular mallet finger deformity. Volar displacement is treated with the joint in extension; the dorsal dislocations employ the extension block principle.

Hand Fractures

Let me say at the outset that more than 90 percent of hand fractures seen in the athlete are manageable by nonoperative means. The goal should be early (within 7 days) unloaded digital motion. This will allow rapid diminution of swelling and present intra- and extra-articular adhesions, thus preserving joint mobility. These objectives can be achieved through the use of adjacent finger strapping (buddy taping) and extension block splinting, in addition to the early unloaded motion of the digits.

Unloaded motion means avoiding stress on the digit, that is, avoiding any power grip exercises for the first few weeks.

Hand fractures may be transverse, oblique, or comminuted. Care must be taken to ensure that excessive shortening does not occur, especially in the proximal phalanx, or the extensor mechanism may not function properly. Two other concerns are malrotation and excessive angulation. Rotation can only be checked with the MP and PIP joints in full flexion, in which position the nail plates should point toward the scaphoid tubercle.

Some angulation is allowed with metacarpal neck fractures (boxers' fractures). In the fourth and fifth metacarpals, 35 to 40° of volar angulation is acceptable because of the mobility of the CMC joints. This is not true of the second and third metacarpals, and angulations beyond 15 to 20° should be corrected. There is no place for the use of plaster casts with the "90-90" position of the MCP and PIP joints. If this is felt necessary because of instability, I would favor the use of percutaneous pins to obtain stability. The fixation can then be augmented with the use of a gutter splint.

The majority of phalangeal fractures are stable in flexion and unstable in extension. One must establish a stable arc of motion for the fracture and then allow motion through that range. It may be necessary to anesthetize the digit and examine the fracture stability under anesthesia. If the fracture is stable through a full range of motion, it can be managed with buddy taping and early motion. If there is a range of instability, extension block splinting is employed. Weekly roentgenograms should be obtained for the first 3 weeks. Phalangeal fractures that require open reduction are those that are unstable through all ranges of motion and those with a large intra-articular component which is displaced or unstable. Once stability has been obtained, early unloaded motion should be started.

TENDON INJURIES IN THE HAND AND WRIST

C. STEWART WRIGHT, M.D., F.R.C.S.(C)

Acute and chronic tendon injuries may occur with many sporting activities. When they do occur, even minor injuries may be disabling to the athlete. All too often, potentially serious trauma to tendons in the upper extremity is not diagnosed and passed off as "sprains" or, if diagnosed, improperly treated, impairing the athlete's performance and causing unnecessary pain. I hope to raise the reader's level of awareness for potential deep structure injury beneath the swollen hand or wrist.

THE WRIST

Flexors

On the flexor surface of the wrist, the tendons most commonly injured are the flexor carpi radialis (FCR) and the flexor carpi ulnaris (FCU). The thumb and digital flexors may also be injured at the wrist, but much less frequently than the wrist flexors. The usual mechanism of injury is a blow against the dorsiflexed wrist (e.g., a fall on the hand or colliding with another player with the arm extended). FCU is the tendon most often injured, and the patient's complaint is pain along the volar ulnar aspect of the wrist and upon palpation of the pisiform. Ulnar wrist flexion against resistance will produce pain. In all of these injuries, a post-traumatic tendonitis must be differentiated from a bony injury and thus radiographic evaluation is necessary.

An injury to the FCR produces pain on the volar radial aspect of the wrist. There may be pain with flexion and extension of the wrist. Again, FCR tendonitis may mimic fractures of the scaphoid or distal radius.

Acute injuries to the FCU and FCR may also produce volar wrist capsule strains and should be treated with volar wrist splinting. Oral anti-inflammatory agents may reduce inflammation and decrease pain. Steroid and local anesthetic injections seldom are used in acute cases, but are reserved for injuries that do not respond to the initial supportive treatment over 4 to 6 weeks. When injections are given, corticosteroids are used and should be mixed with 1 percent Xylocaine. Care must be taken to ensure that the injection is peritendinous and not intratendinous, intravascular, or intraneural. I do not believe that there is a place for more than two or three injections.

When the injections have proved unsuccessful, one must either reconsider the diagnosis or decide whether surgery is appropriate. These injuries should only rarely come to surgery before 6 to 12 months have passed since the traumatic event. The athlete should also have had the benefit of a supervised physical therapy program prior to any considerations of surgery. This not only may improve the symptoms, but also will give the physician some idea of how the patient will cooperate postoperatively.

The incision for releasing the FCR should be kept radial to the tendon to avoid injury to the palmar cutaneous branch of the median nerve. At the same time, care is necessary to avoid injury to the radial artery. The thenar muscles are then reflected to expose the scaphoid tubercle and trapezial crest. Portions of these bony prominences are then resected and the FCR released circumferentially to its insertion. Postoperatively, the patient should begin early wrist motion. With the FCU tenolysis is necessary, as is removal of part or all of the pisiform.

Extensors

Six extensor compartments are housed on the dorsum of the wrist. Tenosynovitis may involve any of the 12 wrist and digital extensors. As with the flexors of the wrist, the extensor injuries may present as acute tears, repetitive trauma, or repetitive stress (overuse).

The most radial extensor compartment houses the extensor pollicis brevis (EPB) and abductor pollicis longus (APL). At the level of the radial styloid these tendons pass under a ligamentous retinaculum approximately 1 cm in length. A tenosynovitis at this level is referred to as DeQuervain's tenovaginitis, after the man who described the condition in 1895. These patients complain of localized pain over the radial styloid which may be confused with arthritis of the carpometacarpal joint of the thumb. The so-called Finklestein's test for DeQuervain's disease refers to increased pain at the radial styloid with the ulnar deviation of the wrist after the thumb has been flexed into the palm.

Treatment of this problem should initially include oral anti-inflammatory agents, a splint that immobilizes all 3 joints of the thumb, heat, and hydrotherapy. The splint is removed for the warm water soaks, but is otherwise worn full time during the acute phase. Local injections of corticosteroid and Xylocaine may be repeated once or twice. Surgery should be employed when there has been a failure of conservative treatment over 12 to 16 weeks.

A longitudinal incision is recommended, but a horizontal one may be used. The most serious complication is damage to the superficial branches of the radial sensory nerve which may number 1 to 3. No patient will thank you if you relieve his tendonitis, but leave him with a painful neuroma. The retinaculum is then divided longitudinally and part of it excised to avoid recurrence. The EPB must be identified as well as the presence of a multiple tailed APL, which is fairly common. There may be multiple compartments, and it is important to release each and to resect any septa. Bony prominences should be rongeured smooth, and postoperatively motion should be started within 7 to 10 days.

The second extensor compartment contains the extensor carpi radialis longus and brevis (ECRL and ECRB). It is usually possible to delineate the two different tendons inserting at the base of the second and third metacarpals. The acute injuries require splinting and oral anti-inflammatory drugs followed by steroid injections for those who do not respond.

Another condition that may be confused with the two previously mentioned is the so-called "intersection syndrome." This occurs on the radial aspect of the wrist, but more proximally than DeQuervain's disease. It occurs at the intersection of the first and second extensor compartment tendons. It has been described in weightlifters, rowers, and canoeists, and has been seen to be associated with hypertrophy of the APL and EPB muscle bellies overlying the tendons of the radial wrist extensors. If conservative means do not resolve the problem, surgical decompression of the sheath of the overlying muscles provides quick relief of symptoms.

The extensor pollicis longus (EPL) is the sole occupant of the third compartment and can become inflamed as it passes around Lister's tubercle on the distal radius. This is an uncommon problem, but when it does occur, it requires early surgical decompression because of the possibility of tendon rupture. Surgery should be considered when there is no response to treatment in the first 4 weeks.

Compartment four contains the extensor digitorum communis (EDC) and extensor indicis proprius (EIP), and compartment five, the extensor digiti minimi (EDM). These tendons all pass underneath the extensor retinaculum and may develop a tenosynovitis at that level. Again, the use of splinting and oral anti-inflammatory preparations is recommended, followed by steroid injection and later by a surgical decompression if necessary. If surgery is needed, a portion of retinaculum should be left intact to prevent bowstringing when the wrist is dorsiflexed.

The extensor carpi ulnaris (ECU) is in the last compartment. ECU tendonitis presents with pain on the dorsal ulnar aspect of the wrist and base of the fifth metacarpal. If this condition requires surgical decompression, the dorsal sensory branch of the ulnar nerve must be protected.

DIGITAL TENDONS

Flexors

A tenosynovitis of the digital flexors—flexor digitorum superficialis (FDS), flexor digitorum profundus (FDP), and flexor pollicis longus (FPL)—may present as swelling and tenderness at the metacarpal phalangeal (MCP) joint level in the palm. When more severe, this can produce the phenomenon of triggering as the flexor tendon moves through the narrowed A1 pulley in flexion and has trouble re-entering the flexor sheath with digital extension. Most of these respond favorably to oral anti-inflammatory preparations early in their course or to corticosteroid injection once triggering begins. For those which do not respond, a trigger finger release may be carried out under local anesthetic. These are best done through a longitudinal incision in the distal palm and the entire A1 pulley incised. Care is taken to preserve the A2 pulley and early motion is started after surgery. In the thumb, the neurovascular bundles are quite volar and the ulnar digital nerve crosses the tendon sheath. These structures must be identified and protected from injury.

Avulsion of the insertion of a flexor profundus tendon (FDP and FPL) is a relatively common injury, especially in athletes. Most occur in the ring digit, but any finger may be involved. It is not uncommon for this injury to be seen late because the significance of the initial injury may not have been recognized. The usual mechanism of injury is an opponent pulling away from a player who has hold of the opponent's jersey or pants. This results in forced extension of the digit while the FDP is maximally contracted, producing avulsion.

These injuries have been divided into three groups. Type 1 is a retraction of the tendon into the palm. This results because of a rupture of the vinculum longus and thus loss of an important part of the tendon blood supply. No active distal interphalangeal joint (DIP) motion is present, and there is usually a tender lump in the palm where the tendon has retracted. These should be repaired within the first week of injury. The tendon must be threaded back through the tendon sheath and reinserted into the distal phalanx with a pullout wire.

In type 2, which is the most common type, the tendon retracts to the proximal interphalangeal (PIP) joint level. This occurs because the vinculum is still intact and prevents retraction of the FDP. Once again, there is no active DIP motion and there is pain and swelling at the PIP level. The tendon blood supply is largely intact, and these tendons have been successfully reinserted as long as 8 to 12 weeks postinjury. Ideally, they are repaired during the first week.

The type 3 injuries include avulsion of a large fragment from the base of the distal phalanx. This is usually large enough to catch on the A4 pulley and prevent proximal migration of the tendon. Once again, no active DIP motion is possible. These require open reduction of the displaced fragment along with reinsertion of the flexor tendon.

When these injuries are seen late, many surgeons believe that they are best left alone unless there is a painful lump in the palm or an unstable DIP joint. The tendon stump may be excised and the DIP joint fused if necessary. Depending on the patient's lack of function, a tendon graft or two-stage tendon repair may be considered as an alternative.

Extensors

Extensor tendon injuries in the hand will be considered at three different levels: the DIP joint, the PIP joint, and the MCP joint.

DIP Joint

At the DIP joint, the so-called mallet finger deformity occurs with avulsion of the extensor tendon at its insertion. This usually occurs when the finger is struck end-on by a football, baseball, or basketball. The tendon at this level consists of a the conjoined lateral bands and it may be injured in four ways. Type 1 is an avulsion of the tendon from the distal phalanx. Type 2 is associated with a dorsal lip fracture of less than one-third of the articular surface. Type 3 has an associated fracture greater than one-third of the articular surfce and it may render the DIP joint unstable. Type 4 occurs in children, and a Salter I or transepiphyseal injury occurs at the base of the distal phalanx. The type 1 injury is by far the most common.

The vast majority of mallet finger injuries can be successfully treated by conservative means. The DIP joint is splinted in extension or slight hyperextension for 6 weeks full-time and then a further 4 to 6 weeks of night-time splinting. There are good commercially available splints or they may be fabricated on an individual basis by the therapist. The DIP joint is immobilized but the PIP joint remains free. This method of treatment may be successful even if started up to 8 weeks postinjury, provided there is still some inflammatory reaction present over the DIP joint. When the associated fracture fragment renders the DIP joint unstable, it may still be possible to do a closed reduction and percutaneous pinning. If this is not successful, then an open reduction of the fragment should be carried out. This is done in association with a transarticular Kirschner wire and should have an external splint for 6 weeks to ensure that the K-wire does not break.

There are many procedures described for repair of the chronic mallet deformity and none has a high success rate. The most reliable operation is a DIP fusion with the joint in 10 to 15° of flexion.

PIP Joint

At this level, the central slip is ruptured and there is progressive volar subluxation of the lateral bands. This results in a flexion deformity of PIP joint because of the unopposed pull of the FDS. Hyperextension of the DIP joint will occur through the pull of the lateral bands and the oblique retinacular ligament and produce the so-called boutonniere deformity. Initially, the PIP joint may appear only in slight flexion and the injury may be missed. It may be 10 to 21 days before the full-blown deformity develops.

Like mallet finger deformities, most boutonnieres may be managed by closed means. This involves splinting the PIP joint in extension, but encouraging flexion of the DIP joint. With the PIP joint splinted, both active and passive exercises are carried out at the DIP joint to help restore normal tendon balance.

Boutonniere deformities discovered late may still be treated by conservative means as late as 8 to 12 weeks after the injury. This may require serial casting or daily monitoring of the splinting to help overcome any PIP flexion contracture that may be present. Chronic deformities at this level are very difficult problems and should be managed by a physician skilled in hand surgery.

MP Joint

Injuries to the extensor mechanism at this level usually involve a longitudinal tear of the saggital band. When this occurs the extensor tendon is able to sublux or dislocate away from the site of injury. Any digit may be involved, but the middle finger is the most common. Also, the radial side is injured more frequently than the ulnar. Physical examination demonstrates inability to fully extend the digit as well as deviation of the digit away from the side of injury.

When this injury occurs without extensor subluxation, it may be treated with splinting alone. Otherwise, acute injuries at the MP joint should be repaired primarily and the joint immobilized for 3 weeks. It is important to ensure that the extensor is centralized over the MP joint. There is usually sufficient tissue for repair, but if deficient, then a portion of juncturae tendinum or a retrograde piece of extensor may be sutured directly into the defect or looped around the lumbrical to realign the extensor mechanism. Any of these latter procedures may be used to correct this injury in its chronic state.

HIP, THIGH AND PELVIS INJURIES

SOFT TISSUE INJURY TO THE HIP AND THIGH

CHARLES R. BULL, M.D., B.Sc.(Med),
F.R.C.S.(C), F.A.C.S., F.I.C.S.

HEMATOMAS

In hockey the missed hip check resulting in a thrust of the knee at a fleeting opponent can often inflict an unpenalized and unrecognized serious injury. The blow taken on the central lateral midthigh area produces a hematoma with moderate initial pain. The injured player is able to continue to participate in many cases and effectively pumps more blood into the hematoma. He can even take an additional injury, compounding the problem. Then, after the 10-minute intermission, he is unable to walk or skate. Untreated, this injury may lead to the complication of *myositis ossificans*, which may leave the individual sidelined with a partially mobile knee for as long as one year in some cases.

Initial Management

The measures that constitute immediate local management—RICE (spelled by the first letter of each measure)—are as follows:

1. *Rest* (R) with the leg on a bench or on pillows at 90—90 degree position of hip and knees. The important thing is to have the foot elevated well above the heart.

2. *Ice pack* (I) in a towel over the hematoma, on the area of maximum pain because there is not usually any bruising initially. The ice pack should be removed every 20 minutes for 20 minutes and then re-applied (20 minutes on; 20 minutes off), and continued to a lesser extent for at least 72 hours. *Do not apply heat.*

3. *Compression* (C) with two or three 6-inch tightly applied tensor bandages. Be careful not to compromise the circulation; monitor the circulation by checking the peripheral pulses frequently. Just elevate the leg. Do not massage it or otherwise exercise it.

4. *Elevation* (E), with the foot elevated well above the heart, for 72 hours. He should remain totally off his feet for this period.

Medications

The use of Papase (*Carica papaya* enzymes) has never been proved effectual and should be abandoned.

Antiinflammatory medications should be given as early as possible, particularly within the first 24 hours, to reduce the swelling and muscle spasm. The antiprostaglandins, such as Anaprox (naproxen sodium), are probably the most effective preparations—2 tablets stat and one three times daily for 7 to 10 days. Antiprostaglandins are recommended because there is a large amount of prostaglandin released immediately at the time of injury, and this is a major factor in causing the initial swelling. Muscle relaxants do not work and theoretically can cause more bleeding in the relaxed muscle. (Alcohol is also contraindicated for the same reason.)

The most important initial management is "recognition of the serious nature of the problem". Thus rest, crutches, bed rest, ice, and elevation should be followed by a surgical assessment.

An initial soft tissue radiograph will delineate a hematoma in one-third of the cases and is worthwhile. One should probably try to grade these hematomatas into first-, second-, and third-degree hematoma, as determined by pain, lack of mobility, degree of swelling, and response to rest.

First- and second-degree hematomas permit 90 degree movement and straight leg-raising. Third-degree hematomas restrict movement to less than 90 degrees and permit *active* knee flexion, but not straight leg-raising. These patients have severe pain in spite of medication and should be hospitalized.

The very serious third-degree injuries are usually fairly obvious. There is severe pain, immobility of the knee in particular as well as the hip, and swelling that increases by 1½ to 2 inches (4 to 5 cm) the girth of the quadriceps by actual measurement. A very tense, large swollen area, 6 to 8 inches in diameter (15 to 20 cm), often can be felt bulging beneath the fascia lata. It feels "different", not truly fluctuant, but much tenser than normal muscle, and there is often an associated large tense synovial effusion in the knee. This can be mistaken for an intrinsic knee problem, but is actually a sympathetic response and the knee itself is normal.

Wydase (Hyaluronidase), steroids, or local anesthetics have been injected into these hematomas in the first 72 hours, but this practice is contraindicated because of (1) increased tendency to infection, and (2) their alteration of the defense mechanism and production of collagen fibers, which in essence would delay healing rather than enhance it.

At 72 hours the repair stage starts and patients with first-degree hematoma should be fairly comfortable. Some swelling is noted, but there should be moderately good mobility and, at this stage, fairly extensive bruising in the classic cases.

The muscle fibers are crushed or torn and the hematoma can be very extensive. The most frequent problem is an *inter*stitial or *inter*muscular hematoma in which the muscle sheath ruptures and the blood and bruising tracks up or down the leg. These are the "good ones", although they do look bad due to extensive bruising.

The "bad ones" are the *intra*muscular hematomas, in which the muscle sheath remains intact and thus the hematoma remains isolated. Absorption is much more difficult. In these cases the periosteum is also often damaged and osteoblasts become available to convert the subperiosteal or intramuscular hematomas into myositis ossificans.

Physiotherapy can push the "good ones" (intermuscular), but the bad ones have to rest to prevent further bleeding and enlargement of the hematomas. Cool whirlpool, range of motion exercises, light cycling, light weights, springs and pulleys, and early walking progressing to light jogging and early skating can be instituted in the good ones.

The third-degree injuries are worse at the end of 72 hours, with unremitting severe pain and increasing immobility, and these should be operated on. Under general anesthesia, a satisfactory 4-inch (10-cm) incision is made laterally through the fascia lata. Careful probing with a Kelly hemostat is then undertaken, and as soon as blood and clot are released, the incision is opened more widely by blunt dissection.

The hematoma usually lies right on top of the bone and can be evacuated and completely removed with the assistance of copious irrigation with Garamycin solution. The fascia lata, the subcutaneous tissue, and the skin are then closed and a Jones bandage is applied from toes to groin. Once the clot has been evacuated, treatment can be the same as for a first-degree injury over the next 7 to 10 days—physiotherapy, ice, sound, progressing to range of motion, but no massage.

Second-degree injuries are puzzling, but when in doubt they should be treated as third-degree injuries. A long 16-gauge or 14-gauge needle introduced into the hematoma in an attempt to aspirate blood seems to be a sensible procedure, but it is not. It is usually hard to find the exact fluctuant area, and often the clot cannot be aspirated. Furthermore, the needle is likely to introduce an infection; once the hematoma is infected, a systemic problem exists, requiring surgical drainage and systemic antibiotics and increasing the danger of long-term complications. Therefore the hematoma is either decompressed satisfactorily in the operating room or treated conservatively.

A missed third-degree injury may come to light at that 7- to 10-day mark, as indicated by a swollen painful thigh and immobile hip and knee. These injuries are often treated with hot baths and are the most likely to develop into myositis ossificans.

I still surgically explore these on occasion. I also prescribe physiotherapy to try to mobilize these people with gentle pool therapy, ultrasound, and management to decrease the swelling, but again no massage, no faradism to stimulate the muscle or increase bleeding, and no isokinetic or isotonic weight program.

The first radiologic signs of ossification, the typical "sandstorm" appearance, are visible about 3 weeks after the injury. As this matures, an anvil-shaped lesion appears. The full-blown myositis ossificans, verified radiographically (Fig. 1), needs no treatment other than rest. Swimming and cycling are permitted, but no running, skating, and the like.

I emphasize that it can take up to 6, even 12, months for this problem to settle completely. I never operate on a fully developed myositis ossificans (fully calcified) because the ossification tends to recur.

The fully developed quiescent case of myositis ossificans allows a normal return to unlimited sports.

Prevention consists in:

1. *Better conditioning* to avoid the missed hip check.

2. *Better warm-ups.*

3. *Stretching exercises* starting from the neck and working down literally to the Achilles tendon, feet, and toes form part of the basis of a sensible warm-up program.

4. *Equipment* should fit properly and should be used even during light practice. The Cooperall reduces hematomas because of its uniform fit and total body padding (Fig. 2).

5. *The rules*—kneeing, spearing, and cross-checking rules—all have to be enforced by the coach as well as the referee.

6. *Protective taping or adhesive*, tensor bandage, or bracing is beneficial on a weakened joint or limb; in current use are "pro" type neoprene sleeves or even pantaloon leg sleeves, for thigh hematomas in particular, which are effective but expensive.

7. *Cautious return*: Beware of further trauma. Basically, the player can skate in a straight line at first, but must not push, twist, or pivot; gradually he progresses to these activities as his strength returns.

8. *Caution regarding massage.* Trainers, physiotherapists, and masseurs have to be very careful in the active phase not to prolong or initiate bleeding or augment tissue damage.

9. *Other methods* of treatment, such as ethylchloride spray (which is probably of no benefit), analgesic balm, and DMSO are contraindicated as they only remove the pain. Pressure or trigger point injection, acupuncture, and TNS Probe are advocated by some and may have some benefit, although to this date it has not been proved.

10. *Strengthening.* After severe injury it takes at least 6 weeks to get into the remodeling phase with

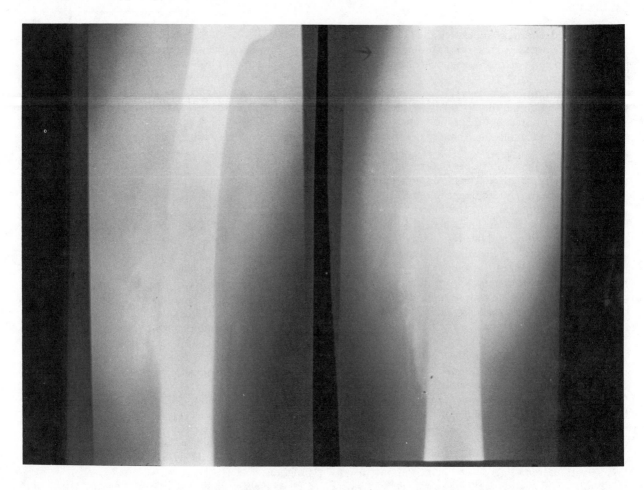

Figure 1   Myositis ossificans subsequent to thigh hematoma.

additional strength. This can be graded clinically from 1 to 6 by the physiotherapist or physician, but it is more realistically graded by Cybex isokinetic equipment. This gives a computerized assessment of the exact strength deficiency and compares it to the opposite leg, as well as quadriceps to hamstrings and fast-twitch to slow-twitch muscle strength. In our clinics, results of these Cybex tests should be 90 percent of normal before the patient returns to the sport.

11. *Additional overall strength training.* Isokinetic training is best, and in the case of the thigh, it should not be only the gastrocnemius and hamstrings, but also the adductors and abductors, evertors and invertors with stereotactic training (jumping over sticks or boxes), and thus the athlete is less apt to restrain the injured limb. This is different from conventional weight training, which is strictly isotonic. The isokinetic strengthening also develops the fast-twitch fibers and creates more overall strength in the limb. This type of training has not been emphasized enough in the past.

HIP POINTERS

Hip pointers are more likely to be self-inflicted by a fall into the boards or goalpost or, less often, a hard cross-check, in lacrosse for instance. Specifically, a col-

lection of blood forms beneath the periosteum in the area adjacent to the iliac crest and involves the muscles and soft tissues above the crest. The hip pointer is a very painful localized swelling with significant localized bruising. However, it is never as serious on a long-term basis as the previously discussed hematomas.

Because long-term problems are very unusual, treatment can be a little less aggressive. However, the same principles apply: (1) RICE, and (2) immediate physiotherapy with sound or interferential, no injections, and usually no operation.

X-ray studies should be done to rule out a fracture or displaced epiphyseal fracture, which requires a much longer immobilization process (6 to 8 weeks). In an uncomplicated hip pointer, a large protective donut type pad can be fashioned over the hip, and in many cases the player can return in 7 to 10 days, although I have known some to take as long as 2 months.

Better warm-up and conditioning are the best preventive measures and better equipment (i.e., the Cooperall) is second in importance.

MUSCLE STRAINS

These can result from indirect or direct injuries. The muscle commonly affected is the antagonist or checking

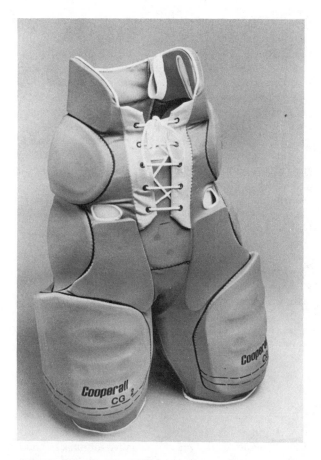

Figure 2 Protective equipment, such as the Cooperall, greatly reduces the incidence of thigh hematoma.

muscle, such as the hamstrings or adductors, and it can occur anywhere in the muscle tendon unit. It is most likely to affect the muscle origin or insertion, but a muscle tendinous junction, muscle belly, or tendon sheath can be involved.

The resultant inflammatory response (tendinitis), in the case of the adductors, causes the "pulled groin". Psoas and rectus muscle involvement are alternative forms of the "pulled groin". In the hamstrings the tendinitis-periostitis picture at the ischial tuberosity characterizes the "pulled ham".

The isolated inner-body muscle strain in the mid-portion of the hamstrings or adductors is usually more responsive to treatment, and with successful treatment, athletes return to their sport in approximately half the time. The same principles of early recognition and caution regarding re-aggravation apply. The cause is often some new stretching exercise or some sport or drill unrelated to the major sport, i.e., off-ice drills such as dancercize or running as an adjunct to hockey. The essential management is to stop these off ice activities.

Physiotherapy is the key here, and a good physiotherapist (massage therapist) can initially decrease a lot of the muscle spasm. Then a strong rehabilitation strengthening program with springs, pulleys, surgical tubing, stair stepping, and side stepping should be added. Progress in the final remodeling-strengthening phase through isokinetic equipment is very worthwhile. (The adductor, abductor machine, for instance, can be used for both speed and endurance.)

Aquabics or pool therapy—running in water, doing the alphabet in water, kicking in water—is quite worthwhile in early phases, but should be followed by a return to short-stride activities such as skating without stretching out the stride or slow running without lifting the leg. *Pain should be your guide*, and obviously anything that hurts should be avoided.

Muscle strains are endemic in the quality runners, and they are usually due to the drills. Hard interval training, such as repeat 50s, 100s, and 200s with unsatisfactory rest breaks, is the culprit. Many national sprinters warm up for an hour prior to doing their interval work.

The A and B drills, which require a hard (goose step) kicking out very quickly or a high-stepping, very quick knee elevation like that of a majorette, can cause these muscle strains and should only be done after a 20-minute basic warm-up and de-emphasized when any type of injury has been sustained.

These muscle and ligament strains can also be satisfactorily classified as first-, second-, and third-degree. The first-degree strains, particularly in sprinters, are often just a type of muscle spasm or strain, and in some cases the sprinter can compete the same day. A calcium lack is a possible etiology, and calcium (Sandoz, 4 ml or 1 teaspoon daily) is a good prophylactic medication in some cases.

The second-degree strain is usually an overuse overtraining injury and can respond quickly to a training alleviation or alteration, e.g., substituting cycling and swimming for running.

The third-degree problems give the athlete pain before, during, and after the sport. They interfere with his life style and everyday activities and are probably associated with a true tear in the muscle, muscle tendon junction, or insertion into the periosteum. Treatment consists of complete rest for as long as 6 to 8 weeks, and in cases of severe adductor or hamstring tendinitis, some quality athletes are kept away from their sport as long as 3 to 6 months; running is prohibited, but judicious cycling and swimming are allowed.

Return to competition should be determined by leg strength. Cybex evaluation can indicate when drills such as cuts, pivots, figure of 8s, hard striding, jumps, and full stretching workouts can be resumed.

A person who is subject to repeated muscle strains needs to have his training schedule re-evaluated. Some athletes experience a "true overuse syndrome", in which their resting pulse is elevated. They are agitated and restless, literally owing to total body exhaustion. They are prone to muscle strains and pulls.

Complete blood work, a zeta sedimentation rate (ZSR), and serum ferritin may show altered chemistry and should be repeated in athletes who are trying to "peak" and are not succeeding.

Principles

1. *It is hard to strain a hot muscle* therefore warm up. The Olympic sprinters warm up for over an hour to run a 50- or 100-meter run.

2. *You cannot tire a young athlete.* Some of the tennis greats can run for half an hour, skip for half an hour, play for half an hour prior to their match. A proper warm up will not tire you; it will enhance performance and prevent injuries.

3. *Sensible Drills.* The only person who has to do olympic weight training is an olympic weight lifter. Thus sensible drills to strengthen and tone up muscles with realistic weights—three sets of 10 or three sets of 30 are indicated. Isokinetic workouts, beating the clock for instance, 20 times in 20 seconds, are also good, but the muscle has to be exercised short of excess fatigue or exhaustion. There is no point in just wearing out a muscle. The principle is to strengthen it.

4. *The best training is the sport itself.* Skating is for hockey players, gymnastics for gymnasts. They are most apt to get hurt in alternative sports or repetitive drills, i.e., repetitive jumping and dunking in basketball or running with ankle weights on.

5. *Routine medications and diet supplements.* Vitamin C is probably needed by individuals in hard training to improve the biochemical environment and regeneration of constantly strained muscles. Calcium can be used in certain cases to decrease muscle cramps. Emphasize a balanced diet, and no other regular medications or supplements are needed.

6. *Avoid muscle overload.* Strengthen muscles, reduce load, alter equipment, improve style.

7. *Chronic problems.* Heat before playing, aspirin before playing, massage with liniment, ultrasound, whirlpool as necessary.

8. *Trigger points* for massage. Good athletic trainers can often remove some of the muscle knots and spasms prior to competition.

9. *Stretch throughout the day,* four times daily for 10 to 15 minutes, to keep muscles relaxed and in tone.

10. *Bone scans* can be used to elucidate the magnitude of the muscle-periosteal injury in some cases, but are usually not indicated.

11. *Other medications.* Spreading or dispersal agents and oral proteolytic enzymes are ineffective. Muscle relaxants usually have no place in muscle strains of the hip and just tire a young athlete. Local anesthesia to freeze the area of muscle strain or spasm to allow the athlete to play is too risky. It is almost guaranteed to increase the injury (to convert a first-degree injury to a third-degree injury).

12. *Steroids.* Local steroids can be used if there is an isolated trigger point or a localized point, such as the adductor tendon origin strain. The steroids are then injected around the pubic tubercle and cautiously instilled beneath the spermatic cord. Steroids should not be introduced into the tendon itself or into the cord, but injected judiciously along the periosteum with a small 25-gauge needle. This can be done in resistant cases and repeated on three occasions one month apart. This must be augmented by physiotherapy. Oral steroids are basically never used in my practice. Topical agents are ineffectual. However, some benefit may be derived from ionophoresis with 5 percent hydrocortisone cream and 5 amps of electronic stimulation placed over a gauze pad for 20 minutes, administered at two day intervals.

13. *Anabolics.* Oral anabolics are considered to have some effect in the healing of a torn muscle, but they are used so indiscriminately for muscle strengthening and training that these nontherapeutic uses of anabolic steroids, or even growth hormones, make their therapeutic use questionable. Thus, even if therapeutic uses are beneficial, to avoid complicity and unfair training aids, one should probably avoid these medications.

14. *Surgery.* I have operated on the adductor tendon to release it from its insertion into the pubis. This is a full adductor tendon release; it is similar to a tennis elbow release in that it allows the pressure to be removed from that area, but results have not been proved. In my hands it has been beneficial in the long-term, very resistant case.

Differential Diagnosis

Lumbar disc herniation with resultant nerve root irritation and sciatica may be mistaken for muscle strain, as may stress fracture of the pubic ramus. Strained rectus femoris muscles can be confused with a stress fracture of the femur or intrinsic pathology in the hip joint itself.

Around the hip joint two major bursal complexes are subject to inflammation in response to athletic activity. The gluteal bursa in the buttock, and the trochanteric bursa over the greater trochanter may both be the sites of a very troublesome bursitis.

The trochanteric bursa is inflamed from the repetitive slipping back and forth across the trochanter of the tensor fascia lata. Common in runners, dancers and gymnasts it may also trouble racquet sports players with pain during activity, local tenderness to pressure may prevent lying on the affected side. The deep gluteal bursae when inflamed are associated with a deep seated buttock discomfort which may simulate referred pain from the back and has to be distinguished from a lumbar disc problem or piriformis syndrome where the sciatic nerve is irritated at its emergence through the greater sciatic notch.

Modification of activity is the mainstay of treatment, physiotherapy with deep heat or ultrasound, anti-inflammatory medication and local steroids also have a place. Occasionally surgical release of the tensor fascia is necessary in refractory cases of trochanteric bursitis and on occasions a piriformis release is necessary in those with a piriformis syndrome but care has to be taken to absolutely rule out a lumbar spine problem.

PARTICIPANT CHARACTERISTICS AND SPORTS PARTICIPATION

Guidance in the selection of a suitable sport for an individual should be an important factor in pregame physicals. Obviously, people who are much too stiff and inflexible should not be allowed to participate in sports where pulled muscles and tendons are a problem. Similarly, individuals with undue joint laxity may be at risk in contact sports. Judicious guidance to the player from his coach, doctor, or parent may help prevent many of these injuries. There should also be avenues for immediate medical referral and satisfactory quality physiotherapy of an immediate nature, followed by long-term complete rehabilitation and counseling regarding reinjury if the morbidity of these common soft tissue injuries is to be reduced.

FRACTURES OF THE PELVIS AND FEMUR

JAMES F. KELLAM, B.SC., M.D., F.R.C.S.(C)

THE PELVIS

Before dealing with the specifics of pelvic fractures an understanding of the pelvis as a functional unit is needed. The pelvis is composed of two innominate bones and the sacrum. These bones in isolation represent no stability. In order for the pelvis to perform its function it is necessary for the innominate bones to be firmly fixed to the sacrum and to themselves. This fixation is obtained posteriorly with the anterior sacroiliac ligaments and the posterior sacroiliac ligaments. The posterior sacroiliac ligaments running from the posterior tubercle of the ilium to the sacrum are the largest and strongest ligaments in the body. The anterior structures of the ilium and the two innominate bones are joined through the symphysis pubis, which is a strong fibrous junction. Pelvic stability is also maintained by strong ligaments running from the sacrum to the ischial tuberosity (the sacrotuberous ligament) and to the ischial spine (the sacrospinous ligament). The lumbar spine also participates in pelvic stability with the iliolumbar ligaments, which run from both transverse processes of the fifth lumbar vertebra to the posterior iliac spines. With these ligaments intact, the pelvis is thus a stable structure able to withstand the forces of weight-bearing through the acetabulum, up the strong thick cancellous and cortical bone of the posterior ilium, and through the sacrum and along the vertebral column. The anterior structures, the pubic rami and ischial rami and symphysis, do not participate significantly in the weight-bearing forces, but act as a strut to maintain the pelvis in its normal anatomic configuration as well as protection for the pelvic contents. The pelvic contents are important to remember in massive pelvic disruptions as they are frequently injured and can lead to bladder, urethral, nerve, and, particularly, acutely hemorrhagic problems for the patient.

Pelvic stability is defined as the ability of the pelvis to withstand physiologic forces applied to it. This means that the posterior ligamentous complexes must remain intact. Pelvic instability represents disruption of the posterior osseous ligamentous complex. This may occur by fractures through the sacrum, sacroiliac dislocations, or a combination of fracture dislocations of the ilium and sacroiliac joint as well as fractures through the posterior iliac wing. This stability can be represented as a spectrum and must be assessed in each individual case.

Stress fractures appear to occur more commonly in women than in men. This may be due to the fact that female bones are somewhat more slender and the pubic symphysis shallower, and to several other anatomic differences which really do not effectively explain this difference. Gait differences during running between male and female may account for some mechanistic differences. The female runner tends to rely on hip extension forces to a greater extent than does the male, so that the female pelvis would be more acceptable to tensile stresses. It is interesting to note that stress fractures in the pelvis appear to be secondary to exposure to tensile stress rather than compression stress. This is noted because of the medial position of the fractures in the pubic or ischial ramus where muscle pulls are occurring during hip extension. This would account for a single fracture occurring in a wing-like structure. The other interesting difference in pelvic stress fractures is that these do not appear to be associated with the usual changes in technique, equipment, or surfaces of running. They do appear to occur within a specific period of time following high-intensity activities, which may represent failure from excessive repetition of muscle contraction.

Incidence of Pelvic Fractures

In order for major pelvic disruptions to occur, high energy must be transmitted through the pelvic ring. This is normally seen in motor vehicle and motorcycle accidents in the civilian population. It may also be noted after falls from heights. Sports are not known for the production of major pelvic disruptions. It is obvious that such high-energy sports as motor car racing, motocross, and rodeo will lead to the potential for major pelvic disruptions. However, in most sports, the participant is well protected and does not suffer massive pelvic disruption. Stress fractures or stable pelvic fractures are more common.

Clinical Presentation

Pelvic fractures can be divided into two groups, stress fractures and major pelvic fractures.

With the major pelvic fracture, the mechanism of injury is obviously one of a high-velocity, high-energy transfer. This acute injury occurs as a sudden event. When first seen, the patient generally is unable to bear weight and is in significant pain in the region of the pelvic girdle. The history should point to the mechanism of injury. Pelvic fractures occur from anteriorly-posteriorly directed forces, forces directed laterally to the pelvis such as a blow over the buttock or greater trochanteric region, as well as vertical shear forces which occur in falls. Further questioning of the patient should bring to light symptoms of associated intra-abdominal or intrapelvic injuries, such as abdominal pain, the inability to void, and neurologic symptoms of numbness, tingling, or weakness in the lower extremities.

Stress fractures usually occur as a sudden onset of discomfort, usually related in the pelvic region. These are seen in people who are runners or are doing repetitive activities which place significantly high stresses across the pelvis over a prolonged period of time. It is important to inquire into the training regimen of the athlete, if there has been a sudden increase in mileage, change in technique, or change in training surfaces and location. It is also important to know when the discomfort occurs: whether with weight-bearing such as walking or only during the athletic event or training.

Physical examination of the pelvis determines the stability of the injury as well as associated injuries. It is imperative to remember that the acute pelvic fracture often is accompanied by hypovolemic shock. The initial evaluation of this patient requires the physician to remember the priorities of resuscitation. Examination of the airway, breathing, and circulatory status of the patient should be done prior to pelvic examination. Stabilization of the patient in hypovolemic shock or with airway problems is imperative. Intra-abdominal bleeding should also be evaluated.

The assessment of the pelvis begins with inspection. One should look for areas of swelling and bruising. Major pelvic disruptions are noted in patients with large flank hematomas, scrotal hematomas, and large hematomas posteriorly over the sacroiliac complex. Deformity of the lower extremity may also be noted. A lateral compression pelvic fracture causes an internal rotation deformity of the lower extremity, and an anteroposterior displaced fracture results in increased external rotation of the lower extremity. A vertical shear fracture causes a leg length discrepancy, the shorter side being on the fracture side. Palpation of the pelvic ring, both posteriorly over the posterior sacroiliac complex and ante-riorly over the pubic rami and symphysis, is imperative to determine areas of tenderness and discomfort. Manually compressing the pelvis by placing the hands on the anterior superior iliac spines and forcing the pelvis inward will reveal an instability or discomfort posteriorly or anteriorly depending on the fracture; forcing the pelvis outward also shows instability. The urethra is inspected for blood, an indication of urethral disruption. In addition, a rectal examination is done in males to determine the position of the prostate. A high-riding prostate or one that is mobile is another indication of urethral tears. Catheterization should not be attempted in these patients until a cysto-urethrogram has been performed to evaluate the urethra. If it is intact, a catheter may then be passed. Further evaluation of the lower extremities for neurologic involvement and vascular involvement should also be done at this time.

Investigations

In order to assess the pelvis radiographically, three views are required. The pelvis is approximately 40° oblique to the long axis of the body. Consequently, an AP film of the pelvis represents an oblique view of the pelvis. This view is necessary to provide an overview of the pelvis and its structures. Two further views at right angles to each other can be obtained. The inlet view is done with the patient supine and the x-ray beam directed from cephalad to caudad at 45° to the long axis of the body. This view permits assessment of posterior displacement, of rotation—whether internal or external, and of the sacrum for fractures. The outlet view, or tangential view, is done at 45° to the long axis of the body with the tube directed from caudad to cephalad. This view allows assessment of the sacrum, sacral foramina, and superior rotation as well as superior migration of the pelvis. These two views, at right angles to each other, fill the criteria of fracture evaluation, especially that of stress fractures. Because of overlap in the AP view, it may be difficult to determine the exact structure that is injured in a stress fracture with only the AP view.

Bone scanning is particularly useful in the athlete who complains of a potential stress fracture. The bone scan is particularly sensitive to areas of increased bone turnover, as occur in stress fracture. If radiographs do not demonstrate a fracture, bone scanning is the next step. The stress fracture is demonstrated on the scan as a well-localized area of increased activity in the area of fracture.

Computed tomography of the pelvis is another useful technique for assessing the pelvis and its displacement, but more so in acute pelvic fractures than in stress fractures.

Tomograms of the pelvis may also be useful in the delineation of stress fractures.

Management

Once a pelvic fracture is diagnosed in an athlete, the major decision in management concerns the stability of the pelvic ring. Stability depends on the degree of disruption of the posterior bony, ligamentous complex of the pelvis. A clinical impression of instability can be verified radiographically. Significant displacement posteriorly in the femoral sacral arch around the sacroiliac joint region of greater than 5 mm to 1 cm represents significant instability. Evidence of avulsion fractures of the transverse process of L5, of the spinous process of the ischium, and occasionally of the origin of the sacrotuberous and sacrospinous ligaments from the sacrum also represent potential instability. The type of fracture pattern is also helpful in determining instability. Impacted fractures in cancellous bone represent a stable situation, whereas a shear fracture or a fracture through cancellous bone in which a gap is noted is potentially unstable. Stable pelvic fractures can be managed on bed rest until comfort is achieved. At this point the patient may be mobilized on crutches, non-weight-bearing on the involved side. During this period functional rehabilitation involving the cardiovascular system and the uninjured side may be carried out within the limits of discomfort for the patient. Pelvic fractures take approximately 6 to 8 weeks to become relatively solid, so that partial weight-bearing may occur. This time period should be judged clinically with assessment of each individual athlete. A stable pelvic fracture may be well united and early rehabilitation of the athlete may be possible within 6 weeks in some circumstances, provided lower extremity deformity, such as rotation or shortening, is not significant.

In the unstable pelvic fracture, anteroposterior compression injuries disrupt the symphysis and open the pelvis like a book. With less than 2.5 cm of disruption through the symphysis, these fractures remain relatively stable and may be managed with some method of closing the book—by internal fixation, external skeletal fixation, or a pelvic sling. A minimum of 6 weeks—more likely 3 months—is required for union to occur with this type of treatment. External skeletal fixation of the pelvis in an anteroposterior stable compression injury is ideal in that it allows a functional rehabilitation of the patient. They may be up with crutches, non-weight-bearing on the involved side, and be able to participate in upper extremity activities. Most lateral compression injuries are stable injuries and may be managed with appropriate bed rest and mobilization. The vertical shear injury is an unstable injury. The end point of all mechanisms results in an unstable fracture that follows the pattern of a vertical shear injury. With a posterior instability, evaluation must be made as to how significant this is. Control of posterior instability is not possible with external skeletal fixation frames, but requires open reduction and internal fixation of the posterior bony ligamentous complex. This type of internal fixation of the pelvis is not without complications. Infection, gluteal muscle necrosis, as well as impingement of the sacral roots with internal fixation devices into the sacrum have occurred. This type of surgical intervention should be done by a surgeon experienced in pelvic fracture treatment. Other methods of treatment of the unstable fracture are combinations of external skeletal fixation and traction. This type of treatment usually requires a 3-month period of bed rest, with 6 to 8 weeks of traction followed by another 6 weeks of recumbency for union of the fracture to occur.

Stress fractures are managed symptomatically. If they occur during weight-bearing and walking, crutch walking or pool therapy may be helpful. If they occur during training, this must be either slowed down or abandoned and other forms of maintenance of the athlete must be instituted. Evaluation of technique, environment, and equipment should be undertaken by consultation among physician, coach, and athlete in order to ascertain why this occurred and what can be done to correct it. The presence of a stress fracture should alert one to other potential problems, such as primary or secondary malignant disease.

The athlete should not return to competitive sports until he is pain-free and has regained strength, endurance, and agility. Otherwise the athlete is at significant risk for recurrent or new injury.

THE FEMUR

Fractures of the femur are a serious problem to an athlete. The femur, the largest bone in the body, is subject to the greatest stress and is surrounded by the major musculature of the lower extremity. At either end of the femur are the two major weight-bearing joints required in all athletic activities: the hip and the knee. The hip is important in that stress fractures of the femoral neck may occur in athletes and thus lead to significant problems if missed or treated inadequately. If femoral shaft fractures are not treated properly, the thigh musculature cannot be maintained in good condition and ultimately affects knee function—through weakness, fibrosis, or secondary joint stiffness. Fractures in or above the knee are discussed elsewhere in this text.

Fractures of the femoral neck, which usually are stress fractures but may be incurred during high-energy sporting activities, can lead to several difficulties, the most serious being the development of avascular necrosis of the femoral head. This blood supply to the femoral head comes from a circle of vessels around the greater trochanteric region, courses up the posterior retinaculum of the femoral neck, and dives into the femoral head at the articular cartilage margin. Fractures of the femoral neck may disrupt this blood supply and thus lead to avascular necrosis and its attendant complications if late segmental collapse of the femoral head occurs. Nonunions and malunions also may occur. The hip requires an anatomic reduction in order that the biomechanics of gait, particularly for running, are maintained. Therefore, if a nonunion or malunion does occur, the athlete will be hindered.

The femoral shaft is enclosed within the major musculature of the lower extremity. Anteriorly the quadriceps, the major extensor of the knee as well as one of the major components of the patellofemoral mechanism, can be injured. Posteriorly, the hamstring groups of muscles are also involved as well as the sciatic nerve.

Thus, femoral shaft fractures involve some form of muscle injury, particularly anteriorly to the quadriceps, and ultimately lead to knee problems through the weakness or loss of function of the quadriceps. Depending on the treatment of femoral shaft fractures, knee stiffness may result. This stiffness, along with shortening and malunion, may be a particular problem to athletes who require their lower extremities for repetitive activities and power activities. In addition to those fractures of the femoral shaft caused by high velocity, stress fractures of the shaft, neck, and proximal area have been reported.

Incidence

Femoral fractures in athletes are extremely uncommon. The usual causes of stress fracture are overuse and change, particularly in marathon runners. It usually occurs in the beginning of training or after a sudden intensification of activity, such as a long run. Non-stress fractures or acute fractures of the femoral shaft have been documented in different contact sports. In a series of hockey injuries only one of 108 fractures reviewed was to the femur. In other reviews, contact sports or high-velocity sports do not show significant femoral shaft fractures, although they do occur sporadically.

Clinical Presentation

The acute femoral neck fracture or femoral shaft fracture usually occurs in isolated incidents with the sudden onset of acute discomfort and pain following a significant transfer of energy to the extremity. This may be through contact or can occur simply through twisting activities. The patient is unable to bear weight and complains of pain at a specific site.

Stress fractures of the femoral neck or medial aspect of the proximal femur usually are gradual in onset. The patient develops pain and discomfort, usually during activity or during a long run. This pain persists and is aggravated by increased activity. It is relieved by rest or non-weight-bearing. This fracture occurs as an acute episode and is not preceded by chronic discomfort. One should be aware that pain in the knee region, particularly on the medial aspect of the knee, may be indicative of hip joint disease. It also appears that stress fractures of the femur occur in the early part of a training routine, because increased stress is placed on the bone before the bone is able to withstand it.

Physical examination of the patient with an acute fracture usually shows the patient lying with an externally rotated leg, with acute pain and discomfort on motion and crepitus at the fracture site. With femoral shaft fractures, significant blood loss may occur, although it is uncommon. In a patient with a stress fracture, the leg usually has normal alignment, but on range of motion examination of the hip, there are decreases in the range owing to pain with rotation and flexion. Pain usually occurs at the extremes. Tenderness at the region of the fracture may be present.

Investigations

The first study consists of an anteroposterior and lateral roentgenogram of the hip or femur. It is important that both the joint above and that below the fracture be examined radiographically, particularly in the acute fracture. Because a stress fracture may not be visible on initial examination of the films, a high index of suspicion is necessary. One should also be aware of other diagnoses that may cause pain in this region (tumors or infection). A stress fracture may be one of two types and it is important to make the distinction. The compressive type which usually is noted at the lower border of the femoral neck, is demonstrated radiographically as increased radiodensity along the fracture site or sclerosis at the fracture line. This type of fracture is rarely displaced unless continued stresses are placed on it. The second type of stress fracture, the distraction fracture, is transverse in direction, is seen in the older individual, and usually occurs at the superior aspect of the neck with a radiolucency. The fracture line develops at right angles to the line of stress and displacement is common.

Acute fractures of the femoral neck are obvious. It is important to determine the amount of displacement. The greater the displacement of the femoral neck fracture, the greater the risk for avascular necrosis and the greater the necessity for an accurate anatomic reduction.

Acute fracture of the femoral shaft should be assessed as well. It is important to determine the type of comminution that is present and thus whether the fracture is stable or unstable. Fractures of the femoral shaft that have more than 50 percent of the cortex intact on both the distal and proximal fragment are stable fractures. The two fragments can be lined up to prevent any axial displacement such as shortening. Comminution is particularly important in the proximal and distal portions. Although 50 percent of the cortex may be intact in the distal fracture, comminution may allow the fracture to slip, depending on the treatment, and thus shorten. If there is less than 50 percent cortical contact between both fractures, the fracture is considered unstable.

Bone scan may be indicated. Radionuclide images of the femoral shaft or femoral neck may be diagnostic in individuals in whom stress fractures are expected but not visualized on the plain radiographs. Tomography may also be necessary to delineate the fracture. This study may be necessary for diagnosis or to determine the extent of the fracture, particularly in the femoral neck, that is, whether the fracture is completely across the neck or incomplete.

Management

In managing the acute fracture, one should initially ascertain that the patient is stabilized. If this fracture has occurred in a high-velocity situation, other associated injuries may be present. Priorities of resuscitation should be honored before treatment of the fracture is begun. This is not a particular problem with stress fractures.

Treatment of a stress fracture involving the femoral neck is based on the nature of the fracture. Compression fractures of the femoral neck, as mentioned, rarely cause displacement if the stresses are removed by appropriate non-weight-bearing, either by crutches or by bed rest. The distraction stress fracture of the femoral neck usually is displaced and should be internally fixed. Any displaced fracture of the femoral neck should undergo internal fixation to allow for anatomic reduction. Most stress fractures are minimally displaced or may be reduced anatomically by means of a closed method using a fracture table. Following this maneuver, they may be internally fixed by means of an appropriate device. Fractures in which anatomic reduction cannot be obtained should be considered for open reduction.

There are many techniques for the fixation of femoral neck fractures. The principle of internal fixation of femoral neck fractures requires a technique that allows for controlled impaction of the fracture, usually by means of a sliding compression screw system. Multiple pin fixation, using smooth pins or cancellous screws, is also a useful technique for the minimally displaced or anatomically reduced stress fracture of the femoral neck. Following reduction and internal fixation of the fracture, the vascularity of the femoral head should be evaluated. It is probably best done at this time by a bone marrow scanning technique using technetium-99m sulfur colloid. It may also be adequately performed with one of the currently used bone scanning agents incorporating technetium-99m. If the femoral head is viable, no further treatment should be considered. However, if the bone scan demonstrates an avascular head, consideration should be given to a muscle pedicle bone graft using the quadratus femoris-based bone-block technique. This may increase the chances of revascularization of the femoral head and fracture union.

Following operative or nonoperative treatment, weight-bearing should not be allowed for approximately 6 weeks. This should be guided basically by the radiographic evidence of fracture union. As the fracture unites, gradual weight-bearing may be reinstituted. Cardiovascular fitness may be maintained by activities that do not allow stresses to be placed across the femur (e.g., swimming or waist-deep water walking or running). These should be incorporated into the treatment as the clinical course permits. Most patients with stress fractures of the femoral neck can resume activities about 6 months after injury.

The treatment of acute femoral shaft fractures should preserve and encourage as much functional return as quickly as possible. The technique of closed intramedullary nailing of long bone fractures is ideally suited for this fracture. This technique, developed by Gerhardt Kuntscher, is based on his principles of fracture care. The first and foremost principle was the restoration and preservation of function, which is imperative in the athlete. This was accomplished by a technique that allowed for fracture immobilization until healing occurred, but at the same time avoiding assault on the fracture site, thus eliminating significant muscle dissection and devascularization of fracture fragments. This

technique also encouraged healing by secondary bony union, particularly with its own internal bone graft from reamings.

This technique is done with a closed reduction of the femoral shaft fracture. When this has been completed on the fracture table, through a small incision over the greater trochanteric region, the greater trochanter is entered in line with the axis of the medullary canal, a guide wire passed across the fracture site, and the medullary canal of the femur is reamed with reamers of progressively increasing size. This allows for the internal aspect of the medullary canal to be made into a tube of a specific size, to permit passage of a nail large enough to immobilize the femur without bending and to allow for impingement between the nail and the internal aspect of the femur. This elastic impingement, which occurs as the nail is driven into the bone, provides the stability if associated with a stable fracture pattern. However, only fractures that are transverse or short oblique in nature are amenable to this closed technique because the nail is a weight-sharing device. It allows the fracture to participate in bone healing and weight-bearing stresses. Because it is close to the central axis of the femur, very few stresses are placed on the nail as far as tension or bending are concerned. There is minimal change in the cortical bone of the femur, and thus the problems of removal of the nail are minimal for recovery.

Recently, the development of a locked intramedullary nail has extended the indications for this technique. A locked intramedullary nail is a cloverleaf nail that has holes at the proximal and distal ends. Through specially designed siting devices, these holes may be filled with locking screws. Fractures that do not have stability (i.e., comminuted fractures, fractures in the distal and proximal third of the femur) may also be treated by the closed intramedullary nailing technique, as may any fracture of the shaft of the femur from within approximately 2 to 3 cm of the lesser trochanter to within 5 cm of the adductor tubercle.

This method of treatment of femoral shaft fractures allows for immediate mobilization of the athlete. The first day postoperatively the athlete may begin quadriceps setting exercises and be encouraged in straight leg-raising. Once straight leg-raising has been accomplished, there is sufficient quadriceps control for the patient to be mobilized onto crutches in a non-weight-bearing or partial weight-bearing mode, depending on fracture stability. If a locking nail has been used and it has been necessary to lock this at both ends, that is a static locked nail, weight-bearing is delayed until bridging callus is noted between the fracture fragments. This usually occurs at 3 months, at which point one of the sets of screws may be removed and full weight-bearing may be commenced to mature the callous. Range of motion exercises of the knee are commenced immediately. Usually by 3 weeks 90 degrees of motion has been obtained and in stable fractures full weight-bearing may be commenced. Union is rapid with this technique. During the initial 6 weeks, cardiovascular fitness may be obtained by non-weight-bearing exercises such as swimming, walking in waist-deep water, and bicycling. Once the fracture has consolidated adequately, further rehabilitation may be commenced. Usually by 12 months, the fracture has fully consolidated and healing has matured to allow the removal of the nail to occur. Nail removal should be undertaken in patients under the age of 50. This is a simple operation requiring several days of hospital admission for nail removal. Following this, the patient may again commence activities in a protected fashion until they are comfortable, usually within 3 to 6 weeks. Removal of the implant should be timed with the athlete's sporting activities. As long a period as possible between nail removal and the recommencement of highly stressful activities should be observed. Usually in 6 to 9 months the femur has regained its strength and full activities can be allowed.

Recent reports of the closed intramedullary nailing technique have shown that a 99 percent union rate with a less than 1 percent infection rate in closed femoral shaft fractures has been obtained. These results are similar to the early results of the locked intramedullary nailing technique. Other methods of femoral fracture treatment are associated with problems that may be particularly difficult for the athlete to overcome. The treatment of femoral shaft fractures in traction is usually associated with significant quadriceps atrophy and weakness as well as a decrease in the range of motion of the knee. Cast bracing of fractures may, as with traction, allow for some decreased quadriceps power, range of motion of the knee, and occasional shortening and malunions. Plate fixation of femoral fractures allows for an anatomic reduction, but does require an open procedure with stripping of the muscle, particularly the quadriceps, which may lead to decreased range of motion and quadriceps weakness. Plate fixation is also associated with refracturing, particularly at the time of plate removal. Although this is low if the fracture is united, there is evidence that the bone underneath the plate may undergo cancellization or become weakened due to the weight-relieving aspects of a plate. To avoid this will require protection of the patient for a 12-month period before stressful activities are resumed.

With femoral shaft fractures, knee ligament injuries and internal derangements of the knee may also occur. This has been noted in up to 25 percent of patients with femoral shaft fractures. Once the fracture has been stabilized, examination of the knee is imperative. If significant knee injuries have occurred, these should be treated appropriately. In this situation it is imperative that the femoral fracture be fixed in order that a knee reconstructive procedure and rehabilitation can be undertaken.

Finally, as far as treatment is concerned, return of the athlete to full activity depends on his ability to regain strength, endurance, and agility.

There are many techniques for the fixation of femoral neck fractures. The principle of internal fixation of femoral neck fractures requires a technique that allows for controlled impaction of the fracture, usually by means of a sliding compression screw system. Multiple pin fixation, using smooth pins or cancellous screws, is also a useful technique for the minimally displaced or anatomically reduced stress fracture of the femoral neck.

Following reduction and internal fixation of the fracture, the vascularity of the femoral head should be evaluated. It is probably best done at this time by a bone marrow scanning technique using technetium-99m sulfur colloid. It may also be adequately performed with one of the currently used bone scanning agents incorporating technetium-99m. If the femoral head is viable, no further treatment should be considered. However, if the bone scan demonstrates an avascular head, consideration should be given to a muscle pedicle bone graft using the quadratus femoris-based bone-block technique. This may increase the chances of revascularization of the femoral head and fracture union.

Following operative or nonoperative treatment, weight-bearing should not be allowed for approximately 6 weeks. This should be guided basically by the radiographic evidence of fracture union. As the fracture unites, gradual weight-bearing may be reinstituteed. Cardiovascular fitness may be maintained by activities that do not allow stresses to be placed across the femur (e.g., swimming or waist-deep water walking or running). These should be incorporated into the treatment as the clinical course permits. Most patients with stress fractures of the femoral neck can resume activities about 6 months after injury.

The treatment of acute femoral shaft fractures should preserve and encourage as much functional return as quickly as possible. The technique of closed intramedullary nailing of long bone fractures is ideally suited for this fracture. This technique, developed by Gerhardt Kuntscher, is based on his principles of fracture care. The first and foremost principle was the restoration and preservation of function, which is imperative in the athlete. This was accomplished by a technique that allowed for fracture immobilization until healing occurred, but at the same time avoiding assault on the fracture site, thus eliminating significant muscle dissection and devascularization of fracture fragments. This technique also encouraged healing by secondary bony union, particularly with its own internal bone graft from reamings.

This technique is done with a closed reduction of the femoral shaft fracture. When this has been completed on the fracture table, through a small incision over the greater trochanteric region, the greater trochanter is entered in line with the axis of the medullary canal, a guide wire passed across the fracture site, and the medullary canal of the femur is reamed with reamers of progressively increasing size. This allows for the internal aspect of the medullary canal to be made into a tube of a specific size, to permit passage of a nail large enough to immobilize the femur without bending and to allow for impingement between the nail and the internal aspect of the femur. This elastic impingement, which occurs as the nail is driven into the bone, provides the stability if associated with a stable fracture pattern. However, only fractures that are transverse or short oblique in nature are amenable to this closed technique because the nail is a weight-sharing device. It allows the fracture to participate in bone healing and weight-bearing stresses. Because it is close to the central axis of the femur, very few stresses are placed on the nail as far as tension or bending are concerned. There is minimal change in the cortical bone of the femur, and thus the problems of removal of the nail are minimal for recovery.

Recently, the development of a locked intramedullary nail has extended the indications for this technique. A locked intramedullary nail is a cloverleaf nail that has holes at the proximal and distal ends. Through specially designed siting devices, these holes may be filled with locking screws. Fractures that do not have stability (i.e., comminuted fractures, fractures in the distal and proximal third of the femur) may also be treated by the closed intramedullary nailing technique, as may any fracture of the shaft of the femur from within approximately 2 to 3 cm of the lesser trochanter to within 5 cm of the adductor tubercle.

This method of treatment of femoral shaft fractures allows for immediate mobilization of the athlete. The first day postoperatively the athlete may begin quadriceps setting exercises and be encouraged in straight leg-raising. Once straight leg-raising has been accomplished, there is sufficient quadriceps control for the patient to be mobilized onto crutches in a non-weight-bearing or partial weight-bearing mode, depending on fracture stability. If a locking nail has been used and it has been necessary to lock this at both ends, that is a static locked nail, weight-bearing is delayed until bridging callus is noted between the fracture fragments. This usually occurs at 3 months, at which point one of the sets of screws may be removed and full weight-bearing may be commenced to mature the callous. Range of motion exercises of the knee are commenced immediately. Usually by 3 weeks 90 degrees of motion has been obtained and in stable fractures full weight-bearing may be commenced. Union is rapid with this technique. During the initial 6 weeks, cardiovascular fitness may be obtained by non-weight-bearing exercises such as swimming, walking in waist-deep water, and bicycling. Once the fracture has consolidated adequately, further rehabilitation may be commenced. Usually by 12 months, the fracture has fully consolidated and healing has matured to allow the removal of the nail to occur. Nail removal should be undertaken in patients under the age of 50. This is a simple operation requiring several days of hospital admission for nail removal. Following this, the patient may again commence activities in a protected fashion until they are comfortable, usually within 3 to 6 weeks. Removal of the implant should be timed with the athlete's sporting activities. As long a period as possible between nail removal and the recommencement of highly stressful activities should be observed. Usually in 6 to 9 months the femur has regained its strength and full activities can be allowed.

Recent reports of the closed intramedullary nailing technique have shown that a 99 percent union rate with a less than 1 percent infection rate in closed femoral shaft fractures has been obtained. These results are similar to the early results of the locked intramedullary nailing technique. Other methods of femoral fracture treatment are associated with problems that may be particularly difficult for the athlete to overcome. The treatment of femoral shaft fractures in traction is usually associated with significant quadriceps atrophy and weakness as well as a decrease in the range of motion of the knee. Cast bracing of fractures may, as with traction, allow for some decreased quadriceps power, range of motion of the knee, and occasional shortening and malunions. Plate fixation of femoral fractures allows for an anatomic reduction, but does require an open procedure with stripping of the muscle, particularly the quadriceps, which may lead to decreased range of motion and quadriceps weakness. Plate fixation is also associated with refracturing, particularly at the time of plate removal. Although this is low if the fracture is united, there is evidence that the bone underneath the plate may undergo cancellization or become weakened due to the weight-relieving aspects of a plate. To avoid this will require protection of the patient for a 12-month period before stressful activities are resumed.

With femoral shaft fractures, knee ligament injuries and internal derangements of the knee may also occur. This has been noted in up to 25 percent of patients with femoral shaft fractures. Once the fracture has been stabilized, examination of the knee is imperative. If significant knee injuries have occurred, these should be treated appropriately. In this situation it is imperative that the femoral fracture be fixed in order that a knee reconstructive procedure and rehabilitation can be undertaken.

Finally, as far as treatment is concerned, return of the athlete to full activity depends on his ability to regain strength, endurance, and agility.

KNEE INJURIES

KNEE PAIN: OVERUSE SYNDROMES AROUND THE KNEE

R. PETER WELSH, M.B., Ch.B., F.R.C.S.(C), F.A.C.S.
CHRISTINE HUTTON, M.B., Ch.B.

Periarticular knee pain can be troublesome to the athlete, diminishing performance and blunting the training effort. With athletic effort overload or overuse syndromes are common. Symptoms may arise from the patellar mechanism, from the quadriceps tendon or the ligamentum patella at its origin and insertion, from the stabilizing retinaculae, from the fatpads deep to the supra- and infrapatellar tendons, or from the synovial lining where it forms plicae or folds which run medially beneath the extensor mechanism and distally along the medial border of the patella to the distal fatpad. In addition, bursae may be aggravated not only prepatellar but also deep to the infrapatellar tendon, as well as beneath the pes anserine tendons on the medial side and the iliotibial tract on the lateral side. Any of these structures may be involved in the genesis of periarticular overuse syndromes around the knee.

Extensor Mechanism Dysfunction

The commonest presenting symptom is that of pain in or around the knee associated with running, jumping, or kicking activities, or with kneeling or crouching. Discomfort is commonly aggravated on ascending and descending stairs; a sensation of instability or crepitus may also be noted. On examination, the only positive findings may be tenderness to palpation around or over the patella and its tendons or to compression of the patella against the femoral condyles. It should be noted that there are no signs of internal derangement, there is no effusion, no loss of range of motion, or ligamentous instability. There may be some mild quadriceps wasting and, occasionally, some retropatellar crepitus, but most commonly the examiner is unable to demonstrate major abnormality and this can lead him to discount the significance of the patient's complaints or to erroneously label the condition "chondromalacia". Both these approaches

do the patient a gross disservice. A specific diagnosis should be made in every instance.

Patellar Tendinitis (Jumper's Knee)

Inflammation of the distal tendon of the quadriceps muscle (suprapatellar tendinitis), of the origin of the infrapatellar tendon (infrapatellar tendinitis), and of the insertion of the infrapatellar tendon (Osgood-Schlatter disease) are all overuse syndromes associated with running and jumping activities. Pain and tenderness are usually localized to the inflamed area. The discomfort tends to develop during the course of the activity and often persists afterwards.

Initial treatment consists of physiotherapy with local ice frictions and ultrasound and of strengthening and, more particularly, stretching of the quadriceps muscle in conjunction with oral nonsteroidal anti-inflammatory medication for 10 to 15 days. As with all tendinitis, aggressive treatment in the early stages is more successful than later treatment in the chronic established condition. The athlete is reassured that no harm is being done to the knee joint and is permitted to continue with sporting activities but in modified form. That is, if the provocative exercise involves springing and bounding, these must be discontinued and running or cycling exercises substituted. In all cases, the intention should be to maintain the athlete's basic fitness while the condition is allowed to recover without continuing provocative stimuli.

In cases refractory to this regimen, local injection of steroid around the tendon and into the underlying bursa may be indicated. The injection of steroid can have a direct, deleterious effect upon the collagenous structures. Injection, particularly of the infrapatellar tendon, should be limited to a maximum of 2 injections spaced at least 6 months apart lest the weakening of the tendon predispose to its rupture.

Surgical Treatment. On occasion, the patellar tendinitis may become so pernicious that the athlete is forced to give up his chosen activity. Under such circumstances, when all conservative treatments have been exhausted, localized tenolysis has been most successful in reestablishing athletic capability.

In this minor procedure through a transverse skin incision, the ligamentum patella is split longitudinally along the direction of its fibers right at the lower pole of the patella. With a sharp dissection, the ligamentum is reflected off the lower pole of the patella over an area of about 2 cm, retaining adequate supporting tissue on both the medial and lateral sides. The tendon may be degenerate, with granulation in the substance of the tendon; this degenerate tendon segment, which is usually quite small, is excised and sent for histologic examination. The exposed portion of the lower pole of the patella is then decorticated with an osteotome and the bed drilled with a fine drill point. Access to the infrapatellar fatpad is also gained; if this is hypertrophied, the redundant tissue is excised. A simple oversewing of the tendon is carried out with resorbable sutures, and the limb is protected in a soft dressing. Splint protection is afforded for 2 weeks; following suture removal, a light exercise program including hydrotherapy and bicycle exercises is commenced. Isometric quadriceps and hip flexor-abductor exercises are maintained; return to running activity is allowed at 6 weeks.

It is not a common indication for surgery, but this simple procedure has been effective in those athletes who have proven refractory to all other measures.

Osgood-Schlatter Disease

Osgood-Schlatter disease is a tendinitis in which the tibial apophysis is involved in the adolescent. Pressures on the sensitive growth area evoke a local discomfort which can become very disabling. The conventional treatment of this condition has included complete immobilization in a cylinder cast in full extension for 6 weeks. However, in most instances, one need not resort to such treatment; the use of an infrapatellar strap worn across the tendon during activity may decrease the pull on the tendon or the tubercle, as happens when a forearm band is used for tennis elbow. The mainstay of management of this condition involves restriction of jumping or bounding activities while the athlete is acutely tender, the use of local ice friction treatments, and diligent application to quadriceps stretching routines. By decreasing the pull on the quadriceps mechanism and making the quadriceps muscle more flexible, the load on the infrapatellar tendon and thus the impact on the tibial tubercle can be greatly reduced. Most athletes can continue their sports activity, but Osgood-Schlatter syndrome tends to be episodic and there may be occasions for weeks at a time where restriction of activity becomes necessary. Most adolescents grow through this condition in the course of 2 to 3 years. However, the condition may continue into late adolescence or adulthood with continuing problems around the tibial tubercle insertion. Use of local steroid injection may settle symptoms, but there are other instances when surgical treatment becomes necessary.

Surgical Treatment. X-ray review of patients with persistent symptoms around the tibial tubercle will often reveal an ossific loose body in the tendon substance where the tibial tubercle apophysis has fragmented and

one of the islands of bone has not united with the parent tibia. This local irritation is remedied by the excision of the loose fragment. A transverse incision at the tibial tubercle insertion followed by a longitudinal split in the tendon identifies the loose body; all fragments and any bursal reactive tissue are excised. The tendon is then oversewn and the leg protected in a soft dressing. Return to activity is allowed as symptoms dictate, but it will usually take 6 to 8 weeks before jumping and bounding activities can be recommenced.

Bursitis

Prepatellar Bursitis

Prepatellar bursitis (housemaid's knee) presents with pain and swelling in the bursal tissue over the anterior surface of the patella resulting from either direct trauma or repetitive irritation. A fluctuating swelling can be aspirated, local steroid injected, and a compression dressing applied. Follow-up care with anti-inflammatory medication and a therapy program with ultrasound will settle most cases. In longstanding cases, it may be necessary to consider surgical excision of the bursa.

Surgical Treatment. A transverse incision enables the prepatellar bursa to be completely shelled out and peeled off the surface of the patella. The tissues are often very extensively scarred and thickened; removal leaves a large space for potential hematoma formation. To control this, the prepatellar subcutaneous tissues should be sewn down to the fascia over the patella to close this space. A suction drain should be left *in situ* for 24 hours and a compression bandage applied for 2 weeks.

Infrapatellar Bursitis

Infrapatellar bursitis is a common accompaniment of infrapatellar tendinitis, associated also with the infrapatellar fatpad syndrome. Local steroid injection into the bursa through the ligamentum patella will usually settle an infrapatellar tendon bursitis satisfactorily. At the time of surgery for infrapatellar tendinitis, this area should be thoroughly inspected for its possible involvement in the pathology.

Iliotibial Band Bursitis

Iliotibial band bursitis is a troublesome inflammation of the bursa underlying the distal portion of the iliotibial tract on the lateral aspect of the knee and results from the friction forces associated with repetitive knee flexion and extension associated with impact loading of the knee, as in jogging. This is a perplexing condition for it presents in an athlete with no previous inkling or indication of harm or injury. It may suddenly smite the athlete even in the course of a race event with a sharp pain over the lateral femoral condyle and become so painful within a space of 100 yards that the athlete is forced to completely discontinue the activity. On walking, the knee seems to spontaneously improve, but as soon as attempts are made to run again, the sharp pain returns. On endeavoring subsequently to run, the athlete will find that he can often run for a short distance only to find the pain appear as suddenly as it had initially. This condition is often confused with internal derangements. A runner must recognize that with this condition he cannot persist in running farther than the threshold of discomfort allows. Maintaining a steady activity level over a reduced distance (even at an increased pace) will often see the condition disappear as mysteriously as it occurred. The use of ice friction treatments, ultrasound, stretching and strengthening exercises, and oral anti-inflammatory medication are all adjunctive therapies often necessary to help alleviate this troublesome condition. On occasion, local steroid injection into the bursa may be indicated and surgical treatment may become necessary.

Surgical Treatment of Iliotibial Band Bursitis. There are class athletes whose condition fails to respond to local measures, modification of activity, and attention to the footwear and gait pattern. Their condition may warrant surgical release of the iliotibial tract and excision of the bursa.

A longitudinal incision is made over the lateral femoral condyle parallel to the upper border of the iliotibial tract. The fascia is incised longitudinally in the direction of its fibers, marking the upper margin of the iliotibial tract and releasing distally to the point of the femoral condyle and proximally for 2 inches. On flexion and extension of the knee, the fascial band will be seen to have been freed and the bursa clearly revealed on flexion. Redundant bursal tissue can then be excised. Sutures are only required in the subcutaneous tissues and skin; a soft dressing is then applied. Light activity can commence when the sutures have been removed, with return to running activity as symptoms allow.

Pes Anserine Bursitis

Pes anserine bursitis is an inflammation of the bursa underlying the sartorius, gracilis, and semitendinosis tendon complex on the medial aspect of the knee. This troublesome condition, that affects cyclists, runners, and swimmers is treated locally with ultrasound and ice frictions, these being the mainstay of therapy. Oral anti-inflammatory medication and local steroids may be necessary. Attention to footwear may be necessary, with particular concern for overpronation in runners. In swimmers, this bursitis can be very troublesome and associated with a medial ligament tendinitis; unless there is modification of the kick technique, this condition may prove refractory and jeopardize the athlete's ability to continue successfully in competitive swimming.

Retinaculitis

Inflammation of the medial and lateral supporting structures presents with pain and tenderness over the retinaculae where they play over the underlying femoral condyles pinching the synovium and evoking pain from this source as a consequence of repetitive loading of the knee. It is important to distinguish this state from a true chondromalacia, for the prognosis is much different. Urgent attention to flexibility exercises, particularly stretching out the quadriceps, is essential to relieve pressures over the femoral condylar margins.

In the genesis of a tighter retinaculum and extensor mechanism, one must comment upon the overzealous closure of the knee after arthrotomy. If the capsule is tightened unduly following a surgical arthrotomy of the knee, there can be a marked increase in the pressures over the condylar margins, increasing pressures on the patella as well. Postsurgical knee pain stems often from this tightening of the capsule, and postoperative stretching exercises for the quadriceps mechanism are therefore a very important adjunct to any surgical intervention in the knee.

Fatpad Impingement Syndromes

Impingement of the patellar fatpads or the synovium can be either acute or chronic in nature. Acute impingement can occur with sudden forced extension of the knee where the structures are caught between the patella or its tendons and the underlying femoral condyle. The mechanism of injury is elicited from the history, with pain and tenderness noted clinically medial and lateral to the patellar tendons or within the joint. The natural course of the injury is to recover fully without intervention.

Chronic impingement syndromes often develop without specific history of trauma. With repetitive activity, the fatpad and synovium hypertrophy and become pinched between the patella and femur where they are subject to repetitive low-grade trauma and become persistently symptomatic. This condition is often confused with chondromalacia patella because of the associated crepitus that is sometimes present. Careful examination differentiates the area of involvement from the patella which remains completely smooth and uninvolved. Haffa's syndrome can become troublesome to the athlete and may even require surgical excision of the hypertrophied tissue for satisfactory resolution.

At the outset, it is important to reduce patella loads with a program of flexibility exercises for the quadriceps muscle group. Avoidance of provocative overloading is most important, and discontinuation of springing activity may be necessary. The athlete with a fatpad syndrome is often found to be engaging only in intermittent activity. It is vital to even out the athletic effort and continue a program of regular, daily activity at a reduced but consistent level of performance. Local ultrasound and ice frictions are sometimes of help; a steroid injection may be tried but is usually ineffective. On occasion, surgical treatment may become necessary.

Surgical Treatment of the Fatpad Syndrome. Arthroscopy of the knee should be performed to rule out completely any associated internal derangement or involvement of the articular surface of the patella. It is possible by arthroscopic technique to trim the infrapatellar fatpad to reduce the impingement between the lower pole of the patella and the femoral condyle. At the same time, a lateral retinacular release should be carried out and is best made through a separate 2-cm incision, exposing the retinaculum on the lateral side. A compression dressing is applied for 5 days before a light exercise routine is commenced. Prior to the advent of arthroscopic surgical technique, an open fatpad excision was carried out, making a small arthrotomy and completely excising the infrapatellar fatpad. Should arthroscopic excision of the fatpad be inadequate, this treatment is still recommended. It should be emphasized that it is only in very rare instances that the fatpad need be excised; however, on occasion, the symptoms can be extreme, as in the case of a pianist who had to give up her chosen profession because of fatpad sensitivity while operating the foot pedals. With excision of the fatpad she returned to her "sport" without further problem.

PATELLOFEMORAL ARTHRALGIA, PATELLAR INSTABILITY, AND CHONDROMALACIA PATELLA

R. PETER WELSH, M.B., Ch.B., F.R.C.S.(C), F.A.C.S.
CHRISTINE HUTTON, M.B., Ch.B.

PATELLOFEMORAL ARTHRALGIA

Of all knee maladies, the patellofemoral derangements pose the greatest difficulty in management. Running and jumping sports put great demands on the patellar mechanism where seemingly trivial imperfections can seriously compromise the athlete's optimal performance. Overt pathology is usually not evident; the spectrum of normal anatomy and physiology so wide that determining the variants predisposing to pain and dysfunction poses a true dilemma to the clinician. The site and origin of pain is often obscure.

Essential to understanding the patellofemoral arthralgias are the concepts of abnormal patellar pressures and abnormal patellar excursion.

The patella is a sesamoid bone lying in the quadriceps apparatus that provides enhanced mechanical advantage to the muscles during extension. The anatomy of the extensor mechanism is such that the patella is subject not only to the forces directed along the line of the quadriceps muscles and the infrapatellar tendon but also to the resultant vectors of these forces.

Factors leading to increases in quadriceps load result in abnormal patellar pressures. The resulting pain is believed to be due to stimulation of nerve endings in the underlying subchondral bone but may also relate to strain in the retinacula or impingement of the fatpad or the synovium which are both richly endowed with nerve elements.

Abnormal Patellar Pressures

Inflexibility of the quadriceps muscles is probably the most common cause of primary abnormal patellar pressures. During the adolescent growth spurt, bone growth may outstrip the rate at which muscle fibers stretch, causing abnormal muscle tightness and excessive compressive forces across the patella. The juvenile is particularly prone to derangement of this type, accounting for many instances of patellofemoral arthralgia in the teenager.

Muscle injury from trauma with hematoma and scar formation may similarly cause abnormal muscle tightness as can also surgical intervention. Indeed, overzealous capsular closure after arthrotomy may significantly tighten the capsule, thereby increasing the patellofemoral pressures, a state likely to worsen with subsequent surgery and produce more scarring. Similarly, with patellar stabilization procedures, these forces may be increased. Lateral retinacular release is therefore an essential adjunct to all surgery performed to reduce these pressures.

Abnormal Patellar Excursion

The line of force of the quadriceps is basically along the line of the shaft of the femur. The physiological valgus of the knee gives an angle Q between the pull of the muscle and that of the infrapatellar tendon. In the normal knee, the natural tendency of the patella to displace laterally is resisted by the medial stabilizing structures, the distal fibers of vastus medialis and the medial retinaculum, and lateral excursion is further limited by the prominent lateral femoral condyle. Genu valgum, excessive external tibial torsion, and pes planus effectively increase the Q angle and the lateral force.

Failure of the medial structures, i.e., lax retinaculum or weak quadriceps, shortening or tightness of the lateral stabilizing structures, and bony anomalies such as flattened lateral femoral condyle also predispose to force imbalance, resulting in lateral tilting or lateral excursion (subluxation or dislocation) of the patella. It is claimed that minimal but persistent recurrent subluxation of the patella is a major contributing factor in the development of chondromalacia patella; a true degenerative change in the articular cartilage may result from alterations in patellar excursion, but patellofemoral pressures and trauma are also important in the pathogenesis of this condition.

The misnomer chondromalacia patella has in the past been applied indiscriminately to cases of patellofemoral arthralgia. This diagnosis should only be applied when there is actual patellar articular cartilage degeneration.

Iatrogenic Arthralgia

Too often the diagnosis of patellar subluxation has led to the overzealous orthopaedic treatment of patients with patellofemoral arthralgia, even though these individuals were not shown to suffer from proven instability of the patellar mechanism. The result can be an aggravation of the discomfort, or worse, a true deterioration of the status of the articular surfaces.

Procedures which tighten the medial structures or draw the patella down also significantly increase patellar pressures and therefore increase the shear forces interacting between the articulating surfaces. The reversal of these changes can be very difficult and may combine articular debridement, retinacular release, and patellar tendon transposition.

Clinical Features

The different forms of patellofemoral arthralgia can be specifically defined. It is important to separate the entities clinically, because the prognosis and treatment are often different. A clear definition of the condition is essential to distinguish these states from true internal derangement.

Quadriceps wasting may occur, and an effusion may be present but is unusual unless there is an associated reactive synovitis. Range of motion and stability of the knee are never affected. Specific sites of pain should be elicited and any local swelling noted. Signs of abnormal patellar excursion and pressure should be documented noting the overall limb alignment; the Q angle and patella position as well as the tightness of the retinacula and the quadriceps muscle group. Crepitus may be from the patella itself but can also arise from the retinacula and fatpads; care should be taken to determine its exact site of origin.

Finally, the status of the feet with regard to heel varus or valgus and the degree of pronation of the forefoot should be noted; these may have an important bearing on patellar responses on load bearing.

Management

Conservative Treatment

Nearly all these syndromes will respond to a conservative approach. On occasion, the provocative activity must be modified; that is, sport must be carried out at a reduced level, coupled where necessary with alterations in technique and form. A change of activity, e.g., from running to cycling, may be necessary, the emphasis being on maintaining basic fitness until the natural history of the process runs its course.

Although physiotherapy treatments with shortwave diathermy and ultrasound are often symptomatically helpful, an intensive individual program of exercise therapy must be maintained. Isometric quadriceps setting and straight-leg raising, followed by progressive resisted exercise over the final 5 to 10 degrees of knee extension are emphasized. Resisted exercises through the full range of motion are avoided because of the excessive compressive forces they apply across the patella. Sequential faradism can be applied if muscle bulk is significantly reduced. Stretching must be equally emphasized in an effort to reduce the loads across the joint and at the same time enhance the strength capability of the muscle group. Orthotics aimed at correcting pes planus and heel valgus may be helpful in cases where such a condition is contributing to abnormal patellar mechanics, particularly in association with genu valgum.

Surgical Treatment

Intensive conservative management for at least six months should precede any surgery; the patient should have been disabled to the point of nonparticipation in work or sport before such treatment is contemplated.

Retinacular Release. The lateral retinaculum is a capsular structure. It is extra-articular, and therefore, an intra-articular arthroscopic procedure makes no sense at all. However, arthroscopy is an essential prelude to this procedure, not only to scan the joint but also to deal with any intra-articular pathology that may be encountered. Having been reassured that the interior of the joint is normal, retinacular release should be carried out extra-articularly in order to preserve the integrity of the synovium.

A skin incision is made 1 cm in length over the lateral aspect of the knee at the junction of the upper and mid-third of the patella. Dissection is continued subcutaneously to expose the capsule and fascial elements. A careful incision of the retinaculum is made and then the capsule is separated from the underlying synovium. The retinaculum and lateral capsule are then released proximally and distally over a 10-cm length, avoiding completely the synovium. Simple skin closure and a pressure dressing are added, and the patient is able to commence an active rehabilitation program two days after surgery.

Fat Pad Excision. With repetitive activity, the fat pad and synovium hypertrophy and become pinched between the patella and femur, where they are subject to repetitive low-grade trauma and become persistently symptomatic. This condition is often confused with chondromalacia patella because of the associated crepitus that can sometimes be elicited. Careful examination differentiates the area of involvement from the patella which is completely smooth and uninvolved. Haffa's syndrome may require surgical excision of the hypertrophied tissue for satisfactory resolution.

The fat pad is a very substantial structure, and although it is possible to nibble away at this with basket forceps and other arthroscopic instruments, this can be very time-consuming and often incomplete. As a first-line treatment it is commendable because of its low morbidity. However, if arthroscopic excision of the fat pad proves inadequate, open excision is considered. A short medial arthrotomy offers excellent visualization of the fat pad which can be excised in its entirety. Because a prearthrotomy arthroscopy has been carried out, it is not necessary to explore the joint further, but zealous cauterization of the bleeding points in the base of the excised area is essential, for the fat pad is an extremely vascular structure.

Synovial Excision. In the suprapatellar area at the superior margin of the intercondylar articular groove, synovial impingement can become extremely troublesome, and local excision of the excessive synovial tissue becomes necessary. Given that preliminary arthroscopy has precluded other pathology, localized synovectomy using arthroscopic instrumentation is relatively easy.

PATELLAR INSTABILITY

Acute Patellar Dislocation

Traumatic dislocation of the patella is an injury which must be treated as any other ligamentous derangement of the knee. It requires a full evaluation to determine the extent of the instability and any other associated injury to the joint. The hemarthrosis should be aspirated before the knee is further carefully evaluated. X-ray studies should include skyline views of the patella and should be carefully evaluated to determine whether there is any associated damage to the articular surfaces, since portions of the articular cartilage and osteochondral fragments may be sheared off when the patella is forcibly dislocated.

Arthroscopy and Conservative Treatment

Arthroscopy should be carried out if there is doubt about the presence of a loose body. By arthroscopic technique, such fragments may be removed from the joint before a stovepipe cast is applied in full extension. After 4 weeks in cast, during which time quadriceps setting exercises and faradic stimulation are instituted, protection is further offered with a patella-restraining brace. Knee mobilization is commenced at this time; return to sports activity can be allowed only when full range of motion and full rehabilitation of the quadriceps, with particularly full flexibility, has been restored.

Open Surgical Treatment

Occasionally, traumatic dislocation is so severe as to shear off a major portion of the articular surface and/or produce a major disruption of the medial retinacular structures. Under these circumstances, it is better to formally open the knee, remove the loose body, and debride the damaged joint surface by shaving the margins and drilling the base. A formal arthrotomy is made medially, releasing the patellar mechanism sufficiently to evert the patella and obtain adequate visualization of the undersurface to deal with any local pathology. An extra-articular lateral release must be carried out, preserving the synovium but relaxing completely the lateral retinaculum and associated capsule along a line parallel to the iliotibial tract distally to the ligamentum patella and proximally outside the vastus lateralis.

Medial capsular plication should reconstitute the medial side without overzealous tightening that would unduly increase pressure on the patella. The repair must be fully tested through a full range of motion and, under direct vision, be seen to be sound and without excessive tension on the repaired area. Hinge-brace protection allowing a 0- to 30-degree range is practiced for 4 weeks, during which time an ongoing program of selective quadriceps faradism to vastus medialis and isometric quadriceps exercises is initiated. After removal from the hinge-brace, a patellar restraining support is utilized for 4 weeks as therapy intensifies with range of motion and flexibility exercises.

Patellar Subluxation

The diagnosis of patellar subluxation is too readily applied to patients with patellar symptomatology and varying presentations of their patellar mechanics. The extremely wide variation of patellar tracking and anatomic variance of the Q angle seen in athletes often makes it difficult to decide where true normal lies. Patellar subluxation should be confirmed only in those patients with demonstrably unstable patellae and a positive apprehension sign.

Nonoperative Treatment

Efforts at rehabilitation are directed in two areas for those with patella subluxation. Attention must be paid to the overall limb alignment and foot mechanics. In those with undue genu valgum or a tendency to overpronation, orthotic support should be considered with a medial heel wedge in a shoe with firm heel counter, the forefoot being aided further with a scaphoid pad and first metatarsal mound.

The knee itself then becomes the focus of further support with a simple elasticized patella-restraining brace for use during sports activity. The exercise program has a twofold thrust: to develop the strength in the muscle groups, and this can be supplemented with faradic stimulation selectively applied to the vastus medialis. However, quadriceps flexibility is the key to reducing pressures on the patella, and a diligent program of stretching exercises must be undertaken if the quadriceps is to function as a better shock absorber. With reduced tensions in this muscle group, there is less tendency for the patella to subluxate laterally, and the clinical situation is greatly enhanced.

Surgical Stabilization for Patellar Subluxation

For those patients with patellar instability without true dislocation who are symptomatically limited in their sports endeavors by a knee that gives way, stabilization by soft tissue reconstruction should suffice. There should be little need for meddling with the tibial tubercle insertion of the ligamentum patella unless there is frank dislocation or true chondromalacic degeneration of the patella.

Arthroscopy of the knee should precede patellar stabilization to ensure that no other internal derangement be overlooked. A combination of a lateral retinacular release and medial capsular plication with vastus medialis advancement will secure the patella without undue tension. The vastus medialis is released as a tongue in its distal portion; after plicating the capsule in a double-breasted fashion, the muscle is sewn down at its fascial margin, overlapping slightly the capsular repair. It should be emphasized that the repair should be completely sound, with the knee able to be passed through a full range of motion before closure. The lateral side is left completely open with an extrasynovial lateral retinacular capsular release. Hinge-brace protection is afforded for 4 weeks allowing a 0- to 30-degree excursion within the brace. Weightbearing should be protected with crutches during this time. The ongoing rehabilitation program is then similar to that for the patient managed conservatively. Return to sport is allowed when optimal range and strength have been achieved.

Patellar Dislocation

True dislocation of the patella requires a major stabilization if the athlete is to return to competitive activity. However, few procedures in orthopaedic surgery are associated with greater morbidity than that seen in patients who have been subjected to unnecessary and injudicious stabilization procedures for supposed instability of the patella. If the patellar mechanism is overtightened or if the patella is drawn down to an unphysiologic location, impaired function with inevitable, rapid, articular deterioration will be the result. The objective of a patella stabilization procedure must be to secure the patella without interfering unduly with the patellar mechanics by tightening the capsule and increasing patellar pressures.

Surgical Stabilization

The essential features of stabilization should release the lateral structures as well as realign the distal insertion of the ligamentum patella.

A good view of the patella can be obtained through a lateral skin incision. This allows for an adequate debridement of any articular irregularity and the drilling of roughened bony areas if necessary. The lateral retinaculum and lateral capsule are released proximally lateral to the vastus lateralis and distally to the ligamentum patella.

The tendon insertion is now gently elevated on a 3-mm thick sliver of bone freed proximally but hinged distally; it can be eased medially in the manner of Elmslie and Trillat on a 5×1.5 cm pedicle of bone. The bed should be prepared medially by gentle decortication with an osteotome and the transposed tendon insertion impacted before being secured with a single screw. Only the lateral synovium is closed; the capsule is left open. A soft dressing is all that is necessary; early mobilization is encouraged with active range of motion and full weight-bearing with crutches commencing on the third postoperative day.

CHONDROMALACIA PATELLA

True chondromalacia patella, where the articular facets of the patella are degenerate with ragged fronded surfaces, can be a difficult condition to deal with.

Conservative Treatment

Avoidance of provocative overload is essential. Therefore, for the chondromalacic patient, jumping sports such as basketball and gymnastics are ruled out. Jogging and skiing are also troublesome, and, for many athletes, much of their training will have to be modified to avoid compounding the insult. Supplemental training with cycling and swimming may be the only way of maintaining form. An enthusiasm for exercise therapy with quadriceps strengthening must be tempered in such individuals, for overloading the quadriceps may well aggravate the condition. It is vital to avoid all resisted exercises, crouches, and deep knee bends. Particularly to be condemned are the traditional quadriceps exercises using weight resistance with the knee extending from a flexed position.

Antiinflammatory medication can be of help if there is a reactive synovitis, enteric-coated ASA being favored because of the chronic nature of the condition. Steroid injection may occasionally help if recurrent effusions prove troublesome; but if the athlete is troubled to this degree, it may be necessary to consider some form of surgical intervention.

Surgical Treatment for Chondromalacia Patella

Arthroscopic Debridement and Retinacular Release. A lateral retinacular release should be combined with any intra-articular debridement and may even precede or follow the joint surgery. The role of arthroscopic debridement has yet to be defined, but certainly with fine scissors, basket forceps, and articular shavers, it is possible to smooth off much of the superficial roughness. Arguments as to the genesis of the chondromalacic state abound, and many contend that such superficial treatments do not address predisposing mechanical abnormalities. This is true, but it certainly offers a great advance over open articular debridement which is mentioned only to be condemned because of its attendant morbidity in terms of the much longer time required for recovery.

Open Debridement and Maquet Patelloplasty. Open debridement alone offers no advantage over a closed procedure. However, when other measures have failed, open debridement combined with an elevation of the tibial tubercle insertion of the ligamentum patella can favorably alter the clinical course of patients suffering from chronic chondromalacia patella.

The approach recommended utilizes a lateral skin incision and complete retinacular and capsular release as described for the patellar stabilization procedure. The patella is everted and a careful debridement is carried out. Full-thickness lesions should be demarcated with vertically cut edges and the malacic cartilage excised. The bed should be drilled through the subchondral plate. Superficial and fibrillated lesions should be shaved down to smooth substance but sound adjacent cartilage should not be interfered with in any way.

The elevation of the tibial tubercle is carried out with sharp osteotomes in a similar manner to that employed for stabilization procedures. The tendon, along with a 3-mm thick sliver of bone, is elevated on a pedicle 1.5 cm wide by 5 cm long. A wedge shaped bone block, 1.5×1 cm is easily taken from the lateral flare of the tibia adjacent to the tibial tubercle insertion. The bone graft is then impacted beneath the elevated tendon where it remains fully secure and needs no extra fixation. Because there is no tibial osteotomy as such, fasciotomy is not required, but the closure is left completely open on the lateral side after closing the synovium. The elevation of the tibial tubercle by 1 to 1.5 cm appears to be sufficient to redistribute forces on the patella. The results of this procedure have greatly surpassed those achieved previously by debridement alone. Because the graft is secure beneath the ligamentum, early mobilization can be instituted. It is essential to maintain motion after the patellar debridement; cast immobilization is contraindicated. Weightbearing is protected with crutches for 4 weeks until the graft has consolidated.

QUADRICEPS AND PATELLAR TENDON RUPTURES

CHRISTOPHER W. SIWEK, M.D.

Injuries to the extensor mechanism of the knee have been recognized and described since the times of Galen. Samuel of England, in 1838, is credited with the first published case of quadriceps tendon rupture in English literature. Treatment of these injuries consisted of immobilization and limited weight-bearing until Lister, in 1878, first practiced suture of the knee extensor. Charles McBurney reported the first successful repair of the quadriceps tendon in North America in 1887. McMaster, in 1933, published his experimental studies on ruptures of tendons and muscles in animals. He concluded that ruptures of the quadriceps and patellar tendons rarely occur through their substance, but rather are sustained at the musculotendinous junction or insertion of the tendon into the bone. During the last half century, several different methods have been described, dealing with repairs and reconstruction of neglected, delayed ruptures of extensor mechanism of knee joint.

MECHANISM AND LEVEL OF RUPTURE

Continuity of the extensor mechanism of the knee is disrupted as a result of sudden, powerful contracture of quadriceps muscle against the weight of the body applied to the affected extremity. The actual moment of tearing occurs when the knee is in a mild flexion, the patella

firmly held against the femoral condyles by the pull of quadriceps muscle and the force continuing.

The mechanism of rupture for quadriceps as well as patellar tendons is the same. The level of rupture is determined by predisposing factors.

It appears to me that the single, most important, factor is the individual's age. The natural physiologic aging process "favors" patellar tendon ruptures in younger individuals below the age of 40 and quadriceps tendon ruptures in those above that age. Males sustain injuries six times more often than females, according to my study. Other predisposing factors include diabetes, rheumatoid arthritis, gout, psoriatic arthritis, hyperparathyroidism, systemic lupus erythematosus, and nephritis. Ruptures of patellar tendons in athletes following multiple knee injections with steroids also have been documented.

EXAMINATION

Ruptures of the quadriceps and patellar tendons are uncommon considering all the trauma that occurs about the knee. The severe hematoma that often accompanies the acute rupture may conceal the important diagnostic signs. Much too frequently, these ruptures are misdiagnosed in the acute stage of knee injury. In my study, 39 percent of ruptures have been missed on the initial examination. Testing of the extensor mechanism should be an essential part of the total comprehensive knee evaluation. It is of utmost importance that an early diagnosis be established in order to ensure good final results. During examination, one must look for loss of active knee extension or inability to maintain a passively extended joint against gravity. If the rupture does not extend through medial and lateral retinacula, the patient may have limited, weak, active extension, but still is not able to maintain the completely extended knee joint against gravity. Lack of complete active extension, accompanied by local tenderness and hemarthrosis, strongly suggests at least a partial tear. Complete ruptures are always associated with a palpable soft tissue defect. The rent is easily identifiable in quadriceps tendon, owing to a larger mass of the tissue. However, it may be difficult to palpate a rent in the patellar tendon at the time of swelling and hemarthrosis. In this situation, one should examine the joint while the patient is sitting on a table with his/her legs hanging down. Examination is done by comparing both patellar tendons. The examiner sits in front of the patient, identifies both patellar tendons by placing his thumbs on them, and asks the patient to slowly extend both knees. The examiner should immediately feel "sudden tension" under the thumb that is over the normal patellar tendon, but this tension is absent on the affected side. Proximally (patellar tendon rupture) or distally (quadricep tendon rupture) a displaced patella may also be observed clinically or radiographically. Old untreated ruptures with partial return of function may be a diagnostic problem. Although partial return of quadriceps function in these cases may occur several weeks after the injury, the disability remains.

QUADRICEPS TENDON RUPTURES

Occurrence

As noted previously, this lesion usually occurs in individuals who are past the fifth decade in age. I have reviewed 117 cases, published from 1880 to 1978, in which the age of the patient was given. There was 69 quadriceps tendon ruptures, and all but four occurred in patients who were 40 years of age or older. In my own study, 78 percent of quadriceps tendon ruptures occurred in the fifth decade of life or later.

The tears are transverse in nature, and they begin in the central portion of rectus femoris, traversing its entire thickness. Only on rare occasions is the tear limited to the rectus femoris; usually it extends laterally and medially, implicating the fibrous expansions of the vastus lateralis and medialis for varying distances. Most of the injuries are observed at the level of the quadriceps tendon attachment to the patella. The margins of the tear are ragged, and tissues are infiltrated with blood. Intratendinous tears do not occur so frequently, and once such a tear is found, a "pathologic tear" should be suspected. Systemic diseases, as previously mentioned, or prior steroid infiltrations should be included in the differential diagnosis.

Microscopic examination of tissue from the rupture site shows local degenerative changes, including a decreased level of collagen in fibers of the tendon, fibrotic degeneration, and infiltration.

Diagnosis

The diagnosis is made readily, provided correct interpretation is given to the clinical features. Frequently, the true nature of the lesion is overlooked because the examiner does not suspect the possibility of a rupture of the quadriceps tendon and depends too heavily on roentgenographic findings, which are not always helpful. The clinical findings are directly related to the extent of tear and the degree of separation of fragments. The cardinal clinical features are a history of stumbling, with the experiencing of severe pain above the knee and subsequent inability to extend the joint.

In complete tears, including synovial membrane, a large hemarthrosis is present. Upon flexion of the knee, the bloody content of the joint is displaced into the suprapatellar pouch and is easily observed as an "abnormal" bulge at the level of rupture. One can palpate a soft tissue defect above the patella. The patella itself may be displaced distally, and it has increased side-to-side motion when compared to the unaffected leg. Roentgenograms may reveal a distally displaced patella, and soft tissue technique may demonstrate the rent itself. If the tear occurs at the tendo-osseous junction, small fragments of avulsed superior pole of the patella appear to be displaced proximally, being retracted with rectus femoris.

Small tears within the rectus femoris alone may be difficult to diagnose. This may be especially true in obese individuals. These patients still have active extension against gravity, but never complete extension. The examiner may reverse the test: rather than asking the patient to extend the joint, he should bring the knee to complete extension and ask the patient to maintain it. In cases of tear, one always notices a "drop" of the leg of varying degrees. During the examination, the patient complains of increased pain in the suprapatellar region owing to quadriceps tension. In some of these diagnostically difficult cases, a CT scan has been helpful in identifying the rupture, its extent, and its location.

Proper diagnosis of small tears can be easily missed. I have observed that this incorrect diagnosis is most often made in the emergency room. Usually, the history and physical examination "fit" into a pattern of "sprained knee", and patient is given some kind of knee splint. Because the knee support allows some mobility, reasonable comfort, and noticeable steady improvement, the patient may continue this incorrect therapy for several weeks. Disappointment comes when the patient cannot regain full quadriceps strength and is unable to climb stairs or walk on an inclined plane without risk of falling. Return to even mild recreational sport activity is impossible.

Treatment

Repair of the defect should be achieved by surgical intervention in all cases of tear of the extensor mechanism. Adequate assessment of the tear should be made in order to achieve proper and lasting repair. Treatment is generally divided into early and late repair. Distinction between these two phases is made more by the amount of retraction of quadriceps, by difficulty of end-to-end approximation, and by the amount of scar tissue formation than by actual time from rupture to repair. These findings vary from case to case. In the past, I have used 2 weeks as a cut-off time between early and late repairs, but in many instances, I was able to do primary repairs with end-to-end suture in tears as old as 3 weeks, and in small tears even older. I would suggest that we use the term late repair when, because of time loss, surgical treatment is more extensive and requires additional reinforcement of suture, other than just end-to-end repair. In my experience, no additional reinforcement has been necessary in early repairs or in cases in which end-to-end approximation is achieved without significant strain and tension.

Preferred Methods for Early Repairs

Techniques of repair may vary according to the level of rupture. If the tear is intratendinous and an adequate amount of tissue is available for approximation, an end-to-end suture repair is sufficient. In cases in which the quadriceps tendon is avulsed from patellar attachment, longitudinal holes have to be drilled in the patella for placement of sutures to secure the repair.

Surgical Technique (End-to-End Repair)

A midline anterior longitudinal skin incision is begun about 10 cm proximal to the superior pole of the patella. In tears involving large portions of medial and lateral retinaculum, the incision may have to be extended proximally for an additional 5 to 7 cm. Distally, the incision ends at the joint level. After dissecting subcutaneous and fatty tissues, the rupture is exposed with its hematoma and ragged edges. All clots are removed and the cavity is well irrigated. The entire quadriceps tendon and the suprapatellar pouch area is examined and damage assessed. The edges of the tendon are trimmed of all devitalized and frayed strands of tissue. If the synovial membrane of the suprapatellar pouch is torn, it should be repaired first. If difficulty in approximation exists, a towel clip should be placed in the rectus femoris tendon at the proximal side of the wound and traction applied distally. A rent in the quadriceps tendon should be closed with heavy absorbable horizontal mattress sutures. Deep layers are closed first; suturing is continued outward through the middle layers of vastus medialis and lateralis to the most anterior tendon of rectus femoris. The suture line is tested under direct vision. The knee is passively flexed to 90° and the repair carefully examined. Subcutaneous and skin closure is done with the knee in 45° of flexion to avoid tight suturing and future tissue contractures, which may delay recovery of range of motion. The entire procedure is done without tourniquet control. The tourniquet is applied, but used only if necessary. An inflated tourniquet causes additional retraction of the proximal fragment and distorts the anatomy of thigh muscles. Meticulous hemostasis is done to avoid hematoma formation.

Surgical Technique (Tendon-to-Bone Repair)

The technique differs slightly in cases of avulsion of the tendon from the superior pole of the patella. An avulsed rectus is less frayed than with an intratendinous rupture. There is always a good thick stump of tendon to work with. Attention should be directed toward debridement and preparation of the patella for acceptance of the tendon and proper placement of holes drilled through the body of the patella. By means of a small curette, the edge of the superior pole is "cleaned" from remaining fragments of tendon and sclerotic bone; damage to articulating surface is avoided. With a drill sized 3/32, three holes are made in the following fashion: A sponge is placed into the floor of the defect to prevent bony fragments from falling into the knee joint. The first hole is drilled centrally, starting at the proximal pole of the patella just superior to the articulating surface. The drill should exit at the lower portion of the body of the patella, making the hole at least 2 cm long; otherwise fracture may occur. A small guide wire may be placed into the hole to ensure parallel placement of two additional holes. The lateral holes should be at least 1 cm away from the central one, but well within the body of the patella. Two separate heavy sutures are placed through the holes and the rectus femoris (Fig. 1). Additional reinforcing sutures are placed through the superior layer of the rectus femoris. The remaining portion of tear within both vastus muscles are closed as described previously. The use of more than three holes in the patella is unnecessary and may weaken the bone. Occasionally, I use Bunnell's pull-out wire to secure the repair for the period of healing.

Late Repair

Neglected cases exhibit marked disability because of lack of stability in the affected extremity. Many of these patients must depend on the use of a cane or a brace in order to walk. The quadriceps muscle becomes contracted and extensive adhesions develop. The edges of ruptured tendon become thickened and sclerotic.

Debridement and excision of devitalized tissue should be the first step in surgical repair. All necrotic tissues at the rupture site must be evacuated in order to have vital substances for approximation. Failure to achieve this may result in poor delayed healing and possibly re-rupture. Release of adhesions, mainly between the quadriceps and the femur, may allow for additional distal displacement of the stump. Meticulous hemostasis must be achieved. If good approximation is

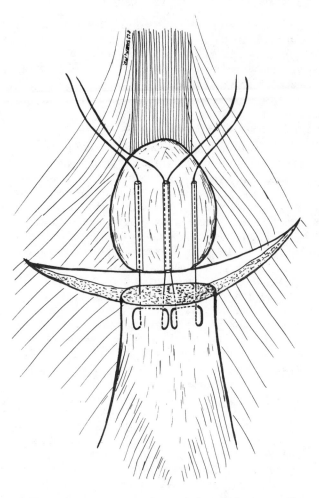

Figure 1 Tendon-to-bone repair of quadriceps tendon rupture. Two separate heavy sutures are placed through the holes in the patella and the rectus femoris.

possible, I prefer to repair by means of the tendon-to-bone technique (already described). Sutures passed through drilled holes make the repair more secure. At this point, after the rent itself is closed, routine testing of suture line by knee flexion is done, and about 90° of flexion should be possible. The surgeon has to bear in mind that excessive tension of the extensor mechanism will cause limited range of motion and may produce painful patellar symptoms, particularly in active sports-oriented individuals.

The next step in late repairs of the quadriceps tendon is reinforcement of the rupture. The least traumatic and most adequate repair is achieved by means of the Scuderi-type inverted V-flap, taken from the rectus femoris and crossed over the suture line. The triangular flap is based 2 cm above the side of rupture, and it covers the entire width of the rectus. A height of 6 to 8 cm is sufficient for the triangle. An even thickness of 3 to 4 mm (about one-third the full thickness of the tendon) is stripped, starting from the apex of the triangle and ending 2 cm above the rupture level. The flap is inverted and tacked down to the distal portion of the extensor mechanism covering the rent. Depending on the quality of the

repair, an additional pullout wire can be used for protection, and it may remain in place throughout the healing process. In late repairs, I prefer to anchor the pull-out wire to the transverse tibial pin rather than place the pin through the patella. In the latter case, demineralization of the patella occurs owing to prolonged disuse, and additional transverse holes may dangerously weaken the patella subjecting it to fractures.

One further step is taken in the repair of a neglected quadriceps tendon rupture when, despite releases, approximation of the edges of the rent is not possible. A lengthening of the quadriceps tendon by the "sliding" method of Codivilla is used. Occasionally, I have reinforced the suture line with wide strip of fascia lata obtained from the same side. This is used instead of the Scuderi inverted V-flap in cases in which the area is already weakened by a quadriceps-lengthening procedure. The reinforcing strip is sutured to the vastus muscles above and to the patella and its medial and lateral retinacula below.

Postoperative Management

Following the operation, the knee is maintained in complete extension. Compression dressings and a conventional knee splint are applied. In less reliable patients, a long leg cast is preferred. Routine wound care is given to the operated site. The patient uses crutches and is allowed "toe touch" for balance only. Quadriceps-setting and leg-raising with assistance are initiated as soon as postsurgical pain and soreness permit. Two weeks after surgery, sutures are removed. The leg is placed in a brace with adjustable hinges at the knee level. Passive range of motion starts 3 weeks after repair and does not exceed 60° until the fifth postoperative week. The patient is allowed partial to full weight-bearing as tolerated, beginning the third postsurgical week. Quadriceps stimulation is used if necessary. The brace is discontinued between the fifth and the seventh week. Judgment regarding the optimal time to discontinue the immobilization is based on the size of the tear and the "soundness" of the repair. Range of motion is continued since full recovery seldom is obtained at this point. Strengthening exercises should include a comprehensive program to regain complete balance of all muscle groups in the leg.

Mild, recreational, noncontact sport activity may be initiated 3 to 4 months after surgery, depending on the severity of the tear. Competitive sports should not be allowed until the full strength of the quadriceps muscle is achieved.

Results

Early repair of the quadriceps tendon, with adequate postoperative physical therapy, gives excellent results. Thirty patients studied by me regained quadriceps strength comparable to that of the opposite leg, and range of motion measured at least 120° (in older patients) or more.

Late repair greatly diminishes the chance of regaining satisfactory function postoperatively. In my study, the main obstacle to better results was limited range of motion. Of six patients who underwent delayed repair, only one regained more than 90° of knee flexion. Five of them had persistent quadriceps atrophy.

Since quadriceps tendon ruptures occur in the older population, the timing of physical therapy after repair is very important. In patients with adequate secure repairs, strengthening exercises and range of motion should begin soon after surgery. In motivated patients, complete recovery can be expected.

PATELLAR TENDON RUPTURES

Occurrence

Rupture of the patellar tendon is very rare and occurs mostly in younger individuals below the age of 40. In the group of 33 patients studied by me, only one sustained injury after the age of 40 (patient was 47); the remaining 32 were under 40. The incidence of patellar tendon rupture is about equal to that of quadriceps tendon rupture, and the mechanism is the same.

Most commonly, the lesion comprises complete avulsion of the tendon from the inferior pole of the patella, and the tear extends into both medial and lateral retinacula. Occasionally, small fragments of bone are avulsed from the patella. A healthy patellar tendon does not rupture through its substance, and if such a lesion is found, one should suspect underlying causes other than the injury. Effects of injudicious steroid injections in young athletic individuals have to be included in the differential diagnosis. Bilateral simultaneous ruptures also are suspect for systemic diseases. There is no mention of such a case in the literature, all reported simultaneous, bilateral ruptures being associated with a variety of "predisposing factors".

I have seen cases in which some longitudinal fibers of the patellar tendon have been detached from the patella and others from the tibial tubercle (Fig. 2), causing severe shredding of the tissue. This "spaghetti-like" effect makes direct suturing impossible, and fascia lata graft is necessary to restore continuity.

Injuries to the distal portion of the patellar tendon are usually associated with avulsion fractures of the tibial tubercle, often preceded by Osgood-Schlatter's disease.

Diagnosis

A detailed history helps to recreate the actual moment of injury, which should strongly suggest rupture of the extensor mechanism. The cardinal sign—lack of active extension—is always present. Proximal migration of the patella is easily noted clinically and radiographi-

cally. In more difficult cases, one could make comparisons to the opposite knee. If swelling obscures the pathology, a test of "sudden tension", as described previously, may be of value.

Treatment

Ruptures should be repaired at the earliest opportunity. In early repairs, surgical technique differs according to the level of injury. Delayed suturing may require additional preoperative or intraoperative procedures. Regardless of the type of injury and the surgical technique used, gentle handling of the tissues is important. The fat pad should remain undisturbed and its normal contact with the patellar tendon preserved since it serves as a very important blood supply to the tendon. Any debridement at the rupture site must be adequate, but careless excision of tissue avoided. Functionally disabling patella baja may result if an excess of tendon is removed.

Actual repair of the patellar tendon, as opposed to quadriceps tendon repair, does not give a sense of "soundness" and security. The patellar tendon is susceptible to longitudinal separations of its fibers, and placement of sutures under excessive traction may cause additional shredding of the tendon. Sutures have to be passed

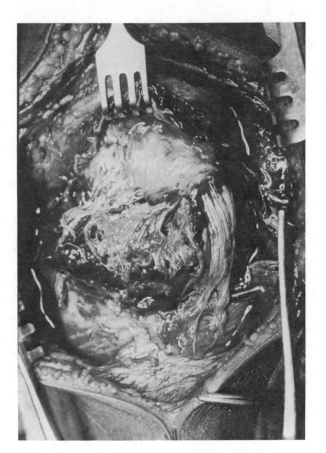

Figure 2 Patellar tendon rupture. Some longitudinal fibers have been detached from the patellar tendon and others from the tibial tubercle, causing severe shredding of the tissue.

through "tight" healthy portions of tendon in a manner that will not cause strangulation of tissue. I routinely use pull-out wires to avoid tension on the suture line and weakening of the repair.

Preferred Methods

Bone-to-Tendon Technique

This repair is a mirror image of the technique described for quadriceps tendon avulsion from the superior pole of the patella.

The skin incision extends from 5 cm above the superior pole of the patella to the tibial tubercle in straight anterior fashion. The entire patellar tendon is exposed and the quality of tissue is noted. The avulsed end of the tendon is debrided by sharp transverse dissection, removing enough frayed fragments to leave a thick wide stump for repair. The main supporting sutures are opposed (Fig. 3). The same technique may be used in cases of fracture of the inferior pole of the patella when comminuted fragments are excised.

Tendon-to-Tendon Technique

As already mentioned, one should suspect "pathologic" rupture when a tear has occurred transverely

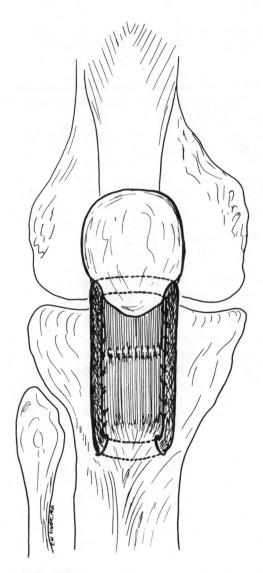

Figure 4 Tendon-to-tendon repair of patellar tendon rupture. The graft is rolled into a cord and passed through both tunnels (see text).

through the substance of the tendon. In these cases, direct mattress suturing is not strong enough to maintain continuity of the tendon, even with the leg immobilized in full extension. Quadriceps contractures may cut the sutures through fragile tendon, causing separation of fragments. On the other hand, more vigorous and more bulky suturing may strangulate the tissue.

I reinforce the suture line with a strip of fascia lata obtained from the same side. The strip has to be three times the length of the ruptured tendon and 1.5 cm wide in order to be sufficient for repair. Two tunnels are made, one at 1.5 cm to 2 cm above the inferior pole of the patella and the second 1 cm below the attachment of the patellar tendon to the tibial tubercle. A high-speed air drill with a 3-mm bur is excellent for shaping the edges of the tunnels. When this instrument is used, "chipping" of bone and fractures are easily avoided. One has to ensure that edges of both tunnels are smooth and round to prevent them from cutting into a fascia lata graft. Before final repair is done, a pull-out wire is passed through the

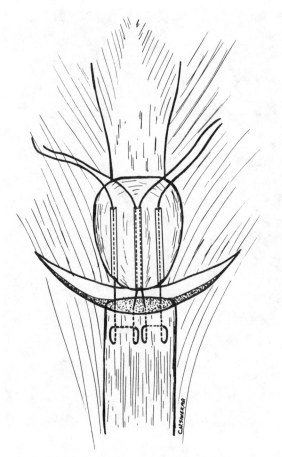

Figure 3 Bone-to-tendon repair of patellar tendon rupture. The main supporting sutures are opposed (see text).

superior pole of the patella, and sufficient distal traction is applied. Wires are anchored to the transverse tibial pin. Excessive traction on the patella is avoided since it may result in a patella baja. The graft is rolled nto a cord and passed through both tunnels (Fig. 4). The entire graft is tucked down to both sides of the patellar tendon. The wound is closed as usual.

Delayed Repairs

Despite delay, primary approximation of fragments is possible in many cases. These ruptures can be treated by one of the techniques described above. In severely neglected cases, preoperative skeletal traction may be necessary to overcome contractures and adhesions of the quadriceps mechanism. Following are indications for preoperative traction: (1) marked clinical and radiographic proximal displacement of the patella, (2) an inability to manually move the patella to its anatomic position (3) a loss of free passive side-to-side motion of the patella (indicative of severe adhesions).

Traction is applied through a 9/64-inch Steinmann pin placed transversely into the patella. The size of the pin largely depends on the size of the patella. To avoid skin tension, the skin is displaced proximally prior to pin insertion, and a maximum of 2 kilograms of weight is applied. It may take a few days to 2 weeks before adequate displacement is obtained. Progress of the traction is checked clinically or radiographically. During the period of traction, the knee is engaged in passive range of motion. This is done most comfortably with the patient lying on the unaffected side.

When satisfactory distal displacement of the patella is achieved, surgical repair follows. After routine exposure of the lesion, a second Steinmann pin is inserted into the proximal tibia. The patella is brought to its anatomic position and maintained thereby wiring both Steinmann pins together. Actual repair of the patellar tendon is done by means of the tendon-to-tendon technique, already described.

A patellar tendon that is not performing its function because of rupture quickly undergoes disuse degeneration and disintegration. In these severe cases, one may have to reconstruct the entire patellar tendon, and I prefer to use the distal tendinous portion of the semitendinosus muscle as a substitute for the patellar tendon. The tendon is looped through transverse tunnels in the patella and proximal tibia and then sewn onto itself. After wound closure, a long leg cast is applied, incorporating both pins.

Postoperative Care

For early repairs with good strong approximation, postoperative management is the same as for early repairs of quadriceps tendon ruptures.

In delayed repairs of the patellar tendon, judgment of postoperative management is based on the extent of rupture, the quality and availability of tissues for approximation, and the actual strength of the suture line at the conclusion of surgery. If pins and wires have been used, they should be maintained for 4 to 5 weeks. Cast immobilization with the knee in full extension is continued for 7 to 8 weeks postoperatively.

In early repairs, mild, recreational, noncontact sports activity may be initiated 3 to 4 months after surgery. Prolonged recovery in delayed repairs may extend this time to 6 months.

Results

In my study, 25 patients had early repairs of patellar tendons. Twenty of them obtained excellent results with full range of motion and strength of quadriceps muscle equal to that of the opposite leg. Four patients were unable to obtain full active extension, even though passive extension was possible. One patient reruptured his patellar tendon 8 weeks following original repair, while attempting to play football on a recreational level.

Results of seven late repairs in my study were directly related to but he had other medical problems which did not allow him to receive a proper course of therapy. In the remaining five ruptures, motion ranged from full extension to 130° of flexion. Good quadriceps strength was regained despite persistent atrophy of thigh muscles.

MEDIAL LIGAMENT INSTABILITY OF THE KNEE

R. PETER WELSH, M.B., Ch.B.,
F.R.C.S.(C), F.A.C.S.

The medial collateral system forms the most vital stabilizer of the medial aspect of the knee, with its deep and superficial ligaments reinforced by strong capsular support and enveloped by the tendons of the semimembranosus and the pes anserinus.

Particularly in contact sports is this complex vulnerable to sharp valgus loading with consequential tearing of these structures. Depending on the position of the knee at the time of injury and the magnitude of the force involved, various elements of the complex may be torn. The ultimate stability of the knee is severely compromised with major tears, and even minor instabilities can markedly inhibit athletic performance.

It is imperative therefore that these injuries be accurately diagnosed and treatment appropriate to the injury administered.

CLINICAL FEATURES

Injury to the medial complex is a traumatic event. Be it from impact loading by an opponent at football or from a fall while skiing, major force applied to the limb is a common feature. If a major injury is sustained with the leg in extension when the capsular ligaments are at their tautest, severe capsular as well as ligament injury will ensue. In extreme instances, the anterior and the posterior cruciate ligaments may also be involved. If the knee is slightly flexed, the medial collateral ligament alone may be injured, but if a rotary component is involved, injury to the anterior cruciate ligament is commonly associated, and damage to the articular surfaces and menisci also is possible.

It is the evaluation of whether or not other structures are involved in the injury that makes injury to the medial collateral ligament so important. In its own right, management of injury to the medial collateral ligament is relatively straightforward, but other associated ligament injury or meniscal disorder may necessitate more direct intervention.

CLINICAL PRESENTATION

Following a valgus strain load of the knee of significant degree, most athletes are incapacitated, but the heavily muscled, highly motivated hockey or football player may endeavor to, and be able to, return to the field of play. This is extremely dangerous and must not be allowed because the compromised knee is now so vulnerable to even minor traumatic incidents that more serious injury can be readily sustained.

On examining the acutely injured knee, the points of maximal tenderness at the media femoral condylar origin over the joint line or at the tibial insertion may give a clue as to the site of the tear.

The early appearance of an effusion suggests hemorrhage into the knee, which may well indicate an associated anterior cruciate ligament disruption or capsular involvement. If the capsule is intact, an acute medial collateral ligament strain may not be accompanied by early effusion, although later (6 to 12 hours), the presence of a reactive synovial effusion is usual. Paradoxically, in case of a massive disruption with anterior cruciate ligament and capsular insult, there may be no obvious intra-articular accumulation because with breaching of the integrity of the capsule, the hemarthrosis escapes from the joint and dissipates in the soft tissues about the knee. Before clinical examination is pursued further, aspiration of any hemarthrosis under local anaesthesia greatly facilitates the further evaluation of the status of the joint and should be routinely performed.

Varus and valgus stress testing with the knee in full extension and in 15 degrees of flexion assesses the stability of the collateral structures. Laxity in full extension confirm capsular disruption and probably associated cruciate injury. The Lachman and MacIntosh tests confirm the presence of any associated anterior cruciate ligament disruption.

The knee should also be examined for any patellar instability, meniscal disorder, or intra-articular injury.

X-ray studies conclude the clinical examination with routine AP, lateral, tunnel, and skyline views to rule out any associated osteochondral fracture or bony injury.

In most minor strains it is possible to assess the basic stability of the knee in the manner just described with assurance that a major injury is not being overlooked.

EXAMINATION UNDER ANESTHESIA

In more severe injuries, in patients presenting several hours after the trauma, in those who are strong and heavily muscled, in those who are anxious and resistant to examination, or in any individual in whom the examiner has any doubts as to the basic stability of the knee, examination under anesthesia should be carried out.

This may be performed under spinal, epidural, or general anesthesia, as long as the patient is kept relaxed and pain-free. The basic examination can then be repeated and a clear evaluation of the stability of the knee achieved. At the same time, stress x-ray studies with the knee stretched open should be done to record the degree of instability; this should always be compared to the uninjured, opposite side. Arthroscopy should also be performed at this time to establish the basic integrity of the internal structures. Simple meniscal or articular lesions can also be treated by arthroscopic technique at this time.

Armed with all information regarding the knee—its ligament status and stability and the status of the interior—the physician can now plan the treatment appropriate to the patient's needs.

MANAGEMENT OF ACUTE MEDIAL COLLATERAL LIGAMENT DISRUPTION

For isolated medial collateral ligament tears, cast immobilization is used. For isolated medial collateral ligament tear with internal derangement, treatment consists of arthroscopic surgery and cast immobilization. For medial collateral ligament disruption and anterior cruciate ligament rupture, surgical repair of both ligaments is required.

Cast Treatment

Cast immobilization is recommended for all medial collateral ligament disruptions in which the medial collateral ligament is injured in isolation. If a meniscal disorder is identified, it should be treated by arthroscopic technique and the leg immobilized thereafter.

It is not necessary to operate on the isolated medial collateral ligament tear. The results of adequate cast immobilization have proved most satisfactory, with the morbidity greatly reduced and a more rapid return to both work and play achieved than when such injury is treated surgically. However, casting must be properly carried out; stove pipe immobilization is worthless. The cast must be full-length, toe to groin, flexed 90 degrees at the knee and internally rotated 15 degrees. This allows the ligament to heal while in its shortest position with tightening of the posteromedial corner. In the athlete under 30 years of age, the cast is maintained for 6 weeks; in those 30 to 40 years of age, for 4 to 5 weeks.

At 3 weeks, a limited number of class athletes have been changed to a cast-brace in the same basic position, but allowing limited extension with a hinge to 60 degrees for the final 3 weeks. This seems to expedite the post-cast recovery and rehabilitation, and cast-bracing will undoubtedly come to play a greater role as our experience expands.

Following release from the cast, the patient becomes mobile for 3 weeks on his or her own, with pool or spa therapy when possible. From 9 weeks on, a full program of rehabilitation is instituted, mobilizing with hydro and cycle therapy, strengthening hip flexors, hip abductors, and hamstring muscle groups as well as the quadriceps. A program of stretching of the adductors, hamstrings, quads, and calf muscle groups follows. Weight-bearing with crutches is continued until extension to 10 degrees is achieved; return to sport is not allowed until a normal gait pattern has been established.

Surgical Treatment

For those with disruption of both the medial collateral ligament and the anterior cruciate ligament, surgical repair is mandatory. This necessitates repair of both ligaments; it is of limited value to repair only the medial collateral ligament when the anterior cruciate ligament is also injured.

Incisions on the anteromedial side should not be extravagantly curved, as this may only compromise venous and lymphatic drainage of any skin flaps. A long, straight, medial incision is favored, starting below the tibial tubercle and extending upward over the vastus medialis. When the knee is flexed, this incision permits easy access to the posteromedial corner of the knee yet allows ready access for removal of a patellotendon graft from the midline. The prepatellar fascia is preserved with the skin flaps and the middle one-third of the ligamentum patella is taken out as a graft for cruciate reinforcement. The technique of cruciate reconstruction is described in the chapter on anterior cruciate ligament disruption, this part of the repair being completed after dealing with any intra-articular pathology and before proceeding with the reconstruction of the medial collateral ligament.

In mobilizing the medial skin flap, it is taken together with the capsular fascia, which is released along the inferior margin of vastus medialis and folded posteriorly. An anterior arthrotomy allows a thorough inspection of the joint, and with folding back of the capsular fascia, the disruption of the capsular and ligament structures can be identified. It is imperative to postively identify the extent of the damage before proceeding further. There is no sense in damaging, by ill-considered dissection, tissues already severely compromised. Having identified whence the superficial portion of the medial collateral ligament has been torn (that is, proximally, distally, or midsubstance) and having determined the extent of the disruption of the deep portion of the ligament, the surgeon can now perform a posterior arthrotomy behind the line of the ligament. In the posteromedial corner, the local trauma can be assessed, including any injury to the semimembranosus or the pes.

A systematic repair follows, sewing up the posteromedial corner, plicating the redundant and stretched tissues, and closing the posterior arthrotomy before proceeding forward to repair the deep and then the superficial ligaments. It may be necessary to reimplant the origin of the ligament to the medial femoral condyle, and this should be embedded in exactly the same location whence it was avulsed. It is permissible to use a staple in this location, but not advised in reinserting the distal portion to the tibia because this part of the ligament has a natural excursion along the medial margin of the tibial plateau, making its insertion more distally deep to the pes. Interference with this insertion by more proximal tethering can lead to a troublesome stiffness of the knee. Finally, the anterior capsulotomy is closed and the capsular and prepatellar fascia drawn over the top to seal the repair.

Cast immobilization and the rehabilitation program proceed thereafter as described for the conservative treatment.

The recovery following such reconstruction is necessarily protracted, and it may be 6 months before full extension is achieved. If at 3 months full flexion has not been achieved, gentle manipulation under general anesthesia is occasionally necessary. The results of major reconstruction in a series of over 50 cases have been most satisfactory, and return to competitive contact sports without bracing the expected outcome.

CHRONIC INSTABILITY OF THE MEDIAL COLLATERAL LIGAMENT

There is no doubt that the opportune time to treat a lesion of the medial collateral ligament is early and not late. The torn anterior cruciate ligament can be substituted for by late reconstruction with reasonably reliable results predicted. However, reconstruction for chronic medial collateral ligament instability is not quite as predictable, and although brace control can be effective, it is no substitute for good primary treatment.

In the case of late treatment, it is once again important to identify an associated ligament instability of the anterior cruciate ligament and any associated internal derangement. Unfortunately, many individuals with chronic medial collateral ligament instability may also be showing degenerative wear changes in the joint and may need an associated debridement or meniscal surgery.

Brace Protection

In those with symptomatic instability of mild to moderate degree, most can be controlled adequately for sports purposes with a Lennox-Hill type brace. This device, with built-in medial rotation control, admirably protects and substitutes for a deficiency of the medial-collateral ligament and is routinely described as a first-line treatment choice.

Surgical Reconstruction

In an unfortunate few, the instability is so marked that insecurity in everyday life is a problem and brace protection a nonviable alternative. For these, a late repair is required, in which case it is necessary to rebuild the whole medial side, both the posteromedial capsule and the collateral ligament structures. Reinforcement may also be necessary, utilizing adjacent tendon structures such as the semimembranosus and the pes tendons.

Again, a straight anteromedial incision is recommended, although if previous surgery has been undertaken, utilization of the scar has to be considered. Separation of the prepatellar and capsular fascia with the skin flaps ensures their viability, and two arthrotomies are made, one anterior and the other posterior to the medial collateral ligament complex. The collateral origin should first be secured in its correct anatomic position. As this is the center of the axis of the knee joint rotation, it should not be moved proximally to an aberrant location. If laxity prevails, the distal insertion can be taken down and reimplantation made distally, not at the joint margin, but at its true position deep to the pes anserinus insertion.

The posterior medial corner is now plicated and any redundancy taken up in closing the posterior arthrotomy. The semimembranosus can be used to reinforce the posteromedial corner and the pes reimplanted proximally to add further stability anteriorly. Finally, the anterior arthrotomy is closed and the fascia reconstituted.

A regimen of cast immobilization and subsequent rehabilitation follows, as has been previously described for the acute repair.

ACUTE INJURY TO THE ANTERIOR CRUCIATE LIGAMENT

R. PETER WELSH, M.B., Ch.B., F.R.C.S.(C), F.A.C.S.

Rupture of the anterior cruciate ligament constitutes a major handicap to those who are athletically inclined. A knee so injured is vulnerable to episodes of "giving way" which may not only seriously compromise athletic performance but also render the knee subject to further major articular insult with meniscal disruption and articular surface breakdown.

It is imperative to identify all such lesions and afford appropriate advice, counsel, and treatment. This does not imply that all ruptures of the anterior cruciate liga-ment should be surgically treated *per primum* since not all cruciate-deficient knees become manifestly unstable. However, athletic performance following injury to the anterior cruciate ligament may well have to be modified, and, should instability of the knee be an ongoing problem, late stabilization may have to be performed. The incidence of secondary articular injuries (meniscal derangement, 54% and serious articular lesions, 38%) encountered in a series of 125 late reconstructions followed up over a 5-year period, leads me to conclude that a more aggressive surgical approach should be undertaken in the athletically active individual.

ACUTE RUPTURE OF THE ANTERIOR CRUCIATE LIGAMENT

An athlete who, propping to cut or leaping to make a shot, feels a sudden "pop" in the knee and an associated sensation of "the knee coming apart" is probably experiencing a tear of the anterior cruciate ligament. This can also occur from direct trauma as in falls in skiing or in contact sports such as football or hockey where an opponent's impact provides a disruptive external force. However, these injuries are more dramatic and the injury is less likely to be overlooked than in the first group of individuals where a seemingly innocuous noncontact presentation is often the catalyst. Both instances present athletes with disruptions of the anterior cruciate ligament that deserve close clinical attention.

Hemarthrosis almost always accompanies such injuries, and the presence of blood in the knee may make the joint difficult to examine. The hemarthrosis should always be aspirated; if necessary, the installation of local anesthetic (20 ml of 1% Xylocaine) can often aid further evaluation of the joint. Under such circumstances, it should be possible with the Lachman test to identify most lesions of the anterior cruciate ligament.

The Lachman test should be carried out gently with the knee in 15° of flexion, grasping the thigh and leg and drawing the tibia gently forward. The Macintosh test provides further confirmation, the pivot shift being elicitable in all cases of anterior cruciate rupture. The key again is gentleness in the examination with the examiner cradling the leg with the knee in 15° of flexion; as the patient relaxes the hamstrings, the tibia will subluxate forward from the femur. If the examiner maintains a gentle longitudinal pressure on the limb and flexes it slightly, a reduction of the tibia will occur. The key to confirming anterior cruciate ligament rupture is the initial subluxation of the tibia; attempts to force a "pivot shift" should not be pursued as this may be resisted by the patient with an acutely injured knee. The major fault in examining the acute knee is the exertion of too great a valgus stress or the overzealous loading of the limb with longitudinal pressure causing the hamstring to go into spasm and totally preventing the tibia from subluxating forward on the femur.

Traumatic rupture of the anterior cruciate ligament, associated soft tissue injury to other structures about the knee, and possible rupture of the medial collateral ligament may make clinical examination difficult without anesthetic. Where there is any clinical doubt, examination under general anesthetic should be carried out with the Lachman and Macintosh tests confirming the diagnosis of anterior cruciate ligament rupture as well as declaring the status of other ligamentous structures.

If a general anesthetic has to be resorted to, it should be standard practice to arthroscope the knee at the same time. The arthroscopic evaluation is carried out not to confirm the tear of the anterior cruciate ligament but to define whether or not there is any other associated intraarticular pathology either to the menisci or to the joint surfaces. This may require patient irrigation of the joint in order to clear the hemarthrosis in order to enable effective visualization. However, it can be extremely misleading to try to define tears of the ligament by direct visualization. With trauma to the tissues in the intercondular area and to the synovium and fatpad, definition of

a cruciate tear may be very difficult. It should be emphasized that confirmation of anterior cruciate ligament deficiency is a clinical observation confirmed by Lachman and Macintosh testing, not by endeavoring to interpret the tangled mess which so often obscures the view within the acutely injured knee.

MANAGEMENT

Having defined a tear of the anterior cruciate ligament, a definite plan of action should be outlined for each athlete based upon the injury, the patient's sporting aspirations, and his work and social circumstances.

Indications for Primary Repair

1. Rupture of the medial collateral and anterior cruciate ligaments is an absolute indication for reconstruction of both ligaments in all athletic patients.
2. All ruptures involving avulsion of the tibial tubercle attachment of the anterior cruciate ligament should be repaired *per primum*.
3. Repair of an isolated anterior cruciate ligament should be undertaken in any competitive athlete with a manifestly unstable knee, that is, with a grossly positive pivot shift instability.
4. Ruptures in young athletes who wish to pursue a competitive sports program and in those older athletes whose work or family commitments allow the time for surgery and full rehabilitation without too great a disruption of their normal lifestyle.

The greyer zone arises when the ligament is torn, but the knee is not grossly unstable. If there is an associated meniscal injury, consider an arthroscopic surgical treatment of the meniscal pathology, and pursue a watch-and-wait policy with regard to the ongoing stability of the knee. If stability proves unsatisfactory, the knee may be stabilized electively as a late procedure.

The Conservative Course

The surgical treatment of the acute anterior cruciate ligament lesion involves a certain commitment on the patient's part. Following the procedure a period of cast and brace protection and non-weightbearing on crutches is required. It may be 3 months before the patient can place his foot to the ground for effective weightbearing and even then a cane may be required for a further month or more. For the young athlete or student this is not too great a hardship. For the older person, work and family commitments may make such limitation of daily activity a social and economic hardship, leading one to consider pursuing a conservative course with a view to undertaking a late stabilization should the knee prove unstable in the long term.

Therefore one must offer an alternative to primary reconstruction. If primary surgical repair is not chosen, or should individuals not present within the first month following injury (beyond which time a primary reconstruction is no longer feasible due to contraction of the injured ligament structures), then a definite program of rehabilitation should be mapped out. Following the immediate injury, rest with splint support is recommended for 3 days. During this time, ice pack application controls swelling, eases pain, and paves the way for an early, active rehabilitation program. Physiotherapy is instituted on the fourth day with heat, pool therapy, and gentle mobilizing exercises. The use of the exercise bicycle is encouraged as strength develops. Strengthening exercises emphasizing the hip flexors and abductors and the hamstrings are added. Quadriceps building is done with isometric strengthening and quadriceps faradism, but resisted exercises are not encouraged. Weightbearing is allowed as comfort permits; by 6 weeks, full mobilization should have been achieved, allowing a graduated return to sporting activity. As the athlete returns to sport, an elasticized knee support is often of great help. This offers support for the stabilizing muscle groups of the thigh and leg and greatly aids the proprioceptive feedback that is often disrupted in ligamentous injuries of this type.

Definite guidance has to be given to patients with a known cruciate ligament injury who are returning to a sports program. Sports such as running, cycling, and swimming are going to cause little problem; skiing, skating, and hockey may be fine because the knee is maintained in flexion. However, sports which involve jumping, leg extension, and propping and cutting may cause problems to the athlete. Basketball, tennis, and baseball may pose difficulties and can predispose to further injury should repeated episodes of "giving way" occur. Under these circumstances, sports should be discontinued and consideration given to late surgical stabilization if an active sporting career is to be further pursued.

I have not found that in the knee suffering from cruciate deficiency stabilizing braces are in any way effective. If the knee becomes unstable, a brace will only protect the knee from further extraneous insult, as in contact sports, but it cannot control the inherent instability enough to allow propping and cutting activities. These patients must consider a late stabilization procedure and then may use a brace to prevent the knee from being further traumatized by extraneous insult.

Primary Surgical Treatment

When the anterior cruciate ruptures, it usually suffers an intersubstance tear, with avulsion of a portion of the ligament from its femoral attachment and propagation of the tear through the body of the ligament, usually to its midportion. In so doing, the rupture causes a complete disruption of the blood supply from the posterior geniculate artery so that direct primary suture of the anterior cruciate is a totally ineffective and futile surgical gesture, mentioned only to be condemned.

Reinforcement is an essential component of pri-

mary anterior cruciate ligament repair. It is essential to provide a supporting scaffold for the replication of the original structure. The only exception is an avulsion of the tibial tubercle attachment of the anterior cruciate ligament. Here, direct accurate relocation of the avulsed fragment is totally successful because the blood supply of the ligament is not jeopardized. During open arthrotomy, it is imperative to completely and accurately relocate the avulsed ligament, impacting the bone into its bed after drawing it into place with two stout sutures. These sutures are passed through two drill holes directed from the proximal tibia up through the bed of the avulsed area; tied in place, the ligament will consolidate in place. Consolidation of its bony insertion will take only 4 to 6 weeks with brace protection.

The majority of cruciate ligament disruptions involve intersubstance tears and necessitate graft reinforcement. The modified Macintosh technique has been used with great success and is my preferred treatment. In a series of 80 repairs carried out over a 5-year period, only six unsatisfactory results were encountered. This procedure can be commended as effective and reliable, provided certain technical points are closely adhered to.

The quadriceps patellar tendon over the top reconstruction is a variation of the Jones repair and can be commended. The middle one-third of the patellar tendon is utilized, taking only partial thickness of the quadriceps tendon above the knee, widening out over the patella to gain sufficient tissue, and then taking only limited tissue below. This is formed into a tube graft with a longitudinal running suture to facilitate later drawing through the knee. Minimizing the interference with the quadriceps mechanism above the knee obviates difficulties from overzealous harvest of tissue and tightening of the suprapatellar tendon complex. Such tightening will otherwise interfere severely with patellar function and can account for postoperative patellofemoral pain, knee stiffness, and impaired range of motion.

The tendon graft is then passed through a drill hole in the proximal tibia, the line of the graft passing up through the bed of the torn ligament. The remnant of the torn ligament is taken as a separate entity on a further suture, enfolding the new graft and thus acting as a scaffold for tissue reconstitution. Beyond 3 to 4 weeks from the time of injury, this stump of original ligament has usually shrunken so as to render this process less assured; an elective substitution procedure is then to be preferred.

The correct positioning of this graft, Macintosh has emphasized, should replicate that of the original ligament which inserts not into but around the back of the lateral femoral condyle. A bed is roughened posteriorly through the intercondylar arch, and the graft and original ligament with drawer sutures is retrieved through a lateral approach made posterior to the intermuscular septum. Further roughening of the back of the condyle prepares the bed for the ligament which is now drawn up over the top of the lateral femoral condyle to the highest point in the intercondylar notch where it is now secured. Flexion-extension mobilization of the knee will have no effect on the length of the ligament, confirming it to be isometrically located. Thus, while cast protection is usually afforded, protective mobilization in a hinge-brace system is equally effective because, in this isometric location, there is no undue unphysiologic tension on the ligament.

Of 80 patients, only six went on to have further problems with instability. The recovery phase following this procedure is protracted, requiring 6 weeks of cast protection, almost 2 months more on crutches, and only by 5 months is independence without a cane achieved. Even at 6 months, a 0° to 5° flexion tendency is often noted; this may slow a return to active sports. Participation in active sports is encouraged as soon as adequate extension is achieved. Of the 80 patients, no athlete was braced afterwards, and return to active sports by 9 months from the time of original injury and treatment was the rule.

CHRONIC ANTERIOR CRUCIATE LIGAMENT INSTABILITY

R. PETER WELSH, M.B., Ch.B., F.R.C.S.(C), F.A.C.S.

Chronic anterior cruciate ligament instability seriously compromises an athlete's performance and poses a threat to the knee in that persistent episodes of uncontrolled subluxation must inevitably lead to internal derangement, including meniscal tears and articular insult. In its fulminant form, a progressive degeneration ensues with bicompartmental post-traumatic arthritis, the arthropathy of cruciate neglect.

CLINICAL FEATURES

In those presenting for late stabilization, the time lapse between acute injury and reconstructive surgery may be many years. In a series of 155 late reconstructions, the time lapse ranged from 1 to 22 years, with a mean of 3½ years. In many such instances, the acute episode may be forgotten or at best remain ill-defined in the patient's memory. In many cases all that can be recalled is a severe knee strain that occurred "some years ago". After a somewhat prolonged recovery phase, in most instances, the athletes return to active sports, and it is only over a period of time that their problem becomes manifest. Many individuals seem able to cope adequately for several years, with only the occasional episode of "giving way". Gradually, however, the knee becomes more insecure, until it finally decompensates and becomes critically unstable, not only for sports activities, but even in everyday life.

It is often at this stage that surgical control is sought; brace control, although it may be adequate for certain sports activities, cannot generally be applied if the knee is unstable at work or in everyday life activity.

Unfortunately, by this stage, further irreparable articular insult may have occurred. In a series of 155 late reconstructions, 38 percent showed major articular lesions, and 54 percent meniscal tears requiring meniscectomy.

It is essential at this stage to identify the nature of a particular patient's knee derangement, defining the cruciate deficiency and any associated meniscal or articular disorder, so that a rational program of management can be planned.

The Lachman test and Macintosh Pivot Shift test, as described in the chapter on the *Acute Injury to the Anterior Cruciate Ligament* form the basis for the clinical confirmation of an anterior cruciate deficiency. Both tests demonstrate the anterior subluxation of the tibia beneath the femur, but the Macintosh Test can be quantitatively more helpful in the chronic situation. The degree of tibial subluxation should be documented, noting if possible whether the lateral plateau presents the more obvious subluxation or whether the medial plateau presents with equal prominence. This has great significance in defining whether or not a lateral substitution repair alone will suffice if the instability is predominantly a lateral phenomenon. When the tibia presents as a whole with major medial subluxation as well, a repair based on the lateral aspect alone will be inadequate, and further reinforcement, both intra-articularly and medially, should be contemplated.

A further examination of the knee should include an assessment of the status of the menisci and articular surfaces and any derangement of patellar mechanics. Finally, it is worth noting the general body type of a patient; those who are "loose-jointed" and "hyperflexible" offer a greater challenge in achieving stability then do the "tight" body types.

CONSERVATIVE MANAGEMENT OF LATE ANTERIOR CRUCIATE LIGAMENT INSTABILITY

It is obvious that not all individuals with a disruption of their anterior cruciate ligament require stabilization. Many individuals can cope adequately in everyday life or modify their work and recreational activities so that their knees are never functionally unstable to them. It is important in this regard to counsel individuals against pursuing recreation that may be unsuitable to their situation. Thus individuals who are involved in jumping sports, such as basketball, football, or baseball, find that when they land with their leg in extension or pivot from the affected side, their knee gives way, and they should really consider giving up that sport or having their knee stabilized. Brace control may be tried, but there is no brace that adequately controls many of these situations which demand loading in extension or pivoting from the affected side.

Surprisingly, sports such as skiing or skating or squash may be possible. As long as a flexed attitude of the knee is sustained, the knee will not subluxate, and sports participation may be continued as long as further internal derangement is not evident.

For those whose knees are insecure, redirection into less provocative sports activities may therefore be a viable alternative. Even so, active strengthening for the knee should be part of the serious athlete's exercise program. Although quadriceps drills are important for strength and durability, these should not overload the patella mechanism, and if anything, extra emphasis should be given to overdeveloping the hamstrings as well as the hip flexors and abductors.

Bracing does have a definite role, and it can be a threefold benefit: (1) to control the knee so that it does not extend fully, thus avoiding potentially unstable situations; (2) to protect the compromised knee from extraneous forces as in contact sports, thus presenting the superimposition of further insult, which might damage further other ligament structures; and (3) to enhance the proprioceptive feedback and muscle control of the extremity, further enhancing the protective responses of the body. The prototype brace and the benchmark against which all other imitations must be compared remains the Lennox-Hill derotation brace. Such braces should endeavor to build in cruciate control restraints and control extension so that the hamstrings remain the effective dynamic group acting across the joint, restraining the tibia in its tendency to anterior subluxation, thus substituting for the deficiency of the anterior cruciate ligament.

However, should a cruciate-deficient knee prove unstable in everyday life, as in stepping down off a curb or turning about, surgical stabilization becomes mandatory. Similarly, for many individuals engaged in sports in whom the anterior cruciate knee proves most unsatisfactory, and for whom alternative treatments have been exhausted, consideration should be given to surgery, particularly if other internal derangement is apparent.

SURGICAL MANAGEMENT OF THE ANTERIOR CRUCIATE DEFICIENT KNEE

It is essential in evaluating a patient's clinical problem that the nature of the instability pattern be fully appreciated before surgical repair is undertaken. The Macintosh test is the single most important test in defining whether the repair can be confined to the lateral

aspect of the joint or whether an intra-articular or medial reinforcement is required.

If subluxation of the whole tibia is apparent, restraint will have to be offered with three-point fixation if a durable repair is to be achieved. The difference between the acute injury and the late situation is that in the chronically unstable knee, the secondary periarticular capsular and tendinous restraints, as a consequence of repeated episodes of subluxation, have been stretched out and attenuated to the point where they no longer support the knee and require substitution.

In devising a reconstruction for a particular patient, examination under anesthetic prior to the surgery affords us an opportunity to reaffirm the pattern of instability present. Arthroscopic evaluation permits a thorough inspection of the interior and detection of any intraarticular disorder that may need concurrent surgical remedy.

SURGICAL REPAIR

Lateral Compartment Pivot Instability

If the instability is that of anterior cruciate ligament deficiency with a lateral pivot shift alone and no medial subluxation, a lateral substitution repair will stabilize the knee completely. Here the objective is to secure the posterolateral corner of the knee. Although it is possible to use three structures—the popliteus, the biceps, or the fascia lata—the modified Macintosh technique is preferred.

Modified Macintosh Technique of Lateral Substitution Repair

Examination under anesthsia confirms the pattern of instability with a purely lateral pivot shift phenomenon, and any intra-articular disorder is treated prior to surgery by arthroscopic surgical technique.

A long lateral incision exposes the iliotibial tract allowing a strip graft 2 cm in width and 20 cm in length to be mobilized. The graft is left attached distally at Gerdy's tubercle, but is folded side to side on itself and fashioned into a tube with a longitudinal running suture, which is left long at the end to act as a drawstring.

The tube graft is now passed deep to the lateral ligament, deep to the popliteus, and deep to the arcuate complex in the posterolateral corner of the knee. A subperiosteal tunnel is fashioned up the back of the lateral femoral condyle and the graft passed in this deep to the intermuscular septum. While the knee is maintained in external rotation and flexion, the ligament graft is secured to the lateral ligament, popliteus, arcuate tendon, and posterolateral capsular structures. The free end of the graft is now passed deep to the arcuate tendon and lateral ligament, paralleling the original course before being folded back on itself and sewn into the posterolateral capsule as further reinforcement. It is possible to close the fascial defect distally, but often the defect must be left wide open proximally.

Postoperatively the patient is maintained in a cast at 90 degrees flexion and 20 degrees external rotation, for 6 weeks in those under 30 years of age, 4 to 5 weeks in those aged 30 to 40 years, and 3 weeks only if over 40 years of age.

Pivot Instability with Complete Tibial Subluxation

In major degrees of anterior cruciate ligament insufficiency, the whole tibia can be subluxated forward on Macintosh testing. In this case, control of the instability must be offered not only laterally, but also medially. At the same time opportunity should be taken to reconstitute the original ligament, if possible, with a graft substitution through the knee.

On the medial side, potential structures to be utilized include the posteromedial capsule, the semimembranosus, and the pes anserinus tendons. The through-the-knee graft can be formed with fascia lata, semitendinosus, or patellar tendon. Again the preferred technique is a Macintosh lateral substitution with iliotibial through-the-knee graft. The medial side is reinforced with a capsular plication and pes anserinus transfer.

Modified Macintosh Technique with Capsular Reinforcement and Pes Anserinus Tendon Plasty

The fascia lata graft harvested in this situation must be some 6 to 8 cm longer in order to be passed from the posterolateral corner of the knee down through the intercondylar notch, through the knee, and into a tunnel in the proximal tibia.

The lateral substitution repair is undertaken, as previously described, with the graft passing deep to the lateral ligament, the popliteus, and the arcuate complex before being passed through a subperiosteal tunnel behind the lateral femoral condyle and lateral intermuscular septum. Secured at these points it is now redirected through the intercondylar notch and down through a tunnel in the proximal tibia, which has been pre-drilled through a further exposure made medially. Having been drawn into its new bed, the ligament is secured to the ligamentum patellae and pretibial fascia.

The medial capsule is opened posteriorly, and any redundancy plicated in order to tighten the posteromedial corner of the joint. The pes anserinus tendons are then mobilized from below upward, and the semitendinosus folded along the proximal tibial margin and secured just below the joint line.

The period of postoperative immobilization is similar to that already noted, but in this instance a cast position is maintained at 90 degrees flexion in neutral rotation.

Surgery for Failed Anterior Cruciate Repair

The above principles apply in those instances in which the knee remains unstable despite previous attempts at repair. The major instability pattern must be clearly identified and three-point fixation achieved with the lateral substitution repair, a through-the-knee graft, and medial plication and pes plasty.

Even after previous surgery for which fascia lata has already been utilized, it is usually possible to harvest enough fascia lata to carry out a lateral substitution repair and tighten up the posterolateral corner. However, it is not possible to bring the fascia through the knee, and in these instances a patellar tendon graft is utilized to reconstitute the intra-articular restraint, the technique employed being similar to that described for the acute repair.

It is in the situation of the multiply operated knee with continuing marked instability that the utilization of artificial ligament grafts may find their place. At this time, however, experience with these biologic repairs described herein has proved most satisfactory and the repairs durable beyond 10 years.

POSTOPERATIVE REHABILITATION

Following removal from the cast, the patient is allowed 3 weeks to loosen the knee on their own and is encouraged to freely mobilize the extremity utilizing, where possible, a spa or whirlpool.

Active physiotherapy is then instituted, with emphasis on first mobilizing the knee with hydrotherapy, cycling exercises, and gentle passive stretching.

Strengthening exercises are subsequently added, emphasizing the hip flexors, hip abductors, and hamstrings, using intially only isometric and faradic stimulation for the quadriceps. Until knee extension is achieved, resisted quadriceps exercises are minimized in order to reduce loading of the patella mechanism, because the development of patellar pain after a period of cast immobilization will only be aggravated by overzealous quadriceps loading. For similar reasons, crutch walking is continued until the knee extends to 10 degrees, usually by the end of the third month, and from this time on, more aggressive strengthening can be undertaken.

Return to sport is allowed when full range and strength have been achieved and a normal running gait pattern established.

Brace protection is offered to those who wish to return to heavy contact sport, but otherwise is not routinely employed.

ARTHROGRAPHY AND ARTHROSCOPY

H. PETER JAMES, M.D., F.R.C.S.(C)

Arthrography and diagnostic arthroscopy provide information about the internal structures of the knee which enhances the clinical diagnosis and significantly increases the diagnostic accuracy in determining the cause of an internal derangement of the knee joint.

ARTHROGRAPHY

The arthrogram identifies meniscal tears, and the skilled arthrographer can provide information which significantly increases the accuracy of the clinical diagnosis. The development of diagnostic arthroscopy of the knee has reduced the need for arthrography, but arthrography of the knee is more cost-effective and less invasive than diagnostic arthroscopy. Using the arthrogram as a screening test allows the clinician to proceed directly to arthroscopic surgery if a meniscal tear is found. In sprains of the medial collateral ligament and painful patellofemoral conditions, the arthrogram is useful in ruling out tears of the menisci so that conservative treatment can be confidently instituted.

DIAGNOSTIC ARTHROSCOPY

Diagnostic arthroscopic examination of the knee reveals the extent and type of meniscal tears, the location and degree of articular cartilage lesions, and the general appearance of the synovial lining. Because of these features, arthroscopy results in a more thorough and detailed examination of the knee than does arthrography. Since the development of arthroscopic surgery, the frequency of purely diagnostic arthroscopy has been reserved for diagnostic problems not identified by arthrography. When a surgically correctable problem such as a torn meniscus is found at arthroscopy, surgeons familiar with arthroscopic surgical techniques proceed immediately to definitive surgical treatment under arthroscopic control. As more surgeons develop arthroscopic surgical skills, the practice of diagnostic arthroscopy followed by open arthrotomy is becoming less frequent and eventually will be discontinued.

Diagnostic arthroscopy under local anesthesia has been shown to be as accurate as arthroscopy under general anesthesia. Under local anesthesia with epinephrine and without a tourniquet, arthroscopic examination of the knee has been routinely performed for the past 5 years at the Orthopaedic and Arthritic Hospital. A recent review of the first one thousand cases showed a diagnostic arthroscopic accuracy of 97 percent. The initial clinical diagnosis approached an accuracy rating of 70 percent. The arthrograms performed by a skilled arthrographer resulted in an accuracy of 92 per-

cent for medial meniscus lesions and 80 percent for abnormalities of the lateral meniscus. When arthrography and arthroscopy were combined, the diagnostic accuracy rose to 99 percent. Diagnostic arthroscopy under local anesthesia is less invasive and more cost-effective than under general anesthesia. All patients are prepared for general anesthesia, and when a surgically correctable lesion is found, arthroscopic surgery is performed under the same local anesthetic, after additional sedation, or with a general anesthesia as necessary for the patient's comfort. Local anesthesia is not used in patients with acute knee injuries or patients with arthritis and multiple joint involvement. Arthroscopy should be deferred until at least one week following arthrography to prevent infection since a significant percentage of synovial fluid samples have yielded positive cultures within one week after arthrography of the knee, without clinical symptoms or signs of infection. The following sections illustrate application of the aforementioned guidelines for using arthrography and arthroscopy in the diagnosis of acute, chronic, and degenerative knee problems.

ACUTE KNEE INJURIES

Following acute injuries of the knee, the degree of injury to the collateral and cruciate ligaments must be identified as soon as possible. When the ligaments cannot be satisfactorily examined with the patient awake, examination under anesthesia is necessary. If instability of the knee is present in two planes (anteroposterior and valgus-varus), arthrotomy and repair or reconstruction of the torn ligaments should be carried out.

If instability is present in only one plane (torn anterior cruciate ligament or torn medial collateral ligament), arthroscopic examination under general anesthesia is performed to clear the hemarthrosis, and examine the menisci and articular surfaces of the joint. If a torn meniscus is found in the presence of medial collateral ligament instability, partial medial meniscectomy or meniscus repair can be done under arthroscopic control immediately, followed by conservative treatment, such as cast bracing for an isolated tear of the medial collateral ligament. The patient in the high-risk, high-activity category, such as a young athlete with an isolated anterior cruciate tear usually requires immediate reconstruction of the anterior cruciate ligament. Arthroscopy is not necessary in this patient since any meniscus lesion can be dealt with at the time of arthrotomy for the anterior cruciate reconstruction. In acute knee injuries, arthrography is not used, and arthroscopy is performed under general anesthesia.

RECURRENT INJURY

Recurrent Injury with a Stable Knee (Intact Ligaments)

Recurrent painful catching, giving way, or locking of the knee is probably caused by a tear of the meniscus once patellofemoral causes have been ruled out. In these conditions, the arthrogram usually confirms the presence of a torn meniscus. If the arthrogram is positive, arthroscopic surgery is usually the best treatment, with either arthroscopic meniscectomy or suturing of the meniscus if a peripheral tear is found. If the arthrogram does not show a torn meniscus and the recurrent symptoms persist, arthroscopic examination is necessary to definitely rule out a meniscus tear and examine the articular cartilage for defects which could mimic the symptoms of a torn meniscus. Occasionally, loose bodies of articular cartilage which do not show on the roentgenogram produce symptoms similar to those of a torn meniscus. If surgically correctable, these lesions can be corrected by means of arthroscopic surgery. Therefore, whether the arthrogram is positive or negative, arthroscopy is usually necessary for recurrent injuries of the stable knee, and arthroscopic surgery is usually definitive. In view of the lesser diagnostic accuracy of the arthrogram, arthroscopy is usually the best investigative tool for these types of knee problems. Arthrography is useful in ruling out meniscus tears only if it is negative and the symptoms do not recur.

Recurrent Injury with Knee Instability (Usually a Torn Anterior Cruciate Ligament)

Recurrent painful instability of the anterior cruciate-deficient knee usually indicates further damage to the secondary supporting structures or the articular cartilage. Often the arthrogram shows a tear in one of the menisci. The arthrogram does not show the articular cartilage defects which frequently occur with recurrent episodes of instability. Since instability due to a torn anterior cruciate ligament is usually painless if the arthrogram is negative, arthroscopic examination is necessary to identify the cause of the pain associated with the instability. Treatment of the recurrent painful unstable knee is primarily directed at the treatment of the anterior cruciate ligament. If functional instability persists in a physically active person, reconstruction of the anterior cruciate ligament and simultaneous open partial medial meniscectomy or meniscus repair is indicated. In a more sedentary person, when functional instability can be controlled with a modification of activities or derotation brace, the pain associated with recurrent instability can usually be relieved by arthroscopically controlled partial medial meniscectomy. Suturing of the meniscus is not successful in the face of a torn anterior cruciate ligament. Occasionally, arthroscopic examination of the articular cartilage and menisci is worthwhile to determine whether the degenerative changes have progressed to the point where anterior cruciate ligament reconstruction would not make a significant difference in the progression of the degenerative arthritic changes.

DEGENERATIVE CONDITION

Degenerative tears of the menisci may occur before there are radiographic changes to indicate degenerative arthritis in the knee. In patients over 35 years of age, degenerative tears of the menisci can occur suddenly with minimal trauma, such as crouching, and are frequently temporarily relieved by rest and anti-inflammatory medication. The symptoms frequently recur without trauma and persist, eventually requiring definitive treatment.

Arthrography of the knee usually is not helpful in degenerative tears of the menisci. The arthrogram usually shows a tear in the meniscus, but gives little information regarding the type of tear, the condition of the surrounding articular cartilage, and the extent of the tear in the meniscus. Since the prognosis for surgery of these degenerative tears is directly related to the amount of articular cartilage degeneration accompanying the meniscus tear, arthroscopic examination is necessary to obtain a true picture of the total degenerative changes in the affected compartment of the knee. Following arthroscopic examination, the torn fragments of the meniscus can be resected under arthroscopic control, and the affected degenerative articular cartilage can be debrided and the joint lavaged to give temporary relief. Arthroscopic examination of the opposite compartment helps in the planning of a subsequent corrective osteotomy if the degenerative changes are advanced and the symptoms recur.

Arthrography is now used as a minimally invasive screening test to rule out tears of the menisci so that early conservative treatment and rehabilitation can be initiated in painful patellofemoral conditions and nonrecurrent one-plane ligament injuries. In recurrent injuries that do not involve the patellofemoral joint, arthroscopic examination is the preferred investigative tool to make an accurate diagnosis and frequently can be followed immediately by definitive arthroscopic surgery.

It is better to look and see than to wait and see.

OSTEOCHONDRITIS DISSECANS, OSTEOCHONDRAL FRACTURES, AND OSTEOARTHRITIS OF THE KNEE

JOHN C. CAMERON, M.D., F.R.C.S.(C)

OSTEOCHONDRITIS DISSECANS

Osteochondritis dissecans of the knee is a condition in which a fragment of bone, adjacent to the articular surface of the knee, is deprived of its blood supply and undergoes avascular necrosis. As new blood vessels invade the necrotic bone, it is gradually replaced by creeping substitution. During this period, the overlying articular cartilage, nourished by the synovial fluid, remains viable. If repeated impact or joint motion causes micro-movement of the fragment, the progress of invading vessels is hindered, and the avascular bone fragment may displace and form a loose body within the knee joint, leaving a defect in the articular cartilage.

The symptoms of osteochondritis dissecans usually occur in the second decade. The most frequent symptom is pain, with associated swelling as well as locking and instability. The symptoms are generally related to physical activity. Many of the patients present with pain associated with an effusion, with no specific history of injury, and on physical examination little is found other than the effusion. X-ray studies are essential for diagnosis. The lesion can occur in decreasing order of frequency in the lateral aspect of the medial femoral condyle, lateral femoral condyle, femoral groove, and patella.

There are many theories regarding the etiology of the lesion, from abnormal secondary centers of ossification in younger patients to impingement against an enlarged anterior tibial spine. Wilson devised a clinical test for osteochondritis dissecans. He noted that patients with osteochondritis dissecans walked with the tibia in external rotation. In carrying out his test with the patient supine, the knee is flexed through 90° and the tibia is internally rotated. The knee is then gradually extended, and at 30° of flexion, sharp pain is elicited. External rotation of the knee immediately relieves this pain.

The management of the lesion in the individual patient is determined by the age of the patient and the size and location, as well as the radiographic appearance, of the fragment. The majority of lesions in younger patients have a favorable prognosis. The skeletally immature patient has a much greater potential for revascularization of the avascular fragment before any damage to the overlying articular cartilage occurs. When patients develop symptoms in the latter part of the second decade, operative intervention is often unavoidable.

The operative management of the condition is determined to a large extent by the integrity of the articular cartilage. If the fragment has separated at an early stage, often the defect will fill in and hardly be noticeable on arthroscopic examination. In these cases, the symptoms are generally due to the loose osteochondral fragment, and can usually be managed by arthroscopic removal of the fragment.

A more difficult decision is necessary in the symptomatic individual with a large lesion and an intact articular surface. If there is a very dense sclerotic margin on the femoral side of the lesion, we carry out a retrograde currettage through a large drill hole starting from the extra-articular surface of the medial femoral condyle. By palpation of the articular cartilage at the time of currettage, we can avoid damage to the articular surface. We currette out as much of the avascular bone and sclerotic margin as possible and replace this with a local bone graft from the femoral metaphysis. This bone graft is packed solidly up to the articular surface in order to provide support. The patient is then kept non-weight-bearing on crutches for 3 months with quadriceps rehabilitation and range-of-motion exercises.

In the patient with osteochondritis dissecans and an intact joint surface with minimal sclerosis about the lesion, internal fixation is utilized. Smillie pins provide fixation for shearing forces, but do not provide any compression across the line of cleavage between the fragment and the distal femur. Recently we have begun to use small scaphoid screws with cancellous threads crossing the cleavage plane to achieve compression of the fragment. Often it is possible to keep the screw placement such that the screw head will be off the major weight-bearing portion of the condyle, adjacent to the intercondylar notch. The screw head should also be countersunk in the articular cartilage. Our results with this treatment have been excellent, and again these patients are kept non-weight-bearing for 3 months. X-ray examination at 3 months is not generally helpful in assessing union, but the patients have remained asymptomatic with progressive weight-bearing after this period.

In most of these patients we have carried out arthroscopic examination under local anesthesia to probe the lesion and to determine the stability of the repair and its support of the articular surface. To date, these examinations have shown maintenance of articular cartilage viability and congruence, as well as restoration of subchondral bony support. Progressive activity, based on absence of symptoms and joint effusion, is then carried out, with a gradual return to normal activities.

OSTEOCHONDRAL FRACTURES OF THE KNEE

One of the more serious causes of acute hemarthrosis of the knee is an osteochondral fracture. The patient presents after a knee injury with a hemarthrosis of rapid onset. If a diagnostic aspiration is carried out, it should be performed under sterile conditions and the aspirate should be examined for evidence of fat droplets. There are three reasons for carrying out aspiration of the knee:

1. To establish a diagnosis, i.e., whether the fluid is blood or excess synovial fluid.

2. To relieve pressure that is causing excessive pain.

3. When swelling restricts movement of the knee to less than 90°.

Hemarthrosis due to an osteochondral fracture usually recurs rapidly after aspiration.

All knee injuries resulting in acute hemarthrosis must undergo x-ray examination. The specific injuries in which diagnosis should be made early are major knee ligament disruption, and intra-articular fractures, including osteochondral fractures. One should be able to diagnose the first group on physical examination. If a satisfactory examination cannot be carried out because of pain, an examination under anesthesia should be considered. In the group of patients with intra-articular fractures, roentgenograms should be taken in multiple planes, AP, lateral, 2 obliques, and a 30° skyline patellofemoral view. In many cases one may see only a small osseous fragment, while the associated articular cartilage fragment is very large.

The majority of osteochondral fractures occur with patellar dislocation. As the patella rides over the lateral femoral condyle, a portion of the articular surface of the patella or the lateral femoral condyle is sheared off and forms an osteochondral loose body within the knee. The amount of bone seen on x-ray examination is often deceptive with regard to the size of the fragment. Occasionally, fragments may be avulsed from the medial border of the patella, and as they remain attached to the patellar retinaculum, they are stable and are not considered loose fragments. Unfortunately this often cannot be determined unless arthroscopic examination is carried out.

The size and source of the osteochondral fragment also may be determined by arthroscopic examination. When the patient is asleep, physical examination of the knee may demonstrate marked crepitus in the area of the lesion. The treatment of the injury depends on the location, size, and comminution of the osteochondral fragment. In general, the smaller and the more comminuted fragments should be removed, and the larger intact fragments should be put back in their bed and internally fixed. The larger the fragment of bone involved, the greater the likelihood of subsequent union. The most troublesome lesions are the highly comminuted fractures occurring on a major weight-bearing surface, such as the patella. Our results with excision and debridement and early continuous passive motion have been encouraging. On repeat arthroscopic examination, most of these lesions are seen to have filled in with fibrocartilage. However, most patients remain symptomatic with pain and effusion when they stress their knee, and seldom do they return to their pre-injury level of function. Rehabilitation of the lower extremity muscles is very important, and consideration should be given to surgical correction of any underlying predisposition to patellar dislocation. Our approach is to rehabilitate the knee after the acute injury before considering elective surgical procedures.

We believe that immobilization of a knee with an osteochondral fracture is detrimental to articular cartilage and that procedures for patellar tendon transfer, which require immobilization of the knee, should be avoided. At the time of anesthesia for the acute injury, accurate documentation of patellar instability should be made and any patellofemoral or lower extremity malalignment noted. In many cases, quadriceps rehabilitation is all that is required for dynamic patellar stabilization. The return of the patient to sporting activities must be slowly progressive and determined primarily by symptoms, such as pain and instability, and physical signs, such as swelling.

OSTEOARTHRITIS OF THE KNEE

Osteoarthritis of the knee in the athlete usually falls into one of several categories: (1) associated with ligamentous instability, (2) postmeniscectomy, (3) post-trauma (secondary to joint surface injury).

Knee ligament instability, particularly anterior cruciate instability, places the meniscus and joint surface under conditions of shear stresses, for which they do not function well. The resultant meniscal tears and joint surface damage often lead to a rapid downgrading in knee function. Because the ligamentous instability must be considered the underlying pathologic condition, it is often necessary to deal with this in order to preserve knee function. In many cases, the patient's symptoms are initially due to his ligamentous instability, but with progressive joint surface damage, his later smptoms may be due to degenerative arthritis. The treatment, either knee ligament repair or osteotomy, is dependent upon the stage of progression of his disease. We believe that early ligamentous reconstruction, in the patient who is symptomatically unstable, usually halts further progression of articular surface damage. The rehabilitation necessary to regain a high level of physical performance is considerable, but many of these patients function surprisingly well in spite of significant joint surface damage. The task of the treating physician or surgeon is then to determine what the primary source of the patient's disability is, whether knee ligament instability or degenerative osteoarthritis.

Consider the following common scenario: The patient with chronic anterior cruciate instability, whose instability goes unrecognized, subsequently has a meniscectomy which may relieve some of his discomfort initially, but does nothing to stabilize his knee. Then, over the course of several years, he develops increasing pain in his knee and, on physical and radiographic examination, demonstrates osteoarthritis.

The patient with posterior cruciate instability, who develops patellofemoral degenerative changes, will deteriorate functionally. However, we have found that maintaining quadriceps function and strength allows many of these athletes to continue to function at very high levels. In assessing the disability in a particular athlete, it is necessary to consider the particular sport in which he is involved. Many sports which involve straight-ahead movement only, without any lateral movement or pivoting, can be carried out without significant problems in the patient with anterior cruciate instability. Therefore, to take an athlete who is functioning at a very high level and subject him to a ligamentous reconstruction is of questionable value. On the other hand, athletes who are involved in sports such as soccer, which involves rapid lateral movement and pivoting, are generally significantly disabled by their instability and, in spite of rehabilitation of their quadriceps and hamstring muscle groups, are unable to regain their former function after anterior cruciate injuries.

The postmeniscectomy patient who has unicompartmental joint surface wear in association with either valgus or varus alignment may be treated by osteotomy. This realignment often transfers sufficient weight to the undamaged compartment of the knee, so that excellent function is restored. Lesser degrees of disability require only continued muscle rehabilitation and anti-inflammatory medications. Unfortunately joint surface wear in this type of patient tends to progress more rapidly when subjected to excessive loads. It has therefore been our policy to discourage patients with osteo-arthritic changes from participating in activities that involve repetitive heavy loading or impact of their damaged knee.

A similar approach is taken in dealing with patients who have posttraumatic arthritis secondary to joint surface injuries, such as intra-articular fractures. In many cases, tibial plateau fractures, if well managed, return to a high level of activity, but one can expect to have a progressive downgrading in performance with increasing surface damage. As these patients progress in their rehabilitation, we often carry out outpatient arthroscopic examinations under local anesthesia in order to determine a prognosis at 6 months and a year following any injury, and also to give the patient some idea as to the activity level toward which they should aim. There is not much doubt that continued impact loading on a damaged articular surface will lead to gradual deterioration. However, if the articular cartilage is relatively undamaged, or is restored, and on arthroscopic examination appears relatively normal, we encourage these patients to gradually increase their activity level, again depending ultimately on their symptoms and signs.

LEG, ANKLE AND FOOT INJURIES

STRESS FRACTURES OF THE LOWER EXTREMITY

JOHN H. OLIVER, M.D., F.R.C.S.(C)

When the forces of daily participation in a sport become excessive, reaction to the accumulated stress can develop in the athlete's anatomic structures. The stress reaction that develops in bones has been termed a "stress fracture". The weight-bearing bones of the lower extremity are common sites of stress fractures in athletes who participate in sports that require the repetitive actions of running or jumping.

Stress fracture is a term describing the reaction to injury in the bone. The fracture is a local manifestation of a syndrome of accumulated stress in the anatomic tissues. As the bone develops a fatigue area of injury, new bone forms in reaction to the fatigue. Besides the reaction in the bone, there is usually reaction in the soft tissue support structures, such as the muscle and tendon aponeuroses. The stress reaction in the bone must be considered to be part of this overall reaction in the local tissues.

Frequent sites for stress fractures are the areas of the lower one-third of tibia and fibula, and the shafts of the metatarsals. However, stress reactions can occur in any area of the lower extremity bones and have been reported in the femoral neck, in the femoral diaphysis, and in the bones of the foot, the talus and calcaneus.

Proper management of an athlete with a stress injury depends on an accurate diagnosis of this injury. Early appropriate steps toward treatment ensure an optimum rate of recovery.

The history of the athlete's activity program often provides clues to the causative factors leading to the injury. The athlete frequently describes symptoms of pain, located at one specific area in the lower extremity, that develops during participation in a certain activity, such as running or jumping. Usually, the athlete has been overtraining or performing the sport activity repetitively. A careful evaluation of the athlete's training program or activity routine will often provide the clue to the cause of the stress injury. In a sport such as running, the athlete may have inadvertently trained too aggressively over a short period of time. This is frequently the case when a runner increases distances prior to a marathon. Occasionally, an athlete may experience a sudden onset of symptoms after a particularly excessive athletic performance. This often is seen in dance-related injuries. A careful review of the athlete's schedule of activities prior to the onset of the symptoms will point to changes that may have occurred in the training program. The athlete may have adjusted his or her training environment. Common examples of this are a change from flat terrain to hills, soft running surface to hard pavement, or soft wood floors to a hard concrete surface. Inadvertently, the athlete may have adjusted training schedules by increasing the time spent at daily practices. On occasion, a change in the sport activity can produce the stress reaction, as seen when an athlete takes up a sport for the first time, without adequate guidance or preparation.

DIAGNOSIS

The cardinal sign is pain experienced with activity. The pain is localized to one area of the lower extremity and occurs whenever the athlete performs the stressful activity. In runners, the pain of a stress fracture usually is experienced soon after the athlete begins running. The pain only remits when the activity is stopped. The area of sensitivity is usually located in the exact region of the stress reaction in the bone. When this area is palpated or pressed, the athlete experiences pain. If the stress reaction has been present for a few days, swelling may be noted in the region, especially in stress fractures of the metatarsals or distal fibula or tibia. Occasionally, the tissues over the stress area may feel warmer to the touch. Pain on weight-bearing on the affected leg may cause the athlete to develop an "antalgic" type of limp.

Generally, by the time an athlete seeks medical advice the diagnosis of stress fracture may be evident on the basis of the history and clinical features. An x-ray examination of the involved bone may reveal a site of increased density, but in the early stages of a stress reaction, the radiograph may show little, if any, noticeable change. In such instances, a technetium polyphosphate bone scan may reveal a site of increased uptake on the scan in the region corresponding to the site of pain. In many instances, the bone scan shows a site of reaction before a change is noticeable radiographically.

MANAGEMENT

After the initial assessment of the injury, the management program for an athlete with a stress fracture involves a treatment plan customized for the athlete and the sport. First and foremost, the athlete must be educated regarding the cause of the stress fracture and the benefit of modified rest to permit healing of the fracture. In most cases, the pain forces the athlete to modify or curtail activities. Occasionally, the athlete persists at sport and inadvertently prolongs the healing course of the stress reaction.

The mainstay of any treatment program is to remove the stressful activity from the athlete's program. Most athletes require a substitute program of activity to provide them with a daily cardiorespiratory workout. Swimming or cycling programs are useful alternative programs. Application of ice directly to the stress area diminishes local swelling and pain. Ultrasound application may promote healing of the injured area.

Each situation in which an athlete has developed a stress reaction must be individually evaluated. The cause for the stress fracture may have been an error in training. If this error is not corrected, the stress fracture often recurs when the athlete returns to the same activity.

Occasionally, the stress fracture has developed in an athlete who has an anatomic predisposition toward injury. Individuals with a particular alignment of the lower legs, such as bow legs or knock knees, may have a tendency to develop stress fractures. Assessment of shoe wear patterns may reveal peculiarities that necessitate correction of the shoe or possibly use of an orthotic. The properly fitted orthotic adjusts the forces directed on the lower extremity, evenly distributing these forces. An all-purpose, ready-made orthotic may be adequate, but a custom-fitted orthotic usually is required for the individual with a persistent problem of stress fracture.

When weight-bearing causes pain, the athlete should avoid stressing the affected limb, perhaps by using crutches. Occasionally, it is necessary to immobilize the lower leg in a cast. A light-weight removable plastic splint-orthosis can achieve proper protection and at the same time permit joint motion.

Ultimately, the goal of all parts of the treatment plan is to return the athlete to sport as quickly and as safely as possible. The timing of the return to sport must be carefully judged so as to avoid recurrence of the injury. If proper precautions of rest and protection from continued stress are followed, 8 to 10 weeks are required to permit healing of the bone injury.

There are specific guidelines which help to determine when the athlete can return to sports. First, the athlete must no longer perceive local pain in the region of the stress reaction or feel discomfort when the area is palpated. Swelling, redness, and warmth should have disappeared. When scheduling the return to the sport, it is wise to advise the athlete to start with a very relaxed training schedule. For a runner, this may mean a training schedule that consists of running on a soft surface, such as a track, for 15 to 30 minutes at a reduced pace, two to three times a week. If there is no pain, the runner may increase the time increment by 10 minutes each run per week for 2 to 3 weeks. Ultimately, the frequency of runs may increase. The aim of the program is to increase the running schedule over a 2- to 3-month time frame.

In a schedule of return to sports involving jumping, the athlete should spend most of the first 2 weeks in a program that mainly consists of running. If running is pain-free, the jumping activities may be attempted for periods of 20 minutes per day. These practice periods can be gradually increased at a weekly rate aiming to return the athlete to the original program over 2 months.

It is important to inform the athlete that stress injuries can recur. On any occasion that the athlete perceives a return of symptoms, the activity level must be adjusted back to a level at which there is no discomfort. If the symptoms return, a careful reassessment of the athlete and the training program is necessary.

EXAMPLES OF STRESS FRACTURES

The most common sites of stress fractures are the diaphyses of the metatarsal bones of the foot. Common symptoms are pain on weight-bearing and swelling over the dorsum of the foot. Ice application over the forefoot and elevation helps to decrease the swelling, and the use of crutches is advisable to decrease all stress of weight-bearing. These stress fractures must be treated with respect. If the athlete returns to activity too soon, the reaction recurs in many cases. A minimum of 6 to 8 weeks is usually required for adequate healing.

Stress fractures of the *distal fibula* often occur at a site just proximal to the level of the ankle joint or at the distal tip of the fibula. These fractures sometimes occur after sudden excessive stress, as when the athlete twists the foot or receives a direct blow to the area. Once the initial symptoms of pain and swelling have diminished, activities that do not involve repetitive stress (e.g., running) may be permitted. Many athletes can return to their sports sooner than 8 weeks, particularly if they avoid sudden or repetitive stresses.

Stress fractures of the *tibia* generally occur in the diaphysial shaft at the level of the middle or distal third. Usually, these fractures develop over a period of a few weeks. The typical case is that of the athlete who has been training aggressively for a competition and, in many cases, has ignored the early painful symptoms. Palpation over the skin area is particularly painful, and in many cases, roentgenograms show evidence of increased density in the region of the stress reaction. Treatment should be aimed at reducing all stress on the site of the injury by the use of crutches and, if necessary, a light-weight plastic below-knee walking orthosis. Fractures in the distal tibia heal readily, usually in 2 to 3 months, if the area is protected from further stress.

Stress fractures of the *femur* are rare, but they do occur in athletes who practice competitively with a daily routine of several hours. The site of the stress reaction is usually the inferior neck of the femur. Symptoms may be subtle at first, consisting only of a dull diffuse ache in the region of the hip joint or groin. Frequently, these athletes have perceived the symptoms to reflect a "simple muscle strain" and have continued the stressful activity. Other symptoms are a decreased range of motion of the hip joint on the affected side and mild discomfort on palpation. Radiographic views, both anterior and lateral oblique, of the affected hip and the opposite hip should be compared. A stress fracture may be visible in the region of the inferior neck, or, as is often the case, the only visible sign may be increased bone density in the region of the neck. If no abnormality is obvious on a conventional radiograph, a bone scan should help to demonstrate increased activity if there is a stress fracture. Treatment involves close supervision of the athlete and total cessation of all stress-provoking activities. If walking is painful, crutches should be prescribed. Usually

swimming does not aggravate the symptoms and is therefore a good alternate exercise activity.

Although extremely rare, *deformity* of the femoral neck has been known to result from a stress fracture. Examination of the athlete may reveal a measurable actual leg length discrepancy and an obvious limp, and radiographs show deformity of the neck-shaft femoral angle when compared to the opposite asymptomatic hip. The treatment depends on the extent of deformity. If the measurable leg length difference exceeds three-fourths of an inch and the femoral neck to shaft angle has been altered significantly, surgical correction may be advisable. Fortunately, the occurrence of deformity with a stress fracture is rare. Usually, the symptoms of pain alert the athlete before accumulated stress causes the bone to deform.

DISORDERS AFFECTING TENDON STRUCTURES ABOUT THE ANKLE

R. PETER WELSH, M.B., Ch.B., F.R.C.S.(C), F.A.C.S.
BRUCE R. HUFFER, M.D.

ACHILLES TENDINITIS AND RETROCALCANEAL BURSITIS

The morbidity of this syndrome has not always been appreciated and treatment efforts have not been rigorous enough to prevent chronicity of what is a most disabling condition to the athlete involved in any running or jumping sport. Indeed in a review of 50 track and field athletes engaged in competitive athletics who were afflicted with this syndrome for greater than 3 months despite treatment measures, 28 or 56 percent never returned to competitive athletics at their pre-injury level and 9 or 18 percent had to give up all sports participation completely.

This condition must be taken seriously and treated much more aggressively than it has been in the past if prolonged morbidity is to be reduced.

Pain occurring about the heel may be a result of several pathologic conditions, often making it difficult to distinguish the exact cause. These can be divided into pathologic conditions directly involving the tendon or the peritendon and painful bursitis about the calcaneal tuberosity.

Achilles Tendon Disease

The tendo Achillis, unlike other tendons such as the peroneals, is not invested by a true synovial sheath but

instead by a film-like peritenon. The tendon itself is made of dense fibrous tissue with little vascularity, but the peritenon is a loose connective tissue with abundant vascularity, prone to an inflammatory response. Achilles tendon disease can be classified into two types: (1) pure peritendinitis, and (2) peritendinitis with tendor degeneration. In pure peritendinitis, only the peritendinous structures are inflamed and thickened, (the term tenosynovitis should be reserved for tendons with true synovial sheaths). If the tendon itself is also involved, not only with an inflammatory reaction but also in a degenerate process, the tendon appears thicker, softer, and a deeper yellow; it loses its normal collagen configuration and shows areas of focal cyst formation. This classification is histologic and clinically it may be difficult to differentiate the exact pathology, but the etiology is common and appears to be related to problems with tissue vascularity. The blood supply to the Achilles tendon is from two sources. One from the muscle proximally passes distally in the tendon to meet in a watershed area some 2–3 cm above the tendon insertion with vessels coursing upward from the os calcis. With activity the Achilles tendon is subject to repetitive stretching and compression of the tendon and its blood supply in this critical watershed area. Here a relative abnormal vascularity persists, predisposing to tendon degeneration, with the associated peritendinous inflammatory response characterizing the clinical presentation.

Bursitis About The Calcaneus

Although numerous bursae have been described about the Achilles tendon and calcaneus, the only consistent anatomic bursa is the retrocalcaneal bursa located between the posterior superior surface of the calcaneus and the tendo Achillis. This bursa may become inflamed and hypertrophied in runners as can that associated with a prominence of the tuberosities of the os calcis, so-called pump-bumps. On rare occasions a bursitis may develop between the Achilles tendon and the skin.

Symptoms

Pain is the symptom that brings the athlete to seek medical attention and it may be located anywhere from the attachment of the Achilles tendon to the os calcis to the musculotendinous junction several centimeters above the tip of the superior calcaneal tuberosity. Initially, pain may only occur early in the run, but in chronic cases, pain may be constant. Particularly troublesome is stiffness on arising in the morning, which may take some hours to "loosen up".

Physical Examination

Tenderness may be noted anywhere along the length of the Achilles tendon. Nodular thickening may be noted, and peritendinous soft tissue swelling may be present. Retrocalcaneal bursitis can often be diagnosed if pain occurs while squeezing the bursal region between the os calcis and the tendo Achillis. Patients are often noted to have tightness of the tendo Achillis and the entire gastrocnemius-soleus complex, and this should be tested for and compared to the noninjured side. Roentgenographic examination is rarely of use, although on occasion a prominence of the superior tuberosity or calcific deposits within the tendon may be noted.

Treatment

As in most overuse syndromes resulting from repetitive stress, reduced loading of the injured part must be imposed. Runners must decrease their distance and should eliminate hill-work. Sprinters and jumpers must refrain from all springing and bounding, and if the tendon is persistently tender, a switch to walking, cycling, or swimming is advised. Soft padding in the hindfoot region of the running shoe may decrease the impact of running on the Achilles tendon, and a slight lift placed into the heel may decrease stress on the tendon. One of the most important aspects of treatment involves the diligent stretching of the triceps surae mechanism before running. Local ice friction treatment can be extremely helpful, and a limited course of ultrasound should be tried (10 to 12 treatments). Further treatments are unlikely to be of enhanced benefit. Anti-inflammatory medicine can be prescribed, but steroid injections are never used because of its weakening effect on tendinous tissue with a likely predisposition to rupture.

A small percentage of patients do not respond to conservative treatment and require exploration. At surgery it is important to precisely define the pathology; in cases of peritendinitis alone a simple tenolysis is effective. However, if the tendon is degenerate, the yellowish necrotic areas of tendon should be excised through a longitudinal incision into the tendon. Revascularization appears to be encouraged by such a procedure, and recovery generally is most favorable. In cases of a chron-

ically inflamed retrocalcaneal bursa, excision of the bursa and underlying bony prominence usually is effective, but it is very important to leave a negative bony impression where there was previously a prominence if recurrence is to be avoided.

Protected weight-bearing with crutches, but with early mobilization of the ankle, is practiced postoperatively. Return to sport may be delayed, and diligent calf-stretching exercises should be practiced throughout the recovery phase.

SUBCALCANEAL PAIN FROM PLANTAR FASCIITIS AND SEVER'S DISEASE

Plantar Fasciitis

Pain originating in the subcalcaneal region is not uncommon in athletes engaged in running and jumping sports. The condition has been given a variety of names including plantar fasciitis, painful heel syndrome, and calcaneal spurs. Pain may arise at the calcaneal tuberosity and origin of the plantar fascia as well as from the subcalcaneal bursa or the heel pad itself, which is comprised of a thick layer of fibrous septae and fat. Pain may also arise in the tendinous origins of the intrinsic foot muscles at their calcaneal attachment or from trauma to the medial heel branches of the calcaneal nerve.

Etiology

The cause of plantar fasciitis is not well understood, but in the athlete the process most likely begins as a strain of the plantar fascia, either as a single injury or, more likely, as a result of repetitive trauma at the point of fascial attachment to the calcaneal tubercle. In the early stages a fibrositis of low chronicity takes place, with tendinous degeneration and an ongoing low-grade inflammatory response which never succeeds in adequately repairing the injury. The calcaneal spur may be part of this response, but it is more generally seen as a physiologic local response of the bone to tension stresses in the plantar fascia.

Occasionally, another cause of pain in this area may be entrapment or trauma to a branch of the medial calcaneal nerve. This branch has been shown to be vulnerable to pressure from calcaneal spurs as well as local irritation and inflammation.

Diagnosis

In general the diagnosis is not difficult to make. The athlete complains of pain when the heel strikes the ground during walking or running, a continuous low-grade pain during the day, and pain and stiffness after use and particularly on rising in the morning.

Clinically one can usually only demonstrate tenderness locally at the attachment of the plantar fascia to the medial process of the tuberosity. Such tenderness is exquisite, aggravated with weight-bearing, and occasionally aggravated by hyperpronation of the forefoot as the plantar fascia is put on stretch.

Treatment

The aggravating insult must be reduced if the athlete is to overcome this condition. Thus impact loading of the heel area has to be avoided, which for the running athlete may mean a switch to cycling or swimming.

Strengthening the intrinsic muscles of the foot as well as the tibialis posterior muscle helps in the support of the longitudinal arch and in reducing tensions in the plantar fascia and intrinsic musculature.

A soft orthosis may be of great help, but its design should serve the following functions: (1) relieve the pressure on the tender area, (2) support the arch, and (3) control the heel. To these ends a simple foam cushion can be used as can a "doughnut" with a hole in the center to reduce loads on the heal area. However, it is better to build this into a heel cup with a varus tilt to direct the heel plant to the outer border of the foot and at the same time reduce tension in the plantar fascia.

Local physiotherapy measures with ultrasound can be strikingly beneficial, and anti-inflammatory medication in high doses for a 2- to 3-week course is often helpful. If a major response is not seen with these measures in the first 2 weeks, the local infiltration of corticosteroid into the tender focus should be undertaken. This can be repeated on two further occasions at 6-week intervals. On rare occasions if symptoms persist to the point where continued sports participation is impossible, consideration may be given to surgical treatment.

The preferred surgical approach utilizes a 3-cm incision placed medially at the junction of the thick plantar skin with the medial aspect of the heel. Dissection must not damage the heel pad, but must separate the tendinous muscle attachment and plantar fascial origin from their calcaneal attachment. A segment of tendon and fascia is excised together with the calcaneal spur if present. Postoperatively, a compressive dressing is applied, the wound always drained, and weight-bearing is restricted with crutches until weight can be borne comfortably on the heel. A very gradual return to activity is allowed, and the recovery can take as long as 3 to 4 months.

Sever's Disease (Os Calcis Apophysitis)

In the adolescent, maturation of the os calcis apophysis, to which the Achilles tendon makes its attachment, may be associated with a dysvascular degeneration with fragmentation of the apophysis. This process, one of the osteochondroses, is akin to Osgood-Schlatter disease seen about the knee at the insertion of the patellar tendon and is similarly associated with local pain and sensitivity to pressure and loads.

Presenting usually in the 11- to 13-year-old age group, the condition is self-limiting, but nonetheless troublesome through the active phase until growth maturation of the os calcis is completed in the early teens. Pain with running and jumping and a constant aching after activity, particularly at night, may necessitate simple anti-inflammatory analgesic treatment with aspirin. Heel cushions and modification of the sports program are necessary until symptoms subside. Confirmation of the process is shown radiographically, with fragmentation of the heel apophysis early and marked sclerosis later as new bone is laid down and the process matures.

FLEXOR HALLUCIS LONGUS STENOSING TENOSYNOVITIS AND OS TRIGONUM SYNDROME

Pain in the posterior aspect of the ankle and hindfoot is relatively common in athletes. Although the symptoms are most commonly attributed to the Achilles tendon, two other conditions cause pain in this area and may be misdiagnosed as "Achilles tendinitis". These conditions are inflammation and stenosis of the tendon of the flexor hallucis longus and os trigonum syndrome.

Flexor Hallucis Longus Stenosing Tenosynovitis

Tendinitis of the flexor hallucis longus is extremely common in ballet dancers, although it is occasionally seen in other sports as well. The flexor hallucis longus tendon, called the "Achilles tendon of the dancer's foot", is often strained as it traverses its fibrous and osseous tunnel on the posterior aspect of the talus between the medial and lateral tubercles. The os trigonum is the name of a separate ossicle in relation to this tendon about which progressive inflammation can lead to a stenosing tenosynovitis. If scarring is severe over time, a "pseudo hallux rigidus" can develop. Partial rupture of the flexor hallucis longus tendon has also been reported. Symptoms of tendinitis include recurrent pain, tenderness, and swelling behind the medial malleolus of the ankle, and sometimes triggering or crepitus. A misdiagnosis of tendinitis of the posterior tibial tendon is often made, and indeed such a condition may coexist with disease of the flexor hallucis longus.

Physical examination reveals localized tenderness over the sheath of the flexor hallucis longus behind the medial malleolus. Sometimes nodules within the tendon can be palpated. Rarely, with an abnormal distal insertion of the muscle fibers on the tendon, a "functional hallux rigidus" can result when the muscle fibers become pulled down into the fibrosseous tunnel. This condition must be differentiated from a posterior impingement syndrome. The pain is usually behind the lateral malleolus in this condition and caused by plantar flexion.

Treatment

Treatment in the early stages consists of rest, anti-inflammatory medication, ice applications, and gentle stretching. Activities that reproduce symptoms should be avoided. Although most cases eventually become asymptomatic with conservative treatment, symptoms occasionally progress and become severe and disabling. In these cases tenolysis of the flexor hallucis longus should be suspected.

Os Trigonum Syndrome

The os trigonum represents the ununited lateral tubercle on the posterior aspect of the talus and occurs in 8 to 13 percent of the general population. Pain originating at the os trigonum is rare in nonathletes, but relatively common in ballet dancers. When the dancer attempts to force plantar flexion beyond its range, the os trigonum is caught between the posterior tip of the tibia and the os calcis. This may result in contusion, extrusion, or fracture of the os trigonum.

The diagnosis is suggested when a dancer complains of pain and tenderness posterolaterally in the ankle, whereas with flexor hallucis longus tendinitis pain and tenderness are medially based. The condition may be misdiagnosed as chronic peroneal tendinitis. However, on careful examination, the location of the tenderness is found to be behind the peroneal tendons, and forced passive plantar flexion reproduces the symptoms. Lateral roentgenograms with full plantar flexion reveal the os trigonum. Relief of symptoms with locally injected Xylocaine confirms the diagnosis.

Treatment

In the dancer the most important aspect of treatment is avoiding any motion that places the ankle in extreme plantar flexion in which posterior impingement occurs. Mild anti-inflammatory medicine and physical therapy, as well as local steroid injections, may be helpful in dancers who are not helped by conservative therapy. Surgical excision may be warranted.

On occasion both stenosing tenosynovitis of the flexor hallucis longus tendon and the os trigonum syndrome occur together. In such situations, when conservative treatment has not been beneficial, combined tenolysis of the flexor hallucis longus as well as os trigonum excision should be carried out. Although surgical treatment can lead to good results, the dancer should be cautioned that full recovery can take as long as 8 months.

PERONEAL TENOSYNOVITIS; TIBIALIS POSTERIOR TENDINITIS AND TENOSYNOVITIS

Stenosing tenosynovitis of the peroneal tendons on the lateral side of the ankle and tibialis posterior on the medial side may be the cause of considerable morbidity in the running and jumping athlete.

Anatomy

The tendons of the peroneus longus and brevis enter a common sheath 4 cm proximal to the lateral malleolus. This sheath encloses them as they pass behind and into a shallow groove in the posterior portion of the fibular malleolus. The brevis tendon continues to its insertion into the tuberosity at the base of the fifth metatarsal while the longus tendon passes under the cuboid into a second sheath formed by the long plantar ligament and cuboid groove. It inserts into the lateral side of the base of the first metatarsal. The peroneals are active evertors of the foot. They contribute to final pronation and push-off in the second stage of walking and also contribute considerably to the stability of the ankle joint. The tibialis posterior passes posterior to the medial malleolus in company with the long flexor tendons to the toes. As it does so it is enveloped by a synovial sleeve and retained by a thick retinaculum before passing to its insertion into the tubercle of the tarsal scaphoid.

Posttraumatic Peroneal Tendinitis (Stenosing Tenosynovitis)

Limitation of normal excursion of the peroneal tendons at the level of the peroneal trochlea after trauma can cause lateral tarsal pain. The etiology can be secondary to trauma to other ankle structures, that is, calcaneal fractures, ankle sprains, subtalar fractures, or fractures of the lateral fibular ridge; acute injury resulting from forced dorsiflexion and inversion may be the initiating cause. The diagnosis is suspected by the patient who complains of pain localized to the lateral aspect of the heel or external malleolar area following injury. The patient notes accentuation of pain when walking barefoot or on rough terrain. On examination there is an antalgic gait, limitation of subtalar motion, and point tenderness over the peroneal tendons. Forced plantar flexion in inversion accentuates symptoms. Injection of several milliliters of local anesthetic into the tendon sheath with relief of symptoms strongly suggests the diagnosis. Peroneal tenography shows either a complete block or constriction of the peroneal tendon sheath at the level of the inferior peroneal retinaculum.

The tibialis posterior may be similarly involved, but with a similar symptom pattern referrable to the medial aspect of the ankle.

Treatment

Conservative treatment includes anti-inflammatory medication and stretching of the parent muscle groups, icing and ultrasound to the local area of inflammation, reduction in the provocative activity, and substitution of a noninjurious exercise program.

Orthotic support can be of great help, but must be carefully customized, the objective being to unload the offended tendon in each case. Thus with a peroneal tendon problem, the ankle should usually be tilted into valgus; with a tibialis posterior problem, the heel should be tilted in varus. However, if local tendon compression is believed to be an etiologic factor, reverse wedges are required. Great care must be exercised in utilizing such devices lest the symptoms be further aggravated.

Local steroid infiltration into the tendon sheath is effective if utilized before the condition becomes chronic. The tendon itself must not be injected and a limit of three injections imposed, for rupture of either of these tendon groups can be disastrous.

Surgical Treatment

Peroneal Tenosynovitis. Rarely is surgical decompression of the peroneal tendons required. If localized tenolysis is carried out, care must be taken to preserve the retinaculum in order to prevent a subsequent tendon subluxation or dislocation.

Tibialis Tenosynovitis. Simple tenolysis is most effective for refractory cases. With release of structures behind the medial malleolus freedom for the tendons to glide ensures relief of pain.

Accessory Tarsal Scaphoid Syndrome

Localized tendinitis of tibialis posterior may be associated at its insertion with the persistent nonunion of an accessory ossicle—the accessory tarsal scaphoid. Generally this condition responds to orthotic support of the long arch and an intensive course of intrinsic and tibialis-strengthening exercises, as well as the general local measures of ice and ultrasound.

However, on occasion, symptoms prove unresponsive, and local excision of the accessory ossicle is indicated. It is essential to carefully incise the tendon longitudinally and shell out the loose bone, leaving the tendon insertion intact. Cast protection is unnecessary, but protected weight-bearing and an arch support are continued until comfort is achieved. Return to sports may take 3 to 4 months.

Dorsal Tenosynovitis

The extensor tendon complex may be involved in dorsal tenosynovitis both anterior to the ankle and over the dorsum of the foot. On occasion midtarsal osteophytes may be associated with early arthritic change and be a predisposing factor.

Should the usual conservative measures, especially avoidance of footwear compression dorsally, be ineffective, a localized tenolysis can be performed. If midtarsal osteophytes are noted in the older athlete, a localized debridement should complement the procedure.

Acute and Chronic Luxations of the Peroneal Tendons

Traumatic dislocation of the peroneal tendons may be seen secondary to skiing accidents. Skiing requires that the peroneal muscles be contracted forcefully whenever the skier is making a turn or is traversing a hill. In such a situation, forced supination of the foot greatly enhances the risk of dislocation. The usual mechanism of injury is the ankle being forced into severe dorsiflexion with the foot slightly inverted, followed by a violent reflex contraction of the peroneals. For the dislocation to take place, the peroneals must go into a violent reflex action. Should the ski tip dive into the snow and become fixed, the patient is thrown forward, causing a dorsiflexion of the ankle, and acute dislocation of the peroneal tendons may ensue.

In the acute situation the diagnosis is suggested by swelling and ecchymosis in a region of the superior peroneal retinaculum, with sharp tenderness in the sulcus as well as along the distal fibula. Because the tendons spontaneously relocate, examination must attempt to reproduce the injury or the diagnosis may be missed. This is done by plantar flexion, eversion, and dorsiflexion against resistance, which will elicit pain and often dislocation.

Chronic subluxation or dislocation is often misdiagnosed as a chronic ankle sprain with the patient complaining of a sense of uneasiness, giving way, or snapping in the lateral aspect of the ankle. The diagnosis is confirmed by demonstrating tendon displacement about a stable ankle mortise. On occasion roentgenograms may show an avulsion fracture of the lateral ridge of the lateral malleolus.

Treatment

In the presence of acute or chronic subluxation, a trial of conservative treatment is advised. Ankle taping and an elastic ankle support generally suffice, and most patients with subluxation only will have little functional loss. Surgery is rarely needed in these situations.

Complete dislocation, either acute or chronic, is more difficult to treat. For the acute situation, conservative treatment consists of a below-knee weight-bearing cast for 6 weeks. Surgery is reserved for those in whom recurrence takes place.

Surgical stabilization is effected by elevating a periosteal flap and folding it posteriorly to envelop the reduced peroneal tendons, thus reconstructing the peroneal retinaculum. It is important to hinge this flap along the posterior margin of the fibula and prevent any anterior glide of the tendon. The stretched retinaculum and sheath can be enfolded superficially, reinforcing the repair, which is cast-protected for 6 weeks.

RUPTURE OF THE ACHILLES TENDON

JOHN M. SULLIVAN, M.B., Ch.B., F.R.A.C.S.

In a top class athlete, rupture of the Achilles tendon can herald demotion to a lower class of performance. However, early recognition of the problem and the institution of a rational treatment program can allow the athlete to return to previous peak function. It may, nonetheless, take 12 to 18 months for this recovery.

Within the sporting world the group at greatest risk is the middle-aged athlete in his fourth decade. The younger supremely fit athlete can be affected, but the pathogenesis is quite different. No sport is particularly spared, and the emphasis on certain sports in some reviews represents often the geographic preponderance of that sport. The more mature racquet ball or basketball player is the most vulnerable. In any series of ruptures reviewed, we see skiers, skaters, runners, jumpers, football players, gymnasts, and soccer players. Females are featured to a lesser degree and the incidence on average is about 10 percent that of males. As more females are accepted into the ranks of professional athletes, the percentage will increase.

PATHOGENESIS

The rupture is usually sudden and unexpected; in some instances it is preceded by a period of discomfort or pain. The exercising athlete is usually about to thrust forward or upward, fully weight-bearing, with the ankle joint changing from a position of dorsiflexion to plantar flexion. As this occurs, the knee joint passes into an extended position, placing the calf muscles on maximum stretch as they are about to explosively contract. Often the athlete is retreating or decelerating, and the contracted or contracting calf is further loaded by a sudden change in direction. Examples of the foregoing mechanisms are (1) the unconditioned athlete coming out of the blocks at the commencement of a race; (2) the basketball player changing direction, jumping, and intercepting the ball; and (3) the racquet ball player lunging for a passing ball. An extreme example of forced dorsiflexion against a contracting calf occurs when the athlete lands awkwardly after a jump or lands unexpectedly in a hole.

A less common situation occurs when a direct blow is received to a taut Achilles tendon.

Steroid injected into the tendon or immediate region may precede the rupture.

The site of rupture is regularly 2 to 8 cm above the insertion of the tendo Achilles. A study of Largergren and Lindholm demonstrated that the area of poorest blood supply falls within this section.

The rupture may be complete or partial.

COMPLETE RUPTURE

The sportsman complains of pain which diminishes over the succeeding hours. Often he describes the sensation of having been "kicked" in the back of the heel, and some may even hear the tendon rupture or describe its tearing. Walking is possible albeit flatfooted.

Diagnosis

This is aided by the history and completed by a careful examination. With a fresh rupture a defect can be seen and palpated. If some hours have elapsed since the rupture, there is swelling, possibly ecchymosis, tenderness, and a palpable defect (through soft hematoma) 2 or more centimeter above the calcaneus. The patient may be able to plantar flex the foot by using the toe flexors. The "squeeze" test of Thompson and Doherty is diagnostic. To perform this test the patient is placed prone or asked to kneel on a stool with the leg relaxed. Squeezing the normal calf produces plantar flexion of the foot. Squeeze applied to the affected leg fails to produce plantar flexion, and this constitutes a positive test result.

A roentgenogram should be done in the athlete. This will show alteration of the soft tissues, but more importantly rules out any bone injuries. On the rare occasion, an avulsion flake may be seen and dictates a different form of management.

Management

Nonoperative management will not be discussed as there is no place for this in the treatment of an athlete. Early, that is prior to surgery, the limb should be elevated and ice applied to the region.

Operative Treatment

The operative procedure is short. Either regional or general anesthesia is employed. The patient is placed prone with a soft roll in front of the ankle. A tourniquet is used.

A medial longitudinal incision is made. The midline should not be crossed in a sinuous manner, and the lateral aspect is avoided to prevent scarring and sural nerve tethering in this area. Full-thickness flaps are raised after incising the deep fascia, and the paratenon is incised longitudinally to allow later closure.

The rupture is exposed and most often is 2 to 8 cm above the calcaneus. The fragmented ends are not excised. The area is irrigated free of blood clot, and with the foot in full plantar flexion, the frayed ends of the tendon are meshed together. The suture technique preferred involves the insertion of four separate looped Dexon sutures (No. 1). Two are placed proximally and two distally (Fig. 1), three to four loops in each suture engaging a varying amount of tendon. These are then

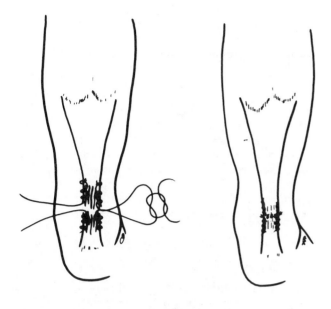

Figure 1 Suture technique.

tied and several opposing sutures supplement the repair across the central tendon. This produces an extremely strong repair and can justifiably allow early passive mobilization without cast immobilization and without weight-bearing. Work on this particular aspect is ongoing (author), and for the present, protected repair will be described.

Argument regarding the effect this suture may have on tendon vascularity may be proffered. To date it has not been seen to be a problem. What is achieved is excellent control of the tendon ends, institution of a durable repair, and the best possible scaffold for healing.

The paratenon is closed with 3–0 Dexon. The tourniquet is deflated, and bleeding is controlled by diathermy. The skin is closed with interrupted 4–0 nylon. Suction drainage is sometimes used, and its routine use would never be condemned.

The leg is placed in a split padded below-knee cast with the foot in plantar flexion just short of the maximum. After three days in bed with the leg elevated mobilization is commenced with crutches. At 2 weeks the cast is removed, sutures are removed, and a new cast applied in a gravity equinus position. A walking platform is applied to level the sole and partial weight-bearing is allowed with the use of crutches. At a total of 6 weeks, the cast is removed and the patient equipped with a 2-cm heel raise.

Rehabilitation

The patient is instructed to wear a raise at all times for the next 4 weeks. Particular stress is placed on caution going upstairs, standing on chairs, or climbing ladders. A specific reminder is made to wear the raised shoe if it is necessary to get up in the night.

Early therapy is aimed at mobilizing the ankle gently and painlessly. Hot whirlpool exposure is extremely beneficial. Swimming and exercycle use with the foot flat on the pedal are subtle encouragements to mobilization. When a heel-toe gait is realized at about the 4-week stage, the raise is removed, and passive stretching can be incorporated into the program. Throughout this period, ultrasound and calf muscle stimulation from the physiotherapist hastens progress. At about 3 months, the athlete is usually able to commence running. At about 6 to 9 months, near-normal function is achieved, but it may take 12 to 18 months to regain peak power take-off. The program does not end here, and the athlete must be instructed on careful warm-up and stretching procedures for both legs.

NEGLECTED COMPLETE RUPTURE

Because of motivation to return to previous peak performance after injury, and a better level of care for the athlete, late diagnosis is not usually a problem. Nonetheless, it does occasionally occur, and its management will be discussed.

Diagnosis

The history tells the story, and the diagnosis is never in doubt. The calf is wasted, the ankle region thickened and tender. The gait is flatfooted, and the "squeeze test" markedly positive.

Operative Treatment

The patient is positioned and tourniquet applied as for treatment of complete rupture. A posteromedial incision is made from the junction of upper and middle thirds of the calf to the posterior and medial side of the tendon insertion at the calcaneus. The deep fascia is divided and the paratenon opened. The rupture is identified and inspected. The very terminal disorganized scar tissue at the tendon ends is excised. Excision is not carried back to normal tissue, as suggested by some authors, as this will leave a very large defect. Once continuity has been re-established, this scar will remodel under tension with the realignment of collagen fibers.

It is unusual to be able to oppose and suture the ends, even with the foot in maximum plantar flexion. However, if this can be achieved, the repair is simple. Otherwise, a sheet of fascia from the gastrocnemius is fashioned (Fig. 2), 10 to 15 cm long and about 4 cm wide proximally. It is carefully stripped off the gastrocnemius by sharp dissection, an attempt being made to leave some fascia covering muscle proximally. This is carried down to 2 cm above the distal end. It is turned over and brought anterior to the distal stump of tendon and rolled around this as a tube. Using O Dexon, the tube is closed, and the proximal end where this flap hinges is sutured. It is unusual to be able to close the donor defect completely, but this is done if possible. If plantaris is present, it is

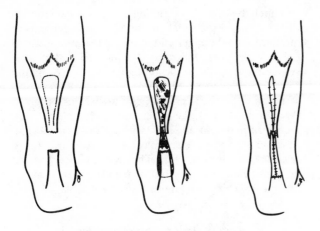

Figure 2 Reconstruction for neglected rupture.

divided distally, opened as a sheet, and placed over the repair as an added sheath to assist in gliding.

The immobilization is as for complete rupture except that the cast is required for 8 weeks. The rehabilitation is similar but more prolonged. Significant morbidity is associated with neglected complete rupture, and a normally functioning unit is difficult to achieve.

PARTIAL RUPTURE

The pathogenesis, as already discussed, must apply in some circumstances. However, partial rupture probably represents an overuse syndrome that occurs in the poorly trained recreational athlete as well as in the intensely trained top athlete.

Pain is the common complaint. It is shooting or tearing in nature (sometimes burning) and is worsened by activity. There may be complaints of stiffness and soreness in the region in the mornings.

Diagnosis

A careful examination is critical. Thickening and nodular formation will often be observed. The ability to stand on tiptoes is unimpaired, except by pain. Impor-

tantly, there is a negative "squeeze" test. Palpation demonstrates further the thickening, nodules, and point tenderness. If the problem is long-standing, calf wasting and weakness can be demonstrated.

Management

In the very acute stages, before disability develops, conservative treatment is worthy of trial. Three weeks in a walking below-knee cast and then physiotherapy with decreased activities for a further 1 month may achieve a good result. Unfortunately, for a great percentage, this regimen fails and the condition becomes chronic.

Operative Treatment

Partial ruptures that have failed conservative treatment and have become chronic are treated surgically. The set-up is as described for a complete rupture. The paratenon is split, and this may be thickened and adherent. In some circumstances, it is best excised. The tendon is palpated and the thickening or nodules delineated. In the area of the rupture a longitudinal split is made in the tendon. This reveals altered structure with loss of the normal tendon sheen and fibrous strand appearance. Depending on the duration of the rupture, there may be hemorrhage with early granulation tissue; there may be yellow streaks or patches of yellow soft tissue interspersed with normal tendon; there may be white firm fibrinoid material blending into normal structure.

The abnormal tissue is excised. If only a small amount of pathologic tissue is excised, the tendon can be closed side-to-side with absorbable sutures. In these circumstances, white O Dexon is used. If a large amount of abnormal tissue is removed but continuity is maintained, the area is reinforced with plantaris. If a section has to be excised, a formal repair and reconstruction is performed.

Postoperatively, a below-knee cast with the foot in neutral is applied when a minimal excision is performed. After one week, the cast is removed and mobilization commences. If a large resection is performed or continuity is disrupted, the casting and rehabilitation is as for the complete rupture.

LIGAMENT INSTABILITY OF THE ANKLE

BERNARD G. COSTELLO, MD., F.R.C.S.(C)

Considering the frequency with which one encounters ankle ligament injuries, ankle instability should be one of the better understood disorders of the entire musculoskeletal system. It is surprising, therefore, that there are still a number of areas of disagreement on the subject of ankle injuries. This review will provide a practical approach to the problem.

From the moment the athlete sustains an injury to the ankle, a pathophysiologic process is set in motion that must be identified, graded, and treated appropriately, in as short a time as possible, to achieve an optimal result.

The vast majority of ankle ligament injuries occur on the lateral aspect of this region. When deltoid (medial) injuries are present, they are commonly associated with lateral malleolar fractures or with major capsular and/or distal tibiofibular ligament injuries.

When an ankle inversion injury takes place, a predictable series of events occurs. With the initial twist injury, if the ankle is immediately righted by the individual, little or no injury occurs. If the corrective response to inversion is unsuccessful, not only do the lateral collateral ligaments (anterior talofibular, calcaneofibular, and posterior talofibular) sustain injury to some extent (grade I to III), but the peroneal muscle group, forced to perform an extremely vigorous isometric contraction against a relatively fixed foot, is also often injured. Failure to recognize and treat this injury is an important cause of chronic "pseudo" instability of the ankle. Finally, proprioceptive conduction seems to be delayed after these injuries, and this can also lead to an apparently unstable ankle. Even in the absence of significant ligament instability, some athletes report that they suffer recurring inversion injuries. The likely reason, in the absence of clear ligamentous instability, is that when inversion occurs, not only is the proprioceptive pathway too slow, but when the message finally reaches the peroneal muscle group to correct the inversion, the muscle itself is too weak to comply.

CLASSIFICATION OF ACUTE INJURY

Ankle sprains are conventionally classified as grade I, II, or III. Grades I and II are minimal and moderate injuries to the ligaments, with variable amounts of pain, swelling, ecchymosis, and loss of function. Neither of these renders the ankle unstable. Grade III injuries, on the other hand, are major disruptions of the ligamentous structures on the lateral aspect of the ankle and produce certain instabilities, which must be identified early in the course of the injury if successful treatment is to be administered.

HISTORY

In most of these injuries, the athlete clearly identifies the mechanism as being inversion and frequently notes that there was a "pop" or a snapping sound at the time of the injury. Loss of function is variable with any one of the three grades and is not fully reliable as an indication of severity of injury.

PHYSICAL EXAMINATION

The physical examination of the injured ankle requires careful and methodical assessment and is not meant to be a random exercise in palpation. Some of the critical areas that must be carefully palpated are the tip of the lateral malleolus, the anterior talofibular ligament area, the calcaneofibular ligament, at least the lateral half of the anterior joint capsule, and finally the base of the fifth metatarsal. Based on this physical examination, one is usually able to grade the injuries accordingly, using the following criteria:

Grade I: No instability, full range of motion, minimal pain and swelling, and usually pain on weight-bearing.

Grade II: Little or no ankle instability, or the presence of a very mild anterior drawer sign. There is a moderate decrease in range of motion as well as moderate pain and swelling. Weight-bearing is usually more difficult than in grade I.

Grade III: The joint is clearly unstable; there is usually severe pain and swelling, with ecchymosis, significant loss of range of movement, and the inability to bear weight.

Apart from the general findings of ligamentous injury, the single most important aspect of the physical examination is the method used to demonstrate the presence of instability. The lateral instabilities of the ankle can either be in an anterior direction (a drawer sign) or a varus instability of the hind foot. The drawer sign is performed by holding the ankle in a neutral position and, with the fingers placed behind the heel, drawing the foot forward in an attempt to sublux the talus slightly in a forward direction. The presence of such a sign indicates disruption of the anterior talofibular ligament. The test for varus instability is performed again with the ankle in a neutral position and the hand placed on the lateral aspect of the heel. The foot is then inverted. If a feeling of instability is present or a "clunk" can be identified as the talus returns to its normal position upon removal of the varus stress, a strong suspicion of varus instability due to injury of the calcaneofibular ligament must be entertained.

RADIOLOGIC INVESTIGATION

A number of radiographic studies are available for ankle ligament injuries, but a frequent dilemma is to appropriately utilize these various investigations. In all but the most minor ankle injuries, routine views should be obtained, including a mortice view of the ankle. If there is clinical suggestion of lateral instability, varus stress views and a lateral view while the drawer sign is being elicited should be obtained. An anterior subluxation of the talus under the tibia is indicative of a disruption of the anterior talofibular ligament. Interpretation of the varus stress test is slightly more complex; however, a tilting of the talus within the ankle mortice of 0 to 7° of varus is indicative of a disruption of the anterior talofibular ligament. A tilt of 7 to 30° indicates increasing severity of injury, up to the point where all of the lateral collateral ligaments are damaged.

Contrast studies are of some value in evaluating the integrity of the lateral collateral ligaments of the ankle. Ankle arthrography, as reported, failed to provide consistently useful information in identifying significant injuries of the lateral collateral ligament system of the ankle. A more recent modification of this technique utilizes a peroneal sheath arthrogram to identify major ligament injury to the lateral aspect of the ankle. If the dye is confined to the peroneal sheath or if a small amount escapes through the sheath but does not enter the ankle joint, this study is considered negative. When the calcaneofibular ligament is torn, the dye passes through the defect in the sheath, into the ankle joint, and then, because the anterior ligament capsule is also often torn, the dye may also pass from the joint itself. If doubt persists after stress views are done, peroneal sheath arthrography may provide a more accurate assessment than ankle arthrography.

PITFALLS

A number of alternate diagnoses should be considered during the course of evaluation of ankle ligament injury. A fracture of the base of the fifth metatarsal may be entirely missed, particularly if routine views of the ankle are ordered without including the foot. Many radiographers exclude the metatarsal bases from an ankle view, and if such a fracture is present and has not been clinically identified through accurate palpation, it will be missed. Osteochondritis dissecans of the talus (osteochondral dome fractures), has been described and should be searched for, as many of them follow an inversion injury.

TREATMENT

Grade I Injury

Grade I injuries of the lateral collateral ligaments of the ankle are considered, for the most part, to be minor injuries. The all-too-frequent routine of an elastic compression bandage, crutches, and advice to elevate the foot, often administered in hospital Emergency Departments, is completely unsatisfactory. The most appro-

priate treatment program for these injuries is the combination of rest, ice, compression, and elevation (RICE). This program is initiated immediately and followed usually for 72 hours, after which the patient is returned to early range-of-motion and weight-bearing, and as rapid a return to normal activity as possible. The use of an adjustable air stirrup splint can be helpful in these cases, particularly in the early stages of return to activity.

Grade II Injury

The best results for partial tears are obtained by early aggressive management. Again, the RICE program is most appropriate, followed by the early use of appropriate physiotherapy modalities to aid in resolution of the soft tissue damage. Range-of-motion exercises and isometrics are begun as soon as pain allows, usually within 48 hours, and the patient is begun on partial weight-bearing at about one week. Many of these injuries are better supported by the use of taping or an Unna boot. The latter is a semi-rigid dressing, supported by an elastic bandage on top, which provides a lightweight and very acceptable support. Standard taping techniques are frequently employed, generally using a Gibney basket weave with a heel lock, after swelling has maximized. If taping is initially employed in the management, it must be an open weave for at least 72 hours to avoid constriction should further swelling occur. The use of a plaster cast for grade II injuries in almost all cases should be condemned. It provides little advantage and does impose upon the injury its own set of consequences (muscle atrophy, stiffness, swelling, and occasionally disuse osteoporosis).

Grade III Injuries

Ligament injuries to the lateral aspect of the ankle resulting in instability involve either the anterior talofibular ligament alone or both the anterior talofibular ligament and the calcaneofibular ligament. Although there may be some place for consideration of nonsurgical management (plaster cast) in major tears of the anterior talofibular ligament alone, grade III injuries to the ankle usually are treated by surgical means. Following direct open repair, a plaster cast is applied for 8 weeks. This is followed by a rehabilitation program similar to that used for grade II injury.

Chronic Instability

Chronic lateral instability of the ankle is a disabling problem. Although nonsurgical methods have been utilized to stabilize the ankle in these cases, using lateral heel wedges (unsuitable for athletic footwear) or various forms of stabilizing ankle wraps, the instability remains a problem.

Various surgical techniques have been utilized to reconstruct chronic lateral instabilities of the ankle. The

Watson-Jones method reconstructs the anterior talofibular ligament only, whereas the Evans procedure utilizes a peroneal tenodesis, again incompletely replacing the damaged structures.

The most logical approach is to employ an operation that is designed to replace both the anterior talofibular and the calcaneofibular ligaments. The modified Elmslie (Chrisman-Snook) procedure serves well in this regard. One-half or occasionally all of the entire peroneus brevis tendon is freed proximally and reflected distally, attaching the peroneus brevis muscle belly to that of the peroneus longus. The tendon is then woven through a tunnel in the area of the damaged anterior talofibular ligament, continued posteriorly through a drill hole in the distal fibula and then distally and attached to the os calcis on its lateral surface, either by a staple or through a tunnel.

In a series reported in 1981, 22 Elmslie reconstructions were reviewed. All patients returned to their original choice of activity following surgery. In my hands, this operation similarly has proved to be very satisfactory in reducing or eliminating both the varus and the anterior drawer instability of the ankle. Postoperatively there is loss of inversion, but this recovers to a limited extent within one year and does not appear to be a major problem for the patient.

METATARSALGIA AND OTHER COMMON FOOT PROBLEMS

R. PETER WELSH, M.B., Ch.B., F.R.C.S.(C), F.A.C.S.

"When the foot aches, the whole body aches!" To the sportsman with pain in the forefoot, the whole athletic performance is indeed compromised, and there are few injuries more frustrating to cope with than these ill-defined and often unresponsive maladies.

CLINICAL ENTITIES

Common foot problems include:

Intermetatarsal ligament strains and intermetatarsal bursitis
Morton's metatarsalgia
Stress fractures
Frieberg's infraction
Metatarsal prolapse and plantar callosities
Sesamoiditis
Bunions and bunionettes
Hallux rigidus
Hammer and claw toes

Intermetatarsal Ligament Strains and Intermetatarsal Bursitis

The running sports impose tremendous loads on the forefoot with impact forces of up to three times body weight at foot-plant and push-off. Intermetatarsal ligament complex is subject to tremendous strain, particularly with the demands of hard surface running, and with aging there is also a gradual splaying of the forefoot, imposing undue stress on this structure. Furthermore, inflammation of the intermetatarsal bursae occurs in response to the jostling motion with running activity, and this results in an ill-defined forefoot pain in the region between adjacent metatarsal heads and necks. Tender to touch, sensitive to loads, this condition may completely preclude running activity.

Morton's Neuroma

Morton's neuroma is a more distinctive entity; symptoms are quite specific, often with a lancinating jab of pain on footfall and an associated neuritis in the form of parasthetic sensations spreading down the adjacent borders of the affected toes in the digital nerve distribution. This condition is defined pathologically as a neuroma, but in reality is due to the bursitic involvement of the neurovascular complex at its intermetatarsal digital bifurcation.

Stress Fractures

Repetitive cycling of any structural element may lead to the development of fatigue fractures. Bone shows such a breach in the rigid cortex of the metatarsal neck area and occasionally near the base of the metatarsal.

In runners and dancers, other sites of these fractures are of course the distal fibular 2 inches above the tip of the lateral malleolus, the tibia about the junction of the proximal and mid one-third, and occasionally in the tibial plateau and the femoral condyle. Very rarely a stress fracture may be seen in the neck of the femur.

The breach in the cortex sets up an intense subperiosteal reaction, which is very painful and does not settle until there is new bone formation sufficient to consolidate the fracture focus. Radiographs may not be positive in the initial stages, and changes may not be observed until periosteal new bone is noted 3 to 4 weeks after injury. A technetium bone scan is often helpful in the early stages in differentiating a stress fracture from a simple intermetatarsal foot strain. The scan is only positive if there is actual bone involvement.

Frieberg's Infraction

A rare avascular necrosis of the metatarsal head, most commonly the second, is occasionally seen as a cause of metatarsalgia. The condition is known as one of the osteochondroses and is in fact akin to Perthes' disease of the hip. The metatarsal head is rendered dysvascular, and then, with regeneration, new bone is laid down on the old scaffold, but not before a fracture or partial collapse of the head distorts the shape of the metatarsal and deranges the metatarsal phalangeal articulation, leading in late stages to degenerative arthritis of the joint.

Metatarsal Prolapse and Plantar Callosities

Abnormal weight-bearing pressures beneath the metatarsal head result in the development of painful callosities. The collapse of the transverse arch of the foot sees the weight borne preferentially on the middle metatarsals instead of the first and fifth. Similarly, the development of an arthritic tendency at the base of the metatarsal may result in loss of flexibility in the foot and abnormal weight distribution across the forefoot without the normal resilience being shown at this level.

With prolapse of the metatarsal head, the prominence of the bone causes abnormal loading on the weight-bearing bursal pad with secondary thickening of the overlying skin, producing a hard callous.

Sesamoiditis

Should the abnormal pressures be maldistributed beneath the first metatarsal head, it is often the metatarsal sesamoids that bear the brunt of the load. Associated sesamoiditis and bursal inflammation may result. Furthermore the sesamoids, which are bones in the tendon of the short flexor of the great toe, are also subject to fracture and developmental abnormalities (they are often bipartite), and in the older individual, they are subject to arthritic change in their articulation with the metatarsal head.

Bunions and Bunionettes

A bunion is a painful bursitis overlying the medial prominence of the first metatarsal head. A bunionette is a similar state on the lateral aspect of the foot in relation to the fifth metatarsal head. In the great toe a bunion may be associated with hallux valgus or hallux rigidus, whereas a bunionette may also be associated with abnormal weight-bearing on the plantar aspect of the foot.

Hammer and Claw Toes

A flexion deformity of the interphalangeal joints of the toes may result in abnormal pressure areas with callous or corn formation overlying the prominence of the angulated joint. A hammer toe is associated with flexion at the DIP joint and extension at the metatarsophalangeal joint. A claw toe maintains a normal articulation at the metatarsophalangeal joint that involves a clawing or flexion deformity at either the PIP or DIP joints.

Hallux Rigidus

A disabling arthritis of the first metatarsophalangeal joint results in gross limitation of first metatarsal joint movement particularly in extension. This markedly limits participation in any of the running or jumping sports for without adequate dorsiflexion, push-off is severely inhibited. Often there is a strong familial tendency in the development of this condition, although it may also arise as a consequence of trauma involving the first metatarsophalangeal joint.

CLINICAL ASSESSMENT

The clinical diagnosis of the aforementioned conditions is, in most instances, obvious. In others, such as hallux rigidus, review of radiographs is required to confirm the extent of the condition, and if doubt exists in defining whether or not a metatarsal neck pain is related to a stress fracture, a technetium bone scan may be required.

In completing the assessment, particular care should be taken on examining the hindfoot, noting the mobility of associated ankle subtalar and midtarsal joints as well as the characteristics of the foot and the heel plant, and whether there is a varus or valgus disposition of the heel which will misdirect the forefoot placement. In all instances, the neurovascular status of the extremities should be carefully evaluated. The foot itself should never be examined in isolation from the rest of the individual. Particular importance is placed in the overall examination, noting the total limb alignment and whether there is a varus or valgus deformity or rotational anomaly of the limb more proximally. Any limb length inequalities should be noted and any rotational abnormality in the hip, femur, or tibia documented. The knee joint function, particularly patellar mechanics, is of vital concern with regards to the functioning of the foot. A tendency to genu valgum with a subluxating patella due to an increased "Q" angle will lead invariably to a displacement of the forefoot with a valgus tendency of the heel at foot-plant, resulting in abnormal hyperpronation of the forefoot.

Finally, in the clinical assessment, any abnormalities of the spine and its development should be noted; for example, scoliosis may affect foot mechanics.

MANAGEMENT OF METATARSALGIA AND FOOT DISORDERS

Management of these conditions may require (1) modification of sports activity, (2) footwear adaptation, (3) use of orthotics and other podiatric appliances, (4) physical therapies, (5) medications, and (6) surgery.

Modification of Sports Activity

Participation in many of the running and jumping sports have to be modified. Acute strains of the forefoot require rest from provocative loading; stress fractures cannot be subjected to more than normal daily walking and must heal completely before running can be resumed. Hallus rigidus may put an end completely to a dancer or jumper's career because of the inability to dorsiflex the great toe joint.

Footwear Adaptation

The footwear must be both protective and supportive, comfortably conforming to the foot. An arch support system should be adequate, but not bulky; of particular importance is the adequacy of heel control, which directs forefoot plant and push-off. Pressure points should be eliminated by stretching at sites of local irritation, or areas of pressure should be bridged so that the sensitive area fits into a relative recess.

Difference conditions dictate particular footwear requirements. With hallux rigidus, a stiff shank or even a rocker bottom sole may be of great assistance, whereas in many sports, a stiff shank may result in excessive loading of the heel at the bone-tendon junction and a predisposition to Achilles tendinitis. Obviously, footwear requirements must be tailored to the needs and condition of the patient.

Use of Orthotics and Other Podiatric Appliances

The role of orthotic supports has unfortunately been grossly overplayed. Nonetheless, customized adaptation of footwear has played a major part in the management of foot disorders.

Orthotics should in most instances be regarded as a temporary aid, just as a back brace aids an acutely injured spine. Most foot disorders suffered acutely are self-limiting, and a soft orthotic may assist by allowing continuance of the sports activity while the healing process occurs. However, once the injury has healed, the device should be discarded. Therefore, it makes no sense for an athlete who has run successfully for perhaps 5 or 10 years to feel that, because of a single foot injury, he must forever persist with an orthotic support in his shoe. Only if an injury proves recurrent and major structural abnormality is seen to benefit from the use of an orthotic should a more permanent device be prescribed.

It should be remembered that an orthotic device occupies space in a shoe and adds weight to the foot, and that by the employment of these aids, even a subtle alteration of foot-plant and push-off must call for compensatory adjustment in the gait pattern elsewhere, at the level of the knee, hip, or spine.

The type of orthotic employed varies according to the condition from which the patient suffers. Orthotics may be of great value in acute long arch strains, in which case an arch support and scaphoid cookie greatly reduce load on the arch structure. A more rigid device is required for the patient with hallux rigidus to restrict pressures on the great toe joint, but such rigidity may throw loads at the heel and cause Achilles tendinitis.

In managing metatarsal problems there is no need for the major building-in of a long arch system into the orthotic; all that is required is a metatarsal pad support beneath the metatarsal neck to elevate and separate the metatarsal heads and reduce their compressive tendency on weight-bearing. This device also may be very effective in the management of Morton's neuroma.

There has been a great tendency to overprescribe orthotics for what is termed the hyperpronated or flat foot. There is such a wide range of what may be considered the normal arch height that to arbitrarily offer orthotics to the flatter-appearing foot totally disregards how that individual may function with that particular foot form. The arbitrary prescription of orthotics in these instances can be more harmful than beneficial, but if injury does prove resistant to other modalities of treatment, and proven benefit is obtained by a soft orthotic device, then prescription of more permanent orthotics should be considered. Otherwise, most orthotics should be used on a temporary basis to assist the athlete through the healing of an injury. It is probably better to further customize the footwear itself than to add redundancy in the form of orthotic devices to the athlete's shoes.

In most instances, soft, resilient orthotics are preferred to the more rigid materials often prescribed. Even though these more rigid materials may prove more durable in regard to the life of the device itself, it is better to have a system that conforms more to the texture of both the shoe and the foot structures than to have a rigid interface between the foot and the shoe.

Other appliances that may be useful are doughnut protective devices over pressure points to prevent friction between the foot and the shoe, e.g., over a bunion or hammer toe prominence. Care must be paid in general to the skin of the foot, with careful attention to any cracks or ulcer areas. A tendency to interdigital fungal infection usually can be handled adequately with topical antifungal agents.

Physical Therapies

As a species, man has lost much of his capacity to individual control of the intrinsic musculature of the foot. Physical therapy aimed at assisting intrinsic function can be of extreme benefit. In this regard, faradic foot baths may be employed to initiate intrinsic response, and teaching of intrinsic exercises may be of considerable benefit.

Passive stretching of deforming digits and stiffening toes is a worthwhile endeavor.

Local measures, such as icing and ultrasound, may have empiric value; if no benefit is obviously arising from their employment, treatment should be discontinued.

Medications

Systemic medication has little place in the management of most of these conditions, but local steroid injections between the metatarsal heads may settle acute bursitis and benefit a Morton's neuroma. Sesamoiditis may also respond to local infiltration. As a general rule in most treatments, if one injection does not help, there seems little justification for continuing treatments of that type, and if one injection works, there is no cause for further treatment.

Surgery

Foot problems of some athletes prove to be both refractory to treatment and sufficiently disabling to preclude any sports participation. These require definitive surgical treatment.

Morton's Neuroma. Local interdigital exploration allows the resection of the involved bursal scar tissue enveloping the bifurcation of the digital nerve and interdigital space. Tourniquet control of circulation greatly aids the dissection in these instances, and a web space incision is favored: this gives a clear view of the whole intermetatarsal space both dorsally and on the plantar aspect.

Frieberg's Infraction. Metatarsal neck osteotomy decompresses the involved metatarsophalangeal joint in addition to easing the weight-bearing load on the affected metatarsal head.

Metatarsal Prolapse and Plantar Callosities. Elevation of the affected metatarsal head by metatarsal neck osteotomy decompresses the lesser and overlying calloused skin. An oblique osteotomy just proximal to the head allows the head to slide up and shorten slightly. Weight-bearing is allowed immediately, but the fracture requires 4 to 6 weeks to unite. The return to sport may be delayed 2 to 3 months by swelling and tenderness.

The patient should be closely observed postoperatively for transfer of weight from one metatarsal to the adjacent metatarsal head, which may necessitate another decompressive osteotomy.

Sesamoiditis. Excision of the sesamoids for nonunion or avascular necrosis or osteoarthritis can be extremely rewarding. Care must be taken to avoid injury to the digital nerves or flexor tendon.

Bunions. If the bunion is associated with hallux valgus, the local excision of the bunion must always be carried out in conjunction with correction of the hallux valgus. In addition, any degree of metatarsus varus should be corrected by metatarsal osteotomy, preferably at the base of the first metatarsal.

Preservation of the intact joint should be practiced whenever possible, and procedures such as the McBride procedure are preferred to excisional remedies such as a Keller procedure.

Bunionettes. The fifth metatarsal head should never be excised in the athlete or a tendency to rolling over and a sense of weakness will always prevail. Instead, in addition to a local bunionette excision, an oblique medializing osteotomy of the neck of the fifth metatarsal allows both correction of the lateral deviating metatarsal head and upward correction of any abnormal weight-bearing pressure point.

Hallux Rigidus. In the athlete, excisional arthroplasty may be necessary, with excision of the base of the proximal phalanx removing sufficient bone to permit adequate dorsiflexion of the joint. Careful capsular reconstruction is essential, but tension on the great toe joint must be minimal at the conclusion of the procedure. The use of interposition material, as with silastic arthroplasty, has little place in the athlete; these materials cannot prove durable to the repetitive load demands of active athletic endeavor.

Metatarsal phalangeal fusion has a definite place in certain individuals. It provides a totally pain-free, strong push-off, but limits the type of footwear that can be used and its success relies on complete mobility of the associated joints at the DIP and the base of the first metatarsal.

Greater morbidity of this procedure, the risk of nonunion, and the necessity for careful technical considerations in obtaining the correct angle of the MTP joint make this a demanding technique. In general, the excisional procedure is favored in dancers and jumpers.

Hammer and Claw Toes. For hammer toes with PIP hyperextension, if the joint remains mobile and the metatarsal phalangeal joint is not subluxated, a flexor to extensor tendon transfer is recommended.

If the PIP deformity is fixed, an IP fusion is preferred; if the MTP joint is concurrently subluxated, a partial excision of the base of the proximal phalanx is added.

For claw toes at the DIP joint, a Jones repair, excising a transverse dorsal elipse of skin, tendon, and a bone wedge at the DIP joint, provides a completely durable correction.

ORTHOTIC SUPPORT FOR THE FOOT

CHARLES R. BULL, M.D., B.Sc.(Med),
F.R.C.S.(C), F.A.C.S., F.I.C.S.

During the past decade running has become popular. With this explosion in the number of runners came sports clinics, podiatrists, orthotists, brace makers, and pedorthists, and the number of running shoe companies went from three to probably fifty. Currently, almost anyone with discomfort in their feet, ankles, knees, hips, or back now wears an orthosis.

Ortho is derived from the Greek word "orthos" denoting straight. Thus orthotics means a pursuit of straightening or correcting. An orthotic device, or orthosis, is similar to a brace or splint, but connotes an attempt to limit, straighten or assist the body in an alignment problem. Orthotic devices for the feet attempt to structurally align the entire lower extremity in order to take pressure off the foot, ankle, shin, knee, hip, and possibly back. The orthotist spends as much time trying to line up the knees and hips as he does correcting the abnormality of the feet. Thus, if he can line up the great toe, patella, and anterior superior spine and have uniform spacing between the ankles and knees he feels successful. An attempt is made to toe out the foot slightly by 15 degrees. This is accomplished through the foot rather than through external rotation of the tibia, and a correction of the valgus or inturned heel is also attempted when the orthotic device is made. The exact location of the mechanical axis of the ankle corresponding to the subtalar joint, allowing for tibial torsion, is a key factor in fashioning orthoses.

These orthoses are basically inserts which can be interchanged from shoe to shoe, but more positive control is possible with caliper bracing, ankle joint stirrups, spring-loaded rods with a ring attachment to the knee.

Orthoses can be prefabricated (ready-made off the shelf) or tailor-made. Most are made of plastic or a Neoprene type of material although they have been made of metal, stainless steel and aluminum, hard plastic, hard and soft rubber, as well as stiffened felt components. Prices vary from a few dollars to as much as $400. The orthoses made by an orthotist under the direction of a physician and molded to the patient's foot at the time of fabrication are inexpensive and continue to be effective for at least 2 years. The podiatrist's orthoses are more sophisticated and more expensive, and they tend to be more effective in difficult cases. They are smaller and better fit the running shoe.

The ready-made orthotics from Spenko or Dr. Scholl (soft rubbery type material) can be satisfactory, although they usually are not. The more substantial plastic skeleton type are better, but do not naturally correct all types of foot abnormalities. The soft tailor-made orthotic with Sorbothane or PVT tends to be a little bulky. It needs a deeper shoe to hold the orthosis and to keep the wearer from falling out of the shoe, but it usually does a very satisfactory job.

The podiatrist's orthosis made by Langer Laboratories of Deerpark, New York can be made from a casting of the runner's foot. The cast is made with care to maintain the foot in neutral position and align with the hind foot in a similar neutral position with some pressure under the fourth and fifth metatarsal heads and the talonavicular joint. This then creates a negative impression of the plantar surface of the foot; Langer then makes a positive plaster cast and fashions the plastic orthosis to that cast. An acrylic heel and anterior post are bonded to this case, and the initial pronation or longitudinal abnormality is corrected. More posting or correction can be done once the orthosis is fitted to the runner by the podiatrist.

We have compared video tapes of runners running with normal foot structure and pronated feet with tapes of runners wearing custom-made orthoses that (1) fit correctly, (2) are undercorrective, and (3) are overcorrective. It is difficult to draw an accurate conclusion from this type of study, but the correction of the pronation usually has to be very accurate or the running gait is made appreciably worse by an incorrect orthotic device.

The orthotic device is of most benefit for foot, ankle, and knee overuse problems such as fasciitis and tendinitis. We doubt that it does much for a true hip problem, and the effect on the back certainly is miniscule. Commonly the patient has pronated feet and valgus heels and knees.

Overweight, poor running style, inexperience—all contribute to an altered footplant. The constant repetitive incorrect plant in running causes accumulated stress on the entire lower limb. Runners comprised 58 percent of the patients receiving orthoses in our sports clinic.

It is important to see an abnormal wear pattern on the running shoe. I set the running shoe itself on a flat surface to see how much it is falling inward. The ideal running shoe should be either neutral or fall outward slightly if the runner plants properly.

I also have the patient stand facing me with his feet parallel and approximately a foot apart to see how much of an arch he has and then have him turn around to see how much valgus deformity there is to the heels. The Achilles tendon should be completely vertical when the patient is standing relaxed. Then the patient lies face down with his heels out over the end of the bed and again the degree of valgus deformity is measured, and forefoot and rearfoot pronation are noted.

I want to emphasize that the mere presence of flatfeet does not necessitate orthotic correction. There are hundreds of runners with flatfeet and no symptoms, many of whom have won every major race in the country. It can be a racial or ethnic factor—the majority of blacks and North American Indians tend to have flat feet, for instance. These people do not need correction unless they are having symptoms of overuse.

PLANTAR FASCIITIS

The plantar fascia is an inflexible band of tough tissue that is prone to inflammation where it originates from the calcaneus. The point is a central focus for maximum stress, and the inflammation often is localized.

Initial treatment with a felt pad or heel lift or with a Sorbothane heel lift is often beneficial, but if the patient has significant pronation which causes an increased stretching and strain on the plantar fascia, suitably designed orthoses probably help decrease the problem. Elevation of the heel in this type of correction distributes more of the forces toward the forefoot. Initially we were taught that the pressures were distributed, with 50 percent of the force of walking or running taken in the heel, and then the force fanned out, with the hallux taking two units of force and each of the other four metatarsals taking one. This concept has changed as a result of biomechanical sensor studies. The consensus is that the heel actually takes more than 50 percent of the weight, and the load transfers down through the second and third metatarsals, leaving less weight or pressure on the first, fourth, and fifth metatarsal areas. Thus the dynamics of correcting plantar fasciitis involve getting a lot of that weight off the heel or area of plantar fascia origin. These patients should be encouraged to wear their orthoses all day long. In difficult cases appropriate physiotherapy, medications, injections, and even surgery are indicated along with the orthosis.

ACHILLES TENDINITIS

This inflammation, which accounts for approximately 11 percent of all the running injuries seen in our clinic, is attributed to micro tears in the tendon causing inflammmation of the adjacent tendon structures (i.e., the vestigial sheath), which can become chronic and even calcifies in rare cases.

Initial treatment consists of rest, cycling, and swimming (but no running), anti-inflammatory agents, and elevation of the heel with felt or Sorbothane pads. The wearing of moderately high heels, such as cowboy boots, may help by (1) causing relative shortening of the Achilles tendon, (2) causing absorption of forces transmitted to the tendon, and (3) resting the tendon and allowing the micro tears to heal.

Varus deformities of the feet have been recognized in runners by the use of high speed films. The average runner lands on the outer heel, and the forces transfer to the outer side of the foot through the mid-stance phase. If he over pronates through this phase, the Achilles undergoes a "whip-like" action in its sequence. Obviously this initiates, aggravates, and perpetuates the tendinitis. Orthotic correction will reduce this type of motion. The gait will have more of a light productive force, and less stress will be transferred to the Achilles.

Once the tendinitis has subsided, the tendon is stretched and the gastrocmemius-soleus complex is strengthened. With this additional strength and flexibility, the runner should be able to plant better and, after a year or two, dispense with the orthosis. I want to emphasize that many orthoses can be used temporarily. At least 6 months is required to settle an acute problem,

and many people improve their running style, strength, and flexibility and thus can dispense with the orthosis after a year or two. This is particularly true in the mature, high-quality runner who has functioned for years without injury. His orthotic device can be used on a temporary basis, and eventually a shoe with a good support, especially a strong heel support, will suffice.

TIB POSTERIOR TENDINITIS

This inflammation occurs at the junction of the posterior tibial muscle and tendon in the midportion of the medial aspect of the leg. It is the most common type of "shin splint" and its most likely cause is "pronated feet". "Shin splints" or inflammation of the shin area (common in runners) can occur in tib posterior or the periosteum overlying the free tibial border (classic location) or in the anterior (lateral) compartment. All three types usually benefit from the use of orthotics.

The muscle functions to help maintain the arch of the foot and to supinate the foot so that it can roll out after footplant. A pronated foot stretches the tendon and muscles, and as the foot pronates through the mid-stance phase, there is an increased force transmitted to the muscle-tendinous junction and into the muscle origin along the tibia. Micro tears result and create inflammation (tendinitis).

An orthotic device will shorten the muscle tendon complex and lessen the necessity to maintain the arch and supinate the foot. Thus there will be less strain as the foot pronates through the mid-phase of the running motion. Correction of foot pronation is probably the most important step in relieving the initial inflammation and preventing recurrence. In some cases, if it is left uncorrected, the condition progresses to periostitis and/or a compartment syndrome or even a stress fracture.

PATELLOFEMORAL SYNDROME

This is the most common problem seen in our sports clinic. The etiology, reason for pain, management, response to treatment, and long-term sequelae are all controversial.

The most realistic cause is a "malalignment phenomenon". The patella travels in the femoral groove, and as the knee flexes beyond 135 degrees or a quarter squat, the compression between surfaces increases.

Ideally the patella tracks symmetrically, but in chondromalacia there appears to be asymmetry. This causes abnormal wear and tear on the patellar surface and thus a softening or roughening, which is manifested clinically by a grating when the patella is moved on the femoral surface. This situation is particularly uncomfortable when the patella is held against a strong quads contraction. What is incomprehensible is that some of the worst clinical cases exhibit minimal signs arthroscopically. Other clinical signs are widened Q-angle, noticeable infacing or squinting of the patella, broad pelvis, femoral antiversion, genu valgus, external tibial rotation, and pronated feet. A correction of the pronated feet by an orthosis will alter the alignment of the leg. This is relative, similar to eyeglasses correcting short-sightedness. Basically, the malalignment returns when the orthoses are not used. Thus tracking will be more efficient and cause less irritation on the patellar articular surface and thereby reduce the pain. Adjunctive treatment includes vastus medialis strengthening and the use of a knee brace for patellar stabilization.

OTHER KNEE PROBLEMS

Pes tendinitis is an inflammation of the pes, which is a confluence of three tendons on the medial aspect of the knee. Because these tendons mesh together so congruently at the knee they are relatively prone to tendinitis, particularly in the presence of genu valgus. An orthotic device tends to transfer the forces laterally and take the pressure off this medial compartment of the knee. Conversely, ileotibial band and popliteus tendinitis are helped by a lateral wedge, which eases the lateral forces in the knee. In many cases, an orthotic device makes this type of problem worse.

VAGUE KNEE PAINS

The best treatment for fat pad syndrome, synovitis, plicae, IDK, and patellar tendinitis is alteration of the running schedule, i.e., decreased hills, decreased speed, new shoes, quadriceps-hamstring exercises to correct an imbalance, increased flexibility, and anti-inflammatory medications.

In a resistant case it is worthwhile to watch the patient run. If he tends to pronate, throw his feet in or out, or have a heavy wide-track Pontiac style, orthoses may help. It is hard to correct the running style in a master athlete. The orthotic devices alter the style subtly, and thereby help to decrease the problem.

CAVUS FOOT

This is almost a contraindication to running. The relatively spastic high-arched foot is very uncomfortable with ordinary walking. It can become unbearable with running. An orthotic device can cushion the impact, but usually cannot create a good mobile running foot.

SUCCESS RATE AND COMPLIANCE

In our study of soft orthotic devices in which 100 patients were reviewed after 1 year, 89 percent felt that the orthoses were of definite benefit; 38 percent limited the use of their orthoses to sports shoes only, while the rest used them in all their shoes; 21 percent stopped using them because the problem had been solved; 69 percent

were still using them after one year; 10 percent stopped using them because they were of no benefit; and 47 percent returned for a check of their orthoses. It is important to check them at the 3- or 4-week point and again after 3 or 4 months to ascertain that correction is satisfactory. Minor adjustments can make the world of difference in their use. In the same series, 9 percent sought the advice of a podiatrist after receiving their orthoses. Probably 10 to 20 percent of runners use orthotic devices. We have prescribed over a thousand in the past 10 years. We wanted to know (1) whether this was necessary, and (2) whether the patient used them. In our series, 69 percent of the 100 patients still used them after one year, and 21 percent discarded them because their problem was solved. Thus we feel orthoses have been beneficial.

Soft orthotic devices are much less expensive than those prescribed by the podiatrist and can be more comfortable. We believe that they can be used on a long-term basis to correct a biomechanical problem.

Studies of the hard orthotics prescribed by the podiatrist often cannot delineate a correction of pronation when the runner is filmed or studied biomechanically. However, orthotic devices do work. Podiatrists have been a definite boon to the runner, often eliminating pain experienced in running. Obviously, the development of quality running shoes has also helped to prevent running injuries.

Orthotics can be applied to other sports. Certainly the use of orthoses in ski boots has been helpful in some cases. Ski boots can also be canted extrinsically to correct a pronated foot. This basically serves the same purpose as an orthosis. Most stop-and-start sports, such as squash and tennis, do not require an orthosis as the unremitting footplant that occurs in running creates a more serious problem. Thus orthotic devices are used in racquet sports, but they are not as necessary or popular.

The principle of orthosis construction, patient selection, and the biomechanical studies of different sports will change markedly in the next few years. Orthotic devices can be beneficial for specific problems, but should be used in conjunction with other methods of treatment. Certainly strengthening programs for the entire lower limb should be instituted when the orthoses are prescribed. In my experience, careful patient selection is the key to proper orthoses use. If patients are made aware of the exact indications for orthoses and are observed closely and instructed in their use, the vast majority of patients should improve. It is only the rare patient with a cavus foot, for instance, who continues to have disability after using the orthoses and cannot tolerate the orthoses. The old time runner from the 1950s and 60s, who had one pair of shoes which he or she discarded when the sole fell off, was guaranteed to have blisters, missing toenails, general aches and pains, which he did not acknowledge to anyone. The modern runner complains if the workout is less than 100 percent. He or she makes use of sports clinics, podiatrists, orthoses, and coaches, and probably runs a lot longer, farther, and faster in comfort. In many cases this is due to the use of orthotic devices.

REHABILITATION AND THERAPY

EXERCISE AND MUSCLE SORENESS

HARM KUIPERS, M.D., Ph.D.
EUGENE JANSSEN, B.S.

Physical activity is generally considered beneficial to physical health, but symptoms of overuse of the locomotor system frequently interfere with such activity. Any part of the locomotor system may be affected, but the part that shows symptoms of overuse most commonly is skeletal muscle.

Muscle soreness and stiffness after exercise occur frequently in untrained people who start a regimen of physical exercise. The better the individual's state of physical conditioning, the more exercise can be tolerated before symptoms of overuse develop. Acute overuse and muscular soreness are also seen in well-trained athletes who perform unaccustomed types of exercise.

CLINICAL FEATURES

The symptoms of moderate acute muscular overuse usually begin after termination of the exercise and reach their maximal intensity 24 to 48 hours later. During the first hours after stopping work, only mild stiffness and discomfort are present; nevertheless, the symptoms are clearly felt if the rest period is followed by renewed activity. Twenty-four hours later, the affected muscles feel sore during any activity and are painful to touch and to stretch. In severe cases, the muscles become swollen and feel hardened to palpation.

The localization of the soreness is strongly dependent on the type of exercise that has been performed. In runners, for instance, soreness and stiffness are seen most frequently in the soleus and gastrocnemius muscles.

Extreme muscular soreness reflects acute overuse, which may occur after protracted heavy exercise, such as running a marathon. It has also been reported in military recruits who perform severe and unusual exercises during their basic training. The clinical symptoms comprise severe delayed-onset muscle pain, soreness, and stiffness which are present not only during exercise, but also in the resting state. The affected muscles are swollen and feel hardened to the touch. The range of motion of adjacent joints may be decreased considerably because of the patient's inability to stretch the affected muscles passively. The symptoms reach a maximum intensity 24 to 48 hours after exercise and gradually decrease over the course of 3 to 7 days. Myoglobinuria, characterized by dark red urine, is observed in a proportion of severe cases; it indicates severe muscular damage and can lead to renal insufficiency. The plasma activity of muscular enzymes such as creatine phosphokinase (CPK), aspartate aminotransferase (AST), malate dehydrogenase (MDH), and lactate dehydrogenase (LDH) are increased considerably in such cases, supporting the diagnosis of muscular damage.

Histologic specimens taken from sore muscles reveal edema, necrosis, and inflammation of the muscle tissue; the combination of tissue damage and myoglobinuria is sometimes described as rhabdomyolysis.

Mild muscle soreness and stiffness may result from both acute and chronic overuse. In the latter case the soreness is mild, being felt particularly at the onset of renewed activity. The affected muscles are somewhat painful to touch and to stretch. In this connection, it is worth mentioning that the medical history of Achilles tendon disorders often starts with mild soreness of the soleus and gastrocnemius muscles.

PATHOPHYSIOLOGIC BASIS OF MUSCLE SORENESS

There are two main theories concerning the pathophysiologic basis of delayed-onset muscle soreness: an increased electrical activity of the muscle fibers and structural changes in the affected muscle.

Spasm Theory

The first theory is based on spontaneous, involuntary contraction of certain motor units (spasm theory). On palpation, the whole of a relaxed muscle may feel hardened and may be painful to the touch, but often there are localized hardened strands. Some investigators hypothesize that these hardened and painful strands consist of involuntarily contracting motor units which suffer local ischemia and resultant pain. The hypothesis was supported by a demonstration of increased electromyographic (EMG) activity in the relaxed state, as recorded by surface electrodes. These findings have been challenged and criticized by others. Investigations from our laboratory using needle electrodes (which allowed registration of single-fiber activity) have shown that the hardened strands are electrically silent when the muscle is relaxed. Based on these findings and the work of other investigators, little support remains for the spasm theory.

Structural Damage

The second theory is based on the premise that exercise induces structural damage in muscle. Several different structures deserve consideration. Some investigators report an increased OH-proline and methylhistidine excretion in urine after severe exercise. This indicates an increased turnover rate for connective tissue. Recent investigations in which eccentric exercise was used to induce muscle soreness confirm that damage to connective tissue can occur, although this is probably not the main cause of muscle soreness, since soreness can also develop after a period of ischemia without the imposition of any mechanical stress.

Recent research has demonstrated structural changes in the muscle fibers. Experiments with eccentric exercise have shown repeatedly that structural damage occurs in the myofibrils. Some investigations also report sarcolemmal damage. These structural changes do not completely explain either the delayed onset of muscular soreness or the delayed enzyme release. Since specimens of muscle obtained from patients with rhabdomyolysis show an inflammatory reaction, it has been postulated that the pain and soreness are related to inflammation. A study performed in our laboratory in which untrained rats were used showed that immediately after submaximal exercise, there were only minor changes in the loaded muscles, such as a disorientation of the myofibrils. Two hours after ceasing exercise, myofibrillar damage was more extensive, and leukocytes had started to infiltrate the affected muscle fibers. The inflammatory reaction reached its peak 24 to 48 hours after work. Thereafter, it subsided, and regeneration was complete within about 2 weeks. A remarkable finding was that the inflammatory and degenerative changes affected only a limited number of muscle fibers, which were randomly distributed through the body of the muscle. The abnormal fibers were focally damaged, as noted on examination of serial sections. The length of the injury varied from 50 to 1500 μ. Since the time sequence of these inflammatory changes matched the subjective symptoms in humans, these findings support the hypothesis that soreness is related to an inflammatory process. Additionally, focal inflammatory changes have been shown in man too, and the time sequence of the mentioned histologic changes is similar to those in rats.

The delayed onset of the inflammatory reaction may explain the delayed release of muscle enzymes and myoglobin; membrane permeability is probably affected adversely by the inflammatory reaction. In a recent study it was found that marathon runners showed a delayed release of muscle enzymes after the marathon with a peak after 24 to 48 hours. A treadmill test 4 and 6 days later elicited a renewed enzyme release, which occurred more quickly and was maximal 5 hours after the test. This suggests that the sarcolemmal permeability recovers in some days, but remains sensitive for a longer period of time.

Mechanical factors make an important contribution to structural damage. Muscle soreness and enzyme release are often observed in runners, whereas in cyclists heavy exertion does not seem to cause either soreness or enzyme release. This may reflect the large mechanical impact stress during running. Protracted exercise is another factor predisposing to muscular damage. By varying the duration of the exercise but keeping the workload constant, we showed that not only the intensity, but also the duration of exercise, determined the extent of structural damage and consequently muscle soreness. It seems that muscle tissue can withstand a certain amount of mechanical stress determined by the combination of duration and intensity, and that loading beyond a certain "threshold" induces structural damage.

In patients with inborn errors of metabolism, muscle soreness occurs easily after relatively mild exercise. The metabolic disturbances may interfere with cellular homeostasis at different levels, evoking both structural changes and an inflammatory reaction.

PLASMA ACTIVITY OF MUSCLE ENZYMES AND MUSCULAR OVERUSE

Muscle enzymes are normally unable to permeate the sarcolemma. An increased activity of such enzymes in the peripheral blood indicates that sarcolemmal permeability has increased. It is thus conceivable to use plasma activity as an indicator of muscular overuse. However, there are many pitfalls to this approach. After normal training, the plasma activity of muscle enzymes may rise without any complaints of muscular origin, whereas muscle soreness may occur without a concomitant increase in plasma activity of muscle enzymes. Although a gross relationship between structural damage, muscle soreness, and increased plasma activity exists, small changes should be interpreted with caution, and a moderate increase of activity may be a physiologic response to exercise. Plasma enzyme data should be regarded as an additional tool, but considerable weight must be given to subjective symptoms of muscular fatigue and eventual soreness. The plasma activity of muscle enzymes alone does not provide adequate guidance for training, and it can easily lead to misinterpretation.

MEASURES TO PREVENT MUSCLE OVERUSE

An important measure to prevent muscle overuse is to increase the amount and the intensity of training gradually, never forgetting a proper warm-up. Changes in the pattern of training (for instance, beginning running after a longer period of inactivity) should be handled with care. The first bout should consist of 20 to 30 minutes of slow running. Elderly people and overweight individuals are advised to precede regular running by a walking program. In order to allow sufficient time for recovery and adaptational changes, running on alternate days is advisable. After some weeks the frequency and speed can be increased. The most common cause of jogging and running injuries and complaints of muscle soreness is lack of patience, since generally people do too much too soon or do not take sufficient rest periods after each training session. Special attention should be paid to footwear and clothing. In runners footwear is most critical in preventing overuse of the locomotor system. In cool conditions (below approximately 15°C), lower limbs should be protected from cooling by appropriate clothing.

Measures to increase recovery should be stressed in training. Cooling down and performing stretching exercises should be an important part of every training session. Although the physiologic basis is incompletely understood, sports practice has shown that regular stretching is a valid means of preventing injuries. Massage of muscles heavily involved in the exercise can also be helpful in preventing or diminishing stiffness and soreness. Self-massage can easily be learned by athletes, and it is an excellent way to prevent injuries. Massage of the calf muscles can be effective in preventing problems with the Achilles tendons, and in people who are susceptible to overuse of the adductor muscles, local massage can prevent pain in the groin region.

TREATMENT OF MUSCLE SORENESS

Although everyone has experienced muscle soreness, its occurrence must be interpreted as a symptom of muscle overuse. In principle the treatment consists of diminishing the amount of work to allow complete recovery. In general, elderly people, weekend enthusiasts, and overweight individuals need a longer period for recovery. Within certain limits a better physical condition results in a faster recovery. Occasional soreness after unusual or long-lasting exercise, however, does not need special attention. In most cases, 1 or 2 days without exercise, or with only mild exercise, will relieve the complaints. Stretching exercises instead of regular training and light massage are recommended. (Stretching should always be preceded by a proper warm up.) If mild soreness and stiffness occur in the course of training, it points to an imbalance between exercise and recovery. Therefore, it is always important to be attentive to the physical

signals of the body. Mild muscle soreness and stiffness noted after waking or during training should be interpreted as overuse. It implies that the amount and intensity of training should be decreased and that special attention should be directed to measures increasing recovery. Experience has taught that low-intensity exercise has a favorable effect on muscle soreness. Additionally, massage and stretching exercises are helpful in accelerating the recovery process. Without any special treatment, muscle soreness melts away in 2 to 4 days; with application of the measures mentioned, the period may be shortened 1 or 2 days. If soreness is sufficiently severe to inhibit exercise, the patient should abstain from training for a couple of days and replace regular exercise by stretching. One should always respect the occurrence of pain during training or stretching. If a dark urine is reported in addition to soreness, rhabdomyolysis with myoglobinuria has to be considered and medical advice and regular control of renal function are recommended. One should also abstain from training. Complaints disappear in about 5 days without any special treatment and thereafter training can be restored gradually. Rhabdomyolysis and myoglobinuria are reported occasionally after a marathon, triathlon, or other long events. Also susceptible are people who are insufficiently conditioned, such as weekend enthusiasts. Insufficient replacement of fluid during the race is a predisposing factor in rhabdomyolysis. Occasional rhabdomyolysis without further complications does not need special treatment except control of renal function. Those who are susceptible should be advised to prepare properly and to drink sufficiently during exercise, especially in hot conditions. In some people, severe muscle soreness and/or myoglobinuria develop on more than one occasion without heavy exertion. This tendency to muscle soreness needs further medical investigation. It may indicate an inborn error of metabolism, as proved to be the case in a number of our patients. In some cases, susceptibility to muscle overuse was associated with histologic evidence of a myopathy. With the increasing number of people who are involved in physical activity, new metabolic disorders will be discovered.

Little is known about the effects of drugs on muscle soreness. Anti-inflammatory drugs are given, but there is no substantial evidence to support their effectiveness. In one study in humans a prostaglandin antagonist (the cyclo-oxygenase inhibitor, ibuprofen) was tested, but it had no influence on the subjective feelings of soreness and on the exercise-induced inflammatory response. Since in most cases muscle soreness is a self-limiting condition and substantial evidence of the effectiveness of drugs is lacking, the application of analgesics and anti-inflammatory drugs in uncomplicated muscle soreness may be questioned.

THE PHYSIOTHERAPIST'S ARMAMENTARIUM

MARY-ANN DALZELL, B.Ph.Th., M.Sc.

Timely and adequate physiotherapeutic treatment of sports-related injuries can significantly reduce the common sequelae of soft tissue disruption and prevent the recurrence of injury. Persistent pain, joint stiffness, muscular spasm, weakness, and inflexibility need not be the "hallmarks of a former athlete". Indeed, the role of the physiotherapist has been developed to focus upon a full restoration of functional capacity prior to reintegration into demanding sports, thereby minimizing long-term complications.

In a clinical setting, the source of referrals for therapy among weekend as well as elite athletes ought to begin in the emergency department, including sports clinic candidates and those presenting in the offices of family practitioners. Implementation of treatment for strains, sprains, severe contusions, and tendinopathies resulting from overuse ideally begins without delay. In the vast majority of sports-related injuries, there are *no indications* for: cast immobilization in the absence of a fracture or an injury needing surgical attention; non-weight-bearing instructions without advice on activity progressions; and anti-inflammatory medications without full rehabilitation of the involved and anatomically related musculoskeletal segments. Likewise, there is generally no time for the medical practitioner to supervise athletes during the various phases of healing and reintegration to full activity. Therefore, the physiotherapist must accept these responsibilities and, in conjunction with the physician, devise an adequate treatment program.

PRINCIPLES OF PHYSIOTHERAPEUTIC TREATMENT

During the acute inflammatory phase of healing, the objectives of treatment are to relieve pain, reduce swelling, increase the local blood supply, debride soft tissues of any necrotic remnants, and protect injured structures. Physical and electrical modalities, such as ice and ultrasound, are capable of accomplishing these tasks in conjunction with anti-inflammatory medications and compression taping. Weight-bearing need be limited only when the involved tissues are directly stressed during the gait cycle. Otherwise, normal physiologic input to the injured structures must be maintained to avoid unnecessary atrophy of muscles and ligaments, while ensuring that cartilaginous lubrication and the neurologic input to joint capsules and proprioceptors are not compromised by disuse. Isometric exercises can be implemented immediately, unless associated with pain. The formerly active individual is more compliant with treatment when encouraged to maintain accustomed levels of conditioning by substituting a sport which does not directly stress the injured tissues. For example, swimming and cycling can be substituted for full weight-bearing activities, while if the upper limb is injured, jogging, cycling, or trunk and lower limb weight-training can be recommended. Any exercises that cause pain, an increase in articular effusion, or muscle spasm must be avoided, as must any exercise that could elongate healing structures during the critical period of collagen deposition.

The duration of the acute inflammatory stage depends on the type of tissue injured and the severity of the induced lesion. Thus progression from the stage of full protection to that of moderate protection is governed by our knowledge of the individual rates and capacities for regeneration of ligaments, muscle, joint capsules, and articular cartilage as well as by clinical signs and symptoms. Graduated stress to the healing structure ensures differentiation of soft tissues in a fashion that will absorb the strains they were designed to accommodate. Gradual re-establishment of full strength, flexibility, and endurance are the primary goals of treatment during this subacute stage.

Prior to discharge, evaluation of the demands that the individual's sport will impose upon the newly healed soft tissues is essential in order to avoid premature overloading. The therapist ensures that proprioceptive reactions, timing, coordination, and power output are restored and, on a periodic basis, reviews training progressions. Decisions whether protective tape, braces, or shoe orthotics are necessary to avoid a recurrence of injury or the development of other related problems must be made in conjunction with the attending physician and the athlete concerned.

In summary, rehabilitation of sports-related injuries must be based upon the response of normal soft tissue to injury and the specific level of training to which the athlete will return. To enhance recovery, therapeutic modalites are chosen in the light of their potential physiologic effects. Thermal modalities, electrical modalities, manual articular mobilizations, and exercise progressions must be selectively used to promote healing, prevent the unnecessary persistence of symptoms after an injury has healed, and prepare the athlete for participation in sport.

UPDATE ON THERAPEUTIC MODALITIES

The use of heat and massage is currently out of favor and cryotherapy and exercise are in favor in relation to their respective effects on the inflammatory process, the relief of pain, muscle spasm, and inflexibility. Traditionally, these thermal and mechanical modalities were used interchangeably, with dependence on their psychologic rather than their physiologic effects. However, recent research has failed to document more than transient responses to heat and massage, whereas ice applications can reduce the local rate of metabolism, vastly influencing neurological structures and priming muscle for work.

Thermal Modalities

The application of superficial heat causes a vasodilatation which persists for approximately one hour after the heat has been removed. At the other end of the temperature spectrum, cooling to temperatures of 3° C induces a reflex sympathetic vasoconstriction, together with a direct vasoconstriction by cooling of blood vessels. Below 2° C, a reflex vasodilatation is evoked to prevent tissue damage. Therefore prolonged ice applications are characterized by alternating vasoconstriction and vasodilatation (the hunting reaction). This reaction is mediated by axon reflexes as opposed to hormonal or blood pressure alterations. In addition, the blood flow and the local rate of metabolism decrease as the temperature of the soft tissue falls. Thus, from a practical perspective, application of ice to an acute athletic injury can prevent excessive bleeding and reduce tissue damage from secondary hypoxia. The duration of application must be consistent with the size of the anatomic segment it is hoped to cool, and with the amount of subcutaneous fat interposed between the skin and the underlying soft tissues. For example, the hand need not be cooled for more than 5 minutes in order to induce a profound temperature decrease, whereas the thigh, which has a layer of subcutaneous fat acting as an insulator, can often tolerate applications of 20 minutes before the intramuscular temperature is significantly reduced.

The neurophysiologic effects of ice are substantial and include (1) a prolonged decrease in muscle spindle activity, (2) facilitation of the H reflex, which monitors alpha motoneuron excitability, and (3) decreased peripheral nerve conduction. Therefore, the muscle hypertonicity and spasm associated with injury can be reduced by cooling the hyperactive spindle organs, which are highly sensitive to temperature changes. Similarly, discomfort can be reduced by cooling the "C" fibers that transmit pain signals. Intermittent ice applications significantly reduce the ingestion of pain medications postsurgically, the effect lasting for up to 3 hours after 15 minutes of cooling. Both acute and chronic pain normally respond to cold, although there are occasional individuals who are hypersensitive to cold applications. This hypersensitivity may be largely psychologic, but it also has some physiologic basis, and must therefore be respected.

Negative reactions to reductions of joint temperatures have also been identified. Joint lubricants increase in viscosity, and the degree of resistance to movement may therefore increase. In addition, proprioceptive nerve fibers quickly lose their sensitivity with cooling impairing skilled motor performance which requires perfect timing and coordination. Therefore, the practice of enveloping injured ankles, knees, or shoulders in ice on the playing field and allowing athletes to continue competing may well place them at a disadvantage, making them more susceptible to further injury.

In a clinical setting, ice massage, cryokinetics, and cryostretch techniques are commonly used. After 5 minutes of ice massage, the intramuscular temperature shows a persistent decrease of 7 to 10°C. This technique decreases muscle spasm via the sympathetic response to surface cooling and also decreases pain in response to counterirritation. Cryokinetics, or the promotion of movement during ice applications, may facilitate muscular contractions owing to the increase in alpha motoneuron excitability mentioned previously. It is most effective when muscles are inhibited by prolonged immobilization or recent injury. The most controversial technique is that of cryostretch, which is intended to increase the extensibility of muscle or joint capsular structures left adherent or inflexible after trauma. Collagen is actually more extensible after warming, and stretching it while cool may well precipitate a rupture. Studies on rat-tail tendon suggest that the ideal method of stretching and maintaining an elongated position consists in a sequence of heat, prolonged stretching, and rapid cooling once the required length has been achieved. This technique has been used clinically with excellent results.

In summary, thermal modalities are not interchangeable. They have precise indications, depending on the therapeutic effects that are required, and can be manipulated by altering the method and duration of application. Generally, neither heat nor ice is used as the sole means of treatment; they are rather a preliminary to electrical modalities and exercise progressions.

Ultrasound

Therapeutic ultrasound is one of the most commonly used physical modalities available to athletes for immediate application in training rooms and follow-up treatment in clinics. It may unfortunately qualify as being one of the most commonly *abused* modalities of treatment as well. Clinically, dosages often remain unmodified despite application to a variety of pathologies. Furthermore, ultrasound has a cumulative effect on both soft tissues and bone which can be destructive unless frequency, duration, and overall number of treatments are closely monitored. The practice of allowing athletes to treat themselves whenever plagued by aches and pains must thus be discouraged.

Both thermal and nonthermal reactions can be produced by ultrasound waves ranging in frequency from 500 to 1500 cycles per second. *Continuous* output generates intense and deep heating reactions. *Intermittent* treatment minimizes heat production and maximizes the mechanical effects of sound waves vibrating within the tissues. Ultrasound waves have an affinity for collagenous tissues and are absorbed to a large extent by cortical bone. Given these variables, dosage intensities and duration depend on (1) the type of injury, (2) the distance of the injured tissue from the skin surface, and (3) the types of tissues interposed between the sound head and the area to be treated.

The conditions that respond most favorably to ultrasound include tendinitis, capsulitis, synovial irritations, periosteal inflammations (shin splints, epicondylitis), and stress fractures. Generally, a continuous output that increases the local blood flow assists in resolution of these chronic inflammatory processes, secondarily increasing the extensibility of collagen and breaking down any adhesions produced in high protein exudates. However, care must be taken not to apply continuous ultrasound directly over an acute soft tissue injury. The intense heating and mechanical vibration may precipitate local hemorrhage and delay the healing process. To avoid these complications, intermittent ultrasound may be used around the periphery of acute lesions; it enhances healing by facilitating diffusion of interstitially accumulated fluids across blood vessel membranes. Moreover, some studies suggest that tissue regeneration can itself be stimulated by the nonthermal reactions of ultrasound.

Electrical Modalities

Electrical modalities which are claimed to accelerate healing and have anti-inflammatory properties include diadynamic and interferential currents. They differ in the type of wave forms generated, the frequency of output, the modulations of current output over application time, and the methods of application. Nonetheless, their effectiveness seems to be relatively independent of the applied electrical wave form characteristics.

Briefly, soft tissue trauma causes an increase in cell metabolism, including the production of H_3O^+ ions. These ions tend to bond to larger molecules and thereby increase in viscosity as well as in concentration. This stagnation of cell metabolism, which is the hallmark of both acute and chronic inflammatory reactions, can be reversed by passing an electrical current through the extracellular fluid. This moves unbound H_3O^+ ions away from cell membranes, into the interstitial fluid, and ultimately into the venous circulation. In combination with thermal or ultrasonic agitation, the bonds of the large molecules created can be broken and normalization of tissue metabolism achieved.

In addition, the electrical modalities have analgesic properties, although in contrast to Transcutaneous Nerve Stimulating (TNS) units, they are not designed to maximize this potential. Thus, if applied shortly after an injury has occurred, not only can the inflammatory reaction be minimized, but the pain can also be reduced. However, caution must be exercised in allowing the athlete to return prematurely to activity. Adequate healing time must be allowed, despite any reduction in symptoms, to avoid recurring problems. This applies to both acute pathologies and chronic overuse syndromes. Generally, an initial period of treatment consists of anti-inflammatory modalities, tendon or capsular mobilizations to prevent adhesions or loss of movement, and maintenance exercises; such techniques precede measures to restore the athlete's strength, flexibility, endurance, and proprioceptive reactions.

Manual Therapy and Exercise Progressions

Manual therapy (which consists of passive peripheral and vertebral joint mobilizations) mimics the accessory articular movements associated with the normal range of physiologic movements. These techniques are used to reduce or eliminate hypomobility due to post-traumatic congestion and retraction of soft tissues; they achieve results far superior to manipulating a joint through its normal range. Following mobilization, active exercises to maintain articular mobility are integrated into the rehabilitation program.

Post-injury, all soft tissues must be able to bear specific loads, have a degree of stretch and elastic recoil, and endure cyclic or repetitive stress. Therefore, the design of exercise progressions to normalize these components of performance requires an understanding of how the pathology affects functional variables, together with an in-depth knowledge of normal biomechanics and kinesiology. For example, a sprain of the medial collateral ligament of the knee is frequently associated with tears of some patellar retinacular fibers which influence the normal tracking of the patella. This may cause the patella to adopt a more oblique position, prematurely engaging the femoral condyles even during full extension. Bracing may hold the patella in place while the retinacular fibers heal, but ultimately reinforcement of the vastus medialis is needed to neutralize the abnormal lateral excursion.

Exercise progression commonly consists of the following sequence: (1) non-weight-bearing exercises to improve strength and endurance—beginning with isometrics and progressing to isotonic and isokinetic exercises, (2) exercises to improve muscular flexibility, (3) partial weight-bearing exercises with concentration upon the load-bearing characteristics of the articulation, (4) full weight-bearing exercises, beginning with work in an isolated range and progressing to reinforcement at the extremes of range, (5) power training at high speeds, using high resistance and a small number of repetitions, (6) functional re-education, including cutting, hopping, take-off, and landing maneuvers, and finally (7) reintegration into a regular athletic training program. Any exercises that cause excessive swelling or persistent pain must be replaced by activities that provide the same degree of work without precipitating any irritation. Alternative positioning, shortening of lever arms which provide weight resistance, or changing the point of application of resistance is frequently sufficient to control exercise-induced problems.

"f" following a page number indicates
a figure, "t" indicates tabular material